SHANG HAN LUN EXPLAINED

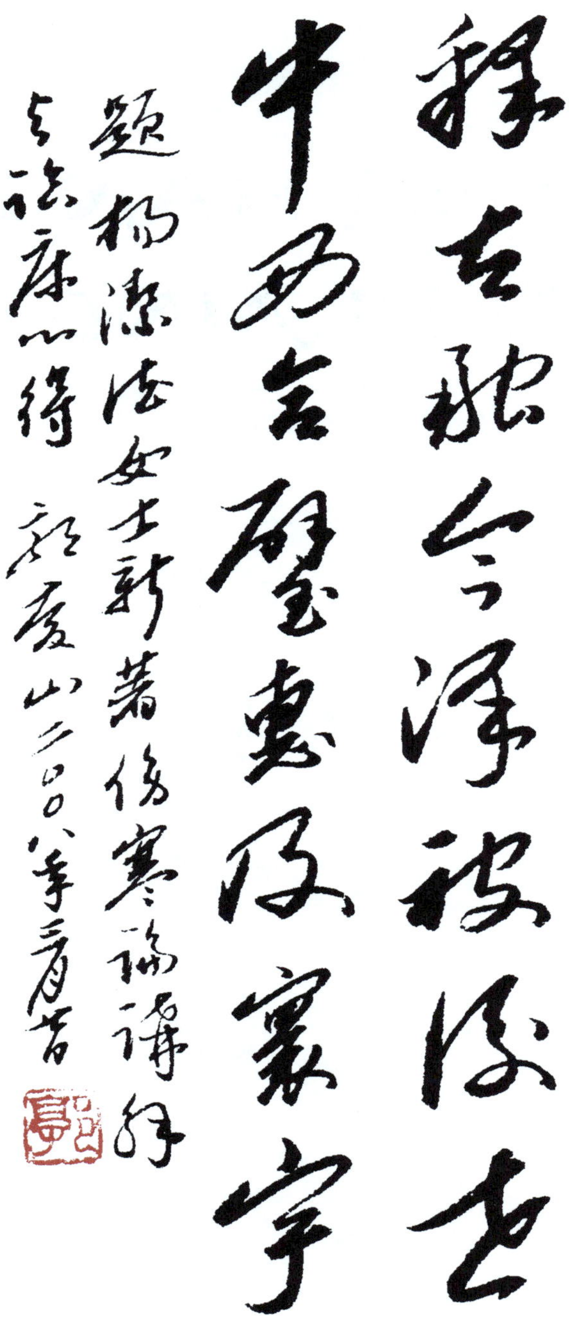

释古融今，泽被后世；中西合璧，惠及寰宇。

"Ancient knowledge expressed today, given to future generations;
East and West in harmony, benefitting the whole world"

Calligraphy by Guo Qing Shan 郭庆山 20 March 2008, in dedication to this book.

SHANG HAN LUN EXPLAINED

A Guided Tour of an Ancient Classic Text
Written By Zhang Zhong Jing in 200 AD
and its Modern Clinical Applications

伤寒论讲解与临床心得

Compiled and Translated by

Greta Young Jie De 杨洁德
Robin Marchment

Churchill Livingstone
is an imprint of Elsevier

Elsevier Australia. ACN 001 002 357
(a division of Reed International Books Australia Pty Ltd)
Tower 1, 475 Victoria Avenue, Chatswood, NSW 2067

National Library of Australia Cataloguing-in-Publication Data

---

Young Jie De, Greta.

Shang han lun explained : a guided tour of an ancient classic text written by Zhang Zhong Jing in 200 AD and its modern clinical applications / Greta Young Jie De and Robin Marchment.

ISBN: 978 0 7295 3881 7 (hbk.)

Includes index.
Bibliography.

Zhang, Zhongjing, fl 168-196. Shang han lun.
Medicine, Chinese—Early works to 1800.
Medicine, Chinese—Formulae, receipts, prescriptions.
Diseases.

Marchment, Robin.

610.951

Publisher: Sophie Kaliniecki
Developmental Editor: Sunalie Silva
Publishing Services Manager: Helena Klijn
Editorial Coordinator: Lauren Allsop
Edited by Wendy Alexander
Cover design by Avril Makula
Cover calligraphy by Professor Guo Qing Shan
Internal design and typesetting by Midland Typesetters
Printed in China by 1010 Printing International Ltd

Contents

CHAPTER 4 SHAO YANG DISEASE

CHAPTER 5 TAI YIN DISEASE

CHAPTER 6 SHAO YIN DISEASE

APPENDICES

Acknowledgements

The authors wish to express their appreciation of the many people who inspired them in their pursuit of knowledge and love of classic literature. Particular thanks go to Greta Young Jie De's teachers, Professor Fu Yan Ling, Professor Hao Wan Shan and Professor Nie Hui Ming of the Beijing University of Chinese Medicine, and heartfelt gratitude goes to Professor Hao Wan Shan for sharing his depth of knowledge and giving this project his support. We would like to pay special tribute to the Shang Han icon, Professor Liu Du Zhou. It was Greta Young's fortune to study under him in 1998 and it was he who was the greatest inspiration in her quest to study Jing Fang. We also give our special thanks to Professor Guo Qing Shan, academic, author, and accomplished calligrapher, for the wonderful brush work in the dedication to this book. Last but not least, we would like to thank our partners for their tolerance of our absence from their lives: Greta's husband Karl Young, for his staunch support in her quest for knowledge of Chinese Medicine, and Robin's husband George Wu for his support in this project.

Note on the case studies

The origins of the facts of many case studies used in this text to illustrate the teachings of *Shang Han Lun* are unknown, or difficult to attribute authoritatively. The cases are published here as they have been written, translated or rephrased by the authors. Other cases are sourced at the point where they appear in the text. Every attempt has been made to trace and acknowledge copyright, but in some cases this may not have been possible. The publisher apologises for any accidental infringement and would welcome any information to redress the situation.

Preface

Shang Han Lun is one of the four major classic texts of Chinese Medicine. It encompasses the medical achievements of the Eastern Han dynasty (25–220 AD) and the period prior to that. It is the first text in Chinese medical history to adopt the Six Channels as a basis for diagnosis and to explain the aetiology and pathological development of externally contracted febrile disease. *Shang Han Lun* has survived the passage of time and this ancient theory and its application to the treatment of disease are still regarded as having great relevance in today's environment.

This book has two objectives. The first is to explain the theory of *Shang Han Lun* and the systematic theory of the Six Channels: the patterns and manifestations and the related treatment strategies. The second is to explain how the principles of *Shang Han Lun* may be applied to disease in our own time.

The 398 original clauses of *Shang Han Lun* have been used as a basis for this text. It follows the conventional channel-by-channel order found in the Ming dynasty's Zhao Kai Mei edition, however, the sequence of the clauses has been further re-arranged for improved clinical relevance. The numbering of the clauses is identical to the Zhao edition and the original sequence of the Zhao edition is included as Appendix 2, and is complete with clauses written in traditional Chinese characters.

In the main text of this book, each clause is cited in the original Chinese followed by a faithful English translation, and is accompanied by an explanation of the aetiology and pathogenesis of the pattern, and a discussion of the formula and its ancient clinical application as well as new concepts and applications. Much reliance has also been placed on *Yi Zong Jin Jian (Golden Mirror of Medical Tradition)* which was commissioned by Emperor Qian Long and compiled in the years 1739–1742. That text comprises ninety fascicles, incorporating both *Shang Han Lun* and *Jin Gui Yao Lue.*

The vast amount of knowledge presented in *Shang Han Lun* is made more easily accessible in this book by the use of headings and summaries which assist the reader to analyse and grasp the concepts: key points are noted in accordance with the spirit of the original clauses; summaries and tables are given to help the reader focus on the essentials; the discussion of each formula and its pattern is followed by case studies that illustrate the clinical application of the original *Shang Han Lun* formulas; and each chapter concludes with a summary of disease patterns, formulas, and treatment principles.

In the process of writing this book, many ancient texts on *Shang Han Lun* were consulted, together with books on modern research. This text incorporates the authors' own case studies as well as case studies from scholars specialising in *Shang Han Lun* based at Beijing University of Chinese Medicine, which is regarded as the key centre for studies in the classics of Chinese medicine. We trust that this text serves to shine a light on what can be a daunting but essential and rewarding foundation classic of Chinese medicine.

Greta Young Jie De 杨洁德
Robin Marchment

About the Authors

Greta Young Jie De was born in Shanghai, China, raised in Hong Kong and now lives in Melbourne, Australia. She is a specialist in the classic literature of Chinese Medicine and is one of its foremost experts, having studied under a number of masters in China for many years. She was awarded a master's degree in Wen Bing by the Beijing University of Chinese Medicine in 1997 and in 2006 was awarded a doctorate of Chinese Medicine in *Shang Han Lun*, also from the Beijing University of Chinese Medicine. These qualifications were obtained under the tutorship of Professors Kong Guang-Yi and Fu Yan Ling. Professor Fu is the official successor of Professor Liu Du Zhou, the revered icon and recognised authority on *Shang Han Lun*. Greta has been a tireless and effective advocate and ambassador in the promotion of traditional Chinese medicine and is a lecturer of Classic Literature at the RMIT University. This book has been a long time in coming and will prove to be a source of inspiration for both students and practitioners of Chinese medicine.

Robin Marchment is a registered herbalist and acupuncturist who runs a private practice and also lectures in Chinese medicine. She has a particular interest in classical Chinese and the classic literature of Chinese medicine. She graduated from Monash University with an honours bachelor degree in European languages and a Diploma in Chinese, and subsequently graduated with a bachelor degree in Chinese medicine at the Australian College of Natural Medicine and an Advanced Diploma in Chinese herbal studies at the Southern School of Natural Therapies. She has also completed internships and further studies in Guangxi and Xi'an. She is the author of *Chinese for TCM Practitioners* and *Gynaecology Revisited: Obstetrics and Gynaecology for Practitioners of Chinese Medicine*.

How to Use this Book

The main text of this book quotes key clauses of *Shang Han Lun* in the original classical Chinese followed by an English translation. The translation stays as faithful as possible to the original whilst retaining a reasonable degree of intelligible flow. This is the tightrope that translators of Chinese must tread: it is a difficult balancing act where choices have to be made between using English which is not easily understood at one end of the spectrum and at the other, simple paraphrasing of the main points. It is unfortunate that many English versions of classic texts tend to paraphrase rather than translate. Sometimes meanings are added, and sometimes important and colourful phrases are omitted. This text has attempted to retain the flavour of the original Chinese in its translation of the clauses, with obscurities then clarified in a separate discussion that follows the translation of each clause.

The main objective of the discussion, however, is not simply to interpret and explain the language of the the original clause, but to analyse the principles proposed in each clause, and explain the pathogenesis of key symptoms and their relevance in terms of differential diagnosis. The discussion of each clause also brings to the reader's attention any historical controversy as to the interpretation of some phrases.

Clinical relevance in the modern setting is demonstrated by presenting case studies and other examples of the application of these classic formulas and their principles in the contemporary treatment of diseases and diagnosis according to the Western scientific model. However, this text by no means claims to be a clinical manual and, as always, the principles of differential diagnosis must be rigorously applied, and no formula should be used simply on the basis of a disease name.

Ancient Han measurements are given as they appear in the original text, and a conversion table can be found in Appendix 9.

This is a vast and complex text, so tools have been provided to penetrate and overcome its difficulties. The following Appendices are included.

Appendix 1: Additional Clauses
Those clauses not included in the main text due to disputed interpretation, dubious origin or uncertain clinical relevance.

Appendix 2: Outline of Clauses in the Sequence of the Zhao Edition
Sequence of the Song dynasty edition of *Shang Han Lun* with clauses written in traditional characters.

Appendix 3: Clause Index
The 398 *Shang Han Lun* clauses listed numerically with the page number on which each clause appears in this book.

Appendix 4: Summary of Formulas and Indications
Summary of all the formulas discussed in *Shang Han Lun* and their application.

Appendix 5: Formula Index
Alphabetical list of all *Shang Han Lun* formulas and their ingredients with clause number(s) in which the formula is described.

Appendix 6: Fu Zi Research
Summary of some recent findings that support the safety of Fu Zi.

Appendix 7: Index to Symptoms and Ailments
An index to facilitate the clinical application of *Shang Han Lun* theory and formulas.

Appendix 8: Glossary
Glossary of terms used in *Shang Han Lun.*

Appendix 9: Weights and Measures
Description of historical weights and measures and their various conversion methods.

Appendix 10: Han Dynasty Time: The Ebb and Flow of the Six Channels
Series of tables and a diagrammatic representation of the interrelationship between the six channels and the time at which they reach their peak flow.

Appendix 11: Heavenly Stems and Earthly Branches
Sequential phases used to reckon time in the Han dynasty.

Appendix 12: Chinese Dynasties and Historical Periods
Chronological table of Chinese dynasties.

Appendix 13: Notable Figures in Chinese Medicine
Notable authors in the history of writings on *Shang Han Lun.*

Appendix 14: References
Detailed list of sources used in the text.

Appendix 15: Herb Names: Cross-reference of Chinese and Pharmaceutical Names
Alphabetical list of herb names by their Pinyin name, cross-referenced to the pharmaceutical name.

Appendix 16: Bibliography
List of texts used by the authors in their study of the classics of Chinese medicine.

緒論

1 Introduction to Shang Han Lun

Development of *Shang Han Lun*

Shang Han Lun (Discourse on Cold Injury) describes the pattern identification and treatment of externally contracted and miscellaneous diseases of internal medicine. It is the earliest medical book written in China still extant which presents a complete theory of disease, its progress and its treatment. It encompasses detailed aetiology, pathogenesis, diagnosis, treatment principles, indicated formulas, their ingredients, directions for decoction and their modifications. It was written during the Eastern Han period (circa 200–210 AD) by Zhang Zhong Jing and was originally named the *Shang Han Za Bing Lun (Discourse on Cold Injury and Miscellaneous Diseases).*

Zhang Zhong Jing, also known as Zhang Ji, was born in Nie Yang (now known as Nan Yang) in the province of He Nan, and lived from about 150 to 219 AD. No detailed bibliographical records remain from that time, but it is known that he studied under Zhang Bo Zu and that he was later renowned as an accomplished practitioner whose academic and clinical skills surpassed those of his teacher, and eventually, his fame equalled that of Hua Tuo, who also lived during the Eastern Han dynasty. This was a tumultuous era when political unrest and constant warfare resulted in the outbreak of a string of epidemics. In the preface of Zhang Zhong Jing's original text, he noted that of his 200 member family, he had lost two-thirds in a ten year period and that seven-tenths of those deaths were attributable to disease which he described as caused by the invasion of exterior cold. For this reason he studied the ancient books of *Su Wen (Plain Questions), Jiu Juan (The Nine Fascicles), Ba Shi Yi Nan (Eighty-One Difficult Issues)* and *Yin Yang Da Lun (The Great Treatise on Yin and Yang)*, subsequently writing *Shang Han Za Bing Lun*, which totalled sixteen volumes.

Lineage of the Song and Zhao Editions

The original text was lost soon after it was written but not, fortunately, before another version was compiled and reorganised by Wang Shu He (Western Jin period, 265–316 AD). Wang Shu He's edition re-arranged the sections of the original *Shang Han Za Bing Lun* which related to externally contracted disease, and compiled them as a separate work; it is this which is now known as *Shang Han Lun*. Subsequently, in the Song dynasty (1127–1279 AD), the sections of *Shang Han Za Bing Lun* relating to other diseases of internal medicine, termed miscellaneous diseases, were reorganised to form the book now known as *Jin Gui Yao Lue* (*Essential Prescriptions of the Golden Cabinet*). There is no longer an extant text of the original Song dynasty edition in China, and today there are two editions of *Shang Han Lun* which are relied upon. The earlier of these, *Zhu Jie Shang Han Lun (Annotations to Shang Han Lun)* by Cheng Wu Ji from the Jin-Yuan period, appeared in about 1144 AD and was the earliest annotated edition. The second version of *Shang Han Lun* used today, and often referred to as the Song edition, is actually the Zhao Kai Mei edition. The original source text was printed with wooden blocks in 1599 and is known as *Zhong Jing Quan Shu* 仲景全书, and is also called the *Song Edition of Shang Han Lun* 宋本伤寒论. This consisted of four books:

1. *San Ke Song Ban Shang Han Lun*
2. *Zhu Jie Shang Han Lun (The Annotated Shang Han Lun)* by Cheng Wu Ji
3. *Shang Han Lei Zheng* by Song Yun Gong
4. *Jin Gui Yao Lue Fang Lun*

The first of these came to be known as the Song version by virtue of the fact that the original Song version no longer existed. Much reliance has also been placed on *Yi Zong Jin Jian* (*Golden Mirror of Medical Tradition*) which was commissioned by Emperor Qian Long and compiled in his reign (1739–1742). It comprises ninety fascicles into which are incorporated both *Shang Han Lun* and *Jin Gui Yao Lue*.

Academic Achievement of *Shang Han Lun*

Shang Han Lun's concept of externally contracted disease and its treatment was seeded in the classics of *Huang Di Nei Jing* (*The Yellow Emperor's Internal Classic*), *Nan Jing* (*The Classic of Difficult Issues*) and *Shen Nong Ben Cao Jing (The Materia Medica Classic)*. However, it was only in *Shang Han Lun* that the relatively abstract theoretical knowledge and generalised clinical observations of those works were developed into a specific body of theory. Basing his theory on the concept of six channel pattern differentiation found in *Su Wen: Re Lun (Su Wen Chapter 31: Discourse on Heat)*, Zhang Zhong Jing identified a range of patterns, which he then analysed and differentiated according to their pathogenesis and symptomatology, describing various pattern changes associated with externally contracted disease. Thus he provided an innovative and comprehensive system of six channel pattern differentiation. *Shang Han Lun* incorporates the theory of yin and yang and the zang fu as outlined in *Nei Jing*, and further develops the theory of the eight guiding principles, and the significance of the channels and network vessels. In addition, it describes in detail the aetiology and pathogenesis of disease, co-ordinating it with the eight treatment strategies of sweating, ejection, precipitation, harmonization, warming, clearing, supplementation and dispersion.

Ultimately, Zhang Zhong Jing produced comprehensive and systematic guidelines for understanding the aetiology and pathogenesis of externally contracted disease and associated treatments, not only developing formulas but also presenting explanations for his herbal modifications, with many formulas from the *Shang Han Lun* still used extensively in the modern day practice of Chinese medicine. Not only did this text provide the foundation for Chinese medical theory, but is regarded as a seminal text which formed the backbone for later developmental theories. One of the most noted of these was *wen bing xue* (warm disease theory) which was developed in the Ming and Qing dynasties. Although both shang han and wen bing theory had their origins in *Nei Jing*, warm disease theory is regarded as a further development of the principles of *Shang Han Lun*.

Definition of Shang Han or Cold Injury

The term 'shang han' has both a narrow and a broad meaning. The narrow concept of shang han is limited to externally contracted disease caused by pathogenic cold or wind cold, whilst the broad meaning refers to all externally contracted disease. The broad concept of shang han (cold injury) is described in both *Nei Jing Su Wen* and *Nan Jing*. The *Su Wen* states, "Now all heat diseases are of the shang han (cold damage) type" and the *Nan Jing: 58th Difficult Issue* states, "There are five types of shang han (cold injury): zhong feng (wind strike), shang han (cold injury), shi wen (damp warmth), re bing (hot disease) and wen bing (warm disease)".

The *Shang Han Lun* text addresses diseases defined by the broad sense of shang han, in other words, both externally contracted disease and other diseases of internal medicine known as miscellaneous disease. However, the main focus is on externally contracted disease caused by pathogenic wind cold, and the various differential patterns. And so it can be said that the main focus is, in fact, on the narrow concept of shang han. The aetiology of externally contracted disease is the six climatic influences of wind, cold, summerheat, damp, dryness and fire. However, the text considers both external and internal factors, the pathogens involved, disease patterns and principles of treatment. Importantly, it must be noted that the concept of shang han in *Shang Han Lun* differs from the modern clinical disease known as shang han, which is equivalent to typhoid fever.

Concept of the Six Channels and Six Channel Pattern Identification

The six channels are the Tai Yang, Yang Ming, Shao Yang, Tai Yin, Shao Yin and Jue Yin and in *Shang Han Lun* they serve to categorise patterns associated with externally contracted disease. The groundwork for the theory of the six channels had been laid down in the *Huang Di Nei Jing* where they were proposed as a basis for the diagnosis and treatment of heat and excess patterns in *Su Wen: Re Lun (Su Wen Chapter 31: Discourse on Heat)* and were further discussed in *Su Wen: Yin Yang Lei Lun (Su Wen Chapter 79: Discourse on the Categories of Yin and Yang)*. However, the diagnosis was generalised and reference to treatment in those chapters was scant, suggesting only that sweating could be used during the first two days and after the third day the disease had entered the interior so purgation could be used, and that meat should be avoided in febrile disease. Furthermore, there was no discussion of deficiency and cold except to say: "Observe deficiency and excess and treat accordingly". The sophisticated theory of *Shang Han Lun* stands in stark contrast to these simple statements: Zhang Zhong Jing proposed a comprehensive theory of classifying disease according to both the three yin and the three yang channels, discussing not only heat and excess, but also deficiency and cold. He defined many patterns within each classification, explaining their pathogenesis and specifying treatment strategies and formulas.

Shang Han Lun's six channel theory covers physiological function and pathological change in the channels and embraces the theories of the channels and network vessels, the zang fu, and qi and blood. By understanding the physiology of the channels, a theory is proposed as to the significance of pathological changes as manifested in signs and symptoms. Six channel pattern identification follows the course of externally contracted disease and identifies its location (exterior or interior), its nature (hot or cold) and explains its pathogenesis. Furthermore, it provides a means to gauge the strength of the zheng qi (antipathogenic qi), the intensity of the disease and, by analysing manifestations during the course of the disease, it also provides a tool to determine the subsequent outcomes or prognosis. Disease in any of the six channels manifests as a pattern which can be differentiated by its signs and symptoms, including, importantly, the pulse. Subsequent identification of the channel involved provides the basis for diagnosis and treatment. In this way, the concept of the six channels in *Shang Han Lun* not only offers criteria for analysis and guiding principles for pattern differentiation, but also provides a framework in which to develop treatment strategies.

There have been many interpretations of six channel pattern identification over the centuries. Some thought it better explained at the level of the zang fu, others thought it more relevant to view the concept at the level of the network vessels, and yet another opinion was to explain it in terms of qi transformation. In fact, all three viewpoints are valid because the six channels are closely related to their corresponding zang fu and associated network vessels, and therefore any pathological manifestation of the zang fu, the network vessels or qi transformation will be reflected in the six channel system.

Categorisation of the Six Channels

There are three yang patterns and three yin patterns, corresponding respectively to the yang and yin channels. The three yang patterns are the Tai Yang, which pertains to the urinary bladder and small intestine channels; the Yang Ming, pertaining to the stomach and large intestine channels; and the Shao Yang, which relates to the gallbladder and san jiao channels. The three yin patterns are the Tai Yin, which relates to the spleen and lung channels; the Shao Yin, which relates to the heart and kidney channels; and the Jue Yin, which pertains to the liver and pericardium channels. The depth of a disease from the most superficial and external to the deepest, most internal, and therefore the most serious, follows the order of Tai Yang, Yang Ming, Shao Yang, Tai Yin, Shao Yin and Jue Yin. A brief description of the patterns follows.

YANG CHANNEL PATTERNS: The most exterior of the channels is **Tai Yang**. This is the first channel affected during the initial stage of externally contracted disease associated with the invasion of pathogenic wind and cold. The manifestations of aversion to cold, fever, headache, a stiff, painful neck and floating pulse all indicate that this is an exterior cold pattern affecting the Tai Yang channel which has caused disharmony between ying (nutrient) and wei (defence) qi.

If the external pathogen penetrates into the interior and transforms into heat, an excess heat phase occurs. There is no longer an aversion to cold, but instead, there is sweating and an aversion to heat. As the disease progresses, damage to body fluids may manifest as thirst. This pattern is classified as **Yang Ming** disease and, if not addressed in time, it can transform into a bowel excess pattern with severe abdominal distension, abdominal pain, tidal fever, sweat streaming from the extremities, a hard stool and a pulse that is submerged and full.

If, during the course of the disease, the pathogenic influence is no longer in the exterior but has not yet penetrated the interior, a struggle results between the zheng qi and the pathogenic qi at the half interior and half exterior level. It manifests with such symptoms as alternating chills and fever, epigastric fullness, pain in the hypochondrium, a bitter taste in the mouth, a dry throat, dizziness, blurred vision, irritability and nausea, all of which are a reflection of constrained liver and gallbladder qi and impairment of the qi dynamic. This is known as **Shao Yang** disease.

Diseases affecting the three yang meridians are generally regarded as excess patterns, because the zheng qi is still intact and is able to offer resistance to the pathogenic qi. Because the location of the disease is relatively exterior and associated with the fu organs, the three yang channel patterns are generally classified as a yang pattern associated with heat and excess in the fu.

YIN CHANNEL PATTERNS: When the pathogen penetrates into the first of the three yin channels, the symptoms of vomiting, diarrhoea, abdominal distension, pain which is alleviated when pressure is applied, and a preference for warmth indicate that the pattern is one of spleen deficiency with depletion of yang qi and an accumulation of cold and damp. This is classified as **Tai Yin** disease.

If the pattern manifests as aversion to cold, an absence of fever, cold extremities, clear and watery diarrhoea, lethargy, a desire to sleep and a pulse that is fine and faint, it indicates deficiency of heart and kidney yang with interior cold. This is classified as **Shao Yin** disease.

If the pattern exhibits upper body heat and lower body cold, excessive thirst, qi surging upward to the heart, vexing heat in the heart, hunger with an inability to eat, vomiting of round worms and continuous diarrhoea, it is classified as **Jue Yin** disease.

Diseases affecting the three yin channels are generally classified as deficiency patterns because of the depletion of zheng qi and general hypoactivity. Because the location of the disease is interior and associated with the zang organs, the three yin channel patterns are generally classified as a yin pattern associated with cold and deficiency in the zang.

Relationship Between Six Channel Pattern Identification and Zang Fu Pattern Identification

Identification according to the six channels provides a systematic framework which can be used to establish the nature and location of the pathogen in externally contracted disease. From this, the diagnosis, principle of treatment and appropriate herbal formula can also be determined. Zang fu pattern identification is based on an understanding of the physiology and pathology the zang and fu. Signs and symptoms serve to identify the disease pattern and provide insight into the location, nature and intensity of the disease.

There is a close link between six channel theory and zang fu theory. The zang fu are at the core of all human physiological function, they are the home of the channels and they are interconnected by means of channels and network vessels. Six channel theory proposes a system where the channels corresponding to the zang fu are paired according to the sequential flow of qi and used as a basis for disease differentiation. A quote from *Ling Shu: Hai Lun Pian (Ling Shu Chapter 33: Discourse on the Seas)* illustrates this: "The twelve channel vessels, internally are connected to zang fu, externally the network vessels are connected to the limbs and joints." Zhang Jie Bing said: "The network vessels are branches of the zang fu; the zang fu are the root of all channels and network vessels. To understand the pathway of the twelve channels is to understand the yin and yang, exterior and interior, qi and blood, excess and deficiency." It follows that the three yang channels reflect pathological change in the fu organs, while the three yin channels reflect pathological change in the zang organs. For example, disease affecting the Tai Yang channel is classified as exterior. If it is not resolved at this level, further penetration via the channel network will affect the transformation function of the associated fu organ of the Tai Yang channel, the urinary bladder, and water amassment will result, manifesting as excessive thirst, difficult urination and a floating pulse.

Relationship Between Six Channel Pattern Identification and the Eight Principles

Eight principle pattern differentiation or 'ba gang bian zheng' is based on the conceptual pairs of yin and yang, exterior and interior, cold and heat, and excess and deficiency. Pattern differentiation according to the eight principles is the net result of analysing data collected by the four examinations, which comprise inspection, listening and smelling, inquiry and palpation. Data obtained from the four examinations forms the basis for identifying the location and nature of disease as well as a means of assessing the relative strengths of zheng qi and pathogenic qi.

The concept of eight principle pattern identification originated in such classics as *Nei Jing* and *Shang Han Lun* with the latter forming the springboard for its later acceptance and development. When six channel pattern identification and the eight principles are used together, they are able to assess not only the location and nature of disease but also its progress and prognosis. These two systems are, in fact, inseparable because the practical application of six channel pattern identification is dependent on differentiating the eight principles of yin and yang; exterior and interior; heat and cold; and excess and deficiency.

Yin and yang represent two polarised stages in the process of transformation of all things in the universe and symbolise two diametrically opposite energies. Ultimate good health is dependent on these two forces being in equilibrium. Disease is the consequence of disharmony between these two elements and, when conducting a diagnosis, it is essential to observe the state of yin and yang. As previously observed, diseases of the three yang meridians are associated with yang, heat and excess, whereas diseases of the three yin meridians are associated with yin, cold and deficiency. *Su Wen: Yin Yang Ying Xiang Da Lun Pian (Su Wen Chapter 5: Great Disourse on the Phenomenon of Yin and Yang)* states: "A good diagnostician observes the complexion and palpates the pulse and first distinguishes between yin and yang". Once the distinction between yin and yang is established, further differentiation can be made between heat and cold, exterior and interior, and excess and deficiency. Disease must be differentiated as to its location: generally speaking, pathogenic involvement of the network vessels is regarded as an exterior disorder, and involvement of the zang fu is classified as an interior pattern.

The selection of the correct treatment strategy is highly dependent on understanding the location of disease. For example, the correct treatment strategy in a Tai Yang exterior pattern is to resolve the exterior with diaphoresis; in a Yang Ming interior pattern, however, the appropriate strategy is to clear internal heat or purge the bowel repletion. For instance, Clause 56 in the Tai Yang chapter says: "If the urine is clear, we know it is not in the interior, it is still in the exterior, one must promote sweating".

Conversely, if there has been no stool for six or seven days and there is also headache and fever, then the pathogen has transferred to the interior and purging is indicated, using Cheng Qi Tang. Where exterior and interior patterns exist simultaneously, the correct strategy is first to release the exterior and then to purge the interior heat. In the treatment of disease, it is essential to understand the correlation of the six channels and the exterior or interior manifestations. Using the wrong strategy can have dire consequences.

Cold and heat are the principles by which the nature of a disease is identified. In terms of their aetiology, disease of the three yang channels pertains to heat and excess whereas disease of the three yin channels pertains to cold and deficiency. Identification of patterns as relating to excess or deficiency helps in the determination of the waxing and waning of disease, where deficiency refers to a deficiency of zheng qi and excess refers to an excess of pathogenic qi. *Su Wen: Tong Ping Xu Shi Lun Pian (Su Wen Chapter 28: Discourse on Deficiency and Excess)* states: "Exuberance of evil qi is excess, depletion of essence qi is deficiency". Thus it can be seen that the eight principles are an integral part of six channel pattern identification and, conversely, the pathomechanism of disease in the six channels is closely linked to the eight principles and the zang fu.

Relationship Between Six Channel Pattern Identification and Identification According to Cause

Pattern identification according to the cause of disease (bing yin bian zheng) is the determination of the cause of disease by examining and analysing its manifestations. Manifestations of disease may have their root in any of a number of causes: the six environmental excesses, the seven emotions, traumatic injury and lifestyle factors such as improper diet or overexertion. The six channel patterns reflect the pathological changes wrought by exterior causes, wind, cold, summerheat, damp, dryness and fire, otherwise known as the six evils or the six exogenous pathogenic factors. In the initial stage, it is pathogenic cold which is the cause of six channel disease.

Tai Yang zhong feng (wind strike) is an exterior deficiency pattern where there is an aversion to wind cold, sweating and a moderate pulse. Tai Yang shang han (cold injury) is an exterior excess pattern with aversion to cold, no sweating and a tight pulse. Both Tai Yang zhong feng and Tai Yang shang han are caused by pathogenic cold but they can be part of a more complex pattern where there is phlegm, fire, water amassment, food stagnation or blood stasis, any one of which may be an aetiological factor in the disease pattern. From this, it can be seen that the concept of diagnosis by aetiology constitutes a critical component of six channel pattern identification.

In *Shang Han Lun*, six channel pattern identification serves as the framework for diagnosis according to aetiology, the channels and network vessels, the zang fu and the eight guiding principles. Subject to the circumstances of an individual disease, any one, or more than one, of those theories can be applied.

Method of Six Channel Diagnosis

In order to utilize the six channel system of pattern identification correctly, there are five key points to bear in mind.

1. The strategy of the six channel system of pattern identification uses the six channels as a means of classifying six different stages of disease caused initially by an externally contracted pathogen. Each channel is characterised by a group of signs and symptoms which is a reflection of the physiology and corresponding pathological changes of that particular channel. Each of the six channels serves as a main category, with each having many sub-categories which are classified as diseases of the related channel. When making a diagnosis according to the method of the six channels, it is essential to identify the channel with which the symptoms and signs are associated.
2. Pathological changes during the course of the disease manifest as changed signs and symptoms. Treatment is then adjusted according to these new manifestations. For example, Clause 25 says: "Having taken Gui Zhi Tang, there is copious sweat, if the pulse is flooding and big, give Gui Zhi Tang as before", whilst Clause 26 says: "Having taken Gui Zhi Tang, after profuse sweating,

there is severe vexation and unresolved thirst, if the pulse is flooding and big, Bai Hu jia Ren Shen Tang governs." The two disease patterns described in these clauses are both associated with the Tai Yang channel and Gui Zhi Tang had been given in both cases. Both mention sweating but the difference is that although in the former there is a surging, large pulse, suggesting an interior syndrome, the absence of thirst shows that the syndrome is still in the exterior. The latter pattern (Clause 26) describes how, after taking Gui Zhi Tang, there is also vexation and thirst, demonstrating a change in the pattern. The symptom of thirst signifies fluid damage due to exuberant heat in the interior, hence it is ascertained that it is no longer in the Tai Yang but in the Yang Ming. The treatment principle must change from promoting sweat, as indicated for Tai Yang syndrome, to clearing heat and generating fluids as indicated for Yang Ming syndrome.

3. In the process of pattern identification, an attempt has to be made to identify similarity or commonality with one of the six patterns, even though the actual pattern may be different from the classic description. Among the complexity of pattern variations, it is necessary to find the common denominator. For example, irrespective of whether the pattern is zhong feng (wind strike) or shang han (cold injury), if the pulse is floating and there is stiffness and pain in the nape and an aversion to cold, then the manifestations are associated with the Tai Yang channel and the principle of treatment is to use acrid warm herbs to release the exterior.
4. The situation of concurrent patterns must be identified, for instance, where some symptoms and signs indicating the Tai Yang pattern are present concurrently with signs and symptoms indicating that the disease has entered another channel. Even though the disease is no longer in the Tai Yang channel, the presence of signs and symptoms typical of Tai Yang channel disease indicates that although the exterior has not been released, the pathogenic influence has entered a deeper channel simultaneously. In such a case, treatment using acrid warm herbs to release the exterior may still apply or may be incorporated with other forms of treatment.
5. The concept of the eight principles is interwoven into the six channels. When diagnosing according to the principles of six channel pattern identification, the eight principles are automatically invoked because without them, the nature and location of the disease can not be determined. The two theories are used in partnership to arrive at an accurate diagnosis and prescribe appropriate treatment.

Six Channel Disease Transmission

Six channel pattern identification studies pathological changes within the zang fu and their associated channels and collaterals, and the progression of disease. If one channel or organ is affected, in time, other channels or organs may also be affected. This concept of disease progression is called transmission or 'chuan bian'. 'Chuan' means 'pass' and the term 'bian' refers to an anomaly in the normal pathway of disease transmission. Another possible interpretation would be 'disease complications'. The following descriptions outline the ways in which disease, which was initially caused by the contraction of exterior cold, may change according to the transmission of the pathogen in six channel pattern identification theory.

1. **Xun Jing Chuan (transmission in the sequence of channels):** When an external pathogen transfers sequentially from the exterior to the interior, from the superficial to the deep level, in the classic sequence of the six channel diseases (Tai Yang to Yang Ming to Shao Yang to Tai Yin to Shao Yin to Jue Yin), it is known as xun jing chuan.
2. **Yue Jing Chuan (transmission by skipping channels):** Where the externally contracted disease does not transmit in the expected order through each of the six channels but skips one or more channels, it is known as yue jing chuan.
3. **Zhi Zhong (direct strike):** Where the external pathogenic factor gives rise to a disease by invading the three yin channels directly and without undergoing the stages of the three yang diseases, it is known as zhi zhong.

4. **He Bing (concurrent disease):** When the symptom complex involves two or three channels concurrently, it is known as he bing. For example, Tai Yang and Yang Ming he bing, Tai Yang and Shao Yang he bing or Tai Yang, Yang Ming and Shao Yang he bing.
5. **Bing Bing (lagover disease):** When the symptom complex of one channel has not yet been resolved and additional symptoms pertaining to another channel appear, it is known as bing bing.

Huai Bing or Transmuted Patterns

Huai bing or a transmuted pattern is an aberration in the course of normal disease transmission and represents deterioration in the disease caused by incorrect treatment, which can be inappropriate application (as a result of wrong diagnosis) or excessive use of such therapies as sweating, emesis or purgation. The mechanism of the deterioration usually relates to damage to zheng qi because of the loss of qi and fluids caused by these treatments. The subsequent interior deficiency allows the pathogen to transmit to a deeper level of the six channel system, creating a more serious and more complex pattern. As said in the *Nei Jing*: "Where zheng qi resides, evil can not enter"; conversely, where there is emptiness, it is exploited by the pathogen, and the disease enters the interior. When this occurs, it is known as adverse treatment, resulting in huai bing or a transmuted pattern. This is discussed in numerous clauses of *Shang Han Lun* for example: Clause 16 "Tai Yang disease for three days, sweating has already been promoted, if there is vomiting, if there is purging, if there is warm needling, the condition is still not resolved, this is transmuted disease, Gui Zhi is not appropriate." Transmuted patterns are an aberration of the six channel patterns but are described in relation to them, as appropriate to their aetiology and pathogenesis. They are also known as 'bian zheng'.

Pattern Differentiation According to Six Channel Theory

Table 1 summarises the diseases of the six channels as diagnosed according to aetiology, pathogenesis and the main signs and symptoms.

Principles of Treatment in Six Channel Disease

The fundamental treatment strategies of diseases associated with the six channels are to:

a) reinforce anti-pathogenic yang or zheng qi;
b) eliminate the pathogenic factor.

Table 2 summarises specific strategies for the diseases associated with each channel. A more extensive description of strategies and treatments is found in the chapters relating to each channel.

Relationship Between Shang Han and Wen Bing

As discussed earlier, the concept of shang han can be defined as either 'broad' or 'narrow'. The broad definition embraces all diseases caused by any exogenous pathogenic factor regardless of whether it is cold or damp or wind or fire, as described in the *Nan Jing: 58th Difficulty* when it states, "There are five types of cold damage: zhong feng (wind strike), shang han (cold injury), shi wen (damp warmth), re bing (heat disease) and wen bing (warm disease). The narrow definition refers only to those diseases caused by exogenous cold or wind cold, as is stated in *Su Wen*: "Now all heat diseases are of the cold injury kind." Although wen bing is contained within the broad definition of shang han and has a connection with shang han theory, they are nevertheless two separate concepts.

During the period that *Nei Jing* and *Nan Jing* were written, both the broad definition encompassing wen bing and the narrow concept of shang han were placed in the same category as externally contracted disease when, in fact, shang han and wen bing are two entirely different types of febrile disease. When *Shang Han Lun* was written, there was a lack of clinical knowledge concerning the aetiology of wen bing and it was only as time progressed that the aetiology and pathogenesis of wen bing were properly understood.

Shang Han Lun was written during the Eastern Han period (circa 196 AD), whilst wen bing theory was developed in a much later period, during the Ming and Qing dynasties. Thanks in part to its early inclusion in shang han theory, and in part to the influence of

Table 1: Pattern differentiation according to six channel theory

	Aetiology	Pathogenesis	Main Symptoms and Signs
Tai Yang disease	Invasion by exogenous wind cold	(1) Disharmony of ying and wei (2) Obstruction of defensive yang qi by cold	Superficial pulse, pain and stiffness in the head and neck, aversion to cold
Yang Ming disease	Tai Yang diseases transmitted to the interior	(1) Hyperactivity of pathogenic heat in the stomach resulting in fluid depletion (2) Unformed heat combined with formed accumulation causing obstruction of fu qi	High fever, profuse sweating, aversion to heat and not cold, flooding pulse Tidal fever, sweat streaming from the extremities, abdominal distension with fullness and pain, hard stool and a sunken and excess pulse
Shao Yang disease	(1) Transmission from other channels (2) Direct attack	Half exterior and half interior due to Shao Yang being the pivoting point of the qi mechanism	Alternating chills and fever, epigastric fullness, loss of appetite which can be accompanied by nausea and vomiting, white tongue coating, restlessness, bitter taste in the mouth, dry throat and wiry pulse
Tai Yin disease	(1) Incorrect treatment of three yang diseases (2) Direct attack	Damage or weakness of spleen yang Direct attack from wind-cold pathogenic factor	Abdominal fullness, loss of appetite, vomiting, diarrhoea, abdominal pain
Shao Yin disease	(1) Transmission from exterior (2) Direct attack due to deficiency	(1) Deficiency of heart and kidney yang qi (2) Obstruction of yang qi by cold	Aversion to cold, preference for lying in curled-up posture, tendency for sleepiness, diarrhoea, vomiting, preference for hot drinks, copious and clear urine, weak and thready pulse
Jue Yin disease	(1) Transmission from other channels; generally the terminal stage of disease (2) Direct attack	Combination of cold and heat	Excessive thirst, feeling of qi rushing to the chest, pain and heat sensation in the chest, feeling of hunger with no desire to eat, diarrhoea and vomiting or vomiting of roundworms

shang han theory over the ensuing centuries, the system of pattern identification in wen bing theory, as developed later, was derived from that expounded in *Shang Han Lun*. Tracing the origins of both shang han and wen bing theories, it is clear that the diagnostic techniques of wen bing are a further development and expansion of the foundation theory of *Shang Han Lun*. It was some centuries later before wen bing finally developed into a system of its own with particularised diagnostic features such as the four aspects (wei, qi, ying, xue) and san jiao pattern identification (upper, middle and lower jiao). Nevertheless the wen bing theories of the four aspects and san jiao were based on many of the concepts of six channel pattern identification as pioneered by Zhang Zhong Jing. This is evidenced in much of wen bing theory, for instance, it is stated in *Wai Gan Wen Re Bing Pian* (*Dissertation on Externally Contracted Febrile Disease*) that, "Diseases of the qi aspect, if not transmitted to the xue aspect, can persist in the san jiao and bear resemblance to diseases of the Shao Yang channel".

To speak of the development of wen bing theory without reference to *Shang Han Lun* is tantamount to talking about water without a spring or a tree without a root. The qi aspect of wen bing theory is comparable to the Yang Ming pattern of *Shang Han Lun*. A further illustration of the correspondence between the two theories is seen in the use of the formula

Table 2: Principles of treatment according to six channel theory

Channel	Diagnosis	Principle of treatment
Tai Yang disease	a) Tai Yang exterior fullness syndrome b) Tai Yang exterior deficiency syndrome	a) Eliminate cold by diaphoresis b) Dispel pathogenic factors from the superficial muscles, eliminate pathogenic wind, regulate ying and wei system
Yang Ming disease	a) Yang Ming channel syndrome b) Yang Ming Fu organ syndrome	a) Clear heat from the Yang Ming b) Purge food stagnation in the fu of the Yang Ming
Shao Yang disease	Pivoting mechanism of Shao Yang is obstructed	Harmonize Shao Yang
Tai Yin disease	Damage to spleen yang by pathogenic cold	Warm the middle and tonify spleen, eliminate cold and parch dampness
Shao Yin disease	a) Cold transformation due to heart and kidney yang deficiency b) Heat transformation due to excess yang as a result of yin deficiency	a) Strengthen yang to dispel cold b) Nourish yin and clear deficiency heat
Jue Yin disease	Heat and cold complex with stomach heat in the middle burner and spleen coldness in the lower burner. Exuberant cold with the possibility of restoring yang qi if given the correct treatment.	Clear heat from the upper jiao and warm cold in the lower jiao

Huang Lian E Jiao Tang in the treatment of Shao Yin disease in *Shang Han Lun*, which is the same formula cited in wen bing to treat heat scorching true yin, thus meeting the wen bing requirement to nourish true yin and clear hyperactive heart fire.

Numerous wen bing xue (warm disease theory) formulas are derived from *Shang Han Lun*. Huang Qin Tang, Bai Hu Tang, Huang Lian E Jiao Tang, Zhi Zi Chi Tang as well as the three Cheng Qi Tang formulas are just some of the many formulae with no modification, frequently cited in the treatment of wen bing. Formulae of wen bing xue which are adaptations of *Shang Han Lun* formulas are Zeng Ye Cheng Qi Tang and Xuan Bai Cheng Qi Tang. Qing dynasty practitioners created new treatment strategies such as clearing heat and relieving toxicity, established the use of aromatic medicinals to transform turbidity, and employed specific medicinals to open the orifices. In addition, new formulas such as Yin Qiao San, Lian Po Yin, Niu Huang Wan and Zhi Bao Dan emerged.

Parallels are often drawn between the treatment strategies proposed respectively by shang han and wen bing theories. At the onset of externally contracted disease with an exterior or wei pattern, both wen bing and shang han theory adopt the treatment principle of releasing the exterior. The critical difference is in the aetiology, with wen bing being caused by pathogenic heat and shang han by pathogenic cold. Correspondingly, acrid cool herbs to release the exterior are adopted by wen bing theory whereas shang han adopts acrid warm herbs to release the exterior and promote sweating. When the pathogenic influence enters the interior and there are such manifestations as fever, thirst, sweating, a flooding pulse or dry accumulation in the bowel with abdominal pain, both shang han and wen bing theories invoke the strategy of clearing heat and purging accumulation. The difference is in the later stages, where wen bing theory focuses mainly on essence, fluid, blood and humour damage and shang han on devastated yang. Hence the corresponding treatment for later stage wen bing disease is to nourish yin and replenish fluid whilst the treatment of later stage shang han disease is based on the restoration of yang qi.

Shang Han and Miscellaneous Diseases

The aetiologies of shang han and miscellaneous diseases differ. Shang han is categorised as disease caused by exterior injury by environmental pathogenic factors; miscellaneous diseases are mainly attributed to internal injury, pertaining to yin and caused by such things as improper diet, emotional stress, phlegm and blood stasis. *Su Wen: Tiao Jing Lun Pian (Su Wen Chapter 62: Discourse on Regulating the Channels)* states: "When evil arises, it relates either to yin or to yang. Disease pertaining to yang is due to wind, rain, cold or summerheat; that pertaining to yin is due to food and drink, an irregular lifestyle or immoderate joy or anger". *Ling Shu: Wu Se Pian (Ling Shu Chapter 49: The Five Colours)* states: "When the disease arises in the interior, first treat the yin, then treat the yang, the reverse will cause deterioration; When the disease arises in the yang, first treat the exterior, then treat the interior, the reverse will cause deterioration." It is clear from these passages that shang han and miscellaneous diseases differ significantly in their aetiology. This is not to say, however, that the two can not manifest simultaneously. Externally contracted disease can activate internal disease or aggravate pre-existing conditions and result in a more complex condition. For example, Tai Yang disease accompanied by asthma as seen in a Gui Zhi jia Hou Po Xing Zi Tang pattern; shang han disease accompanied by water qi beneath the heart, as seen in a Xiao Qing Long Tang pattern and shang han accompanied by heart vexation and palpitations as in a Xiao Jian Zhong Tang pattern. Such examples are numerous in *Shang Han Lun* and show that treatment protocols for the exterior and interior must be differentiated and also take into consideration whether the condition is acute or chronic.

Clinical Application of Six Channel Pattern Identification

The application of the six channel system is not restricted to diagnosis and treatment of externally contracted febrile diseases alone, but can be applied to many disorders of internal medicine, external medicine, gynaecology and paediatrics. *Shang Han Lun* theory has the potential to treat a range of diseases, including cardiac and pulmonary disorders, hepatic and biliary disorders, gastrointestinal disorders and urinary disorders. The application of six channel pattern identification in internal and miscellaneous diseases is based on the following.

AETIOLOGY: The aetiology of disease, which includes qi stagnation, blood stasis, water qi, phlegm fluids, food stagnation, physical exertion and internal injury, is discussed in detail in *Shang Han Lun*. For example, a water qi disorder can be due to yang deficiency resulting in generalised water swelling or oedema, where the treatment prescribed in *Shang Han Lun* is Zhen Wu Tang. However, if the water qi causes oedema from the waist down, the relevant formula in *Shang Han Lun* is Mu Li Ze Xie San. Other patterns described in *Shang Han Lun* are blood accumulation and stasis, with the indicated formula being Tao He Cheng Qi Tang, and the knotted heat and phlegm pattern, which is treated with a formula such as Xiao Xian Xiong Tang.

Many symptoms discussed in *Shang Han Lun* are used as points of reference in contemporary Chinese medicine. For example, in *Shang Han Lun*, a Xie Xin Tang pattern is described as "glomus beneath the heart" or *xin xia pi*.

This is a pattern of heat and cold complex resulting from disharmony of the spleen and stomach. Knowledge of this pattern from *Shang Han Lun* is applied extensively in the diagnosis and treatment of gastrointestinal disorders such as gastritis, diarrhoea and nausea.

PRINCIPLES OF TREATMENT: *Shang Han Lun* discusses in detail the eight treatment methods and their appropriate applications. For example, it outlines the skilful use of diaphoretics in a variety of situations apart from simply promoting sweat in order to release the exterior. Such strategies as: releasing the exterior in order to disperse qi, releasing the exterior in order to transform phlegm fluids, transforming qi in order to disperse water, are only a few examples of treatment protocols outlined in *Shang Han Lun*. Furthermore, some gynaecological disorders can be expressed in terms of six channel theory, for example the strategy of harmonising Shao Yang in the treatment of menstrual irregularity. It should also be noted that particular emphasis is placed on the Three Causes: the cause of season, the cause of region and the cause of the individual constitution. All of these have a bearing on the ultimate treatment.

HERBAL FORMULAS: A range of contemporary diseases encountered in the clinic can be treated by *Shang Han Lun* formulas. Examples of this are Ma Xing Shi Gan Tang in the treatment of pneumonia, Yin Chen Hao Tang for hepatitis, Ban Xia Xie Xin Tang in the treatment of acute gastritis and Bai Tou Weng Tang for bacterial enteritis. A famous Qing practitioner, Ke Yun Bo, once said, "The six channel system in *Shang Han Lun* can be used to address not only shang han disorders but hundreds of diseases." *Shang Han Lun* in fact stands as a guide for the diagnosis and treatment of many contemporary disorders.

Ebb and Flow of Qi in the Six Channels

The ebb and flow of qi in the six channels is significant for the understanding of the exacerbation of disease and also for recovery. The time associated with each of the channels is based on the twelve earthly branches but is not to be confused with the Zi Wu Liu Zhu system. The twelve two-hour periods are: Zi Shi (11pm–1am), Chou Shi (1am–3am), Yin Shi (3am–5am), Mao Shi (5am–7am), Chen Shi (7am–9am), Si Shi (9am–11am), Wu Shi (11am–1pm), Wei Shi (1pm–3pm), Shen Shi (3pm–5pm), You Shi (5pm–7pm), Xu Shi (7pm–9pm) and Hai Shi (9pm–11pm).

The sequence of the six channels starts from Tai Yang, proceeds to Yang Ming, then Shao Yang before entering the three yin channels of Tai Yin, then Shao Ying and finally Jue Yin. There are six periods, each covering six hours and there is some overlapping. The periods do not represent a strict sequential flow but rather the hours during which each channel is at its peak, therefore representing the optimal period for recovery in each channel. Recovery of disease in the three yang channels takes place in the day time, when yang rules, and recovery in the three yin channels takes place from midnight onwards. They are as follows:

- Tai Yang: Si Shi, Wu Shi and Wei Shi (9am–3pm)
- Yang Ming: Shen Shi, You Shi and Xu Shi (3pm–9pm)
- Shao Yang: Yin Shi, Mao Shi and Chen Shi (3am–9am)
- Tai Yin: Hai Shi, Zi Shi and Chou Shi (9pm–3am)
- Shao Yin: Zi Shi, Chou Shi and Yin Shi (11pm–5am)
- Jue Yin: Chou Shi, Yin Shi and Mao Shi (1am–7am).

Decoction Methods

The description of methods and administration of decoction in *Shang Han Lun* and *Jin Gui Yao Lue* constitutes a major contribution to the preparation of herbs in Chinese medicine. All of these specialised cooking techniques are significant for the efficacy of herbal medicine and some of the specifics entail the following.

- Direct boiling in water, which is the most common decoction method.
- Straining and subsequent re-boiling and reducing the liquid in order to concentrate the decoction, as is done for Xiao Chai Hu Tang and Ban Xia Xie Xin Tang.
- Boiling two ingredients separately then straining each and blending them for re-boiling as in Bei He jia Zhi Mu Tang.
- Establishing the duration for decoction based on the time needed for rice to be cooked, as in Fu Zi Geng Mi Tang (*Jin Gui Yao Lue*).
- The steeping of herbs in boiling hot water as in Da Huang Huang Lian Xie Xin Tang and Fu Zi Xie Xin Tang.
- Prior decoction of one or more ingredients, as with Ge Gen in Gen Gen Tang and Ma Huang in Ma Huang Tang.
- Late addition of one or more ingredients as with Mang Xiao in Da Cheng Qi Tang and Mang Xiao and Gan Sui in Da Xian Xiong Tang.
- The separate preparation of an ingredient in order to add it last as with the melting of E Jiao in Huang Lian E Jiao Tang.

- The use of specially prepared water such as worked water (Gan Lan Shui) as in Fu Ling Gui Zhi Gan Cao Da Zao Tang and rain water (Liao Shui) as in Ma Huang Lian Qiao Chi Xiao Dou Tang.
- The use of additional ingredients such as vinegar, wine and honey as in Zhi Gan Cao Tang, Dang Gui Si Ni jia Wu Zhu Yu Sheng Jiang Tang and the use of wine vinegar to soak Wu Mei in preparation for its use in Wu Mei Wan.
- Boiling in an equal amount of water and clear wine as in Zhi Gan Cao Tang.
- Boiling in soured rice water for taxation relapse, as in Zhi Shi Zhi Zi Chi Tang to improve appetite and regulate the stomach qi.

Administration Methods

In *Shang Han Lun* instructions regarding administration are specific and relate to the frequency and time of administration, the dose according to the constitution of the patient, the method and form of administration, and provide advice on when to continue or discontinue the decoction. Such instructions are still relevant in the modern clinical situation, including the following examples.

- *Frequency.* To be taken in a single dose as for Gui Zhi Gan Cao Tang; or to be taken two or three times a day, as for Dang Gui Si Ni jia Wu Zhu Yu Sheng Jiang Tang, Zhu Fu Tang, and most other *Shang Han* formulas.
- *Time.* To be taken at Ping Dan (3–5am), as for Shi Zao Tang; to be taken before meals as for Tao He Cheng Qi Tang and Wu Mei Wan; to be taken throughout the day, as for Huang Lian Tang (three times in the day and twice at night), or Li Zhong Tang (three or four times during the day and twice at night). The time between doses, as in Ma Huang Sheng Ma Tang, where it is the time it takes to cook three dou of rice.
- *Manner.* Taking the herbal preparation with rice water, as in the case of Ban Xia San, taking it with Gan Lan Shui or worked water as in Fu Ling Gui Zhi Gan Cao Da Zao Tang, or following it with hot gruel, as with Gui Zhi Tang when used as a sweat promotion formula, to preserve the stomach qi and enhance sweat promotion; in Shi Zao Tang, the person should be given rice gruel for nourishment as soon as diarrhoea occurs (Clause 152).
- *Dosage.* A larger dose for a robust person and a smaller one for a person of weakened constitution as with San Wu Bai San and Shi Zao Tang.
- *Form.* Herbal preparations can be made into decoctions such as Gui Zhi Tang and Ma Huang Tang, pills such as Wu Mei Wan and Da Xian Xiong Wan, powders such as Wu Ling San and San Wu Bai San, and suppositories and enemas such as Mi Jian Dao and Pig's Bile.
- *Method.* Whether the herbal preparation is to be taken orally, as with most of the formulas, or per rectum, as with Mi Jian Dao, or to be applied topically, as for Gan Cao Jie Geng Tang, where the decoction is held in the back of the mouth so as to treat the throat.
- *Discontinuation.* In formulas such as Da Xian Xiong Tang, Da Cheng Qi Tang, the medication should cease if the bowel moves; with Da Qing Long Tang, if sweat starts to issue; Gua Di San, if vomiting is effected; Mu Li Ze Xie San, if the urination is normal; and Tao Hua Tang, as soon as recovery takes place.
- *Repeat administration.* Da Xian Xiong Wan must be taken until its efficacy is demonstrated by a loose stool, and one further reduced dose of Gan Cao Fu Zi Tang is given when the appetite returns, sweating ceases, and there is vexation.

The Secret of Learning *Shang Han Lun*

Shang Han Lun is an ancient text which has great clinical relevance for contemporary Chinese medicine practitioners. It presents the most comprehensive and systemised body of knowledge on the aetiology, pathogenesis and development of externally contracted diseases and their treatment. The combination of herbs is extraordinarily sophisticated and skilful, and *Shang Han Lun* may be regarded as the richest and most penetrating Chinese medical text ever written. As an ancient medical text which combines both theory and practical applications, it guides practitioners in the treatment of diseases caused by pathogenic cold and provides us with penetrating insights into disease aetiology, diagnosis and treatment strategies which are relevant in the treatment of modern diseases. It offers rich rewards to students and practitioners who extract the essence of this ancient treatment system and use it to full advantage.

太陽

Tai Yang

2

Section One

2.1 OUTLINE OF TAI YANG

Pathway of the Tai Yang Channel

The Tai Yang channel incorporates the foot Tai Yang urinary bladder and the hand Tai Yang small intestine meridians and has an exterior–interior relationship with the Shao Yin channel, which comprises the foot Shao Yin kidney and the hand Shao Yin heart meridians. The external pathway of the foot Tai Yang urinary bladder channel runs from the inner corner of the eye, over the top of the head and down the neck, intersecting the Du meridian before following the spine to the sacrum. From there, it travels down the back of the leg, ending at the tip of the fifth toe. An internal channel runs from the sacrum upwards to the kidneys before homing to the urinary bladder. The luo connecting channel leads to the channel of its yin partner, the kidney, and a divergent channel leads to the heart. Its partner, the channel of the hand Tai Yin small intestine, travels from the little finger to the shoulder, intersects the Du meridian, then crosses the side of the neck and face to meet the foot Tai Yang urinary bladder channel at the inner corner of the eye. An internal channel connects it to the heart.

Physiology of the Tai Yang Channel

The urinary bladder channel is the longest of the channels and because of its connection to all the zang and fu organs, it has the capacity to move qi and blood, supplement yin and yang, nourish the sinews and lubricate the joints. Its pathway traverses the head and courses the entire length of the back and legs, and this extensive domain is the basis of its role in governing the exterior. The *Ling Shu: Ben Zang Pian (Ling Shu Chapter 47: The Organs*) states: "The san jiao and urinary bladder correspond to the interstices and body hair." In *Su Wen: Ling Lan Mi Dian Lun Pian (Su Wen Chapter 8: Confidential Discourse of the Mystical Orchid)* we find: "The urinary bladder is the governor of the metropolis. It stores the body fluids, qi transforms then exits." Which is to say, the urinary bladder, and by inference, the Tai Yang channel, governs a wide range of functions and is also responsible for storing and distributing the fluids which ultimately nourish the skin and hair.

By definition, an exterior syndrome is an invasion by an externally contracted pathogen which affects the exterior and the muscle layer. According to *Shang Han Lun*'s six channel theory, all exterior related disorders caused by pathogenic cold are categorised as a Tai Yang disorder. This is because the foot Tai Yang urinary bladder meridian governs the exterior and acts as the body's first line of defence against pathogenic influences. Any externally contracted pathogen will therefore attack the Tai Yang channel first.

The urinary bladder is one of the six fu and is situated in the lower jiao. Its function of governing the exterior and the skin and interstices is based not only on the extensive range of the associated channels but also on its physiology and its relationship with the kidney. It is paired with the kidney in an exterior–interior relationship via interconnecting collaterals and network vessels and thus has a connection to the primary yang of the kidney. It is the kidney yang which warms and supports the functions of the urinary bladder, entering its channel network to warm and protect the body, where it is better known as wei yang (defence yang) or wei qi (defence qi).

The foot Tai Yang urinary bladder meridian governs the Du Mai, which rules the yang channels. With the support of the qi from the yang channels, the Tai Yang urinary bladder meridian is able to warm and nourish the body and govern the exterior, protecting the body from the invasion of pathogens. Furthermore, the zheng qi from the five zang and six fu is concentrated at the shu xue or transporting points located along the foot Tai Yang meridian as it traverses the back. These transporting points act as a portal for the corresponding zang and fu to nourish and replenish the qi of the foot Tai Yang urinary bladder meridian as it governs the superficial aspects of the body. Conversely, externally contracted pathogens can invade the body through the same network vessels and find their way to the respective organs. In other words, if the exterior disorder is not released from the Tai Yang level, it will transmit into the interior. Therefore, one of the premises of *Shang Han Lun* is that Tai Yang disorders be resolved at the exterior level to prevent the development of more serious pathological manifestations.

In summary, the extensive material base which is provided by the internal organs, enabling the Tai Yang meridian to govern the exterior, comprises: the yang qi of the kidney through its interior–exterior relationship with the urinary bladder, the qi from the yang channels through the urinary bladder channel's connection with the Du meridians, and the qi of the five zang and six fu through the shu transporting points located on the urinary bladder channel. These vital connections help to concentrate the defence yang in the Tai Yang channel, thus supporting its function of protecting the exterior.

Pathology of the Tai Yang Channel

Cold injury is disease caused by externally contracted pathogenic cold. Since the Tai Yang channel governs the exterior of the body, it is commonly the first to be affected. When an external pathogen invades the exterior, it impedes the flow of qi and blood in the Tai Yang channel causing exterior constraint. Because wei qi (defence qi) is disrupted, it can no longer co-ordinate with ying qi (nutrient qi) and this is referred to as a disharmony of ying and wei. The wei qi fails to warm and secure the surface of the body so there is aversion to cold; the constrained qi of the Tai Yang channel causes pain in the neck and head along the course of the Tai Yang channel; because the wei qi rises to the surface to battle the pathogen, the pulse is floating; the struggle between the zheng qi and the pathogen results in fever. This group of signs and symptoms reflects the pathomechanism of Tai Yang and constitutes a Tai Yang exterior pattern.

Tai Yang Disease and Its Transmission Pathway

A number of pathological changes can take place in the course of Tai Yang disease. The changes may be part of the general development of the disease but can also sometimes be attributed to inappropriate treatment. Some examples are:

- The externally contracted cold pathogen may be transmitted via the network vessels from the Tai Yang channel to its associated fu, the urinary bladder, resulting in Tai Yang water amassment.
- If the exterior pathogen is not resolved (whether due to lack of treatment or to inappropriate treatment), a transmuted pattern may arise. Otherwise referred to as huai bing or bian zheng, a transmuted pattern does not possess the characteristic features of Tai Yang disease.
- It is possible for the pathogen to transmit to another channel, without completely leaving the first. This can be seen where the paired relationship between the Tai Yang and Shao Yin channels facilitates the transmission of the pathogen to the Shao Yin channel, resulting in a condition affecting both channels. For example, a pre-existing deficiency of heart

and kidney yang may allow the exterior cold pathogen to transmit inwards, giving rise to devastated yang and exuberant yin. This is true to the adage that Tai Yang is associated with excess and Shao Yin with deficiency.

Tai Yang governs the exterior and acts as a defensive shield for the other channels. If the disease is not resolved, it may transmit from the exterior to the interior; in other words, from Tai Yang to Yang Ming or from Tai Yang to Shao Yang. This phenomenon may take the form of he bing (a combination of patterns in two or more channels) or bing bing (the manifestation of a new channel syndrome before the original channel syndrome is resolved) or even zhi zhong (direct transmission to the yin channels, completely bypassing the three yang channels). The pattern of transmission varies depending on the strength of the zheng qi, the intensity of the pathogen and, above all, the appropriateness of treatment. In general, the pulse sign serves as a guide to determine the transmission pathway.

Key Manifestations of Tai Yang Disease

The signs and symptoms characteristic of a Tai Yang exterior pattern are fever, aversion to cold, headache, a stiff neck and a floating pulse, all reflecting the invasion of wind and cold in the Tai Yang channel. Depending on the constitution of the individual and the relative virulence of the pathogen, there are three differential presentations of the pattern, classified and described in section 2.2 of this chapter.

Classification of Tai Yang Disease

The fact that *Shang Han Lun* has no fewer than 178 clauses relating to Tai Yang disease not only reflects the high incidence of externally contracted disease, but also its potential for transformation into a range of more complex patterns. Apart from the three basic patterns representing the early stage, Zhang Zhong Jing outlines 13 sub-categories detailing complications, and presents a highly developed description of many transmutations which can result from incorrect treatment.

The relative strength of the pathogen, differences in individual constitutions and the duration of disease all have a bearing on the way a pattern develops and on subsequent changes of the disease.

These varying factors result in six categories of disorders associated with the Tai Yang channel:

- channel patterns
- fu patterns
- transmuted patterns
- glomus patterns
- concurrent patterns, and
- patterns resembling Tai Yang.

These categories are explored in detail in sections 2.3 to 2.11 of this chapter.

Treatment of Tai Yang Disease

Tai Yang pattern is associated with the exterior and the corresponding treatment is the use of acrid warm herbs to release the exterior. Formulas such as Ma Huang Tang, Da Qing Long Tang, Xiao Qing Long Tang and Ge Gen Tang are examples of this and in certain circumstances, formulas such as Gui Ma Ge Ban Tang, Gui Er Ma Yi Tang and Gui Er Yue Yi Tang are also employed. For Tai Yang concurrent patterns, the core formula is modified, and the treatment of transmuted patterns is closely based on the manifestations; as exhorted in Clause 16A: "Observe the pulse and signs, know the error committed, treat according to the pattern".

Section Two

2.2 PRINCIPAL FEATURES OF TAI YANG DISEASE

Tai Yang patterns comprise:
- Tai Yang zhong feng (wind strike)
- Tai Yang shang han (cold injury), and
- Tai Yang wen bing (warm disease).

Also described here is the recovery period and its relation to yin and yang patterns. Clause 1 describes the pulse image and key manifestations and characteristics of Tai Yang zhong feng and Tai Yang shang han.

Clause 1

太阳之为病，脉浮，头项强痛而恶寒。

Tai Yang is diseased, the pulse is floating, the head and neck are stiff and painful and there is aversion to cold.

DISCUSSION: Tai Yang disease constitutes the initial stage of externally contracted disease when the pathogen is located in the exterior between the wei (defence) and the ying (nutrient), and the disease is still at the superficial level. The floating pulse is a sign of pathogenic invasion of the exterior. Stiffness of the head and neck indicate Tai Yang disease because the Tai Yang channel passes through that region of the body; the pathogen impedes the normal flow of channel qi, leading to pain and stiffness in the head and neck. Aversion to cold arises because the pathogenic cold has constrained wei yang (defence yang), leading to disharmony of ying and wei. This clause summarises the pathogenesis of Tai Yang disease by describing the manifestations of an invasion by exterior wind cold which impedes the channel qi, constrains wei yang and causes disharmony of ying and wei.

In the past, the pulse and signs cited above were regarded as the golden standard for the diagnosis of externally contracted Tai Yang disease. The clinical reality, however, is that a floating pulse in an externally contracted wind cold pattern is atypical. More often, a rapid, slippery and wiry pulse is encountered, particularly if fever is present, and although there is the mild discomfort or stiffness in the back of the neck, a severely stiff neck is rare. Headache and aversion to cold, however, are typically seen in Tai Yang disease.

Tai Yang Zhong Feng (Wind Strike) Pattern

Clause 2 outlines the pulse and signs specific for Tai Yang zhong feng (wind strike). This pattern is also known as Tai Yang exterior deficiency pattern because the wei yang (defence yang) is contending with the pathogen and is too weak to protect the ying yin and prevent its escape via the pores.

Clause 2

太阳病，发热汗出，恶风，脉缓者，名为中风。

Tai Yang disease, there is fever and sweating, aversion to wind, where the pulse is moderate, it is called wind strike.

DISCUSSION: As stated in *Nan Jing: 58th Difficult Issue*, zhong feng (wind strike) is one of the five categories of shang han (cold injury). Wind is a yang pathogen, and Tai Yang is a yang channel which governs the exterior as a barrier defending against invasion. As the defence yang rises to contend with the pathogenic wind, the struggle between these two yang forces results in fever. The rising defence yang can not perform its function of protecting the ying yin or nutrient fluid and consequently, the ying yin fails to be contained in the interior and discharges outward as sweat. The exterior is insecure, hence the aversion to wind; the moderate pulse is a result of the weak ying yin and the loss of sweat, which is why this pattern is also known as the Tai Yang exterior deficiency pattern. The pathomechanism of this pattern is described by *Shang Han Lun* commentators as strong wei yang (defence yang) and weak ying yin (nutrient yin). Cheng Wu Ji in *Zhu Jie Shang Han Lun* said, "Wind is yang and cold is yin. Wind injures the wei giving rise to fever, sweating and aversion to cold. It is the wei which is attacked by the wind." The treatment principle for zhong feng or wind strike must address, therefore, not only the exterior wind cold, but also the disharmony or imbalance of ying and wei.

The manifestation of disease can be attributed to both internal and external factors. The relative strength of the external pathogenic qi and the body's constitutional zheng qi are major factors in determining the response of the body's defence mechanism. Similar pathogenic influences and diseases can have a different impact on different individuals. Constitutionally strong individuals are seldom affected by cold and an attack by exterior wind cold will manifest as an excess exterior pattern; for the constitutionally weak individual, however, the same wind cold attack will result in a pattern known as an exterior deficiency pattern. This is the key point of differentiation of Tai Yang shang han or cold injury, which is an exterior excess pattern, and Tai Yang zhong feng or wind strike, which is an exterior deficiency pattern. The propensity for one or the other to manifest is highly dependent on the constitution or zheng qi of the person.

COMMENT: Opinions differ as to whether what is referred to in *Shang Han Lun* as Tai Yang wind strike is the same as the clinical condition known as the common cold. Xu Shu Wei said: "The condition now known as shang feng (wind injury) is what the ancient people referred to as zhong feng (wind strike)" (*Xu Shu Wei Shang Han Lun Zhu San Zhong* and *Shang Han Fa Wei Lun*). Zhu Gong said, "The condition now known as wind injury is a condition with headache, fever, a moderate pulse, sweating and aversion to wind" (*Shang Han Bai Wen*). Xu Ling Tai said, "The invasion of pathogenic wind cold manifests as headache, fever, cough and a runny nose. This condition was referred to by ancient people as wind damage" (*Shang Han Lei Fang*).

The conditions of wind strike (zhong feng), wind injury (shang feng) and gan mao (common cold), as described by numerous practitioners in the past, are all caused by externally contracted wind cold and manifest with similar symptoms, with variations mainly attributed to the intensity of the disorder. Dai Yuan Li offered further clarification when he stated, "The mild condition is known as 'gan' or 'affect' and the more serious condition is known as 'shang' or 'injury'" (*Zheng Zhi Yao Jue*). Thus he confirmed that zhong feng (wind strike) as described in *Shang Han Lun* is a more serious condition than that now referred to as gan mao or 'affect manifestation' and which refers to the common cold. So it can be said that shang han (cold injury) and zhong feng (wind strike) are not two separate conditions but rather, two patterns which reflect a difference in intensity of the same condition.

Tai Yang Shang Han (Cold Injury) Pattern

Clause 3 describes the pulse and signs of Tai Yang shang han (cold injury), which is characterised by the yin and yang pulses both being tight.

Clause 3

太阳病，或已发热，或未发热，必恶寒，体痛，呕逆，脉阴阳俱紧者，名为伤寒。

Tai Yang disease, whether there is fever, or there is no fever, there must be aversion to cold, body ache, vomiting, where the yin and yang of the pulse are both tight, it is called shang han.

DISCUSSION: Tai Yang shang han or cold injury is a Tai Yang disease which is caused by pathogenic wind cold constraining the defence yang in the exterior, preventing it from warming the exterior. In this clause, the presence or absence of fever is referring to its onset. There is a direct correlation between the early or late manifestation of fever and the intensity of the pathogen relative to the strength of the constitution. Early manifestation of fever represents invasion of the exterior by pathogenic wind cold where there is a robust response by the defence yang, combating the pathogen. Absence of fever, on the other hand, indicates that the strength of the pathogenic wind cold is relatively greater than that of the defence yang, which is depressed and unable to rise to the occasion. The relative strength of the pathogen as compared with the zheng qi is largely dependent on the constitution of the individual; the vigorousness of the fever being an indicator of the vigour of the zheng qi. At the onset of this disorder, marked fever will be a feature in young healthy individuals but not in older individuals or those with a weaker constitution, when the contraction of wind cold is often accompanied by a low grade fever. This relationship between the intensity of fever and the strength of wei yang or defence yang was described by Ke Yun Bo in *Shang Han Lai Su Ji (Shang Han Revival Compendium)*.

Pathogenic cold is a yin pathogen, which tends to constrain the defence yang, impairing its normal function of warming the body. Because the defence qi is unable to warm the exterior, the patient experiences aversion to cold. The significance of the statement "there must be aversion to cold" is that aversion to cold is an important distinguishing characteristic of Tai Yang disease, and only if there is aversion to cold, can the diagnosis be made. The obstruction of the exterior by the pathogenic cold also impedes the flow of qi and blood, causing pain in the body and tightness in both the proximal and distal positions of the pulse, referred to here as the yin and yang pulses. This tight pulse is typical in Tai Yang shang han, which is an exterior excess cold pattern. A Tai Yang shang han pulse which is both tight and floating is associated with the presence of fever, where the wei yang is pushing the pathogen to the surface. A pulse which is tight but not floating is associated with an absence of fever due to weak or constrained wei yang.

Differentiation of Shang Han and Zhong Feng

Zhong feng or wind strike is caused by the invasion of pathogenic wind which destabilises the defence yang, thereby resulting in the discharge of ying yin. The main manifestations are fever, sweating, aversion to wind and a floating and moderate pulse.

Shang han or cold injury, on the other hand, is caused by the invasion of pathogenic cold which affects the normal function of ying yin and wei yang, thereby causing the defence yang to be constrained. The main manifestations are aversion to cold, fever, absence of sweat, generalised body aches, vomiting and a floating and tight pulse.

The key point for differentiation between Tai Yang shang han and Tai Yang zhong feng is the presence or absence of sweat.

Tai Yang Wen Bing (Warm Disease) Pattern

Clause 6 differentiates between the pulse and manifestations of wen bing (warm disease), zhong feng (wind strike) and shang han (cold injury).

Clause 6

太阳病，发热而渴，不恶寒者，为温病。若发汗已，身灼热者，名风温。风温为病，脉阴阳俱浮，自汗出，身重，多眠睡，鼻息必鼾，语言难出。若被下者，小便不利，直视失溲；若被火者，微发黄色，剧则如惊痫，时瘛疭，若火熏之；一逆尚引日，再逆促命期。

Tai Yang disease, if there is fever and thirst, with no aversion to cold, it is wen bing. If sweat has already been promoted, with the body scorching hot, it is called feng wen. In feng wen, the yin and yang pulses are both floating, there is spontaneous sweating, the body is heavy, there is somnolence, stertorous breathing, difficulty speaking. If there was purging, the urination will not be free, there will be a fixed gaze and loss of continence; if there was fire therapy, there will be slight yellowing, if severe there will be convulsions, periodic spasmodic jerking, as if fumed by fire; one adverse treatment will prolong it, further adverse treatment will hasten the expiry of life.

DISCUSSION: The reference to Tai Yang disease is a reference to externally contracted disease. However, the fever and thirst with no aversion to cold are characteristic of wen bing or warm disease, which includes feng wen or wind warmth, where the attack is one of pathogenic warmth which damages yin fluids. This differs significantly from shang han, where the attack is one of pathogenic cold injuring the yang. The reference to the floating yin and yang pulses is a reference to the fact that exuberant pathogenic heat is surfacing towards the exterior, which is the cause of the spontaneous sweating. The heat damages qi and the depleted qi combined with a lack of fluids to nourish the channels gives rise to a sense of heaviness in the body. If the heat harasses the spirit there will be somnolence, fire will condense fluids into phlegm and the upsurge of wind will carry the phlegm upwards misting the mind and obstructing the orifices, causing stertorous breathing and unintelligible speech.

The initial stage of shang han is marked by an aversion to cold and no thirst; fever may or may not be present and sweating may be promoted. In contrast, the initial stage of wen bing is marked by fever, thirst and no aversion to cold, and the appropriate treatment is the administration of acrid, cool herbs to release the exterior. Sweating, purging and fire therapy are absolutely contraindicated. If any of these are used, the result will be a transmuted pattern with severe yin depletion, which may further fuel the heat. The incorrect promotion of sweat with acrid, warm herbs will serve as a catalyst to transform heat to fire: after the loss of sweat, the fever will be exacerbated and the body will be scorching hot to the touch.

If incorrect purging is adopted, there will be further loss of fluids which will result in inhibited urination. The depleted essence will no longer nourish the eyes and this, combined with the disturbance of the heart spirit, results in a forward staring gaze. Incorrect purging, especially when excessive, can also ultimately lead to faecal incontinence. If fire therapy is adopted to further promote sweating, the exacerbated fluid loss will be catastrophic; the fire will burn out of control, fuming the liver and gallbladder and causing yellowing of the skin and sclera. More severe toxic heat can give rise to endogenous liver wind, which can result in convulsions or occasional jerking of the body. Even one incorrect treatment will lengthen the duration of disease, but a repetition of any adverse treatment could lead to death. This clause warns practitioners of the critical importance in correct diagnosis and treatment of wen bing. Particular care must be taken in differentiating wen bing from shang han because the early stage of wen bing affects the lungs and a slight aversion to cold can sometimes be experienced and the thirst is only a mild thirst. (Excessive thirst indicates an interior pattern.)

Historical commentators differed in their interpretations of wind warmth (feng wen). You Zai Jing put forward the theory that feng wen was caused by pathogenic wind and warmth (*Shang Han Guan Zhu Ji*). Zhang Xu Gu proposed that feng wen is the result of incorrect treatment which has given rise to endogenous liver wind, and on that basis was called feng wen (*Shang Han Lun Ben Zhi* and *Yi Men Bang He*). These two opinions differ on two levels: firstly as to aetiology and whether the condition is caused by an exterior pathogen or by incorrect treatment; and secondly, as to whether the term 'wind' in the name of the pattern refers to exterior or interior wind. In accordance with the interpretation of Clause 6 as outlined above, the authors subscribe to the theory that feng wen is the result of the incorrect treatment of wen bing, causing its transformation into a transmuted pattern. It is important to note that the 'feng wen' alluded to in Clause 6 is entirely different from the "newly contracted feng wen" described by the wen bing specialists in the Qing dynasty.

Differentiation of Disease According to Yin and Yang

Clause 7 differentiates externally contracted diseases according to whether they stem from yin or from yang, and on that basis, determines when recovery is likely to take place.

Clause 7

病有发热恶寒者，发于阳也；无热恶寒者，发于阴也。发于阳，七日愈。发于阴，六日愈。以阳数七、阴数六也。

If the disease has fever and aversion to cold, it stems from yang; if there is no fever and aversion to cold, it stems from yin. That which stems from yang, recovery is in seven days. That which stems from yin, recovery is in six days. This is because yang numbers seven and yin numbers six.

DISCUSSION: Fever and aversion to cold are a means of identifying the nature of the disease and its clinical significance. Fever is a reflection of the struggle of the zheng qi against the pathogen, and in the course of externally contracted disease, the presence or absence of fever enables the practitioner to determine the strength of that struggle. Fever with an aversion to cold is described as stemming from yang because it demonstrates strong zheng qi which is engaged in a vigorous battle to oust the evil. The fever is a result of the zheng qi's strength as it manages to gain the upper hand, and the cold represents the presence of the evil in the exterior. If the strength of the zheng qi is diminished, it is unable to put up such a strong fight, and there will be no fever. The aversion to cold remains as long as the pathogen is present in the exterior. For this reason, the absence of fever is described as stemming from yin.

In *Shang Han Lun Tiao Bian*, Fang You Zhi said: "Tai Yang disease is characterised by aversion to cold and if aversion to cold is accompanied by fever, it is Tai Yang zhong feng. Wind is a yang pathogen and defence qi is also yang. Thus, it can be said that the disease stems from yang." *Yi Zong Jin Jian (Golden Mirror of Medical Tradition)* said: "The initial stage of Tai Yang disease with fever and aversion to cold is said to arise because of defence yang; whereas the initial onset of Tai Yang disease with aversion to cold but no fever is said to arise as a result of nutrient yin." There are three interpretations of this concept:

1. Whether a disease stems from yang or from yin can be used as a guide to pattern identification of all externally contracted disease.
2. Disease stemming from yang relates to Tai Yang disease and that stemming from yin relates to Shao Yin disease. For example, in *Wai Tai Mi Yao* (*Essential Secrets from the Imperial Library)* it is said: "In disease which stems from yang, adopt the strategy of releasing the exterior; in disease which stems from yin, adopt the strategy of warming the interior. Gui Zhi Tang is indicated to release the exterior and Si Ni Tang is indicated to warm the interior."
3. Disease which stems from yang relates to disease of the three yang channels and that stemming from yin relates to disease of the three yin channels. Qian Huang in *Shang Han Shuo Yuan Ji* said: "Disease stemming from yang involves the yang channels, while disease stemming from yin involves the yin channels." *Su Wen: Yin Yang Ying Xiang Da Lun (Su Wen: Great Disourse on the Phenomena of Yin and Yang)* states: "When yang dominates, fever will manifest and when yin dominates there will be aversion to cold."

Reliance on the symptoms of fever and aversion to cold in order to classify disease as pertaining to yin or to yang is a somewhat simplified method of pattern identification and far from absolute. Accurate diagnosis depends on thorough analysis of more than just one or two symptoms. This becomes clear when we compare similar manifestations which occur in different patterns. For instance, a Tai Yang pattern can present with aversion to cold and no fever in the early stage, as can a Yang Ming channel pattern. Only by thorough analysis and accurate pattern identification can an appropriate treatment strategy be devised.

The calculation of recovery of yin and yang type externally contracted disease in Clause 7, based on yin (even) and yang (odd) numbers, originated from Fu Xi the legendary ruler of the ancient book, *He Tu Luo Shu* (*River Charts and the Book of Luo*). Seven is an odd number pertaining to yang and six an even number pertaining to yin; however, this somewhat esoteric method of predicting recovery has not been shown to be clinically useful.

Section Three

2.3 TAI YANG CHANNEL PATTERNS

In Tai Yang disease, there are six categories of patterns:

- channel patterns
- fu patterns
- transmuted patterns
- glomus patterns
- concurrent patterns, and
- patterns resembling Tai Yang.

This section (2.3) describes the manifestations and treatment of Tai Yang channel patterns. The other pattern categories of Tai Yang disease are then addressed separately in sections 2.4 to 2.11 of this chapter.

In Clause 12, Tai Yang disease channel patterns are further differentiated into Tai Yang zhong feng (wind strike) and Tai Yang shang han (cold injury). Pattern identification relies on the observation of the pulses and signs described below. Successful treatment is dependent upon understanding the contraindications and modifications.

2.3.1 Tai Yang Zhong Feng or Gui Zhi Tang Pattern

The term Gui Zhi Tang pattern refers to both the clinical manifestations and the treatment protocols of Tai Yang zhong feng (wind strike), otherwise known as an exterior deficiency pattern.

Clause 12

太阳病中风，阳浮而阴弱，阳浮者，热自发，阴弱者，汗自出。啬啬恶寒，淅淅恶风，翕翕发热，鼻鸣干呕者，桂枝汤主之。

Tai Yang zhong feng, yang is floating and yin is weak, where yang is floating, there is spontaneous fever, where yin is weak, there is spontaneous sweating. Huddled aversion to cold, wetted aversion to wind, feather-warm fever, with a snuffly nose and dry retching, Gui Zhi Tang governs.

GUI ZHI TANG: Gui Zhi (bark removed) 3 liang; Shao Yao 3 liang; Zhi Gan Cao 2 liang; Sheng Jiang (sliced) 3 liang; Da Zao (broken) 12 pieces. The ratio of Gui Zhi to Bai Shao must be 1:1 in order to harmonise ying and wei. Any change in this ratio will alter the function of the formula. Traditionally, Zhi Gan Cao most often referred to dry-roasted Gan Cao, but in modern times, it is usually prepared stir-fried with honey or vinegar.

DIRECTIONS: Break the first three ingredients into pieces, add to the rest of the ingredients in a pot and decoct in 7 sheng (1.4 L) of water. Reduce to three sheng and strain. Take 1 sheng at a moderate temperature followed by 1 sheng of hot, thin gruel to reinforce the effect of the decoction. Cover the body with a blanket for a time until the whole body is damp from light sweat. These instructions must be adhered to. Taking hot gruel and covering the body with a blanket after taking the decoction warms the body and ensures a generalised mild sweat.

The sweat must not be made to flow too freely or recovery will not take place. If the disease is resolved after the first dose, the medication must be discontinued but if there is no sweating, then another dose must be given. If the disease is severe, shorten the interval between doses and administer the three doses in a half day. Observe the patient carefully throughout the day and if, after finishing one pack, the symptoms are still present, repeat. Up to three packs can be given if there has been no sweating. The patient must abstain from foods which are raw and cold, rich and greasy, and also meat, liquor, dairy products, foods with a bad odour and the five acrids, which are scallion, Chinese chive, leek, garlic and asafoetida *(Ben Cao Gang Mu)*.

DISCUSSION: Clause 12 describes a Tai Yang zhong feng pulse where yang is floating and yin is weak. Here, yin and yang refer to the pressure used in pulse taking: light pressure and a floating pulse is yang, whilst heavy pressure and a deep pulse is yin; and so this simply means a floating and moderate pulse. Another interpretation relates to pathogenesis, where floating yang indicates exuberant yang and weak yin refers to deficient nutrient yin. Zhang Zhong Jing said:

"Floating yang is spontaneous fever and weak yin is spontaneous sweating". This is another way of saying that the invasion of pathogenic cold in the exterior has caused the defence yang to rise to the exterior to resist the pathogen, so the pulse is floating, and sweating has depleted the yin fluid, which is reflected in a pulse weak at the deep level. Huddled aversion to cold, implying that the person huddles in order to keep warm and fend off the cold, wetted aversion to wind, referring to a more marked aversion to wind when wet, and feather-warm fever, indicating just a slight rise in temperature, are the primary symptoms of Tai Yang zhong feng. A snuffly nose and dry retching are secondary symptoms of Tai Yang zhong feng, and are due to the affect of pathogenic wind cold on the lung and stomach qi.

Gui Zhi Tang is the guiding formula for Tai Yang zhong feng. It harmonises the nutrient and defence qi, releases pathogens from the muscle layer by promoting sweat, nourishes the yin and regulates the yang. The chief herb is Gui Zhi, which is acrid, dispersing and warm, thus freeing the defence yang and releasing the pathogen from the exterior. The deputy is Shao Yao which is sour and cold, so by nourishing the yin, harmonises the ying and wei.

Yi Zong Jin Jian (Golden Mirror of Medical Tradition) states: "The combination of Gui Zhi, the chief herb, with Shao Yao promotes sweating and at the same time astringes sweat; Shao Yao, the deputy, combined with the chief herb Gui Zhi, harmonises ying and regulates wei; Sheng Jiang assists Gui Zhi in releasing the pathogen from the muscle layer; Da Zao assists Shao Yao to harmonise ying and augment yin; Gan Cao regulates all the herbal ingredients."

Clauses 2 and 12 both discuss the pulse and symptoms associated with Tai Yang zhong feng. Ke Yun Bo, a Qing dynasty annotator of *Shang Han Lun,* identified the main symptom complex of Tai Yang zhong feng as follows: "Headache, spontaneous sweating, fever, aversion to cold, snuffly nose, dry retching etc. Only one sign is needed to indicate that this is the pattern, they do not all have to be present. But a weak pulse and spontaneous sweating are the main manifestations" (*Shang Han Lai Su Ji*). Clinical observation shows that the three pertinent points associated with Tai Yang zhong feng are: (1) a weak constitution, (2) a pulse that is floating, moderate, deficient and weak, and (3) fever, aversion to wind cold and spontaneous sweating.

In *Shang Han Lun*, Gui Zhi Tang is cited for a range of conditions: Tai Yang zhong feng pattern; spontaneous sweating due to disharmony of ying and wei; Tai Yang pattern when the pathogen is still in the exterior after the promotion of sweat or purgation; Tai Yin exterior syndrome. *Jing Gui Yao Lue* also uses Gui Zhi Tang in the treatment of nausea and vomiting during pregnancy, and for Tai Yang zhong feng in the postpartum period.

Ancient Application of Gui Zhi Tang

- *Nan Yang Huo Ren Shu (Nan Yang Book to Safeguard Life)* states that Gui Zhi Tang can be used for people residing in the north-west region of China. For people residing around the area south of Huai River and north of Yangtze River, Gui Zhi Tang can be used during the winter and early spring. If used during the late spring and before the summer solstice, where Gui Zhi Tang is indicated, add 3g of Huang Qin. This was known as Yang Dan Tang (阳旦汤); after the summer solstice, add 15g of Zhi Mu and 30g of Shi Gao or add 3g of Sheng Ma. If the patient has a weak constitution and is cold, no modification is required.
- *Shang Han Lai Su Ji (Shang Han Revival Compendium)* states: "Gui Zhi Tang is indicated for spontaneous sweating, nocturnal sweating, malaria and dysentery". *Wen Bing Tiao Bian (Systematic Differentiation of Warm Disease)* advocated the use of modified Gui Zhi Tang to treat wind cold and numerous other externally contracted febrile diseases where there was aversion to cold.

Modern Application of Gui Zhi Tang

- *Epidemic influenza.* Gui Zhi Tang with the addition of Huang Qi in the treatment of influenza which follows a Gui Zhi Tang pattern.
- *Postpartum fever and spontaneous sweating.* Gui Zhi Tang with the addition of Huang Qi, Dang Gui, Suan Zao Ren, Wu Wei Zi.

- *Joint pain.* If the pattern is related to cold with no swelling and redness of the joint and there is exacerbation of pain in cold weather, Gui Zhi Tang with the addition of Fu Zi can be used. For a hot pattern, Gui Zhi Bai Hu Tang can be used.
- *Morning sickness.* For a pattern characterised by fatigue and discomfort in the stomach, Gui Zhi Tang with the addition of Sha Ren, Bai Zhu, Dang Shen, Fu Ling can be used. For disharmony of liver and spleen, use Gui Zhi Tang with Su Ye, Zhu Ru, Huang Lian. For phlegm damp, add Sha Ren, Chen Pi, Fu Ling.
- *Urticaria.* If the pattern is characterised by itchy skin, spontaneous sweating, aversion to wind and a floating and moderate pulse, use Gui Zhi Tang with the addition of Fang Feng, Jing Jie, Chan Tui.
- *Rhinitis with sensitivity to cold.* Use Gui Zhi Tang with the addition of Ting Li Zi, Chan Tui.
- *Externally contracted wind cold manifesting with fever, aversion to cold, headache, nasal congestion, a floating pulse and a thin white tongue coat.* Use Gui Zhi Tang with Jing Jie 5–10g, Lu Gen 5–10g, Mao Gen 5–10g.

Case Study

Common Cold

Extracted from: Shang Han Lun Tang Zheng Lun Zhi

A 28-year-old male had contracted a cold at the beginning of autumn. He presented with a fever, headache and was clammy to touch. His pulse was floating and moderate and his tongue was moist with a thin, white tongue coat. One pack of Gui Zhi Tang was prescribed, with directions to give it in three doses over the day until it brought out a sweat, with each dose being followed by a bowl of hot rice porridge, and the patient being covered with a rug. The first two doses failed to bring out a sweat but after the third dose, he came out in a mild sweat, slept through the night and was fully recovered in the morning.

Case Study

Skin Rash

Source unknown

A 31-year-old woman presented with a dry, itchy, pale red rash covering her chest, arms and throat. She had had the rash ever since bush walking some weeks before. Her menstrual cycle varied from 27 to 30 days, her face was pale with pale red spots on her cheeks and she also complained of spontaneous sweating during the day in response to little or no exertion. She was sensitive to the cold and avoided going outdoors. Her pulse was soft and the tongue pale red with a thin white coat.

Diagnosis: Disharmony of ying and wei, blood deficiency and wind in the channels.

Treatment principle: Harmonise ying and wei, nourish blood, expel wind from the skin.

A modification of Gui Zhi Tang was prescribed: Gui Zhi 10g; Bai Shao 12g; Da Zao 6 pieces, Sheng Jiang 5g; Jing Jie 8g; He Shou Wu 15g; Chuan Xiong 6g; Dan Shen 8g; Zhi Gan Cao 5g (five packs).

She returned after one week showing about 70% improvement. A further five packs were given, with the addition of Huang Qi 15g to augment the qi and stabilise the exterior.

Additional Indications for Gui Zhi Tang

In addition to the key indications of pain and stiffness in the neck and head and a floating pulse, Gui Zhi Tang can be prescribed for associated disorders such as the following.

- Zhong feng presenting with headache, fever and sweating, which is differentiated from a Yin Qiao San pattern by a moderate floating pulse and aversion to wind.
- Persistence of the zhong feng pattern past the expected duration, due to the virulence and tenacity of a pathogen, and where the patient also suffers from vexation.

These and other patterns indicated for Gui Zhi Tang are described below.

Tai Yang Zhong Feng with Headache, Fever and Sweating

Clause 13

太阳病，头痛，发热，汗出，恶风，桂枝汤主之。

Tai Yang disease, the head aches, there is fever, sweating, aversion to wind, Gui Zhi Tang governs.

DISCUSSION: The Tai Yang channel governs the exterior, rules ying and wei and protects the body against pathogens. When cold invades the body, the Tai Yang channel takes the full force of the attack. Because the Tai Yang channel traverses the head, headache is one of the main manifestations. The struggle of the zheng qi against the pathogenic cold gives rise to fever, the pathogenic cold constrained in the exterior causes the skin interstices to be insecure, resulting in sweating, and impedes the flow of wei yang, causing aversion to wind. This clause describes the characteristic Tai Yang zhong feng symptoms of headache, fever, sweating and aversion to wind. Gui Zhi Tang regulates ying and wei, releases the pathogen from the muscle layer and promotes mild sweat. This clause further expands the indications for Gui Zhi Tang, emphasizing pattern identification as the core issue with the presence of sweating being the key differential factor between zhong feng (wind strike) and shang han (cold injury). The pathomechanism of fever and sweating is explained in connection with Clause 95, below.

Headache is a symptom of all three yang channels patterns and differentiation is as follows.

In Tai Yang headache, the pain is localised in the back of the head and along the neck; in Yang Ming headache, the pain is at the front of the head, particularly across the forehead and is described as a distending pain; Shao Yang headache is usually bilateral and characterised by pressure or tension.

Clause 95

太阳病，发热出汗者，此为荣弱卫强，故使汗出，欲救邪风者，宜桂枝汤。

Tai Yang disease, there is fever and sweating, this is because the nutrient is weak and the defence is strong, so by causing sweat, there will be relief of evil wind, Gui Zhi Tang is appropriate.

DISCUSSION: In this clause, rong, the alternative name for ying is used to refer to nutrient qi. Under normal physiological conditions, wei is yang and circulates outside the vessels, and ying is yin, circulating within the vessels. This is described as ying and wei in perfect harmony. In the event of pathogenic attack, the wei yang rises up to contend with the exterior pathogen and this struggle manifests as fever. Because the wei yang is locked in battle with the pathogen at the surface, it fails to perform its normal function of guarding the interior and this leads to the issue of sweat from the ying. This explains the reference in the clause to sweat being caused by weak rong (ying) and strong wei, where strong wei describes not only the strong action of the defence yang but also implies the presence of a strong pathogen. The focus of this clause is on fever and sweating as identifying symptoms of Tai Yang zhong feng, and it describes the pathogenesis of Tai Yang zhong feng as weak ying and strong wei in the face of an invasion of pathogenic wind. The treatment principle is to dispel pathogenic wind and Gui Zhi Tang is the indicated formula.

Persistent Attack of Tai Yang Zhong Feng

Clause 24

太阳病，初服桂枝汤，反烦不解者，先刺风池、风府，却与桂枝汤则愈。

Tai Yang disease, initially having administered Gui Zhi Tang, but there is vexation with no resolution, first needle Feng Chi and Feng Fu, then give Gui Zhi Tang and there will be recovery.

DISCUSSION: Gui Zhi Tang is the indicated formula for a Tai Yang zhong feng pattern. If, after the first dose, the exterior remains unresolved and the patient is vexed or restless, it could be assumed to be due to incorrect treatment, but this is not so because no change of pulse is noted in the clause. The vexation is a result of the presence of a virulent pathogen, met in battle by the zheng qi, which has been reinforced by the administration of Gui Zhi Tang and stimulated into action. However, its valiant efforts are unsuccessful at first, and additional treatment is required to clear the channel. In this case, the advice is to needle Feng Chi (GB 20) and Feng Fu (Du 16) to expel the pathogenic wind. After the acupuncture, Gui Zhi Tang should again be given to effect full recovery. This is a classic example of the combination of acupuncture and herbal treatment.

There are differing theories as to why the initial dose of Gui Zhi Tang fails to resolve the pathogen and gives rise to vexation. Chen Xiu Yuan believed that Gui Zhi Tang can treat the disorder of the muscle and interstices but not the channel disorder (*Shang Han Yi Fang Ji Zhu* 伤寒医方集注). In *Shang Han Lei Fang,* Xu Ling Tai proposed that the pathogen is lodged in the pathway of the Tai Yang channel and it is this which causes vexation. In *Shang Lun Pian,* Yu Jia Yan suggested that hot gruel may not have been taken with the Gui Zhi Tang. In *Shang Han Lun Tiao Bian,* Fang You Zhi proposed that the vexation was a manifestation of the struggle between the zheng qi and the pathogen and a sign that the patient was about to sweat and recover.

The occurrence of such symptoms as vexation, an oppressed sensation in the chest or shivering following the administration of Gui Zhi Tang, can be a sign of a transmuted pattern caused by incorrect treatment. However, as in this case, they can also be testament to correct medication and Fang You Zhi's interpretation is the one which concords with the theory expressed in Clause 95.

Gui Zhi Tang in the Treatment of Exterior Deficiency

Clause 42 explains that Gui Zhi Tang is indicated in exterior deficiency patterns because of its function of promoting sweat. Clauses 44 and 45 discuss the adverse effects of purging, and confirm that even after sweating and purging, if the exterior remains unresolved, Gui Zhi Tang is still indicated. Clauses 53 and 54 explain the phenomenon of spontaneous sweating.

Clause 42

太阳病，外证未解，脉浮弱者，当以汗解，宜桂枝汤。

Tai Yang disease, where the exterior pattern is unresolved, with the pulse floating and weak, it must be resolved by sweating, Gui Zhi Tang is appropriate.

DISCUSSION: In a Tai Yang exterior pattern, there will be fever, headache and aversion to cold, but the pulse may be either floating and tense or floating and weak or moderate. A tense, floating pulse characterises an exterior excess pattern, where Ma Huang Tang is the indicated formula. The point made by this clause is that one must diagnose according to the pulse. In this clause, the weak pulse is synonymous with a moderate pulse in that they both indicate deficiency. Therefore, the floating weak pulse in Clause 42 shows that the pattern is one of exterior deficiency, which is a Gui Zhi Tang pattern, and not one of exterior excess, which is a Ma Huang Tang pattern. This differentiation is critical. It is inappropriate to promote excessive sweating in a deficiency pattern and Gui Zhi Tang must be used to promote a mild sweat only in order to avoid damaging the qi. A moderate and weak pulse is associated with insufficient or damaged zheng qi and if Ma Huang Tang were administered, yin and yang would be damaged. This clause reminds us that spontaneous sweating is not the only indicator of a Gui Zhi Tang pattern, and that the pulse should also be observed.

Clause 44

太阳病，外证未解，不可下也，下之为逆，欲解外者，宜桂枝汤。

Tai Yang disease, the exterior pattern is unresolved, one should not purge, purging would be adverse, if you wish to resolve the exterior, Gui Zhi Tang is appropriate.

DISCUSSION: The standard strategy of treatment for an exterior pattern is to release the exterior, not to purge, which is appropriate only in an interior pattern. Clause 44 explains that purgation is contraindicated where the exterior pattern is unresolved and, it would, in fact, have unwelcome outcomes. It further stipulates that where an exterior pattern is unresolved, Gui Zhi Tang is the appropriate formula to use to release the exterior. Where there is constipation, the situation can be misleading and care must be taken to make the correct diagnosis. If an exterior pattern is also present, the exterior must be resolved first by promoting sweat. Purgation can only be used once the exterior pattern is resolved, and failure to follow this golden rule can result in a transmuted pattern, and is therefore considered to be adverse treatment.

Purging is absolutely contraindicated in a simple exterior pattern; in a complex pattern affecting both the exterior and the interior, the strategy is to release the exterior before purging. However, one must act as the situation dictates and differentiate the relative urgency of the exterior as compared to the interior in order to determine the most appropriate treatment strategy.

Exterior Pattern Unresolved by Sweating

Clause 45

太阳病，先发汗不解，而复下者，脉浮者不愈。浮为在外，而反下者，故令不愈，今脉浮，故在外，当须解外则愈，宜桂枝汤。

Tai Yang disease, initial sweating does not resolve it, and where there is then purgation, the pulse will be floating and there is no recovery. Floating means it is in the exterior, but contrarily, there was purgation, so it does not bring recovery, currently the pulse is floating, then it is in the exterior, one must resolve the exterior then there will be recovery, Gui Zhi Tang is appropriate.

DISCUSSION: Clause 45 describes the situation where the initial promotion of sweat fails to resolve the exterior Tai Yang pattern, and following that, purgation is used; the pulse remains floating and there is still no recovery, explaining that the floating pulse shows the pathogen is still in the exterior, and so incorrect purging will not bring recovery. However, because the pulse is still floating, we know that the pathogen has not fallen into the interior. It is still an exterior pattern which can be resolved only by releasing the exterior, and so Gui Zhi Tang should be used. Because the earlier therapies of sweating and purgation have damaged qi and fluids, Ma Huang Tang is inappropriate, and Gui Zhi Tang must be used because it treats an exterior pattern where there is underlying deficiency.

In order to establish if the exterior syndrome still prevails, two points can be considered: Clause 44 simply says that where the exterior is not resolved, Gui Zhi Tang should be used to release the exterior; Clause 45 advises first to ascertain whether the exterior syndrome is present by the pulse sign and then, if the pulse is floating, to give Gui Zhi Tang. Clauses 44 and 45 both advocate the use of Gui Zhi Tang and both place emphasis on a floating pulse as a means of confirming that the pathogen is still in the exterior. It could be inferred that as long as the pulse is still floating, sweating can be promoted; however, a floating pulse is a feature of various patterns and can not be used in isolation to diagnose an exterior syndrome. Other signs and symptoms must be analysed in order to reach an accurate diagnosis.

Vexation Following Sweating in Shang Han

Clause 57

伤寒发汗已解，半日许复烦，脉浮数者，可更发汗，宜桂枝汤。

Shang han already resolved by sweating, after about half a day, there is again vexation, where the pulse is floating and rapid, one may promote sweat, Gui Zhi Tang is appropriate.

DISCUSSION: In Tai Yang shang han or cold injury, the promotion of sweat should bring about recovery and the pulse should be normal again. However, if, a few hours after the promotion of sweat, the patient feels vexed and the pulse is floating and rapid, this shows that the exterior syndrome has not been fully resolved and the patient has relapsed. Sweating must again be promoted, but not excessively, and so Gui Zhi Tang is appropriate.

Confusion can arise in the reading of this clause because generally speaking, a floating pulse indicates an exterior pattern but vexation combined with a rapid pulse is a sign of interior heat and could easily be interpreted as a sign of transformation of exterior cold into interior heat. There are two explanations. The first is that after the promotion of sweating, the exterior syndrome has not been fully resolved and a residual pathogen remains which, after a few hours, transforms into exterior heat, causing the patient to feel vexed. The second possibility is that sweating has left the patient deficient and so, after a short time, a further attack by the exterior pathogen takes place. However, irrespective of whether the vexation is due to a residual pathogen or a further attack of an exterior pathogen, as long as there are signs of an exterior pattern, sweating can be promoted. This clause thus reinforces a key issue, which is that sweating is the correct strategy to resolve an exterior pattern when there is supporting evidence to confirm the diagnosis.

Gui Zhi Tang Following Purgation in an Exterior Pattern

Purging is often advocated in febrile disease caused by pathogenic heat and warmth, but where there is an exterior pattern caused by pathogenic wind and cold, purging is contraindicated. In *Shang Han Lun*, purging is advocated in only two circumstances: the first is for Yang Ming fu excess, and the second is an emergency measure to preserve yin when there is exuberant heat. Clause 15 describes the treatment for a Tai Yang pattern where purging was wrongly administered.

Clause 15

太阳病，下之后，其气上冲者，可与桂枝汤，方用前法。若不上冲者，不得与之。

Tai Yang disease, after purgation, where the qi surges upward, one can give Gui Zhi Tang, in accordance with the earlier method. If there is no upsurge, it must not be given.

DISCUSSION: A Tai Yang pattern must be resolved by sweating. Purging can cause the pathogen to fall inward. The reference to qi surging upwards describes a subjective sensation and it is suggested that the presence or absence of this sensation can be used as a gauge to determine whether the exterior pathogen is in the exterior or has fallen inward. If, after the incorrect use of purgatives, the exterior pathogen has not fallen inward, then this shows that the zheng qi is strong enough to vie with the pathogen and so the pathogen can still be released via the promotion of sweat. The upward surging of qi in this situation indicates that the defence qi is mounting a struggle against the pathogen in the exterior level. Therefore, Gui Zhi Tang is the most appropriate formula.

Disharmony of Ying and Wei with Spontaneous Sweating

Clause 53

病常自汗出者，此为荣气和，荣气和者，外不谐，以卫气不共荣气谐和故尔。以荣行脉中，卫行脉外，复发其汗，荣卫和则愈，宜桂枝汤。

Where the disease has constant spontaneous sweat, this means that nutrient qi is harmonious, when the nutrient qi is harmonious, the exterior is in discord, because the defence qi is not in concord with the nutrient qi. Because nutrient qi moves within the vessels, defence qi moves outside the vessels, further promotion of sweating, the nutrient and defence will harmonise then there will be recovery, Gui Zhi Tang is appropriate.

DISCUSSION: The word disease is not restricted to disease caused by exterior wind cold. Recurrent spontaneous sweating is attributed to disharmony of ying and wei, and the mechanism of that disharmony is explained as a discord or disruption of defence qi, which then can not co-ordinate with the nutrient qi. The physiology of these two forces comprises the nutrient qi moving inside the vessels and being secured by the defence qi moving outside the vessels. Meanwhile, the defence qi is nourished by the nutrient qi, thus stabilising it, whilst the defence qi also stabilises the nutrient qi, preventing it from discharging outward. There is strong interdependence between the two.

The primary issue is the failure in co-ordination between the nutrient qi within the vessels and the defence qi outside the vessels. The act of sweating caused by the administration of Gui Zhi Tang causes the ying yin (nutrient yin) to issue outwards and connect with the wei yang (defence qi), which has been ushered to the surface in its effort to combat the pathogen; the two then meet and again interact. This is one explanation of why the mild sweating promoted by Gui Zhi Tang can harmonise ying and wei. However, the principal explanation resides in the fact that Gui Zhi Tang supports both the defence yang and the nutrient yin, thus dispersing the pathogen and astringing the yin, augmenting the deficiency, and harmonising wei yang and ying yin. It should be noted that when Gui Zhi Tang is used for the purpose of promoting sweat in order to release the exterior, the original instructions must be followed and it must be taken with hot gruel and the patient covered with a blanket to facilitate the production of a mild sweat. However, when the primary objective is to harmonise ying and wei, it should be taken without those measures.

Xu Ling Tai in *Shang Han Lei Fang* states: "There is a marked difference between spontaneous sweating and the promotion of sweating. Spontaneous sweating shows that nutrient and defence qi are not harmonious, whereas the action of promoting sweat is a means to facilitate their harmonious co-ordination. Spontaneous sweating is a sign of deficiency which further depletes zheng qi; the therapeutic promotion of sweat is to expel pathogens".

There are two situations where there is spontaneous sweating due to disharmony of ying (nutrient) and wei (defence) qi, as follows.

1. *Invasion of pathogenic wind.* It is the pathogenic wind which is the cause of the disharmony in ying and wei. Gui Zhi Tang promotes sweating in order to expel the pathogenic wind and stops spontaneous sweating by harmonising ying and wei.
2. *Disharmony between ying (nutrient) and wei (defence) with spontaneous sweating is a feature in the absence of wind strike.* In this situation, the main function of Gui Zhi Tang is to harmonise the nutrient and defence qi, thereby securing the exterior and stabilising the sweating. To strengthen the effect of securing the exterior and thus preventing spontaneous sweating, it can be combined with Yu Ping Feng San (Huang Qi, Bai Zhu, Fang Feng). For prolonged spontaneous sweating with cold extremities, Gui Zhi Tang plus Fu Zi can be used.

At the time *Shang Han Lun* was written, the only references were to Shao Yao and there was no differentiation between Bai Shao Yao or Chi Shao Yao. However, we now know that Bai Shao tonifies blood and yin, astringes yin and so augments ying. Chi Shao, on the other hand, cools and invigorates blood, cools liver fire and is therefore dispersing, and can assist in the expulsion of the pathogen. When Gui Zhi Tang is used in the treatment of spontaneous sweating or sweating due to menopausal syndrome, Bai Shao should be used.

Case Study

Spontaneous Sweating
Gui Zhi Tang Pattern
Extracted from Shang Han Lun Yi Shi

A merchant had suffered with spontaneous sweating for over six months. He had been given astringent herbal remedies to stop the sweating but they were of no avail. He subsequently consulted a famous practitioner by the name of Wang Zhen for treatment of his disorder. After going through the enquiry, the doctor realised that the patient did not suffer from fever or aversion to wind but only from spontaneous sweating. His pulse was weak. He was given Gui Zhi Tang and recovered after five days.

Treatment of Periodic Fever with Spontaneous Sweating

Clause 54

病人藏无他病，时发热自汗出而不愈者，此卫气不和也，先其时发汗则愈，宜桂枝汤。

The patient's zang have no disease, where there is occasional fever and spontaneous sweating but without recovery, it means defence qi is disharmonious, promoting sweat in advance will bring recovery, Gui Zhi Tang is appropriate.

DISCUSSION: By specifying that the zang or yin organs are not affected, this clause confirms that the pattern is an exterior one. There is occasional or periodic fever and spontaneous sweating in the absence of any other disorder. The basis of the pattern is disharmony of the wei qi. The clause advocates that sweating should be promoted 'in advance', by which it implies that sweating should have been promoted before the manifestation of fever or sweat. The rationale behind this is that the ying (nutrient) and wei (defence) lack stability and Gui Zhi Tang can bring them into harmony by promoting sweat, but that it is preferable to do so before the disease has already progressed to where there is fever and sweating, as the further loss of sweat can damage the zheng qi.

Gui Zhi Tang not only releases the pathogen from the muscle layer, but can also stop spontaneous sweating. The reason Gui Zhi Tang can both promote and also stop sweating, is that when it is used as a sweat promoting formula, hot thin gruel is taken with it to enhance sweating. When it is used as a formula to stop spontaneous sweating, the mechanism is not by astringing the sweat but rather by preventing leakage of the ying yin through its action of harmonising the ying and wei, thus treating the sweating at its source.

Gui Zhi Tang Contraindications

Gui Zhi Tang is contraindicated in cases of: i) exterior excess; ii) depressed damp in the interior; and iii) exuberant interior heat.

Exterior Excess

Gui Zhi Tang is indicated for exterior deficiency where there is disharmony between the ying and the wei. It is therefore inappropriate for an exterior excess pattern, where the indicated formula is Ma Huang Tang.

Clause 16B

桂枝本为解肌，若其人脉浮紧，发热汗不出者，不可与之也。常须识此勿令误也。

Gui Zhi Tang is basically to resolve the muscle layer, if the patient's pulse is floating and tight, where there is fever and no sweat, it can not be given. One must bear this in mind to avoid making a mistake.

DISCUSSION: This clause describes the main function of Gui Zhi Tang as being the resolution of the muscle layer, which is achieved by mildly promoting sweat and regulating ying and wei. This contrasts with Ma Huang Tang, which releases the exterior by strongly promoting sweating and dispelling wind cold. If the patient's pulse is floating and tight and there is fever and an absence of sweating, then it is a shang han exterior excess pattern and Ma Huang Tang is indicated in order to promote a heavy sweat and expel the wind cold from the exterior. The basic Gui Zhi Tang function of regulating ying and wei will be inadequate. If Gui Zhi Tang is used instead of Ma Huang Tang in an exterior excess pattern, it will fail to dislodge and expel the cold pathogen because its sweat promotion function is weak. Consequently, the blockage of pathogenic cold in the Tai Yang will be exacerbated, as will the constraint of the wei yang. Not only is the exterior not resolved, but it will be aggravated and may deteriorate into a transmuted Da Qing Long Tang pattern, with vexation, but no sweating or yellowing. For this reason, Zhang Zhong Jing exhorts the practitioner not to make that mistake.

Depressed Damp in the Interior

The heavy consumption of alcohol leads to damp and heat being constrained in the interior and Gui Zhi Tang is contraindicated.

Clause 17

若酒客病，不可与桂枝汤，得之则呕，以酒客不喜甘故也。

If there is drinker's disease, one should not give Gui Zhi Tang, doing so will cause vomiting, this is because drinkers do not tolerate sweetness.

DISCUSSION: In someone who consumes large amounts of alcohol, there is a propensity for damp and heat to accumulate in the middle jiao. Because Gui Zhi Tang contains warm, acrid and sweet herbs, it has the potential to aggravate the heat and damp, and so, in a drinker with heat and damp stagnating in the interior, caution must be exercised in the prescription of Gui Zhi Tang, even where zhong feng (wind strike) has been properly diagnosed. Acridity exacerbates heat and sweetness augments damp. So if Gui Zhi Tang is given to a patient suffering from interior heat and dampness, it may further congest the already stagnant spleen and stomach, and a reversal of stomach qi will ensue, manifesting as vomiting. For this reason, it is said that drinkers do not tolerate sweetness.

The expression 'drinkers' disease' (酒客) has two possible interpretations. Some commentators interpret it as drinkers who are affected by Tai Yang zhong feng, whilst others interpret it as a sub-category of Tai Yang zhong feng, where alcohol consumption has generated damp heat, giving rise to disharmony of ying, wei, qi and blood, manifesting as headache, fever, nausea and vomiting and spontaneous sweat. However, this academic differentiation has little effect on the clinical implications. Regardless of whether the patient is a drinker suffering from an attack of zhong feng (wind strike) or the patient is simply a drinker with an underlying pattern of damp heat, Gui Zhi Tang is deemed unsuitable without significant reduction or total omission of Gan Cao and Da Zao, which are sweet and tend to foster the accumulation of damp.

For drinkers suffering from Tai Yang zhong feng, Gui Zhi Tang can be modified not only by reducing or eliminating Da Zao and Gan Cao, but also by the addition of herbs such as Ge Hua and Zhi Ju Zi, in order to clear heat and drain damp. Appropriate alternatives are Ge Gen Qin Lian Tang or Xiao Chai Hu Tang. The main thing is to understand that unmodified Gui Zhi Tang is unsuitable for those whose alcohol consumption is immoderate, even when they are correctly diagnosed with Tai Yang zhong feng.

Exuberant Interior Heat

Gui Zhi Tang is acrid and warm and therefore contraindicated where there is interior heat.

Clause 19

凡服桂枝汤吐者，其后必吐脓血也。

Whenever Gui Zhi Tang is taken there is vomiting, following which there is vomiting of pus and blood.

DISCUSSION: Because Gui Zhi Tang is an acrid, warm formula, it will exacerbate any pre-existing interior heat. Vomiting after the administration of Gui Zhi Tang signals that it was incorrectly prescribed and we can understand that a pattern of severe interior toxic heat must have been present if following that, the vomit actually contains blood and pus. The toxic heat sears qi and scorches blood, causing disharmony in ying and wei. This pattern can mimic Tai Yang zhong feng and if, by mistake, Gui Zhi Tang is used, the subsequent further injury to body fluids will lay the foundation for the exacerbation of interior heat and cause vomiting of pus and blood.

Summary of Gui Zhi Tang Contraindications

- Shang han exterior excess pattern with a floating and tight pulse and pre-existing constrained damp heat, such as found in those who drink alcohol to excess.
- A person with pre-existing interior heat.
- A Tai Yang pattern where, after purgation, there is no upsurge of qi, indicating the yang qi has sunken inwards.
- A Tai Yang pattern where incorrect treatment has caused transmutation and resulted in 'huai bing' or 'transmuted disease'.

Gui Zhi Tang Modifications

Modified Gui Zhi Tang can be used in the treatment of concurrent patterns, where the main symptoms of Gui Zhi Tang are present, but additional symptoms are concurrently observed. These are:

i. Tai Yang zhong feng with inhibited Tai Yang channel qi (Gui Zhi jia Ge Gen Tang Pattern);
ii. Tai Yang zhong feng with wheezing (Gui Zhi jia Hou Po Xing Zi Tang Pattern);
iii. Tai Yang zhong feng pattern with mild wheeze resulting from inappropriate use of purgation (Gui Zhi jia Hou Po Xing Zi Tang Pattern);
iv. Tai Yang zhong feng pattern with damage to yang qi following excessive promotion of sweat (Gui Zhi jia Fu Zi Tang Pattern);
v. Tai Yang mild pattern with fullness in the chest and slight aversion to cold following inappropriate purging (Gui Zhi qu Shao Yao Tang pattern);
vi. Tai Yang severe pattern with fullness in the chest and slight aversion to cold following inappropriate purging (Gui Zhi qu Shao Yao jia Fu Zi Tang pattern);
vii. Tai Yang pattern with damage to nutrient qi following the promotion of sweating (Gui Zhi xin jia Tang Pattern);
viii. Tai Yang Pattern with inhibited channel qi and water accumulation (Gui Zhi qu Gui jia Fu Ling Bai Zhu Tang).

Gui Zhi jia Ge Gen Tang Pattern

(Tai Yang zhong feng with inhibited Tai Yang channel qi.)

Clause 14

太阳病，项背强几几，反汗出恶风者，桂枝加葛根汤主之。

Tai Yang disease, the neck and back are stiff and taut, however where there is sweating and aversion to wind, Gui Zhi jia Ge Gen Tang governs.

GUI ZHI JIA GE GEN TANG: Ge Gen 4 liang; Shao Yao 3 liang; Gan Cao 2 liang; Sheng Jiang (sliced) 3 liang; Da Zao (broken) 12 pieces; Gui Zhi (bark removed) 2 liang; Ma Huang (nodes removed) 3 liang.

DIRECTIONS: First boil Ma Huang and Ge Gen in 1 dou (2 L) of water, boiling until reduced by 2 sheng (400 mL). Strain and add the rest of the ingredients. Simmer, reducing to 3 sheng and strain again. Take 1 sheng of the decoction warm and cover the patient with a blanket to produce a mild sweat. There is no need to drink hot gruel. The rest is as per standard Gui Zhi Tang methods and contraindications.

DISCUSSION: For a diagnosis of a Tai Yang pattern to be made, there must be a stiff neck and headache. However, the pathway of the Tai Yang channel is not limited to the neck and head, but travels the length of the back. The area governed by Tai Yang is extensive and includes the whole back. Therefore, if the pathogenic wind travels further along the channel, inhibiting the flow of qi and blood, the sinews and muscles will be affected and there will be stiffness of the whole back. The use of the Chinese word 反 should be carefully noted. This can be translated variously as 'however', 'instead', 'conversely', 'contrarily' or 'perversely'. In all cases, the implication is that this word is introducing some situation which is unexpected, given what has just been stated. Its use in this clause implies that although we expect the manifestations of a Tai Yang pattern to be a stiff neck, headache and the absence of sweat, it is instead manifesting as sweating and aversion to wind. Thus we understand that this is not a pattern of exterior excess, but one of exterior deficiency, where wind, not cold, is the primary obstructing pathogen. In Tai Yang zhong feng with a tightness and stiffness in the neck and shoulders, Gui Zhi Tang is used to release the pathogenic influence from the muscle layer and dispel wind; the addition of Ge Gen disperses and expels the pathogen from the Tai Yang channel i) by releasing the pathogen from the muscle layer, unblocking the channel and freeing the constrained qi, ii) by raising the yang qi to more effectively target the upper body and neck, iii) by expelling wind and assisting Gui Zhi to release the exterior, and iv) by generating fluids to nourish the channels.

In accordance with *Shang Han Lun* theory, Tai Yang zhong feng with sweating should be treated with Gui Zhi Tang and Tai Yang shang han, where there is no sweat, should be treated with Ma Huang Tang. If Ma Huang Tang is used where there is sweating and aversion to wind, this is contrary to the principle of *Shang Han Lun* in regard to Tai Yang disease: Gui Zhi Tang jia Ge Gen is the correct formula and Ma Huang is contraindicated in that pattern.

In the Song edition of *Shang Han Lun*, Gui Zhi Tang was recorded as including the herb Ma Huang 3 liang. This is, however, generally disregarded, because according to Lin Yi, Ma Huang is not included in Gui Zhi Tang and this is supported by *Jin Gui Yu Han Jing*. The contraindication of Ma Huang in the presence of sweating further substantiates the exclusion of Ma Huang.

Modern Application of Gui Zhi Ge Gen Tang

- Early stage of measles with an indistinct expression of rash.
- Chronic attack of the common cold due to pathogenic cold.
- Stiffness of the neck caused by twisting or sleeping in the wrong posture or from exposure to draft.
- Urticaria, headache and hypertension.
- Headache and hypertension.

Case Study

Frozen Shoulder

Extracted from Shang Han Shi Jian Lun by Chen Rui Chun

A 54-year-old male had suffered from left shoulder pain for a period of two years, with occasional remission in the warmer weather. His condition worsened when the weather turned cold and he was not able to lift his left hand. His blood pressure was normal and his pulse was moderate and forceful. His tongue was pale with a thin, white, slippery tongue coat.

Gui Zhi jia Ge Gen Tang was prescribed: Gui Zhi 10g; Bai Shao 10g; Ge Gen 15g; Dang Gui 10g; Jiang Huang 10g; Zhi Gan Cao 5g; Sheng Jiang 3 pieces; Da Zao 3 pieces.

He took one pack a day for five days, after which his condition improved: there was less pain and he slept better at night. His pulse was moderate and forceful and his tongue was moist with a thin, white coat. He was given another 15 packs of the same formula.

Discussion: Frozen shoulder is a painful condition severely restricting range of motion. Gui Zhi jia Ge Gen Tang can be used with the following modifications. For wind manifesting with pain of unfixed location, add Fang Feng, Qin Jiao, Wei Ling Xian; for blood stasis, add Dang Gui, Tao Ren, Chuan Xiong; if there is qi and blood deficiency, add Huang Qi and Ji Xue Teng.

Gui Zhi jia Hou Po Xing Zi Tang Pattern

(Tai Yang zhong feng accompanied by wheezing.)

This is one of two patterns associated with wheezing, where the wheezing can be pre-exisiting, as described here, or can be due to incorrect purgation, as described opposite.

Clause 18

喘家作桂枝汤，加厚朴，杏子佳。

Wheezing patients presenting with Gui Zhi Tang, adding Hou Po and Xing Ren is good.

GUI ZHI JIA HOU PO XING ZI TANG: Gui Zhi (bark removed) 3 liang; Zhi Gan Cao 2 liang; Sheng Jiang (sliced) 3 liang; Shao Yao 3 liang; Da Zao (broken) 12 pieces; Hou Po (fried with bark removed) 2 liang; Xing Ren (skin and tips removed) 50 pieces.

DIRECTIONS: Boil the ingredients in 7 sheng of water (1400 mL), reducing to 3 sheng. Strain and take 1 sheng, warm. Cover the patient with a blanket so as to produce a mild sweat.

DISCUSSION: This clause describes a patient with a chronic wheeze who has contracted a Gui Zhi Tang pattern. Because the lung qi is already weakened, it is unable to put up resistance and when pathogenic wind cold constrains the exterior, it further impairs the lung qi, giving rise to congestion and wheezing. Gui Zhi Tang disperses exterior wind cold and harmonises the ying and wei. Hou Po transforms phlegm cold and together with Xing Ren, disseminates and descends lung qi. In this way, they both work to stop the lung congestion and wheeze.

The key points of diagnosis are: (1) aversion to wind and spontaneous sweating, which are characteristic of a Tai Yang zhong feng exterior deficiency pattern, with the additional symptoms of coughing and wheezing; (2) a thin white tongue coat and a floating, moderate pulse, and (3) the absence of interior heat signs. Gui Zhi jia Hou Po Xing Zi Tang is indicated for an acute exacerbation of chronic bronchitis or bronchial asthma which presents with fever, aversion to cold, sweating, cough, a white tongue coat and a pulse that is moderate and floating. It is particularly effective for infantile bronchitis and broncho-pneumonia.

Case Study

Chronic Asthma

Extracted from Huang Wen Dong Yi An, Shanghai Science and Technlogy Press 1977

A 61-year-old woman had suffered from wheezing and chronic asthma for more than ten years. The episodes were characterised by cough, white sticky phlegm and wheezing, where the patient had to sleep upright. They were interspersed with periods of remission. She also suffered from a poor appetite, fatigue, spontaneous sweating, and back pain. Her tongue was pale with a thin, greasy coat and her pulse was thready and slippery.

A modified version of Gui Zhi jia Hou Po Xing Zi Tang was prescribed: Gui Zhi 4.5g; Sheng Gan Cao 4.5g; Hou Po 3g; Xing Ren 6g; Su Zi 9g; Zi Wan 15g; Chen Pi 6g; Qian Hu 6g; Hui Xiao Mai 15g.

After three packs her condition improved and she could sleep lying down. She was given another 15 packs of the same formula to consolidate treatment.

Gui Zhi jia Hou Po Xing Zi Tang Pattern (alternative application)

(Tai Yang zhong feng pattern with mild wheeze resulting from inappropriate use of purgation.)

This is a second application of Gui Zhi jia Hou Po Xing Zi Tang pattern where, after purging in Tai Yang disease, the exterior remains unresolved and there is wheezing.

Clause 43

太阳病，下之微喘者，表未解故也，桂枝加厚朴杏子汤主之。

Tai Yang disease, where there is mild wheezing after purgation, then the exterior is not resolved, Gui Zhi jia Hou Po Xing Zi Tang governs.

DISCUSSION: A Tai Yang pattern should be treated by releasing the exterior. Clause 43 describes a situation where purgation was wrongly used, giving rise to a transmuted pattern.

There are three scenarios following inappropriate purgation:

1. The zheng qi remains intact. This is demonstrated by an upsurge of qi and the exterior pattern is unresolved.
2. The zheng qi is damaged and the pathogen falls inward, manifesting as chest bind, glomus beneath the heart or diarrhoea.
3. The zheng qi is not damaged but the exterior pattern remains unresolved. The exterior symptoms of fever and aversion to cold are accompanied by a reversal of lung qi, manifesting as mild wheezing.

Gui Zhi jia Hou Po Xing Zi Tang is the formula cited in both Clauses 18 and 43; however, each represents a different pattern with a different pathogenesis. Clause 18 describes a situation where wheezing is a pre-existing disorder: Tai Yang zhong feng has been contracted by a person who happens to be an asthma sufferer and so the treatment addresses the acute condition, which is the exterior pattern. In Clause 43, on the other hand, the wheezing is newly acquired: it is the result of adverse treatment and is the manifestation of a transmuted pattern and the new symptom has to be addressed as well as the wind cold pattern. Gui Zhi jia Hou Po Xing Zi Tang addresses both the exterior pattern and the wheeze and so is suitable in both cases.

Gui Zhi jia Fu Zi Tang Pattern

(Tai Yang Zhong Feng pattern with damage to yang qi following excessive promotion of sweat.)

When there is excessive promotion of sweat in a Tai Yang zhong feng pattern, yang qi is damaged, and the exterior is not resolved. The required strategy is to release the exterior and restore yang.

Clause 20

太阳病，发汗，遂漏不止，其人恶风，小便难，四肢微急，难以屈伸者，桂枝加附子汤主之。

Tai Yang disease, sweating is promoted, followed by incessant leaking, the person is averse to wind, has difficult urination, where the four limbs are slightly tense, there is difficulty bending and stretching, Gui Zhi jia Fu Zi Tang governs.

GUI ZHI JIA FU ZI TANG: Gui Zhi (bark removed) 3 liang; Shao Yao 3 liang; Zhi Gan Cao 3 liang; Sheng Jiang (sliced) 3 liang; Da Zao (broken) 12 pieces; Fu Zi (fried with skin removed and broken into eight pieces) 1 piece.

DIRECTIONS: Boil the ingredients in 7 sheng of water, reducing to 3 sheng. Strain and take 1 sheng warm. The patient should then rest as per the general instructions for Gui Zhi Tang.

DISCUSSION: This clause is based on the fact that formulas such as Gui Zhi Tang, Ma Huang Tang and Ge Gen Tang should produce a slight streaming sweat all over the body but may, after sweating is promoted, result in an incessant, leakage of sweat. This is a sign that the yang qi has been damaged and so, despite the sweating, the exterior pattern can not be resolved. This is known as lou han or leaking sweat, which can lead to the development of a transmuted pattern.

Sweat is produced by the transformation of fluids, which is dependent on yang qi; so incessant sweating has the propensity to damage not only the yin fluids, but the yang qi as well. In this clause, the symptom of aversion to wind is not just listed with other symptoms, but is emphasised in the separate statement, "the person is averse to wind". This indicates that the aversion to wind in this pattern is more distinct than that normally seen in a Gui Zhi Tang pattern, and this is because excessive sweating has caused significant damage to yang qi. In consequence, there emerges a transmuted pattern characterised by deficiency of the exterior yang, which is then unable to secure the interstices; thus there is a continuous leakage of sweat. The subsequent damage to the yin fluids results in urination difficulty; because the depleted fluids fail to nourish the limbs, they are stiff and do not bend or straighten easily. These symptoms confirm the pathogenesis of excessive sweating having damaged the yang qi, giving rise to further sweating and the severe depletion of yin fluids.

Because the root of this disorder is the excessive loss of body fluids resulting from deficient yang failing to secure the exterior, the treatment must focus primarily on supporting yang, not on nourishing yin. Gui Zhi Tang harmonises ying and wei, and Fu Zi warms the channels and restores yang. Once the yang qi is restored and the exterior is resolved, then the sweating will stop and yin will be preserved and the symptoms relating to fluid loss will be resolved.

Ancient Application of Gui Zhi jia Fu Zi Tang

- *Qian Jin Yao Fang (Thousand Ducat Important Formulas)*: For the treatment of postpartum deficiency presenting with incessant sweating, inhibited urination and stiffness of the limbs with restricted movement, Gui Zhi jia Fu Zi Tang can be used. The dosage of Fu Zi is 2 pieces.
- *Lei Ju Fang Guang Yi*: For a Gui Zhi Tang pattern with aversion to wind or stiff limbs with pain, Gui Zhi jia Fu Zi Tang is indicated.

Modern Application of Gui Zhi jia Fu Zi Tang

- Common cold with aversion to cold and incessant sweating where there is a pre-existing constitutional yang deficiency.
- Stiff limbs, an aching body and aversion to cold where the promotion of heavy sweat has damaged the yang qi.

- Bi syndrome or arthritis where there is stiffness of the joints and aversion to cold.

Gui Zhi Tang warms the channels, disperses cold and harmonises ying and wei. Fu Zi dispels cold and stops pain. This formula can be modified with additional herbs as follows. Ma Huang to magnify the function of dispersing cold and freeing the blocked yang. Huang Qi to augment qi and engender yang. Dang Gui to tonify and invigorate blood and to counteract the drying and dispersing properties of Gui Zhi and Fu Zi. If the patient suffers from generalised heaviness of the lower limbs, Qian Nian Jian and Huai Niu Xi can be added. For lumbar pain, add Xu Duan, Gou Ji and Sang Ji Sheng. For dampness, add Cang Zhu and Yi Ren.

Case Study

Stiff Limbs

Extracted from Shang Han Jiu Shi Lun

A patient contracted Tai Yang disease and after the promotion of sweat, he suffered from incessant sweating, aversion to wind, inhibited urination and stiff limbs. The pulse was floating and big. A floating pulse denotes wind and if it is also big, it indicates deficiency. The symptoms mirrored those described in Clause 20 and so Gui Zhi jia Fu Zi Tang was prescribed. After three doses, the sweating stopped and Shao Yao Gan Cao Tang was given to consolidate treatment.

Gui Zhi qu Shao Yao Tang Pattern

(Mild Tai Yang pattern with fullness in the chest and slight aversion to cold following inappropriate purging.)

This is used in the treatment of Tai Yang disease with inappropriate purgation manifesting with a hasty pulse and fullness in the chest.

Clause 21

太阳病，下之后，脉促，胸满者，桂枝去芍药汤主之。

Tai Yang disease, after purgation, the pulse is hasty, where there is fullness in the chest, Gui Zhi qu Shao Yao Tang governs.

GUI ZHI QU SHAO YAO TANG: Gui Zhi (bark removed) 3 liang; Zhi Gan Cao 2 liang; Sheng Jiang (sliced) 3 liang; Da Zao (broken) 12 pieces.

DIRECTIONS: Boil the ingredients in 7 sheng of water, reducing to 3 sheng. Strain and take 1 sheng warm.

DISCUSSION: This is a Tai Yang exterior pattern where inappropriate purging has adversely affected the chest yang. The qi dynamic is affected, resulting in fullness in the chest and a hasty pulse. A hasty pulse or cu mai (促脉), also known as a skipping pulse, refers to a rapid and irregular pulse which can indicate extreme heat agitating qi, heart fire, heart qi deficiency or the obstruction of the flow of qi and blood. In Clause 21, the hasty pulse is a reflection of the penetration into the chest of the pathogenic heat which stirs qi and also impairs the flow of qi and blood in the chest. One interpretation is that the zheng qi is still able to contend with the pathogen and it is the ensuing struggle which causes the pulse to be hasty. A second explanation is that the hasty pulse is a reflection of the impaired ability of the yang qi to contend with the pathogen, in which case, the pulse would also be weak.

The pathogen is no longer in the exterior but has followed its innate tendency to move inwards and has been transmitted to the chest. Because the lungs are the "lid of the zang" they are the first of the yin organs to be affected when a pathogen transmits inwards; and because of their location in the chest, the qi of the chest, known as ancestral qi or zong qi, is also affected. Gui Zhi qu Shao Yao Tang is an acrid, sweet and dispersing formula which unblocks the chest yang. The omission of the Shao Yao is highly significant: it is cool, sour and astringent, and therefore has the potential to inhibit Gui Zhi's function of dispersing the chest yang.

Gui Zhi qu Shao Yao jia Fu Zi Tang Pattern

(Severe Tai Yang pattern with fullness in the chest and slight aversion to cold following inappropriate purging with damage to yang qi).

This is used in the treatment of Tai Yang disease following inappropriate purgation which manifests as fullness in the chest and a slight aversion to cold. It represents a more severe condition than the Gui Zhi qu Shao Yao Tang Pattern described above.

Clause 22

若微寒者，桂枝去芍药加附子汤主之。

If there is slight cold, Gui Zhi qu Shao Yao jia Fu Zi Tang governs.

GUI ZHI QU SHAO YAO JIA FU ZI TANG: Gui Zhi (bark removed) 3 liang; Zhi Gan Cao 2 liang; Sheng Jiang (sliced) 3 liang; Da Zao (broken) 12 pieces; Fu Zi 1 piece.

DIRECTIONS: Boil the ingredients in 7 sheng of water, reducing to 3 sheng. Strain and take 1 sheng warm.

DISCUSSION: This clause should be read in conjunction with Clause 21, which precedes it. The "slight cold" mentioned in Clause 22, is generally seen to be an additional symptom to those described in the previous clause and is therefore interpreted as an aversion to cold. Thus, this clause describes a pattern which is the result of inappropriate purging in a Tai Yang disorder, and in addition to the aversion to cold mentioned here, there is also chest fullness and a hasty pulse. The inappropriate purging has not merely impaired the flow of the yang qi in the chest, but has damaged the yang qi, hence the aversion to cold. Because this pattern represents damage to yang qi, and not simply constrained yang qi which is not flowing, the indicated formula is Gui Zhi qu Shao Yao Tang, where the addition of Fu Zi not only warms and unblocks the channels to facilitate the flow of qi and blood, but also restores the yang.

The patterns described in Clauses 21 and 22 have in common the impaired flow of chest yang, but differ in that the pattern described in Clause 22 manifests with 'slight cold', which is a reflection of deficient yang. From this, we can understand that Cause 22 describes a situation where the purgation has caused significant damage to yang qi. Because the pattern described in Clause 21 is characterised by depressed chest yang, with no significant deficiency of yang qi, the strategy is to diffuse the blocked yang using herbs which are acrid and dispersing. Clause 22, however, refers to a situation where there is yang qi deficiency as well as depressed chest yang, and so the strategy is to warm and restore the yang qi as well as unblocking the depressed chest yang.

Gui Zhi qu Shao Yao jia Fu Zi Tang re-vitalises the chest yang and transforms exuberant yin, and is therefore indicated in the treatment of blocked chest yang where yang qi is not diffusing. In the clinical situation it can be used to treat such symptoms as an oppressed sensation in the chest, palpitations, cough or dyspnoea associated with yang deficiency and blocked chest yang, and is useful in the treatment of coronary disease where there is deficient yang and exuberant yin.

Case Study

Chest Bi

Extracted from Shang Han Qie Yao

A 46-year-old male construction worker complained of having an oppressed sensation in the chest for many years. From time to time he experienced chest pain which was worse in cold weather. Other symptoms were cough and shortness of breath. His pulse was submerged, wiry and moderate and his hands were cold. He had clear copious urination and his tongue was pale with a slippery, thin, white coat.

The diagnosis was depressed chest yang with a disharmony of qi and blood, and Gui Zhi qu Shao Yao jia Fu Zi Tang (12 doses) was prescribed to warm and tonify the heart yang and dispel cold.

Gui Zhi xin jia Tang Pattern

(Tai Yang pattern with damage to nutrient (ying) qi following the promotion of sweating.)

Clause 62

发汗后，身疼痛，脉沉迟者，桂枝加芍药生姜各一两人参三两新加汤主之。

After promoting sweat, there is aching and pain in the body, where the pulse is submerged and slow, Gui Zhi jia Shao Yao Sheng Jiang Ge Yi Liang Ren Shen San Liang xin jia Tang governs.

GUI ZHI XIN JIA TANG: Gui Zhi (bark removed) 3 liang; Shao Yao 4 liang; Zhi Gan Cao 2 liang; Ren Shen 3 liang; Da Zao 12 pieces; Sheng Jiang 4 liang.

NOTE: The full name for this formula is Gui Zhi jia Shao Yao Sheng Jiang Ge Yi Liang Ren Shen San Liang xin jia Tang, which may be translated as: 'Gui Zhi plus 1 liang each of Shao Yao and Sheng Jiang with 3 liang of Ren Shen newly added Decoction'.

DIRECTIONS: Boil the ingredients in 1 dou 2 sheng of water (2.4 L), reducing to 3 sheng. Strain and take 1 sheng warm. This is Gui Zhi Tang with extra Shao Yao, Sheng Jiang and Ren Shen.

DISCUSSION: Clause 62 describes damage to ying qi caused by the loss of fluids associated with diaphoresis. Consequently, the muscles and sinews are not nourished and there are aches and pains in the muscles and joints. Body aches and pains are associated with a Tai Yang exterior pattern where they are ascribed to the obstruction of the channel qi by pathogenic cold. However, here, the pulse is not floating but submerged, and the aches and pains represent a Gui Zhi xin jia Tang pattern.

After sweating has been promoted to relieve the exterior pathogenic cold, the body aches should abate. The persistence of the aches and pains, accompanied as they are with a pulse which is slow and submerged, shows that the condition is no longer the same. A submerged pulse indicates an interior pattern, while a slow pulse indicates a deficiency of qi and blood. This tells us that this is no longer an exterior pattern but a pattern of qi and blood deficiency where the sinews and muscles are not nourished. The strategy is to regulate ying and wei, augment qi and nourish blood and ying. Gui Zhi Tang jia Shao Yao nourishes ying and blood; Ren Shen tonifies qi and blood; Sheng Jiang assists Gui Zhi jia Shao Yao Tang in its action of dispelling the cold within the ying qi.

There has been some discussion as to whether the exterior is resolved or not. Cheng Wu Ji maintained in *Zhu Jie Shang Han Lun* that if the body aches persist after the promotion of sweat, it indicated an unresolved exterior pathogen and that the submerged slow pulse indicated insufficiency of blood, thus suggesting that the exterior pathogen is not totally resolved and that the zheng qi is damaged. An analysis of the ingredients, however, shows that the main focus of this formula is on augmenting qi, nourishing yin, tonifying blood and harmonising ying. From this, together with the presence of a submerged and slow pulse, it can be concluded that the exterior pattern is already resolved.

KEY POINTS OF DIAGNOSIS: (1) The pathogenesis is an insufficiency of ying qi failing to nourish the sinews and muscles. (2) The chief clinical manifestations are aches and pains in the body and a pulse that is submerged and slow. Other possible signs and symptoms are fatigue, shortness of breath and a pale tongue. Although this formula can be used in an exterior pattern with body aches where there is an underlying deficiency, it is more suitable for body aches and pains accompanied by a slow submerged pulse, indicating an insufficiency of ying qi.

There are five indications for Gui Zhi xin jia Tang.

1. Aches and pains due to damaged nutrient qi being unable to nourish the sinews.
2. Tai Yang zhong feng in a person with a weak constitution and an insufficiency of qi and blood, regardless of whether sweat has been promoted.
3. Bi syndrome accompanied by an exterior deficiency, as evidenced by spontaneous sweating.
4. Aches and pains associated with deficiency in the postpartum period.
5. Low grade fever associated with a deficiency of qi and blood.

Case Study

Postpartum Muscle Pain

Extracted from Robin Marchment's Case Studies

A 32-year-old woman had given birth to her second child four weeks previously. She spent three days in hospital. On returning home, she overtired herself cooking and cleaning and caring for the two children and her husband. She was also breast-feeding the baby. Although the weather was mild, she often found herself with beaded sweat all over her body, and would dress in light clothing and either splash cold water over herself or use an electric fan to keep cool. About one week after returning home, she started to experience lower abdominal pain and her back, legs and arms also ached. She felt chilled when she went outside, although she also sometimes felt overly warm and still perspired for no apparent reason. Her face was pale, her appetite poor and her stool was a little dry. Her tongue was pale and the pulse was deep, weak and thin.

The diagnosis was disharmony of ying and wei and a deficiency of qi and blood. The formula chosen was Gui Zhi xin jia Tang to harmonise ying and wei and tonify qi and blood. Huang Qi and Dang Gui were added to enhance the functions of supplementing qi and blood and to stabilise the exterior. After one week, the chills and spontaneous sweating were virtually gone and the aching had eased. After a further ten days, all symptoms were relieved and she was given Ba Zhen Tang to maintain her health and prevent relapse.

Gui Zhi qu Gui jia Fu Ling Bai Zhu Tang Pattern

(Tai Yang Pattern with inhibited channel qi and accumulation of water.)

Clause 28

服桂枝汤，或下者，仍头项强痛，翕翕发热，无汗，心下满微痛，小便不利者，桂枝去桂加茯苓白术汤主之。

Having administered Gui Zhi Tang, or if there was purgation, the head and neck are still stiff and painful, feather-warm fever, absence of sweating, fullness and slight pain below the heart, where the urination is not free, then Gui Zhi qu Gui jia Fu Ling Bai Zhu Tang governs.

GUI ZHI QU GUI JIA FU LING BAI ZHU TANG: Shao Yao 3 liang; Zhi Gan Cao 2 liang; Sheng Jiang (sliced), Bai Zhu, Fu Ling 3 liang each; Da Zao 12 pieces. This is Gui Zhi Tang with the omission of Gui Zhi and the addition of Fu Ling and Bai Zhu.

DIRECTIONS: Boil the ingredients in 8 sheng of water, reducing to 3 sheng. Strain and take 1 sheng warm. When urination is no longer inhibited, recovery will take place.

DISCUSSION: When Clause 28 states, "the head and neck are still stiff and painful" after Gui Zhi Tang or purgation, it clearly implies that those symptoms were already present before treatment, and have persisted after the administration of Gui Zhi Tang. Their persistence shows that it is not a Tai Yang zhong feng pattern. However, despite the feather-warm fever, absence of sweating, and pain and fullness in the epigastrium, it is not an interior excess pattern either. The statement in the directions for decoction and administration accompanying that clause, "When urination is no longer inhibited, recovery will take place" is an important indicator that the symptom regarding inhibited urination is the key to the diagnosis. This is a pattern where the impaired flow of qi in the Tai Yang channel affects the flow of qi in its associated organ, the urinary bladder, which in turn results in the retention of urine, or water accumulation, in the urinary bladder.

The indicated formula is Gui Zhi qu Gui jia Fu Ling Bai Zhu Tang, which drains damp by strengthening the spleen. Gui Zhi is omitted because there is no exterior pathogen; Fu Ling is added to promote urination and drain damp; Bai Zhu is added because it strengthens the spleen and promotes urination; Sheng Jiang harmonises the spleen to assist in the transformation of water and its warm acrid properties help to disperse the water and relieve the epigastric distension. Shao Yao assists in the elimination of water by dispersing the knotted water bind and, assisted by Zhi Gan Cao, eases the epigastric pain; Zhi Gan Cao and Da Zao nourish the spleen to transform water.

There has been considerable debate as to whether the condition described in Clause 28 is an exterior condition. The majority of past commentators were in agreement that it was a concurrent pattern of an exterior syndrome accompanied by water qi. In *Shang Han Lun*

Ben Zhi, however, Zhang Xu Gu believed that it was not an exterior pattern, nor was it associated with water qi. He proposed that it was a pattern where obstruction of the san jiao resulted in a surge of spleen and stomach qi within the network vessels. The authors feel that neither of the above interpretations offers a satisfactory explanation and that, in fact, it is the water qi which inhibits the Tai Yang channel qi, affecting the qi of the urinary bladder and causing inhibited urination. It is the inhibited urination which is the key point of diagnosis. The water qi described in Tai Yang is due to an unresolved exterior pathogen which has entered the urinary bladder, knotting with water and causing water retention. This is to be differentiated from water retention due to spleen and kidney yang deficiency.

There has also been considerable debate as to whether it is Gui Zhi or Shao Yao which is omitted. The main theories are:

1. Ke Yun Bo believed the formula should be Gui Zhi qu Gui jia Fu Ling Bai Zhu, as described above.
2. *Yi Zong Jing Jian* suggested that it should be Shao Yao, not Gui Zhi, which is omitted in this formula, making it Gui Zhi qu Shao jia Fu Ling Bai Zhu Tang.
3. Cheng Wu Ji said that the formula should be Gui Zhi Tang jia Fu Ling Bai Zhu, which is to say, neither Gui Zhi nor Shao Yao should be omitted.

The authors feel that Ke Yun Bo's proposal is the most logical as this formula is also indicated for 'shui ji' (水悸) or palpitations due to water qi or 'shui pi' (水痞), which is stagnation of water qi giving rise to water glomus beneath the heart. The accumulated water, which forms the glomus, accounts for the inhibited urination, the submerged and wiry pulse and a wet, swollen tongue with a thin or scant white tongue coat.

Case Study

Water Qi

Extracted from Shang Han Qie Yao

A famous Shang Han practitioner from Beijing known as Chen Shen Wu once treated a patient suffering from fever. The fever persisted even after repeated administration of Chinese herbs. When asked about his condition, the patient told the practitioner that he suffered from inhibited urination, epigastric fullness and generalised discomfort. His pulse was submerged and wiry and his tongue was wet and swollen. Dr. Chen said the fever was due to water accumulation and depressed yang qi. Rather than treat the fever, he focused on eliminating the water qi. The patient recovered after three decoctions.

Summary of Gui Zhi Tang Modifications

1. Tai Yang syndrome with a stiff, tight neck and back, accompanied by sweating and aversion to wind: Gui Zhi Tang jia Ge Gen Tang.
2. Asthma sufferers who contract a Gui Zhi Tang pattern, or where wheezing or panting follows inappropriate purging: Gui Zhi Tang jia Hou Po Xing Zi Tang.
3. Where Tai Yang disease was treated by sweating which has led to continued incessant sweating or leaking sweat: Gui Zhi jia Fu Zi Tang.
4. Where Tai Yang disease was treated with purgation which resulted in a hasty pulse and fullness in the chest: Gui Zhi qu Shao Yao Tang. If there is also an aversion to cold: Gui Zhi qu Shao Yao jia Fu Zi Tang.
5. After the promotion of sweat, there are body aches and pains and the pulse is submerged and slow: Gui Zhi xin jia Tang.
6. After the promotion of sweat, the disease remains unresolved and there is epigastric fullness and pain accompanied by inhibited urination: Gui Zhi qu Gui jia Fu Ling Bai Zhu Tang.

The formulas described above can be further modified to treat an exterior pattern whether or not it is accompanied by water qi. The selection of herbs for appropriate modifications will depend on the presentation of the individual patient.

2.3.2 Tai Yang Shang Han or Ma Huang Tang Pattern

The term Ma Huang Tang pattern refers both to the clinical manifestations and the treatment protocols of Tai Yang shang han (cold injury) or exterior excess pattern.

Clause 35

太阳病，头痛发热，身疼腰痛，骨节疼痛，恶风,无汗而喘者，麻黄汤主之。

Tai Yang disease, there is headache, fever, body pain and back ache, the joints are aching and painful, where there is aversion to wind, no sweat and wheezing, Ma Huang Tang governs.

MA HUANG TANG: Ma Huang (nodes removed) 3 liang; Gui Zhi (bark removed) 2 liang; Zhi Gan Cao 1 liang; Xing Ren (skin and tips removed) 70 pieces.

DIRECTIONS: First boil Ma Huang in 9 sheng (1.8 L) of water, until reduced by 2 sheng. Skim off the foam before adding the other ingredients, then boil until reduced to 2.5 sheng (500 mL). Strain and take 8 ge (160 mL). Cover the patient with a blanket to produce a mild streaming sweat. It is not necessary to give hot gruel.

NOTES:

1. The reason for removing the nodes from Ma Huang was that they were thought to reduce the sweat promotion function of Ma Huang. In *Ben Cao Jing Ji Zhu*, Tao Hong Jing said: "Ma Huang with the nodes removed is to stop sweating". Zhang Xi Chun suggests in *Yi Xue Zhong Zhong Can Xi Lu* that Ma Huang with nodes substantially reduces the sweat promotion function and removing the nodes, facilitates sweat promotion. Today Ma Huang is used with the nodes intact to moderate sweating.
2. The dosage of Ma Huang must be greater than that of Gui Zhi and Gan Cao, otherwise the function of promoting sweat and releasing the exterior is compromised. In *Shang Han Guan Zhu Ji*, You Zai Jing said: "Gui Zhi and Gan Cao are considered to be assistants but in fact, their function is to moderate the diaphoretic function of Ma Huang and if the dosage of Gui Zhi and Gan Cao is greater than that of Ma Huang, they will counteract Ma Huang's function of promoting sweat".
3. Removing the scum at the end of the initial decoction of Ma Huang prevents vexation in the patient. Modern research has shown that the scum of decocted Ma Huang has a stimulatory effect on the sympathetic nervous system, causing increased heart rate, vexation and elevated blood pressure.

Key points to bear in mind when using Ma Huang Tang

- The ratio of Ma Huang, Gui Zhi and Gan Cao must be 3:2:1.
- Ma Huang Tang has a strong diaphoretic effect and is indicated only for an externally contracted wind cold excess pattern with no sweating.
- The formula is not recommended for prolonged use.

DISCUSSION: The key symptoms of Tai Yang shang han are: headache, fever, body pain, back ache, joint pain, aversion to wind, absence of sweat and wheezing. These are the 'eight Ma Huang symptoms'. A detailed explanation of Ma Huang Tang pattern symptoms can be found in the discussion accompanying Clauses 1, 3 and 35.

The pathogenesis of Tai Yang shang han is an exterior attack on the Tai Yang channel by pathogenic cold which constrains wei yang (defence yang) and stagnates ying yin (nutrient yin). Pathogenic cold obstructs the flow of qi in the channels, causing a headache and stiff neck, and retards the flow of ying and blood which then fails to nourish the sinews, causing generalised pain in the body and joints. The damage to yang qi by the cold pathogen affects defence yang and its function of warming the surface of the body and so there is aversion to cold. The exterior constraint also affects the defence yang's function of regulating the pores, so they too are blocked, and there is no sweat. The lungs govern the skin and hair, they rule the exterior and are 'the lid of the zang'. They are therefore the first of the zang organs in the line of attack. When an attack of exterior wind cold disrupts their function of descending and dispersing qi, there will be wheezing. The floating pulse of Tai Yang shang han is a reflection of the defence yang rising to expel the exterior pathogen; the tight pulse reflects the constricting properties of pathogenic cold. The treatment strategy is to promote sweating in order to expel the cold pathogen and to disseminate lung qi in order to calm the wheezing.

Aversion to cold can be classified as either yin or yang, as explained in Clause 7, which says: "Disease with fever and aversion to cold stems from yang; no fever and aversion to cold, stems from yin." Absence of sweat can also be differentiated: yang deficiency with no sweat is characterised by cold limbs due to reversal cold and clear, copious urination. Fluid and yin deficiency with no sweat, on the other hand, is characterised by thirst, scant urination and a scant tongue coat. Finally, water retention with no sweat is characterised by epigastric distension, oedema and inhibited urination. The absence of sweat associated with Ma Huang Tang is ascribed to pathogenic cold constraining the exterior and is accompanied by fever, aversion to cold and a floating and tight pulse.

Ancient Application of Ma Huang Tang

- *Shang Han Lai Su Ji (Shang Han Revival Compendium)*: Ma Huang Tang is indicated in the treatment of bi syndrome caused by pathogenic wind, cold and damp.
- *Shang Han Da Bai* (*Clarification of Shang Han Lun*): Ma Huang Tang is advocated for Tai Yang channel disorders characterised by aversion to cold, fever, headache, a floating pulse and no sweating. Ma Huang and Gui Zhi expel the pathogen from the ying and wei, allowing it to exit via the skin pores. Xing Ren is added to descend and disperse lung qi in order to relieve the constraint of lung qi caused by the pathogenic wind, and thus alleviate the wheeze or cough. Zhang Zhong Jing used this formula to treat patients in the the northern regions suffering from Tai Yang channel disorder. Zhu Gong, in *Lei Zheng Huo Ren Shu (Classification of Safeguarding Life)* stated that, when treating patients from the southern province of Zhe Jiang, where dampness prevails, Ma Huang Tang should be modified with the addition of Shi Gao and Huang Qin; if there are signs indicative of a Shao Yang pattern, Chai Hu should be added; if there are signs of a Yang Ming pattern, Ge Gen should be added; for inhibited urination, Che Qian Zi should be added; and in the summer and early autumn, Ma Huang and Gui Zhi should be substituted with Qiang Huo and Du Huo.

Modern Application of Ma Huang Tang

- *Common cold or epidemic influenza.* Indicated when these represent an exterior excess pattern caused by pathogenic cold characterised by fever, aversion to cold, headache, nasal blockage, absence of sweat and a floating, tight pulse.
- *Nephritic oedema.* Indicated for yang water due to externally contracted wind cold (yang water is an excess pattern characterised first by swelling of the face and then accompanied by aversion to cold, fever and cough).
- *Inward fall of infantile measles.* Ye Ju Quan used a modified version of Ma Huang Tang with Huang Qin and Bai Shao in the situation where the measles rash suddenly disappears and there is vigorous fever, absence of sweat and wheezing.
- *Chronic bronchitis.* Indicated where there is a wind cold exterior excess pattern.
- *Acute rheumatoid arthritis due to wind-damp.*
- *Facial paralysis.*
- *Acute and chronic rhinitis.*

Case Study

Shang Hang Exterior Excess

Extracted from Shang Han Lun Tang Zheng Lun Zhi

A 50-year-old male had caught a head cold walking to work. During the night, his fever had reached 39.8°C. He had a marked aversion to cold with shivering but no sweat. His body ached and he had an incessant cough. The tongue coat was thin and white and his pulse was floating, tight and forceful.

The diagnosis was Tai Yang shang han exterior excess and he was prescribed Ma Huang Tang (Ma Huang 9g; Gui Zhi 6g; Xing Ren 12g; Zhi Gan Cao 3g). The first dose brought on a mild sweat, brought relief to the coughing and eased the other symptoms. The treatment was consolidated by repeating the same formula, omitting Gui Zhi and adding Su Ye. The condition was resolved.

Pulse Signs for Sweat Promotion

Clause 51

脉浮者，病在表，可发汗，宜麻黄汤。

Where the pulse is floating, the disease is in the exterior, one should promote sweat, Ma Huang Tang is appropriate.

Clause 52

脉浮而数者，可发汗，宜麻黄汤。

Where the pulse is floating and rapid, one should promote sweat, Ma Huang Tang is appropriate.

DISCUSSION: The style and structure of *Shang Han Lun* incorporates the pulse sign, the pattern and the treatment strategy. Where the pattern takes precedence, in order to focus on the pattern, the pulse is not mentioned. Conversely, in Clauses 51 and 52, the focus is on pulse, and the indication for the use of Ma Huang Tang is explained by the pulse sign. However, Ma Huang Tang can not be prescribed on the basis of the pulse alone. This is exemplified in Clause 50, which stipulates that treatment can not be determined simply because the pulse is floating, and when considering the pulse, the exterior pattern must be diagnosed on the basis that the pulse is floating in the cubit position, but does not indicate a deficiency condition by being slow, moderate or submerged. Although Clauses 51and 52 above both indicate the use of Ma Huang Tang when there is a floating pulse, it is of course essential that other symptoms such as headache, fever, aversion to cold and absence of sweat be present before prescribing it.

Nose Bleed Patterns

Clause 46

太阳病，脉浮紧，无汗发热，身疼痛，八九日不解，表证仍在，此当发其汗。服药已，微除，其人发烦目瞑，剧者必衄，衄乃解。所以然者，阳气重故也。麻黄汤主之。

Tai Yang disease, the pulse is floating and tight, no sweat, fever, body aches and pains, unresolved after eight or nine days, the exterior pattern is still present, then one should promote sweat. After having taken the herbs, there is slight relief, the patient is vexed and the eyes closed, if it is serious, there will be spontaneous bleeding, only through bleeding is there resolution. The reason for this being, the yang qi is heavy. Ma Huang Tang governs.

Clause 47

太阳病，脉浮紧，发热，身无汗，自衄者愈。

Tai Yang disease, the pulse is floating and tight, fever, there is no sweating, spontaneous nose bleed will bring recovery.

Clause 55

伤寒脉浮紧，不发汗，因致衄者，麻黄汤主之。

Shang han, the pulse is floating and tight, sweat is not promoted, resulting in nose bleed, Ma Huang Tang governs.

DISCUSSION: There are two ways in which a Tai Yang exterior excess pattern can be resolved if the pathogen has not fallen inwards; one is by way of sweating and the other is by way of nose bleed. These three clauses each represent a different situation leading to nose bleed associated with a Tai Yang shang han exterior excess pattern.

1. Clause 46 describes a situation where the Tai Yang shang han exterior excess pattern is still unresolved after eight or nine days. This is evidenced by a floating tight pulse, absence of sweat, fever, and body pain. Promotion of sweat by the administration of Ma Huang Tang is still indicated. After the initial dose, symptoms ease but the patient feels vexed. This is interpreted as a sign of the condition being mild. This is because, where the disease is mild, the medication stimulates the interior yang qi, enabling it to contend with the pathogen in a bid to expel

it, which it does by bleeding via the nose. For this reason, the manifestation of vexation can also be interpreted as heralding nose bleed. The stimulated yang qi also results in photophobia, which is the reason for the eyes being closed. The statement "the yang qi is heavy" is interpreted variously as yang which is constrained and therefore weighted down and heavy, and as yang which is severe, as in an exuberant heat pathogen.

2. Clause 47 describes a Tai Yang shang han exterior excess pattern where there is fever, a floating and tight pulse and the absence of sweat. This is resolved by a nose bleed without the use of medication.
3. Clause 55 describes a Tai Yang shang han exterior excess pattern with a floating, tight pulse, fever, aversion to cold and the absence of sweat. The nose bleed is a result of failure to adhere to the correct treatment protocol of promoting sweat; the exterior pathogen is then constrained in the Tai Yang channel. Because it is unable to exit via sweating, it falls inwards causing interior heat and the chaotic flow of blood.

Nose bleed associated with a Tai Yang shang han exterior excess pattern may either resolve the pattern or not. Where it resolves the exterior pattern, there are two explanations: i) Without medication, the nose bleed itself has effected resolution of the exterior pathogen, and ii) medication has been given which stimulates the yang qi, causing the nose bleed and thus effecting resolution. In the first instance, the nose bleed has effectively substituted sweating as a means to resolve the exterior. This is known as 'red sweat', alluding to the fact that sweat and blood are of the same source. Where the nose bleed does not resolve the exterior pathogen, then Ma Huang Tang is used to release the exterior.

In conclusion, it is essential to determine the circumstances under which treatment to promote sweat and release the exterior is required.

a) After the nose bleed, the exterior pattern persists and the pulse sign remains the same. As long as the pattern is one of exterior excess with no sweating, Ma Huang Tang is used. This is because the nose bleed alone can not effectively dispel the pathogen. In *Shang Han Yi Fang Ji Zhu,* Chen Xiu Yuan stated; "If, in a shang han excess pattern, with a pulse that is floating and tight, there is nose bleed and there has been no promotion of sweat, the dripping of blood from the nose is, by itself, not effective in resolving the exterior syndrome and Ma Huang Tang governs".
b) After the nose bleed, before prescribing Ma Huang Tang, it must first be ascertained that the pattern has not transmuted to heat in the ying and xue aspect, and also that the blood is not exhausted. It must also be ascertained that it is not an exterior deficiency pattern, identified by sweating, when Gui Zhi Tang should be used instead.
c) Where there is no interior heat indicated by clear urination, Ma Huang Tang should be used.
d) If the nose bleed is due to pathogenic wind heat, then neither Ma Huang nor Gui Zhi Tang is suitable. *Yi Zong Jin Jian (Golden Mirror of Medical Tradition)* comments: "After nose bleed, if the body is cool, then the condition is resolved. If unresolved, Sheng Ma Ge Gen Tang and Xi Jiao Di Huang Tang are indicated to expel pathogenic heat in the blood." Xu Ling Tai comments in *Shang Han Lei Fang*: "After nose bleed, the use of acrid warm herbs to promote sweating is tantamount to holding onto the firewood to extinguish fire. Instead Hei Gao Tang (Sheng Di, Jing Jie Shui, Lian Qiao, Fu Shen, Chuan Bei, Sheng San Zha, Chan Yi, Dan Shen, Sheng Gan Cao, Xi He Liu) should be used. The aim of this formula is to release the exterior and simultaneously preserve yin.

Transmuted Patterns After Nose Bleed

If the condition is characterised by a scorching fever, a rapid pulse and a crimson tongue with a dry, yellow tongue coat, then there is pathogenic heat in the ying and xue aspects. Therefore, Xi Jiao Di Huang Tang is indicated to clear ying heat and cool blood.

Clause 37

太阳病，十日已去，脉浮细而嗜卧者，外已解也。设胸满胁痛者，与小柴胡汤；脉但浮者，与麻黄汤。

Tai Yang disease, ten days have passed, where the pulse is floating and fine and the patient is sleepy, the exterior pattern has resolved. In the event of chest fullness and pain in the hypochondrium, give Xiao Chai Hu Tang; where there is only a floating pulse, give Ma Huang Tang.

DISCUSSION: If ten days passes where Tai Yang disease has not been resolved, it indicates a longer enduring condition and there are three possible scenarios.

1. If the pulse has changed from floating and tight to floating and fine and the patient is sleepy, it presages recovery.
2. If after ten days, the patient suffers from fullness in the chest and pain in the hypochondrium, then the disorder is in the Shao Yang and Xiao Chai Hu Tang is indicated.
3. If after ten days, the pulse is still floating and tight, indicating persistence of the exterior pattern, then Ma Huang Tang can be given to release the exterior.

NOTE: Sleepiness must be clearly differentiated. The somnolence mentioned in Clause 37 is the sleepiness and restfulness of recovery, where the patient is tranquil and relaxed. The somnolence of Shao Yin disease, which is described as a desire to sleep, refers to fatigue and lethargy. It is associated with a deficiency of yang and is accompanied by a pulse which is faint and fine. The somnolence of Yang Ming disease is accompanied by a clouded spirit, vigorous fever, thirst and a big, flooding pulse, and is associated with interior excess heat.

Summary of Ma Huang Tang Applications

Ma Huang Tang is indicated for externally contracted wind cold causing constraint of defence yang and stagnation of ying yin. Its key signs and symptoms are: aversion to cold, fever, absence of sweat, wheeze, body aches and pains (headache, lumbar pain, joint pain) and a tight pulse. In Clause 3, both yin and yang pulses are described as being tight, where the yin pulse refers to the proximal position (chi mai) and the yang pulse to the distal position (cun mai). In effect, this is describing a pulse where all three positions (cun, guan and chi) are tight. The key point of diagnosis differentiating a Ma Huang Tang pattern from an exterior deficiency pattern is the absence of sweat.

Ma Huang Tang Contraindications

Ma Huang Tang is contraindicated in cases of i) exterior excess with yin deficiency; ii) kidney yin deficiency with heat in the bladder; iii) insufficency of yin blood; iv) a current history of haemorrhage; v) spontaneous, nocturnal or excessive sweating; vi) spleen yang deficiency with cold in the middle burner.

Exterior Excess with Yin Deficiency

Clause 83

咽喉干燥者，不可发汗。

Where the throat is parched and dry, one should not promote sweating.

DISCUSSION: The throat is the gate to the lungs and the entrance to the stomach, and it is where the hand Tai Yin and foot Shao Yin channels traverse. If the yin essence is in abundance, then the throat is nourished. However, if yin fluid is deficient, in particular the yin of the lungs and kidneys, the throat will be dry. If yin fluids are depleted, manifesting as a dry throat, it is contraindicated to use herbs which are acrid and warm in order to promote sweating, even in a Tai Yang exterior pattern. This is because the loss of sweat can further damage the yin essence, potentially causing a deficiency of heat in the interior. Although there is no recommended alternative treatment strategy, Qian Jin Wei Rui Tang (Yu Zhu, Bai Wei, Ma Huang, Du Huo, Xing Ren, Chuang Xiong, Qing Mu, 6g each; Shi Gao 15g) can be used.

Kidney Yin Deficiency with Heat in the Urinary Bladder

Clause 84

淋家，不可发汗，发汗必便血。

In patients with dysuria, one should not promote sweat, the promotion of sweat will cause bloody urination.

DISCUSSION: The urinary bladder and kidney possess an exterior–interior relationship: chronic frequent, painful urination can be a manifestation of kidney yin deficiency with heat in the urinary bladder and, conversely, heat in the urinary bladder has a tendency to damage kidney yin. If sweating is promoted by the use of warm and acrid herbs, the heat generated can cause a chaotic flow of blood in the urinary bladder, manifesting as haematuria. The correct treatment for patients with dysuria is as follows.

- For bladder heat associated with kidney yin deficiency and frequent urination, thirst, vexation, and a fine and rapid pulse, Zhu Ling Tang can be used.
- For excess bladder heat not associated with yin deficiency, Ba Zheng San can be used.
- For patients with dysuria suffering from an externally contracted pathogen, a cool acrid formula or a modification of Xiao Chai Hu Tang can be given.

Insufficiency of Yin Blood

Clause 85

疮家，虽身疼痛，不可发汗，汗出则痉。

Patients suffering from sores, even if there are body aches and pains, one should not promote sweat, if sweat is promoted there will be tetany.

DISCUSSION: Patients with a history of body sores are considered to be deficient in yin blood. If they contract an exterior excess disease, acrid, warm herbs which promote sweating are contraindicated because they further damage blood, which could precipitate tetany as a result of deficient yin blood failing to nourish the sinews.

The pathomechanism of body sores is ascribed to two factors: a) damage to yin blood, which is then unable to nourish the sinews and so also gives rise to aches and pains in the body, and b) an attack of pathogenic wind cold obstructing wei yang and constraining yin ying, which causes not only body sores, but also aches and pains in the body. Therefore, in treating a shang han pattern in patients with sores, not only should formulas such as Ma Huang Tang be avoided because of their potential to induce a strong sweat and damage the yin blood, but herbs which nourish blood or harmonise ying and wei, as may be fitting, should be prescribed. Xiao Jian Zhong Tang with the addition of Huang Qi or Ren Shen is one appropriate formula, and some practitioners have suggested that the strategy should be to relieve toxicity and also include such herbs as Jing Jie and Fang Feng. Suggested formulas are Jing Fang Bai Du San (Qiang Huo, Du Huo, Chai Hu, Qian Hu, Zhi Qiao, Fu Ling, Ren Shen, Jie Geng, Chuan Xiong, Jing Jie, Fang Feng, Gan Cao) and Xiao Chai Hu Tang with the addition of Shan Zhi Zi, Dou Chi, Jin Yin Hua.

Patients with Haemorrhage

Clause 86

衄家，不可发汗，汗出必额上陷，脉急紧，直视不能眴，不得眠。

In patients with nose bleed, one should not promote sweat, if there is sweating the forehead will be sunken, the pulse will be urgent and tense, the gaze will be straight and fixed, unable to sleep.

Clause 87

亡血家，不可发汗，发汗则寒栗而振。

Patients with devastation of blood, one should not promote sweat, the promotion of sweat will cause cold shivering and shaking.

DISCUSSION: Body sores, frequent nose bleeds or other external haemorrhage and blood collapse are all associated with an insufficiency of yin blood. So acrid, warm herbs which are not only drying in nature, but can also promote sweating are contraindicated. This is because sweat and blood are of the same source and the loss of fluids caused by sweating will further damage ying and blood.

Nose bleeds are ascribed to heat in the yang channels causing blood to flow recklessly. Prolonged or recurrent nose bleeds may lead to yin and blood deficiency. Therefore, in patients with a history of frequent nose bleeds, even where an exterior pattern is present, acrid, warm herbs to promote sweating are contraindicated. The further depletion of yin blood due to diaphoresis can exacerbate pathogenic heat, producing the manifestations of "a sunken forehead, an urgent, tight pulse, a fixed forward stare and insomnia". These are manifestations of depleted yin essence.

Blood collapse is the result of serious haemorrhage. Qi is the commander of blood, upon which blood relies for its circulation, whilst blood is the residence and nurturer of qi. Because of this inter-dependence, blood collapse can lead to qi deficiency, and the administration of acrid, warm herbs is contraindicated. The appropriate strategy is to augment qi and nourish blood, whilst obtaining a mild sweat. Examples of appropriate formulas are: Cong Bai Qi Wei Tang (Cong Bai, Ge Gen, Dou Chi, Sheng Jiang, Mai Dong, Di Huang, and Lao Shui or worked water) and Xiao Chai Hu Tang with the addition of Sheng Di, Ge Gen, or other herbs suitable for modification.

Spontaneous, Nocturnal or Excessive Sweating

Clause 88

汗家，重发汗，必恍惚心乱，小便已阴疼，与禹余粮丸。

In patients with sweating, sweat is again promoted, there will be absentmindedness and mental derangement, yin pain after urination, give Yu Yu Liang Wan.

DISCUSSION: Patients who have suffered excessive sweating will tend to be deficient in qi and blood and any further diaphoresis will cause serious depletion of these vital substances. Such symptoms as absentmindedness or derangement are a sign of transmutation, and are manifestations of significant deficiency, where the heart shen is not nourished and supported. The heart and small intestine have an interior-exterior relationship. If the heart yin and blood are deficient, this may in turn affect the fluid of the small intestine, resulting in yin pain after urination, which refers to pain in the lower urinary tract.

The original formula for Yu Yu Liang has been lost. Earlier versions of *Shang Han Lun* advocated a single herb, namely Duan Yu Yu Liang (煅禹余粮). There are several variations in later annotations: Wang Ri Xiu suggested 3 liang each of Yu Yu Liang, Chi Shi Zhi, Sheng Zi Pi (生梓皮) and ½ sheng of Chi Xiao Dou ground into powder and formed into honey pills the size of a bullet, which were to be taken morning and evening with water. A supplementary formula was advocated in *Gu Ben Shang Han Za Bing Lun*: Yu Yu Liang 4 liang, Ren Shen 3 liang, Fu Zi 2 pieces, Wu Wei Zi 3 ge (which is a handful in solid measure), Fu Ling 3 liang and Gan Jiang 3 liang all ground into a powder and formed into honey pills the size of the fruit of Wu Tong (梧桐), which is the Chinese phoenix or parasol tree, often quoted in poetry. Twenty pills were to be taken daily. More recently, it has been suggested that a suitable formula would be a combination of Sheng Mai San and Liu Wei Di Huang Wan.

Spleen Yang Deficiency with Cold in the Middle Burner

Clause 89

病人有寒，复发汗，胃中冷，必吐蛔。

A patient has cold, promotion of sweat is repeated, the stomach will be cold, there will be vomiting of roundworms.

DISCUSSION: In this clause, the cold the patient is suffering from is deficiency cold of the spleen and stomach. If the patient then contracts exterior pathogenic cold, the correct strategy would be to warm the interior and release the exterior pathogen. Diaphoretic therapy is incorrect because it will cause further damage to the spleen and stomach yang, ultimately giving rise to full cold in the stomach. The exuberant yin will then cause a reversal of stomach qi, manifesting as vomiting. Where the patient has roundworms (a common condition in bygone years), the cold will cause them to seek a warmer place in the body, and as they move upwards to the warmth of the upper body, they will also be expelled from the body with the vomiting. The recommended formula is Li Zhong Tang plus Wu Mei Wan, to warm the interior and expel the parasitic infestation.

Clause 49

脉浮数者，法当汗出而愈。若下之，身重心急者，不可发汗，当自汗出乃解。所以然者，尺中脉微，此里虚，须表里实，津液自和，便自汗出愈。

Where the pulse is floating and rapid, there should be sweating with recovery. If there is purgation, with heaviness in the body and palpitations; one should not promote sweat, there will be spontaneous sweating then resolution. The reason for this being, the cubit pulse is faint, this is interior deficiency, the exterior and the interior must be replete, the body fluids harmonise spontaneously, so that spontaneous sweating will bring about recovery.

DISCUSSION: Generally, the early stage of a shang han or cold injury pattern is characterised by a tight floating pulse where aversion to cold is the predominant symptom and fever is mild. Here, the pulse is floating and rapid, indicating the predominance of fever. The strategy is the promotion of sweat to release the exterior and if, in an exterior pattern, purgation is used instead, the pathogen may fall into the interior, damaging the internal qi, leading to symptoms of fatigue and a sensation of heaviness in the body. This deficiency of qi and blood can affect the heart; when the heart qi is unstable, there will be palpitations and restlessness. For these reasons, where there has been incorrect purgation, caution must be exercised in promoting sweating even if an exterior pattern is present.

The deficiency of qi and blood is reflected both in the symptoms and in the pulse. The faintness of the cubit pulse specifically indicates deficiency of kidney yang, and Zhong Jing's assertion that the exterior and interior must be replete simply means that one has to wait for the restoration of zheng qi to bring about harmonisation of qi and body fluids. There will then be spontaneous sweating and the condition will be resolved. There are some circumstances where purgation might have been used legitimately, and in seeking restoration of the zheng qi, the following should be borne in mind.

1. The first option is to use dietary means rather than medical herbs. Once zheng qi is restored, it will expel the pathogen by way of spontaneous sweating.
2. When using medicinals to support the zheng qi, one should consider such formulas as Xiao Jian Zhong Tang in order to tonify deficiency and regulate ying and wei. This follows the basic principle of treating a shang han deficiency pattern by promoting sweat and supporting the middle. The two reasons for deficiency are pre-existing constitutional deficiency or incorrect treatment which has damaged the interior qi.

Clause 50

脉浮紧者，法当身疼痛，宜以汗解之。假令尺中迟者，不可发汗。何以知然？以荣气不足，血少故也。

Where the pulse is floating and tight, there should be body aches and pains, it is appropriate to promote sweat for resolution. Should the cubit pulse now be slow, one should not promote sweat. How do we know the reason? It is because the nutrient qi is insufficient, blood is scarce.

DISCUSSION: The tightness in the pulse is typical of a Tai Yang shang han exterior excess pattern, where pathogenic cold has caused constraint in the exterior, disrupting the harmony of ying and wei, and resulting in generalised aches and pains. Ma Huang Tang is indicated to expel the pathogen by the promotion of heavy sweat. However, if the typical shang han pulse is absent and instead, the cubit pulse is slow, indicating kidney deficiency, then there is an interior deficiency of ying and blood. We are told that it is because the patient had a pre-existing deficiency of ying and blood and, in such a case, it is contraindicated to promote sweat without also nourishing yin and blood. Disregard of this principle would result in the stealing of sweat and the consequent devastation of blood.

Summary of Ma Huang Tang Contraindications

Ma Huang Tang is the guiding formula for a Tai Yang shang han exterior excess pattern characterised by the absence of sweat and by tightness in both the yin and yang pulses, where the objective is to release the exterior, expel the pathogen and disperse pathogenic cold by sweating. However, the use of Ma Huang Tang is restricted to excess conditions, and the promotion of sweat is prohibited in deficiency, particularly where there is insufficiency of yin fluid or deficiency of yang qi, because sweating will further deplete the yin and the yang.

There are nine clauses associated with Ma Huang Tang contraindications. The first seven describe the symptoms which contraindicate the promotion of sweat and the last two describe the contraindicating pulse signs. Diaphoresis is contraindicated in the presence of the following symptoms: a dry throat, dysuria, frequent sweating, body sores, haemorrhage, blood collapse and cold in the stomach. The contraindicating pulse signs are: a faint or slow cubit pulse, reflecting deficiency of qi and blood.

Ma Huang Tang Modifications

The three Ma Huang Tang modifications associated with Tai Yang shang han exterior excess are: i) Ge Gen Tang (Ge Gen jia Ban Xia Tang is discussed later in Clause 33); ii) Da Qing Long Tang and iii) Xiao Qing Long Tang. The symptom complex of the patterns associated with these Ma Huang Tang modifications have in common the core symptoms of Tai Yang shang han, with each pattern featuring one or more additional symptoms which identifies it. For instance, the severely stiff neck and back of a Ge Gen Tang pattern. These additional symptoms are the hall-mark of a concurrent pattern.

Ge Gen Tang Pattern

Clause 31

太阳病，项背强几几，无汗恶风，葛根汤主之。

Tai Yang disease, the neck and back are stiff and taut, absence of sweat and aversion to wind, Ge Gen Tang governs.

GE GEN TANG: Ge Gen 4 liang, Ma Huang (nodes removed) 3 liang; Gui Zhi (bark removed) 2 liang; Sheng Jiang 3 liang; Zhi Gan Cao 2 liang; Shao Yao 2 liang; Da Zao (broken) 12 pieces.

DIRECTIONS: First boil Ma Huang and Ge Gen together in 1 dou (2 L) of water until the water is reduced by 2 sheng. Skim off the foam, add the rest of the ingredients, then simmer until reduced to 3 sheng. Strain and take 1 sheng warm. Cover the patient with a blanket to promote a mild sweat and follow the directions for Gui Zhi Tang with regard to rest and contraindications.

DISCUSSION: The exterior is constrained due to pathogenic wind cold blocking the pores and affecting the proper flow of Tai Yang channel qi. The key points of diagnosis are absence of sweat and aversion to wind cold. Ge Gen Tang is Gui Zhi Tang with the addition of Ma Huang and Ge Gen. The chief herb is Ge Gen, whose function is to expel wind cold, release the exterior, raise the clear yang, generate fluid and nourish the sinews. It is these last three functions in particular which make it effective in treating stiffness of the neck and back. Combined with Ma Huang, it opens the pores, promotes sweating and releases the exterior. Shao Yao and Zhi Gan Cao work together to harmonise the ying and relax the sinews. Sheng

Jiang and Da Zao regulate the wei and support yin.

Ge Gen Tang must be differentiated in its application from Gui Zhi Tang jia Ge Gen and from Ma Huang Tang:

1. Both Ge Gen Tang and Gui Zhi Tang jia Ge Gen are used for Tai Yang channel qi constraint characterised by a stiff neck and back. The former contains Ma Huang and is indicated in an exterior excess pattern with a floating tight pulse and an absence of sweating. The latter does not contain Ma Huang and is indicated in an exterior deficiency pattern with sweating and a floating moderate pulse.
2. Both Ge Gen Tang and Ma Huang Tang are used for Shang Han exterior excess patterns. Wheezing is a characteristic feature of a Ma Huang Tang pattern and is not present in a Ge Gen Tang pattern; Ge Gen Tang pattern has no wheezing but is primarily characterised by a severely stiff neck and back, which is the key indication for Ge Gen Tang.

Ancient Application of Ge Gen Tang

- *Jin Gui Yao Lue:* Ge Gen Tang is advocated for the treatment of Tai Yang disease characterised by an absence of sweat, scant urination, an upsurge of qi to the chest, a clenched jaw, an inability to speak and hard tetany.
- *Qian Jin Fang:* Jie Ji Tang (解肌汤), which is Ge Gen Tang with the omission of Gui Zhi and Sheng Jiang and the addition of Huang Qin, was advocated for the treatment of pathogenic wind constrained in the muscle.

Modern Application of Ge Gen Tang

- Chronic bronchitis.
- Early stage pneumonia.
- Frozen shoulder.
- Bi syndrome due to pathogenic wind-damp.
- Postpartum lumbar pain due to pathogenic wind.
- Trigeminal neuralgia.
- Facial paralysis.
- Sciatica.
- Early stage tetany.

Bai Shao Ge Gen Tang was used in a clinical trial for the treatment of 42 cases of cervical spondylosis. The base formula was: Bai Shao 45g, Ge Gen 20g, Zhi Ma Huang 3g, Gui Zhi 9g, Gan Cao 6g. Modifications were as follows:

- For numbness of the limbs, Quan Xie and Sang Zhi were added.
- For a severe long-term condition with restricted limb movement, Tao Ren and Hong Hua were added.
- For severe neck pain, Qiang Huo, Ru Xiang and Mo Yao were added.
- For vertigo and headache, Tian Ma, Chuan Xiong and Gan Di Long were added.

The treatment regimen comprised one pack per day for a course of between 25 and 40 days. The result was that 26 cases out of 42 had substantial relief (*Jiang Su Zhong Yi* 1990; 10:29).

> **Case Study**
>
> **Gastroenteritis**
>
> ***Extracted from Si Chuan Zhong Yi 1987; 1:18***
>
> A 4-year-old boy had contracted a cold two days earlier, and the previous day he had abdominal rumbling with several episodes of diarrhoea. Other symptoms were aversion to cold, fever, nasal discharge, a poor appetite, a pale red tongue with a thin, white tongue coat and a floating, rapid pulse. There was no sweating.
>
> The diagnosis was an exterior wind cold pattern with diarrhoea. The treatment principle was to disperse cold and release the exterior. He was prescribed Ge Gen Tang as follows: Ge Gen 12g, Ma Huang 5g, Gui Zhi 6g, Bai Shao 10g, Da Zao 3 pieces, Sheng Jiang 2 pieces. After one day, the frequency of the diarrhoea was reduced from several times to only twice in the day and the exterior pattern was resolved. He was given one more dose to consolidate the treatment.

Da Qing Long Tang Pattern

> **Clause 38**
>
> 太阳中风，脉浮紧，发热恶寒，身疼痛，不汗出而烦躁者，大青龙汤主之。若脉微弱，汗出恶风者，不可服者。服者则厥逆，筋惕肉瞤，此为逆也。

Tai Yang zhong feng, the pulse is floating and tight, there is fever and aversion to cold, body aches and pains, with no sweat but with vexation, Da Qing Long Tang governs. If the pulse is faint and weak, where there is sweating and aversion to wind, one should not take medication. Medication will cause desertion reversal, the muscles will jerk and the flesh will twitch, it is an adverse treatment.

Clause 39

伤寒脉浮缓，身不疼，但重，乍有轻时，无少阴证者，大青龙汤发之。

Shang han with a pulse which is floating and moderate, the body does not ache, there is only heaviness, from time to time there is a sense of relief, in the absence of a Shao Yin pattern, Da Qing Long Tang promotes.

DA QING LONG TANG: Ma Huang 6 liang; Gui Zhi (bark removed) 2 liang; Zhi Gan Cao 2 liang; Xing Ren (skin and tips removed) 40 pieces; Sheng Jiang (sliced) 3 liang; Da Zao (broken) 10 pieces; Shi Gao (the size of a hen's egg).

DIRECTIONS: First boil Ma Huang in 9 sheng of water, reducing by 2 sheng. Skim off the foam then add the other ingredients. Simmer and reduce to 3 sheng. Strain and take one sheng warm to produce a mild sweat. In the event of copious sweating, apply warm rice flour to the outside of the body. The medication must be discontinued as soon as sweat is produced, as continued administration will result in excessive sweating followed by yang exhaustion, characterised by aversion to wind, vexation and insomnia.

DISCUSSION: The reference in Clause 38 to Tai Yang zhong feng is actually a reference to Tai Yang shang han, as can be seen by the pulse being floating and tight and the absence of sweat. The correct treatment is Ma Huang Tang and the reference to medication is a reference to Ma Huang Tang. The vexation mentioned in Clause 38 is an indication that the exterior pathogenic cold has not been released, and that the constrained yang qi has transformed into heat which is harassing the heart. If Ma Huang Tang is used, it will promote sweating and disperse cold but not address the transformed interior heat. The phrase 'Da Qing Long Tang promotes' implies the use of that formula in order to promote sweat and resolve the disease. Da Qing Long Tang has the function of diffusing and expelling the heat generated by the constrained yang, and thus effectively releases the exterior whilst clearing interior heat. However, if the pulse is faint and weak and there is aversion to wind, Da Qing Long Tang is contraindicated because the faint, weak pulse represents an interior yang deficiency and the aversion to wind indicates either a deficiency of ying and wei or, alternatively, a deficiency of ying alone, where wei is strong and ying is weak, which is another way of saying that ying and wei are in disharmony. Weakness of ying refers to its inability to contain the strong wei yang and, as a result, the strong defence yang rises to the surface to vie with the exterior pathogen. If Da Qing Long Tang is used for a patient whose pulse is weak and faint and who is averse to wind, then the excessive loss of sweat has the potential to exacerbate the deficiency and cause yang collapse with 'desertion reversal'. This refers to cold limbs caused by desertion of yang, accompanied by muscle twitching. Therefore, it is considered to be an inappropriate or adverse treatment.

Clause 39 describes a Tai Yang shang han pattern where there is a change in the pulse from floating and tight to floating and moderate, and where the body ache is replaced by a sensation of heaviness. This indicates that the exterior pathogenic cold has slowly transformed into interior heat without having left the exterior. The constraint of yang qi by the exterior pathogen disturbs the qi dynamic, resulting in a sensation of heaviness, which is relieved intermittently as the pathogen attempts to enter the interior. The assertion in Clause 39 that there is no Shao Yin pattern is made to emphasise the fact that a Da Qing Long Tang pattern must be differentiated from Shao Yin yang deficiency, which is also characterised by irritability and heaviness of the body.

Da Qing Long Tang is a variation of Ma Huang Tang where the dose of Ma Huang is increased and where Shi Gao, Sheng Jiang and Da Zao are added. The high dose of Ma Huang (6 liang) makes this the most potent of the sweat promotion formulas. Shi Gao clears interior heat and in combination with Ma Huang, releases the constraint of yang qi. The addition of Gan Cao and Da Zao bolsters the source of sweat. Da Qing Long Tang resolves constrained heat in the exterior and vexation in the interior. This effect is described as "the rising of the dragon with the downpour of rain": hence the name Da Qing Long Tang. Where there is a faint and weak pulse and aversion to wind, Da Qing Long Tang is contraindicated.

Ancient Application of Da Qing Long Tang

- *Yi Xue Zhong Zhong Can Xi Lu (Genuine Medical Records with Reference to the West)* used Da Qing Long Tang in the treatment of wen bing (febrile diseases due to pathogenic warmth) with the substitution of Bo He for Gui Zhi.

Modern Application of Da Qing Long Tang

Da Qing Long Tang and its numerous modifications are used in Chinese contemporary medicine for the treatment of acute febrile disease with vigorous fever, such as the common cold, epidemic influenza, epidemic encephalitis (wind cold pattern), chronic bronchitis and pneumonia. The use of Da Qing Long Tang is based on the following.

- Ma Huang must be decocted first and the scum removed.
- It must be taken warm in three doses.
- A slight streaming sweat must be achieved.
- Due to the fact that this is a potent sweat promotion formula, in the event of copious sweating, warm rice powder should be applied to the outside of the body to minimise sweating. (Warm rice powder can be substituted by talcum powder.)

NOTE: Modifications can be made according to the individual condition of the patient. Where cold predominates, the dosage of Ma Huang and Gui Zhi should be relatively larger than that of Shi Gao; conversely, where heat predominates, the dosage of Shi Gao should be increased and the dosage of Ma Huang and Gui Zhi reduced. For high fever with irritability, the dosage of Shi Gao can be anything from 30 to 60g.

Case Study

Externally contracted pattern with vigorous fever

Extracted from Zhong Yi Za Zhi 1966; 3:23

A 36-year-old male had been sick for three days and presented with a high fever of 39.5°C. There was irritability, headache, a generalised ache in the body, absence of sweat, a rapid floating pulse and a thin, white tongue coat.

He was prescribed a formula based on Da Qing Long Tang: Ma Huang 4.5g , Zhu Ru 4.5g, Xing Ren 9g, Sheng Shi Gao 30g, Sheng Gan Cao 3g, Gui Zhi 4.5g, Zhu Ye 30 pieces, fresh Lu Gen 20g. After one pack, the fever and aversion to cold abated but he presented with a cough. A second pack was prescribed with the omission of Ma Huang and Gui Zhi and the addition of Jie Geng and Sang Ye 4.5g each. He recovered after the second pack.

Case Study

Exterior cold combined with an interior heat pattern

Extracted from Shang Han Lun Yi An Xuan Ping by Shen Yan Nan

Guang Dong Zhong Yi 1963; 2:38

A 60-year-old male presented with sudden onset of fever with no sweating, fatigue and a clouded spirit. He had complained to his family of vexation and body pain. His condition was misdiagnosed as a Shao Yin pattern and he was treated with warming herbs such as Gan Jiang and Fu Zi. Dr. Shen was consulted. The patient's pulse was floating and slightly rapid and both his feet felt warm. The diagnosis was Da Qing Long Tang pattern.

The pathogenesis was wind cold constraining the exterior and causing body pain. Constrained heat in the interior manifested as irritability and fever. Da Qing Long Tang was used to release exterior cold and clear interior heat. The formula prescribed was a modification of Da Qing

Long Tang: Sheng Shi Gao 30g, Ma Huang 9g, Gui Zhi 9g, Xing Ren 9g, Sheng Jiang 9g, Zhi Gan Cao 6g, Da Zao 5 pieces.

In view of the patient's age, it was thought that excessive sweating brought on by the warming herbs (Fu Zi and Gan Jiang) of the earlier formula could have contributed to the yang collapse, and so he was asked to take the decoction every 2 hours for a total of three doses with directions to discontinue the medication once he started to sweat. After the three doses, a streaming slight sweat was produced and the condition was resolved.

Xiao Qing Long Tang Pattern

Clause 40

伤寒表不解，心下有水气，干呕发热而咳，或渴，或利，或噎，或小便不利，少腹满，或喘者，小青龙汤主之。

Shang han with an unresolved exterior, water qi below the heart, dry retching, fever and cough, or thirst, or diarrhoea, or dysphagia, or the urination is not free, lesser abdominal distension, or wheezing, Xiao Qing Long Tang governs.

Clause 41

伤寒心下有水气，咳而微喘，发热不渴；服汤已，渴者，此寒去、欲解也；小青龙汤主之。

Shang han, there is water qi below the heart, cough and a slight wheeze, fever without thirst; having taken the decoction, if there is thirst, the cold is going and is about to resolve; Xiao Qing Long Tang governs.

XIAO QING LONG TANG: Ma Huang (nodes removed) 3 liang; Shao Yao 3 liang; Xi Xin 3 liang; Gan Jiang 3 liang; Zhi Gan Cao 3 liang; Wu Wei Zi ½ sheng; Ban Xia ½ sheng.

DIRECTIONS: First boil Ma Huang, in 1 dou of water (2 L), until reduced by 2 sheng, then skim off the foam, add the rest of the ingredients and simmer until reduced to 3 sheng. Strain the decoction and take 1 sheng warm.

MODIFICATIONS: If there is thirst, add Gua Lou Gen 3 liang. If there is mild diarrhoea, omit Ma Huang and add a piece of Rao Hua (*Wikstroemia canescens*) the size of a chicken's egg, which has been dry fried until the colour turns red. If there is dysphagia, omit Ma Huang and add one piece of roasted Fu Zi. If there is fullness in the lesser abdomen, omit Ma Huang and add Fu Ling 4 liang. If there is wheezing, omit Ma Huang and add Xing Ren ½ sheng, having first removed the skin and tips. It should be noted that Rao Hua does not treat diarrhoea and Ma Huang treats wheezing. The statement in relation to these herbs seem to be anomalous and there is doubt as to whether this was Zhong Jing's intention.

There are five modifications of Xiao Qing Long Tang. Four of these omit Ma Huang. The question is, Ma Huang and Xing Ren both treat wheezing and cough. So why did Zhong Jing substitute Ma Huang with Xing Ren to treat wheeze? Let us first examine the indication of Xiao Qing Long Tang in the treatment of wheezing. Clause 40 shows that Xiao Qing Long Tang is indicated for exterior cold with interior water accumulation, where pathogenic cold water qi is assailing the lung. Where wheezing is due to non-dissemination of lung qi, then Ma Huang is the herb of choice. However, the cause of wheezing in a Xiao Qing Long pattern is the accumulation of phlegm fluids which obstruct the descent of lung qi. The treatment principle therefore, is to descend lung qi and so Xing Ren is chosen. Where the principal feature is non-descent of lung qi, Ma Huang is avoided because it diffuses the lungs and has an ascending affect.

Xiao Qing Long Tang has been used effectively in the treatment of emphysema. Modern research of Ma Huang has shown that one of its principal constituents, ephedrine alkaloid, increases the heart rate and constricts the blood vessels and is therefore inappropriate for emphysema patients. In *Jin Gui Yao Lue*, Xiao Qing Long Tang with the addition of Shi Gao is used for the treatment of lung swelling, where there is wheezing due to water accumulation with interior heat. In other words, Xiao Qing Long Tang with modifications can be used to treat miscellaneous disease characterised by wheezing and cough due to pathogenic phlegm damp in the lungs (*Shang Han Lun Lin Chuang Ying Yong Wu Shi Lun – Fifty Clinical Applications of Shang Han Lun* by Pei Yong Qing).

DISCUSSION: The pathogenesis of a Xiao Qing Long Tang pattern can be summarised as an accumulation of water in the chest and epigastrium caused by an attack of pathogenic cold. An exterior pattern is understood to include the symptoms of aversion to cold, absence of sweat, and body pain, as typified by a shang han exterior excess pattern. Water qi below the heart refers to phlegm cold damp harassing the stomach, where it can give rise to a reversal of stomach qi and cause vomiting. If water qi harasses the lung, the reversal of qi will manifest as cough. Water qi follows the ascent and descent of qi, resulting in various symptoms, depending on the zang affected, and include diarrhoea (water qi affecting the intestines), dysphagia (water qi affecting the qi dynamic), inhibited urination (water qi impairing transformation) and wheezing (water qi obstructing the descent of qi). In Clause 40, the term lesser abdomen is used in its general sense and refers to the lower abdomen.

Xiao Qing Long Tang is a modification of Ma Huang Tang where Xing Ren is omitted, the dose of Zhi Gan Cao is increased, and Shao Yao, Ban Xia, Xi Xin, Gan Jiang and Wu Wei Zi are added. Ma Huang promotes sweating and releases the exterior, diffuses lung qi and calms wheezing and at the same time promotes urination. The combination of Ma Huang and Gui Zhi enhances the function of dispersing pathogenic cold to free the constrained yang qi. Gan Jiang and Ban Xia warm the middle and transform the water qi under the heart. Xi Xin is hot and acrid; it releases the exterior, expels cold, warms the interior and resolves phlegm damp. In order to prevent injury to yin and qi by the acrid and warm herbs, the increased dose of Zhi Gan Cao strengthens the middle and supports the zheng qi. Shao Yao and Wu Wei Zi are both sour: Shao Yao conserves the liver yin and Wu Wei Zi astringes the yin of the kidneys.

Key Points in the Application of Xiao Qing Long Tang

- For an acute attack of wheezing caused by wind cold, increase the ratio of Gan Jiang to Wu Wei Zi to enhance the warming and dispersing effect; for a chronic wheezing disorder, increase the dosage of Wu Wei Zi to enhance the action of astringing the lung qi.
- The combination of Ma Huang and Gui Zhi has a potent diffusing and ascending action. Therefore, if the wheezing is severe, Ma Huang should be replaced by Xing Ren. This is because Xi Xin and Ma Huang are both strongly dispersing, whereas Xing Ren has a descending action, thus directly addressing the reversal of lung qi to calm the wheeze. The famous Qing dynasty practitioner, Ye Tian Shi, seldom used Ma Huang and Xi Xin together to treat wheezing.
- For the weak and invalid patient, particularly one with heart and kidney disease, this formula must be used with caution. This is because Xiao Qing Long Tang is indicated for the treatment of exterior cold with interior accumulation of phlegm fluids and its warm, dispersing properties have the potential to injure yin and stir yang. This can give rise to such symptoms as a flushed face, palpitations, wheezing or a stifling sensation in the chest. Excessive stirring of yang qi can also cause nose bleed or deficiency desertion.
- Xiao Qing Long Tang is contraindicated for long term use, because its potential to injure yin and stir yang can lead to a transmuted pattern. It is suitable for acute conditions only and can be followed by Ling Gui formulas such as Ling Gui Zhu Gan Tang, Ling Gui Wei Gan Tang or Ling Gui Xing Gan Tang to consolidate treatment.

Summary of Xiao Qing Long Tang Applications

Xiao Qing Long Tang is indicated for externally contracted pathogenic wind cold with congested fluids and water qi under the heart.

KEY SIGNS AND SYMPTOMS: (1) Water qi is reflected in the patient's facial complexion in the form of 'water marks', which are pigmentation spots on the cheeks or around the eyes. (2) The water qi pattern is further evidenced by a watery tongue coat and a dusky complexion or swelling beneath the eye lids. (3) The patient expectorates copious, white, foamy, watery phlegm. (4) The condition is aggravated in the winter and eases during the warmer weather. (5) Other symptoms can include shortness of breath, oppressed sensation in the chest and orthopnoea. (6) A wiry pulse.

Ancient Application of Xiao Qing Long Tang

- *Jing Fang Shi Yan Lu* (*A Record of Tried and True Classic Formulas*) states: "For severe cases of fever and headache with a strong aversion to cold, increase the dose of Ma Huang and Gui Zhi. For milder fever with a slight aversion to cold, reduce the dose of Ma Huang and Gui Zhi or even substitute Dou Chi for Ma Huang and Su Ye for Gui Zhi. For a severe accumulation of phlegm and water qi, increase the dose of Gan Jiang, Xi Xin, Ban Xia and Wu Wei Zi."
- *Shang Han Lun Lin Chuang Shi Yan Lu* (*A Record of Shang Han Lun Clinically Tried and True Formulas*) states: "If the pattern is accompanied by fever and irritability, add Sheng Shi Gao. For an asthma pattern associated with deficiency, use Xiao Qing Long Tang with the addition of Ge Jie".

Modern Application of Xiao Qing Long Tang

Xiao Qing Long Tang can be used in the treatment of epidemic influenza, acute and chronic bronchitis, bronchial asthma, emphysema, pneumonia and whooping cough where the pathogenesis is exterior wind cold with interior phlegm fluids. For the treatment of whooping cough, Xiao Qing Long Tang can be used modified with the addition of Xing Ren and Sang Bai Pi (*Hu Nan Yi Xue Za Zhi* 1977; June issue).

Case Study

Exterior cold and interior water retention

Extracted from Shang Han Shi Jian Lun by Chen Rui Chun

A 47-year-old male had suffered from wheezing for over ten years. Recently a head cold triggered a severe attack, where he was not able to lie down in bed. He coughed up copious thin, watery sputum. The aversion to cold was not pronounced but his appetite was poor. His tongue was dull with a greasy white coat and his pulse was floating, thready and rapid. There were audible wet rales from both lungs.

He was prescribed a modifed version of Xiao Qing Long Tang: Zhi Ma Huang 5g; Gui Zhi 5g; Wu Wei Zi 6g; Xi Xin 3g; Dang Shen 10g; Fa Ban Xia 10g; Bai Shao 10g; Su Zi 10g; Kuan Dong Hua 10g; Sheng Jiang 3 pieces; Zhi Gan Cao 6g.

After six packs, the symptoms eased but at night there was still an occasional cough with white, watery sputum, and his stool was soft, his pulse was moderate and wiry and his tongue was wet and slippery. A modification of Liu Jun Zi Tang was then prescribed: Dang Shen 15g; Bai Zhu 12g; Fu Ling 15g; Xi Xin 2g; Wu Wei Zi 6g; Chen Pi 10g; Zhi Gan Cao 6g; Sheng Jiang 3 pieces; Fa Ban Xia 10g; Su Zi 10g; Kuan Dong Hua 10g. After six packs, all symptoms were resolved.

Discussion: Xiao Qing Long Tang is indicated for accumulation of phlegm fluids with pathogenic cold in the lung because it warms the lungs and transforms phlegm. However, once the external condition is resolved, it is advisable to tonify the spleen and lungs in order to consolidate the treatment.

Case Study

Asthma

Extracted from Xin Yi Yao Za Zhi 1974; (11):5

A 9-year-old girl had had bronchial asthma since the age of six, suffering frequent upper respiratory infections, particularly during the winter and spring seasons. Western medication managed to alleviate her symptoms but there were recurrent asthmatic attacks. Her complexion was pale and her face slightly puffy, her breathing was rapid, her lips were cyanosed and at times she was unable to lie flat. Her hands and feet were cold, there was no sweating, her tongue coat was white and slippery and her pulse was wiry, taut and slightly rapid. She was prescribed three packs of a modification of Xiao Qing Long Tang: Zhi Ma Huang 4.5g, Di Huang 9g, Rou Gui 1.5g, Zhi Gan Cao 3g, Fa Ban Xia 6g, Wu Wei Zi 3g, Xi Xin 3g, Shu Fu Zi 6g, Dang Gui 6g, Sheng Jiang 4.5g, Ze Xie 6g. After the three packs, her wheezing subsided.

Summary of Ma Huang Tang Modifications

Modified Ma Huang Tang patterns include the Ge Gen Tang pattern, Da Qing Long Tang pattern and Xiao Qing Long Tang pattern, all of which represent an exterior excess pattern with no sweating. A Ge Gen Tang pattern is characterised by a stiff neck and back; a Da Qing Long Tang pattern is characterised by irritability and a Xiao Qing Long Tang pattern is characterised by water qi under the heart.

2.3.3 Tai Yang Mild Exterior Depression

Tai Yang mild exterior depression is a pattern which remains within the definition of an exterior pattern but refers to a situation where the exterior constraint has affected the interior without actually having fallen inwards. This results in dual symptomatology of the exterior and the interior and is represented by three patterns.

1. Gui Zhi Ma Huang Ge Ban Tang pattern;
2. Gui Zhi Er Ma Huang Yi Tang pattern; and
3. Gui Zhi Er Yue Bi Yi Tang pattern.

Where there is a mild exterior pattern with constrained yang, it is not appropriate to use Gui Zhi Tang or Ma Huang Tang for the promotion of sweat, and yet slight sweat promotion is still indicated. Hence the modified formula of Gui Zhi Ma Huang Ge Ban Tang is used. Gui Zhi Er Ma Huang Yi Tang is even milder than Gui Zhi Ma Huang Ge Ban Tang and is used where the condition is milder again. Gui Zhi Er Yue Bi Yi Tang is a formula indicated for a pattern of Tai Yang mild exterior depression which is in the process of transforming into interior heat, hence the addition of a small dose of Shi Gao.

Gui Zhi Ma Huang Ge Ban Tang Pattern

Clause 23

(一) 太阳病，得之八九日，如虐状，发热恶寒，热多寒少，其人不呕，清便欲自可，一日二三度发。(二) 脉微缓者，为欲愈也；(三) 而脉微而恶寒者，此阴阳俱虚，不可更发汗、更下、更吐也；(四) 面色反有热色者，未欲解也，以其不能得小汗出，身必痒，宜桂枝麻黄各半汤。

(1.) Tai Yang disease, for eight or nine days, malaria-like symptoms, fever and aversion to cold, more fever less cold, the person does not vomit, urine and stool are normal, occurring two or three times in a day. (2.) Where the pulse is slightly moderate, this is imminent recovery; (3.) and where the pulse is faint with aversion to cold, this is deficiency of both yin and yang, one should not further promote sweating, nor purging, nor vomiting; (4.) and where the complexion is a hot colour, there is no imminent recovery, this is because the patient can not raise a mild sweat, the body will itch, Gui Zhi Ma Huang Ge Ban Tang is appropriate.

GUI ZHI MA HUANG GE BAN TANG: Gui Zhi (bark removed) 1 liang 16 zhu; Shao Yao, Sheng Jiang (sliced), Zhi Gan Cao and Ma Huang (nodes removed) 1 liang each; Da Zao (broken) 4 pieces; Xing Ren (blanched in hot water, skin and tips removed) 24 pieces. Note that this formula name can be translated as "Half each of Gui Zhi (Tang) and Ma Huang Tang", but in total, the decoction is actually ⅓ of those two formulas combined.

DIRECTIONS: First boil Ma Huang in 5 sheng of water (1 L), simmering and bringing to the boil once or twice, then skimming off the foam before adding the other ingredients. Simmer until reduced to 1 sheng 8 ge (360 mL). Strain and drink 6 ge (120 mL) while warm. This formula constitutes 3 ge each of Ma Huang Tang and Gui Zhi Tang combined together and the whole 6 ge should be drunk at one time. The patient must rest afterwards as with the instructions for Gui Zhi Tang.

DISCUSSION: Clause 23 is better read as four separate statements. The first statement describes a Tai Yang disorder which was contracted eight or nine days earlier, and so we know that it is not in its initial stage. There is both fever and aversion to cold where fever predominates, and the alternating heat and cold occurring two or three times a day resembles the alternating fever and chills of malaria. However, in this case, the alternating episodes of fever and chills represent the waning of the exterior pathogen in the face of intact zheng qi. Although the alternation of chills and fever is reminiscent of a Shao Yang pattern, the absence of vomiting shows that the stomach qi is harmonious and the pathogen has not entered Shao Yang. The fact that the stool and urination are normal shows that the pathogen has not entered Yang Ming. The disorder, therefore, is still a Tai Yang exterior pattern.

The second, third and fourth statements describe three possible developments of mild exterior depression. The second statement tells us that when a pulse which was floating and tight has changed to one which is slightly moderate, the zheng qi is about to return and recovery is imminent. In the third statement, the faint pulse and aversion to cold refer respectively to an interior and exterior deficiency, and therefore a deficiency of both yin and yang. This alludes to an exterior yang deficiency affecting the Shao Yin and manifesting as a concurrent pattern of Tai Yang exterior and Shao Yin interior. In this case, it is essential to support the zheng qi; reliance on diaphoretic, purgative or emetic strategies will further deplete the zheng qi and cause deterioration of the condition. The fourth and final statement describes the patient as having a face the colour of heat, in other words, red, and being unable to raise a sweat. The inability to perspire is a sign of constrained yang in the exterior, and is the reason for the face being red. From this it is clear not only that the pathogen is unresolved, but also that resolution of the exterior is unlikely, since sweat will not issue. The itching skin is also a sign of exterior constraint, where the pathogen is locked in the muscle layer and is unable to exit via sweating. Resolution must be sought in the promotion of mild sweat and Gui Zhi Ma Huang Ge Ban Tang is the formula which should be prescribed.

Gui Zhi Ma Huang Ge Ban Tang is a combination of the two formulas Ma Huang Tang and Gui Zhi Tang, where the ingredients are reduced, producing not double the dose, but only one-third of the total dose of those two formulas. Thus, it is a relatively mild formula which promotes a mild sweat. The role of Gui Zhi Tang is to regulate the ying and wei, whilst Ma Huang Tang opens the skin pores to promote sweating. Shao Yao is sour and Gan Cao is sweet, so together they counter the acridity of Ma Huang and Gui Zhi, thus ensuring the sweating is not excessive.

Case Study

Itchy skin

Extracted from Shang Han Lun Yi An Xuan Ping by Shen Yan Nan Guang Dong Zhong Yi 1963; 3:39

A 44-year-old woman suffered from itchy skin every autumn and winter, particularly when she was exposed to wind. The condition had persisted for the past six years. Western diagnosis had suggested it was due to an allergy, however, anti-histamines had brought no relief. When the itching occurred, the patient experienced greater sensitivity to wind than usual. Her pulse was floating and her tongue was pale. She was given three doses of Gui Zhi Ma Huang Ge Ban Tang and after coming out in a slight sweat, her condition improved. There was no recurrence of the disorder in the following year.

Gui Zhi Er Ma Huang Yi Tang Pattern

Clause 25

服桂枝汤，大汗出，脉洪大者，与桂枝汤，如前法。若形似虐，一日再发者，汗出必解，宜桂枝二麻黄一汤。

Having taken Gui Zhi Tang, there is copious sweat, if the pulse is flooding and big, give Gui Zhi Tang as before. If the disease resembles malaria, occurring again during the day, sweating will resolve it, Gui Zhi Er Ma Huang Yi Tang is appropriate.

GUI ZHI ER MA HUANG YI TANG: Gui Zhi (bark removed) 1 liang 17 zhu; Shao Yao 1 liang 6 zhu; Ma Huang (nodes removed) 16 zhu; Sheng Jiang (sliced) 1 liang 6 zhu; Xing Ren (skin and tips removed) 16 pieces; Zhi Gan Cao 1 liang 2 zhu; Da Zao (broken) 5 pieces. Note that this translates as "Two Parts Gui Zhi One Part Ma Huang Tang" but in fact, the actual dosage is 5/12 of the original Gui Zhi Tang recipe combined with 2/9 of the original Ma Huang Tang recipe.

DIRECTIONS: First boil Ma Huang in 5 sheng (1 L) of water, letting it simmer and bringing it to the boil once or twice before skimming the foam and adding the other ingredients. Simmer again, reducing to 2 sheng and strain. The patient should take 1 sheng immediately while warm, and take a second dose later the same day. Originally, two parts Gui Zhi Tang and one part Ma Huang Tang were combined to make a total of 2 sheng. Nowadays, the combination of these two formulas uses reduced dosages and is decocted to make 1 sheng. The patient should rest afterwards as per the standard directions for Gui Zhi Tang.

DISCUSSION: Gui Zhi Tang is the correct formula for Tai Yang zhong feng (wind strike); however, the effect of Gui Zhi Tang is to produce a light streaming sweat over the whole body. If, after the administration of Gui Zhi Tang, there is copious sweating, this shows that it was used incorrectly and has failed to resolve the disease, resulting in a pulse which is no longer moderate and floating but is flooding and big. However, the pattern remains the same: it is still a Tai Yang zhong feng pattern and the treatment is still Gui Zhi Tang. An alternative situation arises when, after the administration of Gui Zhi Tang, there develops a malaria-like condition with repeated bouts of intermittent fever and chills. This is evidence of a residual pathogen which, although unresolved, is nevertheless a milder condition than the Gui Zhi Ma Huang Ge Ban Tang pattern. Therefore, Gui Zhi Er Ma Huang Yi Tang is used to regulate ying and wei. The formula is composed of Gui Zhi Tang at 5/12 the original dosage, combined with 2/9 the original dosage of Ma Huang Tang. This is the same principle as adopted in Gui Zhi Ma Huang Ge Ban Tang with a dosage which is smaller still. The recommendation is to administer the decoction 1 to 2 hours before an anticipated bout of alternating fever and chills.

Case Study

Chills and fever

Extracted from Xin Bian Shang Han Lun Lei Fang,

China Science & Technology Publishing House

A 12-year-old girl had contracted an attack of wind cold at the beginning of spring, presenting with headache and fever. The fever had receded slightly after home medication had caused her to break out in a heavy sweat. However, it returned again the next day, manifesting as alternating chills and fever resembling malaria, and it was accompanied by aversion to cold. Her pulse was floating and slightly rapid and her tongue coat was thin, white and moist. It was deemed that the pathogen was still lodged in the exterior following the heavy sweating, and that Zhong Jing's Gui Zhi Er Ma Huang Yi Tang should be used to promote a mild sweat to expel the pathogen.

Formula: Gui Zhi 5g, Bai Shao 5g, Sheng Jiang 5g, Zhi Ma Huang 3g, Zhi Gan Cao 3g, Xing Ren 3g. After one pack, the patient came out in a light sweat and the condition was resolved.

Gui Zhi Er Yue Bi Yi Tang Pattern

Clause 27

太阳病，发热恶寒，热多寒少，脉微弱者，此无阳也，不可发汗，宜桂枝二越婢一汤。

Tai Yang disease, there is fever and aversion to cold, there is more fever and less cold, where the pulse is faint and weak, this is an absence of yang, one should not promote sweat, Gui Zhi Er Yue Bi Yi Tang is appropriate.

GUI ZHI ER YUE BI YI TANG: Gui Zhi (bark removed), Shao Yao, Ma Huang, Zhi Gan Cao 18 zhu each; Da Zao (broken) 4 pieces; Sheng Jiang (sliced) 1 liang 2 zhu; Shi Gao 24 zhu (crushed and wrapped in cotton gauze). Note that the formula name translates as two parts Gui Zhi (Tang) and one part Yue Bi Tang.

DIRECTIONS: First decoct Ma Huang in 5 sheng of water. Let it simmer, bringing it to the boil once or twice and skimming the foam before adding the other ingredients. Simmer until reduced to 2 sheng then strain. The patient should take 1 sheng warm. Originally, Gui Zhi Tang and Yue Bi Tang were combined equally and reduced to 1 sheng. Nowadays, the combined formula comprises two parts Gui Zhi Tang and one part Yue Bi Tang and the decoction is only reduced to 2 sheng.

DISCUSSION: Tai Yang disease is normally characterised by fever and aversion to cold. The important differential characteristic of this pattern is the predominance of fever over the symptom of aversion to cold. This is because the prolonged constraint of pathogenic cold is about to transform into heat. However, the symptom of aversion to cold remains, showing that there is still residual pathogenic cold. The faint, weak pulse differentiates this pattern from one of an exterior excess pattern where the pulse is floating and tight, and so it is said that "this is an absence of yang", by which it is meant that it is not a Shang Han exterior excess pattern. The implication of the phrase, "one should not promote sweat" relates precisely to the fact that this is not a yang pattern of exterior excess but a mild pattern of exterior constraint, where strong sweat must not be promoted and yet mild sweating is still required.

In its discussion of transmuted disease where there is both external and internal deficiency, Clause 153 uses the phrase, 无阳则阴独, which may be translated as "no yang just yin alone". This refers to the absence of exterior signs in the presence of interior signs and is used by Cheng Wu Ji to indicate that it is not a Shang Han exterior excess pattern. In the pattern described in Clause 27, there is exterior pathogenic constraint with gradual transformation to heat in the interior, and therefore Ma Huang is inappropriate.

This formula is the combination of Gui Zhi Tang and Yue Bi Tang in the ratio of 2:1. It is a formula which simultaneously releases the exterior and clears interior heat. Gui Zhi Tang regulates ying and wei whilst Yue Bi Tang expels the constrained interior heat. *Shang Han Lai Su Ji (Shang Han Revival Compendium)* compares Yue Bi Tang with Ma Xing Shi Gan Tang, where the former contains Sheng Jiang and Da Zao but not Xing Ren. Gui Zhi Er Yue Bi Yi Tang can be used to treat a concurrent pattern of Tai Yang and Yang Ming characterised by a predominance of fever over chills and an absence of sweating.

Modern Application of Gui Zhi Er Yue Bi Yi Tang

This formula can be used to treat early stage arthritis with intermittent fever and chills, aching or pain in the body and limbs, urticaria, bronchitis, the common cold and tonsillitis. Modifications include the following.

- *Upper respiratory tract infection and bronchitis.* Add Huang Qin, Jie Geng and Xing Ren to clear lung heat and transform phlegm.
- *Tonsillitis.* Add Jie Geng and She Gan to diffuse lung qi and disinhibit the throat.
- *Oedema associated with acute nephritis.* Add Chi Xiao Dou and Yu Mi Xu to promote urination and reduce swelling.
- *Proteinuria.* Add Sheng Huang Qi and Shi Wei to augment qi and promote urination.
- *Haematuria.* Add Bai Mao Gen and Lian Qiao to cool the blood and stop bleeding.
- *Leucocytosis.* Add Bai Jiang Cao, Pu Gong Ying and Jin Yin Hua to clear heat and relieve toxicity.
- *Urticaria.* Add Sheng Di, Chi Shao, Mu Dan Pi and Chan Yi to clear heat, cool the blood, dispel wind and stop the itch.

Case Study

Externally-contracted pattern with vigorous fever

Extracted from Shang Han Lun Hui Yao Fen Xi

A 20-year-old woman became chilled when caught in the rain three days earlier. The previous day she had awoken with a headache, aversion to cold, chills and fever with chills predominating, and a cough with the expectoration of white, sticky phlegm. On the day of the consultation, she still had a headache and her temperature was 38.2°C. The aversion to wind and cold persisted and she was sweating. Her phlegm had become a rusty colour, her throat was dry and sore. She felt thirsty but had no particular desire to drink and her appetite was poor. She also had lower back pain which she had suffered from since the birth of her child the previous February. Her limbs were cold and she was very thin; her stool and urination were normal; her tongue was pale red with a thin, yellow coat and her pulse was slippery and rapid.

The diagnosis was an attack by pathogenic cold and dryness with disharmony of ying and wei. She was prescribed a modified version of Gui Zhi Er Yue Bi Yi Tang: Gui Zhi 3 qian, Bai Shao 3 qian, Ma Huang 2 qian, Xing Ren 2 qian, Gan Cao 2 qian, Sheng Jiang 2 qian, Sheng Shi Gao 8 qian, Hong Zao 3 pieces. After one pack, her symptoms disappeared with the exception of the back pain, for which Ren Dong Lu Lu Tang was then prescribed.

Summary of Tai Yang Mild Exterior Depression

Gui Zhi Ma Huang Ge Ban Tang, Gui Zhi Er Ma Huang Yi Tang and Gui Zhi Er Yue Bi Yi Tang are all modified versions of Gui Zhi Tang, which is the guiding formula to use when the promotion of a mild sweat is indicated. Gui Zhi Ma Huang Ge Ban Tang promotes sweat more strongly than Gui Zhi Er Ma Huang Yi Tang; and Gui Zhi Er Yue Bi Yi Tang contains Shi Gao and is indicated for pathogenic cold slowly transforming into interior heat. Modern research has shown that both Gui Zhi Tang and Yue Bi Tang are anti-pyretic, antitussive, anti-inflammatory, pain relieving and, due to their diuretic effect, are also effective in reducing oedema. (*Yi Fang Xin Xian,* Shanghai Science & Technology Publishing House, 1996, p. 51).

Section Four

2.4 TAI YANG FU PATTERNS

Tai Yang disease can transfer to the interior via the channels and network vessels and affect its fu organ the urinary bladder. The pathogen can knot with water in the urinary bladder or with blood in the lower jiao. This entrapment of water or blood in the interior gives rise to two Tai Yang fu patterns: Tai Yang water amassment or xu shui, and Tai Yang blood amassment or xu xue.

2.4.1 Tai Yang Xu Shui or Water Amassment

Wu Ling San Pattern

Clause 71

（一）太阳病，发汗后，大汗出，胃中干，烦躁不得眠，欲得饮水者，少少与饮之，令胃气和则愈。（二）若脉浮，小便不利，微热消渴者，五苓散主之。

(1) Tai Yang disease, after the promotion of sweat, there is profuse sweating, the stomach is dry, there is vexation and an inability to sleep, if there is a desire to drink, give a small amount of water, it will cause the stomach qi to harmonise then there will be recovery. (2) If the pulse is floating, the urination is not free, with a slight fever and insatiable thirst, Wu Ling San governs.

WU LING SAN: Zhu Ling (skin removed) 18 zhu; Ze Xie 1 liang 6 zhu; Bai Zhu 18 zhu; Fu Ling 18 zhu; Gui Zhi (bark removed) ½ liang.

DIRECTIONS: Grind all five ingredients into a powder and mix well. Take one square spoon (approx 6–9 g) of the mixture with rice water (water taken from the pot as the rice is cooking) three times per day. Drink plenty of warm water and follow the same directions for Gui Zhi Tang in order to promote a sweat, and recovery will follow.

DISCUSSION: This clause describes the aetiology and pathogenesis of water amassment and its two treatment strategies, one being the drinking of water and the other, the administration of the herbal formula, Wu Ling San. It is better read as two sentences as marked above. The first sentence discusses the situation where acrid herbs have been used to promote sweat in order to resolve the exterior, and this is followed by further copious sweating. The subsequent loss of fluids results in dryness of the stomach, and the damage to yin also gives rise to vexation and insomnia. The appropriate response is simply to replenish the lost fluids and restore stomach yin by taking small but frequent sips of water. The second sentence juxtaposes the exterior sign of a floating pulse and the interior symptoms of inhibited urination and thirst, which are manifestations of water retained in the interior. This is because the pathogen has been transmitted along the Tai Yang channel to its fu, the urinary bladder, disrupting the transformation of qi. The failure to transform qi and transport fluids has not only caused inhibited urination but has also given rise to thirst. These two symptoms of inhibited urination and insatiable thirst are key diagnostic features of Tai Yang water amassment, which is also characterised by a thin, white and slippery tongue coat.

Zhu Ling is sweet and bland and frees the waterways. Its action of transforming qi and promoting urination is enhanced by Fu Ling. Ze Xie eliminates damp by promoting urination and also drains fire. Bai Zhu dries damp by strengthening the spleen; Gui Zhi not only releases the exterior, but also promotes urination by warming and freeing the obstructed yang to support the transformation of qi. The instruction to take the Wu Ling powder with warm rice water and then to drink plenty of warm water, has the same objective as the hot gruel in Gui Zhi Tang. The standard directions for Gui Zhi Tang must also be followed in order to support the function of the relatively small dose of Gui Zhi and produce a light sweat and release the exterior.

Clause 72

发汗已，脉浮数，烦渴者，五苓散主之。

Having promoted sweat, if the pulse is floating and rapid, with vexation and thirst, Wu Ling San governs.

DISCUSSION: Clause 72 should be read in conjunction with Clause 71 in order to understand that it is continuing to describe various outcomes following diaphoresis. Here, the pulse has changed from the floating, moderate pulse characteristic of Tai Yang, to one which is floating and rapid. The floating rapid pulse shows that the exterior pathogen has not been eliminated. The vexation and thirst are manifestations of the exterior pathogen having penetrated into the interior via the Tai Yang channel. Clause 72 should be read as a sequel to Clause 71, which also discusses the symptom combination of a floating pulse and thirst. The obstruction caused by the pathogen has caused inhibited urination due to non-transformation of qi in the urinary bladder. The choice of Wu Ling San as the guiding formula tells us that there is water accumulation.

Clause 74

中风发热，六七日不解而烦，有表里证，渴欲饮水，水入则吐者，名曰水逆，五苓散主之。

Zhong feng with fever, for six or seven days is unresolved and there is vexation, there are exterior and interior patterns, thirst with a desire to drink, if drinking causes vomiting, it is called water reversal, Wu Ling San governs.

DISCUSSION: When the fever of Tai Yang zhong feng has persisted for six or seven days, and there are symptoms of vexation and thirst, it means that the exterior pathogen has entered into the Tai Yang urinary bladder via the network channels. Because it has affected both the channel and the fu organ, both exterior and interior patterns are present. In this clause, the exterior pattern is evidenced by the fever and would also be accompanied by aversion to cold, and the interior pattern by the retention of water implied by the use of Wu Ling San. The symptoms of thirst not eased by drinking, vexation, and inhibited urination form the key identifying symptom complex of Tai Yang water amassment. The regurgitation of water after drinking indicates a more serious condition because it means that the failure of qi transformation in the lower jiao and subsequent accumulation of water in the urinary bladder has affected the stomach's descending function, giving rise to 'shui ni' or the reversed flow of water. From this, it can also be inferred that urination would be inhibited. Although this represents a more severe disorder, the pathomechanism is the same as that of the pattern described in Clauses 71 and 72 and the appropriate treatment is therefore Wu Ling San.

Comparison of Wu Ling San with Xiao Qing Long Tang and Bai Hu jia Ren Shen Tang

There are two main points of differentiation in the clinical application of Wu Ling San, Xiao Qing Long Tang and Bai Hu jia Ren Shen Tang.

1. Both Wu Ling San and Xiao Qing Long Tang are indicated for an exterior pattern with interior water accumulation manifesting as inhibited urination and thirst. The former addresses impaired transformation of qi in the urinary bladder whilst the latter addresses water qi under the heart. Thirst and inhibited urination are primary symptoms in the identification of a Wu Ling San pattern but are secondary to the identification of a Xiao Qing Long Tang pattern, where they may or may not be present. Further, whilst a Wu Ling San pattern presents with copious sweating, there is no sweating in a Xiao Qing Long Tang pattern.
2. Both Wu Ling San and Bai Hu jia Ren Shen Tang patterns are characterised by thirst; however, in the case of Wu Ling San, the exterior syndrome remains unresolved as is reflected in the floating rapid pulse, whereas in the Bai Hu jia Ren Shen Tang pattern, there is no exterior syndrome and the pulse is flooding and big. In the Wu Ling San pattern, the thirst is ascribed to non-distribution of fluid, whereas the thirst associated with Bai Hu Tang is a reflection of the consumption of fluids by excessive sweating and vigorous fever.

Ancient Application of Wu Ling San

- *Shang Han Zong Bing Lun* states: "In Shang Han, when the pulse is floating and moderate and the limbs are warm it is a Tai Yin pattern. If there is inhibited urination, the person will suffer from yellowing, and Wu Ling San with the addition of Yin Chen governs." The direction is for Yin Chen to be decocted separately and reduced to a concentrated liquid which is taken with Wu Ling San (in its powdered form) three or four times daily. The pathogen will then be excreted via urination.
- *Ji Yang Gang Mu* states: "Wu Ling San can be used in the treatment of watery diarrhoea, interior dampness and inhibited urination."
- *Shang Han Xu Lun* states: "Wu Ling San, omitting Gui Zhi and adding Huang Qin, can be used for febrile disease where there is fever and thirst, dark, scant urination, a normal bowel movement and a floating pulse."

Modern Application of Wu Ling San

Wu Ling San has a potential for broad application in the treatment of contemporary disease diagnoses. Such diseases include acute and chronic nephritis, infectious hepatitis, liver cirrhosis with ascites, acute and chronic colitis, urinary infection, congestive cardiac disease and oedema associated with heart and kidney disease. Suggested modifications are as follows.

- *Nephritis.* For oedema with scant urination, add Da Fu Pi, Che Qian Zi, Huang Qi, Shan Yao, Jin Yin Hua.
- *Neurogenic urinary frequency.* For frequent or painful urination in the absence of infection, Wu Ling San with the addition of Fu Pen Zi may be used.
- *Cystitis.* For frequent, burning urination, use Wu Ling San with the addition of such herbs as Mu Tong, Qu Mai, Che Qian Zi, Dan Zhu Ye, Zhi Gan Cao, Sheng Di.
- *Acute colitis.* For frequent watery diarrhoea with scant urination, Wu Ling San may be used with the addition of Ge Gen, Huang

Qin, Huang Lian, Zhi Gan Cao and Yi Yi Ren. Where there is heat, omit Gui Zhi. For chronic colitis with watery diarrhoea, combine Wu Ling San with Li Zhong Tang.
- *Post-partum urinary retention.* Use Wu Ling San with the addition of Wu Yao.
- *Vertigo due to water retention.* Use Wu Ling San with the addition of Gan Cao and Ge Gen.
- *Ascites.* Wu Ling San combined with Zhen Wu Tang with the addition of Huai Niu Xi (Fu Zi 30g to be decocted first for one hour, Chi Bai Shao 30g).

NOTE: Traditionally, Wu Ling San is a powder and it should be taken with rice water or warm water in order to achieve a slight sweat. In the contemporary use of Wu Ling San as a decoction, the liquid should not be too concentrated and the dosage of Ze Xie must be increased.

Case Study

Frequent Urination

Extracted from Shang Han Wu Shi Lun: A Case Study by Pei Yong Qing

A 21-year-old woman had suffered from frequent urination for over a month and was at times unable to control her bladder. Urine analysis was normal. Her tongue coat was thin and white and her pulse was submerged. The Chinese medicine diagnosis was impaired transformation of qi in the urinary bladder. She was prescribed six packs of Wu Ling San, after which she recovered fully.

Case Study

Glomus Beneath the Heart

Extracted from Shang Han Wu Shi Lun by Pei Yong Qing

A 38-year-old man had suffered for over seven months from a subjective sensation of obstruction in the stomach region. There was no pain on palpation and it had been diagnosed as chronic superficial gastritis. He had taken patent Chinese formulas such as Xiang Sha Yang Wei Wan and Jian Pi Wan in pill form, which, whilst giving temporary relief, had not resolved the condition. His bowel movement was normal and his urination scant. His tongue was swollen with a thin, slippery tongue coat and his pulse was submerged and wiry.

The Chinese medicine diagnosis was glomus beneath the heart due to water accumulation known as water glomus or shui pi and the treatment principle was to transform qi and promote urination. A modification of Wu Ling San was prescribed: Fu Ling 30g, Gui Zhi 10g, Bai Zhu 10g, Zhu Ling 15g, Ze Xie 18g, Hou Po 3g, Chen Pi 3g. After three packs, his symptoms eased and he was given a further six packs to consolidate the treatment. Following that, the patient was given Jian Pi Wan to strengthen the spleen. He recovered fully.

Note: Wu Ling San is the governing formula for Tai Yang water amassment, described in Clause 156 as water glomus. Diagnosis was based on the inhibited urination, the watery tongue and slippery tongue coat, and the submerged, wiry pulse. Sheng Jiang can be added to enhance water elimination.

Case Study

Gastroenteritis with Vomiting and Diarrhoea

Extracted from Shang Han Wu Shi Lun by Pei Yong Qing

A 20-year-old woman presented with fever, vomiting, diarrhoea and acute abdominal pain. She had had a temperature of 37–39°C for several days. Her complexion was dull and she complained of thirst and of difficulty in passing urine. Her tongue was swollen and large with a white, slippery tongue coat and her pulse was wiry.

The Chinese medicine diagnosis was Huo Luan with water accumulation. Wu Ling San was prescribed: Fu Ling 30g, Zhu Ling 15g, Bai Zhu 12g, Ze Xie 15g, Gui Zhi 3g. After four packs the vomiting and diarrhoea cleared. Xiang Sha Liu Jun Zi Tang was prescribed for another week to consolidate the treatment.

Note: Huo Luan is similar to the Western diagnosis of gastroenteritis. It is attributed to eating the wrong food or to retention of damp heat in the interior. Wu Ling San is used to transform qi and disinhibit water. If cold signs predominate, Fu Zi Li Zhong Tang and Zhen Wu Tang can be combined. If heat signs predominate, Liu Yi San and Ge Gen Qin Lian Tang can be used.

Case Study

Epilepsy

Extracted from Shang Han Wu Shi Lun by Pei Yong Qing

A 43-year-old woman presented with muscle spasm which extended from the left leg to the upper body and head on the left-hand side. She also had a severe headache and stiff neck and her speech was impaired, as was the vision in her left eye. She had a history of epilepsy and for the past two years had suffered from gastric prolapse and Meniere's syndrome and was receiving treatment for those conditions. A CT scan had revealed that she had an osteoma of the frontal bone measuring 1.2 x 1.5 cm and it was thought that this could be the cause of her epilepsy. Surgery was recommended. The patient did not wish to have surgery and sought treatment with Chinese medicine. At the time of her consultation, there was excessive salivation, her tongue was swollen and the coat was white and slippery. Her pulse was wiry and rapid and her urination scant.

Wu Ling San was prescribed: Fu Ling 30g, Gui Zhi 9g, Bai Zhu 9g, Zhu Ling 15g, Ze Xie 30g. After one pack, urination returned to normal and she was given six further packs to consolidate the treatment. Three years later, she accompanied her daughter for treatment of a menstrual disorder and reported that since the medication, there had been no further epileptic seizures.

Note: According to Chinese medicine, the accumulation of phlegm fluids and blood stasis form part of the pathogenesis of epilepsy. Dr Pei had encountered many such patients in his practice and had used Wu Ling San with certain modifications, always using a large dose of Ze Xie. The key points for diagnosis are inhibited urination, a watery and slippery tongue, and a submerged and wiry pulse.

Fu Ling Gan Cao Tang Pattern

Clause 73

伤寒汗出而渴者，五苓散主之；不渴者，茯苓甘草汤主之。

Shang han with sweating and thirst, Wu Ling San governs; with no thirst, Fu Ling Gan Cao Tang governs.

FU LING GAN CAO TANG: Fu Ling 2 liang; Gui Zhi (bark removed) 2 liang; Zhi Gan Cao 1 liang; Sheng Jiang 3 liang.

DIRECTIONS: Boil the ingredients in 4 sheng of water, reducing to 2 sheng. Strain, divide into three doses and take warm.

DISCUSSION: Clause 73 compares the patterns of Wu Ling San, where water is knotted in the lower jiao, and Fu Ling Gan Cao Tang, where there is water accumulation in the middle jiao. The Wu Ling San pattern is characterised by thirst and inhibited urination, whereas the Fu Ling Gan Cao Tang pattern is characterised by uninhibited urination with no thirst. The sweating is due to the exterior pattern not having been resolved but, for clinical purposes, Wu Ling San can be used regardless of whether there is an exterior pattern or not. Here, the pathogen has followed the Tai Yang pathway, knotting with the water in the urinary bladder to cause inhibited urination. The accumulation of water obstructs the qi dynamic and the distribution of fluids, giving rise to thirst. If, however, following the promotion of sweat, the stomach yang is damaged, water retention in the middle jiao may result. In this case, there is no thirst or inhibited urination and, instead, Fu Ling Gan Cao Tang should be used. Fu Ling disinhibits water by promoting urination; Gui Zhi warms the yang to disperse fluids; Sheng Jiang also warms and disperses and, together with Gan Cao, harmonises the middle. This formula is designed to warm the stomach and disperse water.

Clause 127

（一）太阳病，小便利者，以饮水多，必心下悸；（二）小便少者，必苦里急也。

(1) TaiYang disease, where urination is free, because of drinking much water, there will be palpitations below the heart; (2) where urination is scant, there will be discomfort and urgency in the interior.

DISCUSSION: Both Clause 127 and Clause 73 describe the differential symptoms of water accumulation in the middle and lower jiao. The first statement in Clause 127 describes uninhibited urination, thus eliminating the involvement of the lower jiao, and also describes palpitations, which are a result of the ingestion of water in quantities too large for the stomach to receive and process. The subsequent accumulation of water knots with the stomach qi, giving rise to palpitations in the epigastric region or 'below the heart'. Water accumulation in the lower jiao, on the other hand, is associated with the non-transformation of urinary bladder qi, and the second statement in Clause 127 describes the resulting scant or inhibited urination, which is accompanied by lower abdominal urgency and discomfort.

Reading between the lines of Clause 127, one can deduce that the aetiology of Tai Yang water amassment is an exterior pathogen which has not been resolved at the exterior level, but has travelled through the Tai Yang channel, ultimately reaching the urinary bladder. The subsequent impairment of its transformation function results in water amassment in the lower jiao, manifesting with inhibited urination and thirst. The main points are as follows.

- *Thirst.* If there is thirst, Wu Ling San is indicated. In the absence of thirst, Fu Ling Gan Cao Tang should be used.
- *Urination.* If urination is uninhibited, there is water amassment in the middle jiao. If urination is scant, there is water amassment in the lower jiao.
- *Location.* If symptoms are located below the heart, it is a middle jiao pattern. If they are in the lesser abdomen, it is a lower jiao pattern.

Xie Xin Tang and Wu Ling San Patterns

Clause 156

本以下之，故心下痞，与泻心汤。痞不解，其人渴而口燥烦，小便不利者，五苓散主之。

Due to purging, there is glomus below the heart, give Xie Xin Tang. The glomus is not resolved, the person is thirsty and there is a dry mouth and vexation, where urination is not free, Wu Ling San governs.

DISCUSSION: Glomus is a subjective sensation of localised fullness or blockage. It is the result of obstruction and is variously attributed to knotted heat below the heart, water amassment in the urinary bladder, or the stagnation of qi and water in the middle jiao. The standard treatment for glomus below the heart is the Xie Xin Tang group of formulas and if Xie Xin Tang fails to resolve glomus, it is because it is not due to heat knotted below the heart. The symptoms of thirst, vexation and a dry mouth indicate that the water accumulation is not in the middle jiao; the inhibited urination confirms that the water amassment has knotted in the lower jiao, and this is known as water glomus. To resolve the glomus, the water must be eliminated. The strategy is to transform qi and disinhibit water, for which the formula is Wu Ling San. The urination associated with kidney yang deficiency is an ambiguous issue. There are two possibilities: the first is where deficient yang fails to warm and transform fluids, resulting in inhibited or scant urination; the second possibility is where inadequate yang is unable to control water, resulting in frequent or copious urination, as described in Clause 316.

Key points for the diagnosis of water glomus are: thirst, a dry mouth, vexation, inhibited urination, a sense of blockage, a swollen tongue and a wet, slippery tongue coat. The indicated formulas are Wu Ling San and Shi Zao Tang. Tang Rong Chuan (also known as Tang Zong Hai) said: "Glomus can be due to water, fire, deficiency and qi. Shi Zao Tang is indicated for a water glomus excess pattern and Wu Ling San is indicated for a water glomus deficiency pattern" (*Xue Zheng Lun* 血证论 (*Treatise on Blood Patterns*).

Comparison of Xie Xin Tang, Wu Ling San and Fu Ling Gan Cao Tang

Clause 156 is better understood when read with reference to Clause 149, which describes a Ban Xia Xie Xin Tang pattern. In *Shang Han Lun*, Xie Xin Tang is the conventional treatment for glomus below the heart associated with spleen yang deficiency. If, after giving Xie Xin Tang, the condition is not resolved, and there is vexation, thirst and inhibited urination, then Wu Ling San is indicated. The formation of glomus can be attributed to several factors. Apart from pathogenic heat knotted below the heart, it can be due to the accumulation of water in the urinary bladder resulting from the impaired qi dynamic of the middle jiao failing to transform and distribute fluids, where stagnant qi and water cause obstruction, giving rise to glomus. In addition to glomus, Clause 156 describes a dry mouth, vexation, and inhibited urination, which are all manifestations of water amassment, and thus Wu Ling San is given. However, if the loss of sweat damages the stomach yang and, as a result, water accumulates in the middle jiao, then there will be neither thirst nor inhibited urination and, instead, Fu Ling Gan Cao Tang should be used.

Summary of Water Amassment Patterns

The aetiology of Tai Yang water amassment is the invasion of an exterior pathogen transmitting to the urinary bladder and impairing its transformation function. The main symptoms are a floating or floating and rapid pulse, inhibited urination, a slight fever, vexation, thirst, reversed flow of water after drinking, and water glomus with abdominal urgency. The governing formula is Wu Ling San, which frees the obstructed yang, disinhibits water and addresses both the exterior and the interior. If the water amassment is not in the lower jiao but in the stomach, then there is no thirst, the urination is not inhibited, and there are palpitations below the heart. Fu Ling Gan Cao Tang is the formula of choice to warm the stomach and disperse the pathogenic water.

2.4.2 Tai Yang Xu Xue or Blood Amassment

Tao He Cheng Qi Tang Pattern

Clause 106

太阳病不解,热结膀胱，其人如狂，血自下，下者愈。其外不解者，尚未可攻，当先解其外。外解已，但少腹急结者，乃可攻者，宜桃核承气汤。

Tai Yang disease is not resolved, heat knots in the urinary bladder, the person seems deranged, blood descends spontaneously, descent brings recovery. Where the exterior is not resolved, one should not attack yet, one must first resolve the exterior. Having resolved the exterior, but there is tense knotting in the lesser abdomen, then one should attack, Tao He Cheng Qi Tang is appropriate.

TAO HE CHENG QI TANG: Tao Ren (skin and tips removed) 50 pieces; Da Huang 4 liang; Gui Zhi (bark removed) 2 liang; Zhi Gan Cao 2 liang; Mang Xiao 2 liang.

DIRECTIONS: Boil the first four ingredients in 7 sheng of water, reducing to 2½ sheng. Strain, add Mang Xiao and bring to the boil again for a minute or so. Take five ge (100 mL) warm three times a day. A slightly loose stool should follow.

DISCUSSION: This clause describes the pathogenesis and treatment of Tai Yang blood amassment. The cause is an exterior pathogen which has transformed into heat, travelled along the channel to the lower jiao and subsequently knotted with the blood. The reference to heat knotting in the urinary bladder may be interpreted more generally as knotted heat and blood in the lower jiao. The psychological disturbance is a result of the heart shen being disturbed by the knotted heat and blood. The lesser abdomen here refers to the lower abdomen. The tense knotting describes spasm, distension and hard glomus pain ascribed to the knotted heat and blood stasis in the lower jiao, which obstructs the flow of qi and blood. The phrase: "blood descends spontaneously, descent brings recovery" refers to bleeding from the lower jiao, either in the urine or the stool. It is also an indication of the severity of the blood amassment, which can be relieved only by the passing of blood, thereby not only eliminating the stasis caused by the pathogenic heat, but also providing an exit for the pathogenic heat itself. To address the exterior first before treating an interior pattern is a fundamental principle in treating a concurrent exterior and interior pattern. Therefore, if there is an unresolved exterior pattern in the presence of blood amassment, then one must release the exterior before purging.

Tao He Cheng Qi Tang is Tiao Wei Cheng Qi Tang (Da Huang, Mang Xiao, Gan Cao) with the addition of Tao Ren and Gui Zhi. Da Huang, which is bitter and cold, combined with Mang Xiao, which is salty and cold, drains heat, softens hardness and purges the knotted heat and blood. As a single herb, Da Huang can eliminate blood stasis but this function is significantly enhanced when it is combined with Tao Ren. Gui Zhi is acrid and warm; it warms the channels and promotes the movement of qi. Its chief function in this formula is not to release the exterior but to free the obstructed yang and promote the flow of qi and blood. Zhi Gan Cao harmonises the stomach and also moderates the potency of the other herbs. The overall action of the formula is to purge heat and break blood stasis in the treatment of knotted stasis and heat in the lower jiao.

There have been various interpretations of the concept of knotted heat in the urinary bladder. Shen Jin Ao in *Shang Han Lun Gang Mu* 伤寒论纲目 *(Guide to Shang Han Lun)* maintained that it referred only to blood accumulation in the bladder. In *Shang Han Shuo Yuan Ji,* Qian Tian Lai believed it referred to blood accumulation in the colon. Ke Yun Bo proposed that it was blood accumulation in the lesser abdomen and Tang Rong Chuan put forth the theory that it was blood amassment in the chamber of blood. A more recent interpretation suggests that it could refer to blood accumulation either in the uterus or the digestive tract, however the authors believe that the concept of blood accumulation in the urinary bladder and lesser abdomen is the most appropriate interpretation. The pathogenesis of this pattern is the knotting of heat and blood in the lower jiao causing blood stasis. It can also be interpreted as heat knotting with pre-existing stasis. The key symptoms are intense tension and pain in the lesser abdomen, disturbance of the spirit, uninhibited urination and a submerged and choppy pulse.

Key points to bear in mind when using Tao He Cheng Qi Tang

1. Gui Zhi plays a significant role in this formula because although Tao Ren has a strong blood transforming function, it does not move the blood. Gui Zhi on the other hand promotes the movement of blood but can not transform stasis. Together they are able to invigorate blood and transform stasis.
2. The dosage of Mang Xiao should be smaller than the dosage recommended in the original text. If there is normal bowel movement with no heat signs, the dosage can be reduced or it can be deleted altogether.
3. The decoction should be taken before meals; in other words, on an empty stomach. The traditional directions for taking herbal decoctions are that if the disorder is above the diaphragm, the medicinal should be taken after food and if the disorder is below the diaphragm, it should be taken before food.
4. This is a potent formula and it is not indicated for long term use. It should be administered with great caution to invalid, elderly or pregnant patients.
5. After the decoction, there should be mild diarrhoea and patients can sometimes experience slight abdominal pain.

Ancient Application of Tao He Cheng Qi Tang

- *Shang Han Zong Bing Lun:* Tao Ren Cheng Qi Tang is indicated for postpartum retention of lochia.
- *Fu Ren Liang Fang Da Quan:* Tao He Cheng Qi Tang is indicated in the treatment of blood stasis characterised by tension and

pain in the lesser abdomen, difficult bowel movement or delirious speech, a parched throat with no desire for drinks, generalised yellowing, uninhibited urination, or knotted blood in the chest which resists pressure, or fever and chill, delirium and disturbance of the spirit.

- *Ji Yang Gang Mu*: Tao He Cheng Qi Tang is indicated in the treatment of diarrhoea with a tarry stool, abdominal pain and tenesmus with knotted heat and blood stasis.

Modern Application of Tao He Cheng Qi Tang

- Stasis-related headache, vertigo, abdominal pain, constipation; febrile disease with scant urination; gynaecological disease such as dysmenorrhoea, amenorrhoea, postpartum retention of lochia, abdominal mass. It is also indicated for cerebral injury, trauma and schizophrenia.
- Stasis-related manic behaviour and postpartum disturbance of the spirit accompanied by hardness and fullness in the lesser abdomen. The disorder is resolved when medication is followed by a tarry stool.
- Haemorrhagic fever. The People's Hospital in Hua Dian County, Ji Lin province recorded the use of Tao He Cheng Qi Tang in the treatment of 58 cases of haemorrhagic fever during the scant urination phase.
- Migraine accompanied by a flushed face, thirst and constipation. Tao He Cheng Qi Tang can be used with the addition of Quan Xie 6g and Jiang Chen 6g to facilitate the penetration of the network vessels.
- Hypertension with a flushed face accompanied by distending pain in the abdomen and constipation.
- Trauma with external injury. Add Gui Wei, Chuan Xiong, Chi Shao, Hong Hua, Su Mu, Niu Xi.
- Amenorrhoea due to blood stagnation. Add Dang Gui, Chuan Xiong, Chi Shao, Hong Hua, Xiang Fu.
- Dysmenorrhoea due to stasis. Add Bai Shao, Xiang Fu, Yan Hu Suo.

Case Study

Uterine Fibroid

Extracted from Xin Zhong Yi 1987; (9):45

A 50-year-old female patient suffered from a return of uterine bleeding a year after her menstruation stopped. The bleeding was intermittent, the blood was thick and dark with clots, and there was a distending pain in the lower abdomen. She was diagnosed as having a uterine fibroid and a hysterectomy was recommended. The patient declined surgery and chose to be treated by Chinese medicine. She was slightly overweight, and had a dusky complexion. The uterine fibroid was easily palpable, and the uterus was the size of a four month pregnancy. Her tongue was dull with stasis spots and a thin, white tongue coat. Her pulse was submerged and thready. The diagnosis was disharmony of the Chong and Ren vessels with stasis obstruction of the uterus. The formula used was a modification of Tao He Cheng Qi Tang: Tao Ren 30g, Da Huang 10g, Zhi Qiao 10g, Gui Zhi 15g, San Leng 15g, Gan Cao 6g. After an initial three packs, there was a reduction in the uterine bleeding. A further thirty packs were given, at the end of which, the bleeding was resolved and an ultrasound of the uterus showed no abnormality.

Case Study

Haematuria Associated with Immune Thrombocytopenia

Extracted from Shang Han Wu Shi Lun by Pei Yong Qing

A 56-year-old woman presented with haematuria. She had mild lower abdominal discomfort but no pain or urgency. She had attended the hospital out-patients' unit for treatment four days earlier but there was still blood in her urine which caused her to be anxious and agitated. Other symptoms were palpitations, fatigue and vertigo. She was on no other medication. There was no previous history of haemorrhage and the evening before the haematuria occurred, she had eaten carp for dinner. There was purple bruising on both her wrists; she had a pale complexion, purplish lips, a dull, and purplish tongue with a thick, yellow coat and a wiry, rapid pulse. Her temperature was 37.1°C; pulse rate 96/min; blood pressure 70/45 mmHg.

Urine analysis showed the presence of red blood cells and protein; haemoglobin levels were well below normal; the red cell count was at the lower end of the normal range and the white cell count was elevated.

The diagnosis was bleeding due to blood stasis and blood heat and Tao He Cheng Qi Tang was prescribed to cool and invigorate the blood and transform the blood stasis in order to stop the bleeding: Tao Ren 15g, Gui Zhi 3g, Sheng Da Huang 6g, Yuan Ming fen 6g (to be mixed with decoction), Sheng Gan Cao 6g, Dan Shen 15g, San Qi Fen 3g. After one pack, the abdominal distension and pain eased. The formula was then modified by reducing Da Huang to 1.5g and adding Shui Zhi 10g, Niu Xi 15g and Sheng Di 15g (five packs). At the end of this course of medication, the urine analysis was near normal. A further 16 packs were given, omitting Mang Xiao, reducing Da Huang to 1g and adding Dang Shen 18g, Huang Qi 18g and Dang Gui 15g (16 doses).

Note: Haematuria is one of the symptoms of thrombocytopenia, which is a disease where thrombocyte (platelet) levels are low, resulting in sporadic bleeding into the tissues causing purpura. Immune thrombocytopenia is associated with the presence of anti-platelet antibodies (IgG). The main treatment principle is to cool and invigorate the blood and stop the bleeding. The meal of carp on the night before the haematuria started could have triggered an allergic reaction and the production of antibodies. It has been suggested that the Chinese treatment strategy of cooling and invigorating blood is effective in the treatment of allergic reaction disorders. The above case study of haematuria is not characterised by frequent, urgent and painful urination but accompanied by discomfort in the lesser abdomen. This mirrors *Shang Han Lun*'s definition of blood amassment, involving the intestines and urinary bladder. Clause 106 shows that "heat in the urinary bladder" actually refers to the lower jiao.

Di Dang Tang Pattern

Clause 124

太阳病六七日，表证仍在，脉微而沉，反不结胸，其人发狂者，以热在下焦，少腹当硬满，小便自利者，下血乃愈。所以然者，以太阳随经，瘀热在里故也，抵当汤主之。

Tai Yang disease for six or seven days, the exterior pattern is still present, the pulse is faint and submerged, but there is no chest bind, where the person is deranged, due to heat in the lower jiao, the lesser abdomen will have hard distension, where the urination is spontaneously free, the descent of blood will bring recovery. The reason for this being, having followed the Tai Yang channel, the stasis heat is in the interior, Di Dang Tang governs.

DI DANG TANG: Shui Zhi (dry-fried) 30 pieces; Meng Chong (wings and legs removed and dry-fried) 30 pieces; Tao Ren (skin and tips removed) 20 pieces; Da Huang (sprinkled with wine) 3 liang.

DIRECTIONS: Boil the ingredients in 5 sheng of water, reducing to 3 sheng. Strain and take 1 sheng warm. If there is no diarrhoea, another 1 sheng dose should be taken.

DISCUSSION: The aetiology of this disorder is similar to that described in Clause 106. Both disorders (Tao He Cheng Qi Tang and Di Dang Tang patterns) are the result of a Tai Yang exterior pathogen entering the interior by following the channel pathway, eventually knotting with blood to cause stasis. The faint and submerged pulse indicates that the pathogen is no longer in the exterior; the hard distension in the lower abdomen shows that this is a more serious condition than that described in Clause 106, and the patient may report that in addition to the distension, there is pain and spasm. The disorder is in the blood aspect and so differs from water amassment in that the heat is knotting with blood, not water. Normal and uninhibited urination shows that there is no water bind in the urinary bladder, and so it may be concluded that it is blood amassment. It is therefore said that the patient will recover after the passing of blood and Di Dang Tang is suitable because it moves blood and eliminates stasis. Shui Zhi and Meng Chong break blood and target the stasis; Tao Ren transforms stasis and Da Huang drains heat and eliminates stasis. The combined effect of these four herbs has a very strong effect in breaking and transforming the knotted blood, and eliminating it by leading it downwards.

Key points to bear in mind when using Di Dang Tang

- If stasis persists after one decoction, a second decoction can be given.
- This formula is not recommended for long term use and is generally contraindicated for invalid, elderly or pregnant patients. If prescribed, it must be done with extreme caution.

Modern Application of Di Dang Tang

- For chronic prostatitis due to kidney deficiency with symptoms of inhibited urination, a distending sensation in the lesser abdomen, lower back pain, tinnitus, insomnia, constipation or spermatorrhoea with a pulse which is submerged, fine and choppy, and a tongue which is pale with a thin coat: add Shan Yu Rou, Shan Yao, Sheng Shu Di, Dan Shen, Huang Qi, Chi Shao, Rou Gui.
- For chronic prostatitis due to accumulated heat in the bladder with symptoms of a scorching sensation in the urethra, yellow urination, hard distension in the lower abdomen, a parched throat, thirst, constipation, a pulse which is slippery and wiry or deep and strong, and a red tongue with a yellow, greasy coat: add Zhi Mu, Huang Bai, Qu Mai, Liu Yi San.
- For amenorrhoea due to excess heat and stasis, with pain in the lower abdomen, a yellow vaginal discharge, a rapid pulse and a yellow tongue coat: add Huang Bai, Bai Jiang Cao.

Clause 125

太阳病，身黄，脉沉结，少腹硬，小便不利者，为无血也。小便自利，其人如狂者，血证谛也，抵当汤主之。

Tai Yang disease, the body is yellow, the pulse deep and knotted, the lesser abdomen is hard, where urination is not free, it is not blood. The urination is spontaneously free, where the person seems deranged, it is certainly a blood pattern, Di Dang Tang governs.

DISCUSSION: Yellowing or jaundice is commonly attributed to damp accumulation, where urination is inhibited. Clause 125 differentiates yellowing due to damp from that due to blood stasis, on the basis of the urination, not being inhibited, but 'spontaneously free', which means it is free of its own accord and not because of some form of diuretic therapy. There are two pertinent issues. The first is the significance of the pulse image in diagnosing blood stasis: it is deep, indicating an interior disharmony, and knotted, which describes the intermittent beat generally caused by stagnant qi and blood. However, as shown by the first statement, a deep, knotted pulse does not always indicate blood amassment, but can indicate some other form of internal obstruction. The second issue is the yellowing or jaundice, which is not always due to damp accumulation, but can be ascribed to blood stasis in the interior impeding the distribution of ying qi. Apart from the important differentiation of urination being inhibited or not, yellowing due to blood retention and yellowing due to damp heat present differently. Yellowing due to blood retention is characterised by a dull, yellow complexion and mental disturbance. Yellowing due to damp heat is characterised by a bright yellow complexion and vexation. Simply stated, the key differential points for diagnosis of blood amassment are uninhibited urination and manic behaviour. The phrase "it is certainly a blood pattern" is confirmation that this is a pattern of blood amassment as opposed to damp accumulation, and the indicated formula is Di Dang Tang to purge stasis.

Di Dang Wan Pattern

> **Clause 126**
>
> 伤寒有热，少腹满，应小便不利，今反利者，为有血也，当下之，不可余药，宜抵当丸。
>
> Shang han with heat, lesser abdominal fullness, it should be that the urination is not free, where now on the contrary it is free, this is blood, it should be purged, one should not add herbs, Di Dang Wan is appropriate.

DI DANG WAN: Shui Zhi (dry-fried) 20 pieces; Meng Chong (wings and legs removed and dry-fried) 20 pieces; Tao Ren (skin and tips removed) 25 pieces; Da Huang 3 liang.

DIRECTIONS: Pound the ingredients into a powder and form into 4 pills. Boil 1 pill in 1 sheng (200 mL) of water, reducing to 7 ge (140 mL). After taking the pill, there should be blood in the stool within twenty-four hours. If there is no blood passed in the stool, another dose should be taken.

DISCUSSION: In Clause 126 the lesser abdomen refers simply to the lower abdomen, and heat with lesser abdominal fullness in a Tai Yang shang han pattern refers to an accumulation of water in the urinary bladder, where we expect urination to be inhibited. If, however, the urination is uninhibited, then it is not a pattern of water amassment but of blood amassment, and so the strategy is to break the blood and expel the stasis. The pattern described in Clause 126 is characterised by abdominal fullness rather than hardness, and is also marked by the absence of derangement or shen disturbance. This shows that the knotted heat and stasis is relatively milder than that of the Di Dang Tang pattern. The heat is less severe than the Tao He Cheng Qi Tang pattern and the stasis is comparatively milder than that in the Di Dang Tang pattern. For this reason, pills are prescribed because they are milder and therefore more appropriate. The ingredients are the same as Di Dang Tang but the dosage of Shui Zhi and Meng Chong is reduced by one-third and five extra pieces of Tao Ren are added, and thus the conversion of the formula to pill form is not just about the method of preparation, but the formula is actually reduced in potency. The statement "不可余药" can be translated as "no extra herbs" and has two interpretations: the preferred interpretation is that no other herbs should be added, however, some interpret it as meaning that the decoction should be drunk without leaving anything.

The differentiation between 'water amassment' and 'blood amassment' hangs on the symptom of urination and whether it is inhibited or not. In practice, however, one can not adhere absolutely to this principle and must use discretionary judgement. In *Wen Yi Lun* 温疫论 *(Discourse on Febrile Epidemic Disease)*, Wu You Ke mentioned that there were cases of blood amassment where inhibited urination was a feature, and it would seem that the location of the knotted blood and heat in the lower abdomen is significant in that regard. In some circumstances, blood amassment may affect normal urinary function, causing inhibited urination. Generally speaking, however, blood amassment in the lower abdomen, including the uterus and large intestine, will not be characterised by inhibited urination.

Modern Application of Di Dang Wan

- *Endometriosis.* Di Dang Wan with the addition of Chuan Lian Zi, Yan Hu Suo, Wu Ling Zhi, Qu Mai, Bian Xu 10g each.
- *Migraine headache.* Di Dang Wan with the addition of Chai Hu, Bai Shao, Dang Gui, Chuan Xiong, Bai Zhu, Gan Cao.

Summary of Tai Yang Blood Amassment Patterns

The cause of Tai Yang blood amassment is ascribed to pathogenic heat entering the interior via the Tai Yang channel, ultimately combining with blood in the lower jiao. Treatment strategies depend on the relative severity of the heat and the blood stasis. Tao He Cheng Qi Tang is indicated for a pattern where there is more heat than stasis; Di Dang Tang is indicated for a pattern where stasis is more severe than heat and where there is uninhibited urination, hardness and pain in the lower abdomen and mental derangement. Di Dang Wan is indicated for a milder condition characterised by lower abdominal fullness and a submerged and faint or submerged and knotted pulse. It must be noted that Tao He Cheng Qi Tang targets a newly manifested condition whilst Di Dang Wan is more appropriate for a chronic condition.

Section Five

2.5 TAI YANG DISEASE TRANSMISSION

Tai Yang disease can resolve without transmission or it can transmit to another channel, with the speed of transmission either fast or slow. The outcomes of Tai Yang disease depend on the relative balance of the patient's zheng qi and the strength of the pathogen. In order to identify transmitted disease, one must first thoroughly comprehend the basic signs and symptoms of untransmitted Tai Yang disease, with one of the chief criteria in identifying transmitted disease being the pulse, which is a key element in pattern differentiation. The original text states clearly that if there are no manifestations of Yang Ming or Shao Yang disease, then transmission has not taken place. The significance of identifying transmission is that it allows pre-emptive treatment such as needling the foot Yang Ming to prevent the complications of transmission. Unresolved Tai Yang disease not only has the potential to transmit to other channels, but may also change into a transmuted pattern. There may be complex presentations of both interior and exterior disease or an overlay of acute and chronic disease, with manifestations of both the root and the tip of the disease. This section guides the practitioner in choosing the sequence of treatment for these various presentations, by differentiating between true and false patterns of heat and cold, and setting criteria for the identification of a recovery pattern.

Clause 4

伤寒一日，太阳受之，脉若静者，为不传；颇欲吐，若躁烦，脉数急者，为传也。

Shang han for one day, Tai Yang is affected, where the pulse is calm, it means no transmission; there is an urge to vomit, if there is agitation and vexation, where the pulse is rapid and urgent, there is transmission.

Clause 5

伤寒二三日，阳明、少阳证不见者，为不传也。

Shang han for two or three days, there is no sign of a Yang Ming or Shao Yang pattern, there is no transmission.

DISCUSSION: The first target of an exterior pathogen is the Tai Yang channel and Tai Yang shang han (cold injury), which includes zhong feng (wind strike), represents newly contracted disease. These two clauses explain how to determine whether transmission to another channel has taken place.

In Clause 4, Zhong Jing proposes the pulse signs as a guide. This is because the pulse reflects subtle pathological changes and so can herald changes in the progress of disease. A calm pulse describes a pulse which is neither rapid nor urgent and is assumed to be unchanged, and to still be floating. From this we may deduce that the pathogen is still in the Tai Yang exterior and there is no transmission. A change in the pulse image to rapid or urgent, on the other hand, would indicate imminent transformation of the pathogen into interior heat. Nausea, here described as an urge to vomit, is generally associated with the transmission of the exterior pathogen into the Shao Yang channel. The symptoms of agitation and vexation reflect exuberant yang heat in the interior, a hallmark of the formation of interior heat in the Yang Ming. These symptoms, therefore, all indicate that the Tai Yang exterior pathogen is about to enter the interior.

Clause 5 explains that because the disease is in its initial stages, it is still in the Tai Yang channel and has not migrated to the Yang Ming or Shao Yang. Since these two channels are the next in line in the standard sequence of transmission, the determination of whether transmission has or has not taken place is made on the basis of the presence or absence of signs or symptoms associated with those channels.

Clause 4 highlights the pulse and symptoms of interior transmission; Clause 5 clarifies the channels involved, thus expanding the terms of reference for identifying transmission based on signs and symptoms. The pulse and symptoms described in Clauses 4 and 5 form the basis for both the treatment principle and herbal prescription. However, additional observation for subtle changes in the condition is essential to avoid inappropriate or wrong treatment.

Clause 8

太阳病，头痛至七日以上自愈者，以行其经尽故也。若欲作再经者，针足阳明，使经不传则愈。

Tai Yang disease, where there is headache for over seven days with spontaneous recovery, it is because the pathogen has passed through the channels. If it is about to transmit to another channel, needling foot Yang Ming will cause it not to transmit and there will be recovery.

DISCUSSION: In Tai Yang disease characterised by headache, it is assumed that there is also aversion to cold, and fever. The reason they are not mentioned in this clause is simply to avoid repeating what is said in Clause 7. Stiffness and pain in the neck are key symptoms of Tai Yang disease and varying severity can reflect the waxing and waning of the condition. If there is no sign of transmission after seven days of Tai Yang disease, it is possible that the body's defence mechanism is strong enough to expel the pathogen and recovery will be spontaneous. However, after approximately seven days, if there is no sign of recovery, one must suspect that the penetration of the pathogen into the interior is imminent. The objective of needling the Yang Ming channel is to stimulate and strengthen the zheng qi in order to prevent further penetration of the pathogen. Needling the foot Yang Ming is generally accepted as referring to the acupuncture point Zu San Li (St 36), which augments qi and blood and strengthens the zheng qi. Supplementary needling of Fu Yang (UB 59) can be used to expel the pathogen from the Tai Yang and enhance the overall effect.

Clause 10

风家，表解而不了了者，十二日愈。

Patients suffering from wind, where the exterior is resolved but not thoroughly, will recover in twelve days.

DISCUSSION: Clause 10 describes the situation of spontaneous recovery without the use of medication. The point being made is that although medicine can hasten recovery, the body's self-regulatory immune mechanism also plays a role. In regard to this issue, there are three points to keep in mind: first, that externally contracted disease is generally self-limiting; second, that in treating illness, particularly an exterior wind pattern, one should be mindful not just of expelling the pathogen, but also of supporting the zheng qi; and third, the approach of supporting the zheng qi with dietary therapy in order to promote spontaneous recovery without using medicinal treatment.

Section Six

2.6 TREATMENT OF TAI YANG TRANSMUTED PATTERNS

A transmuted pattern represents deterioration in the condition, where there have been changes or transmutations in the nature of the pathogen and the channels and organs affected. It is most commonly a result of adverse treatment or no treatment at all.

Clause 16A

太阳病三日，已发汗，若吐、若下、若温针，仍不解者，此为坏病，桂枝不中与之也。观其脉证，知犯何逆，随证治之。

Tai Yang disease for three days, sweating has already been promoted, if there is vomiting, if there is purging, if there is warm needling, and there is still no resolution, this is transmuted disease, Gui Zhi is not appropriate. Observe the pulse and signs, know the error committed, treat according to the pattern.

DISCUSSION: This clause draws attention to the fact that Tai Yang disease should resolve within three days of appropriate diaphoretic treatment in its initial stage. The implication of the persistence of Tai Yang disease following the promotion of sweat is that inappropriate remedies were used, specifically, inducing vomiting, using purgatives, and the excessive application of warm needling to promote sweat. It should be noted here, though, that the primary objective of warm needling is to warm the channels and disperse cold; it was the fire needle (烧针) which was used to promote sweat. Therefore, although Zhang Zhong Jing used the term 'warm needle', it is possible that the intended reference was 'fire needle'.

The inappropriate use of emetic, purgative or diaphoretic therapies constitutes adverse treatment because any of these has the potential to cause the condition to deteriorate into what is known as huai bing or a transmuted pattern. The inference of these terms is that they represent adverse changes in the disease pattern, and are virtually always the result of inappropriate or incorrect treatment. From the fact that sweating has not brought resolution, it is inferred that adverse treatment has been employed and a transmuted pattern has arisen. It can therefore no longer be treated as Tai Yang disease, and Gui Zhi Tang should therefore not be used. The final statement in the clause is a direction to the practitioner to understand where they went wrong, then to observe the pulse and the symptoms carefully in order to treat the pattern correctly. There are two implications in this statement: one is to follow this advice in order to avoid the same mistake in the future, and the other is to make sure of accurate diagnosis in order to treat the transmuted pattern correctly. Differential pattern diagnosis is the essence of Chinese medical diagnostic theory and without it, correct and appropriate treatment can not be given.

Order of Treatment for Exterior, Interior, Acute and Chronic Conditions

Clause 90

本发汗，而复下者，此为逆也；若先发汗，治不为逆。 本先下之 而反汗之，为逆；若先下之，治不为逆。

Where there should be sweating, but instead there is purgation, this is adverse; if sweating is promoted first, the treatment is not adverse. Where there should be purgation first, but instead there is sweating, it is adverse; if purging is used first, the treatment is not adverse.

DISCUSSION: In describing the prescribed treatment sequence for a concurrent exterior and interior pattern, the *Nei Jing* states: "If the condition starts in the exterior and goes to the interior, first treat the exterior and then the interior; if the condition starts in the interior and goes to the exterior, first treat the interior and then the exterior". Clause 90 describes the standard treatment principle for an exterior condition which has also affected the interior, where the exterior must first be resolved by sweating before clearing heat from the interior. Nevertheless, it must be emphasised that each individual case must be considered on the basis of the presenting signs and symptoms, and whether the condition is acute or chronic must also be taken into account.

Clause 94

太阳病未解，脉阴阳俱停，必先振栗，汗出而解；但阳脉微者，先汗出而解；但阴脉微者，下之而解。若欲下者，宜调胃承气汤。

Tai Yang disease is not resolved, the pulses at yin and yang both stop, first there will be shivering and sweat then resolution. Where the yang pulse alone is faint, first there will be sweat then resolution; where the yin pulse alone is faint, purging will bring resolution. If purging is desired, Tiao Wei Cheng Qi Tang is appropriate.

DISCUSSION: Where Tai Yang disease is unresolved, we expect to find the pulse floating in all positions. The reference to the pulses at yin and yang stopping refers to the pulses at the cubit and cun positions respectively, which are submerged and hidden. This is not due to an internal disharmony but to exterior pathogenic constraint in the Tai Yang, which has also affected the flow of qi and blood, resulting in a pulse which can no longer be palpated. Where zheng qi is severely constrained, it can result in a sudden and vigorous reaction against the pathogenic qi which manifests as shivers and sweating. Successful contention of the zheng qi against the pathogenic qi will manifest as fever; if sweat then ensues, the disease will be resolved. The faint yang pulse mentioned in the second sentence refers to a change in the cun pulse from hidden to palpable. Since the yang or cun pulse represents the exterior, it can be interpreted that it is an exterior pattern, where sweating is required to release the exterior and bring resolution. In this case, Gui Zhi Tang can be used. Conversely, the reference to a faint yin pulse refers to the pulse in the proximal position, which represents the interior. The change in the cubit or proximal pulse from hidden to faint reflects the change in the location of the disease from the exterior to the interior, causing interior constraint. Therefore, the correct treatment is to use Tiao Wei Cheng Qi Tang to resolve the interior pathogenic constraint by harmonising the interior and purging the constrained heat.

If there is shivering but no sweat, then the patient's zheng qi is weak, and the essential strategy is to support the zheng qi. This is generally achieved by alternating Gui Zhi Tang with herbs to support yin, yang, qi or blood. In this way, the source of sweat is fortified, the exterior can be released and recovery is hastened.

Shivering and sweating, often referred to as shivering sweat, is a symptom often mentioned in both shang han (cold injury) and wen bing (warm disease). It is encountered in the course of certain epidemic febrile diseases and whilst in many cases it will lead to resolution, it can in some cases cause deterioration. For this reason, it is important to observe the patient's pulse and symptoms. Where a shivering sweat is followed by abatement in the fever and a calm pulse, then the exterior has been resolved and recovery will take place. However, if a shivering sweat is followed by vexation and cold extremities due to the desertion of yang, it is a matter of urgency to rescue the devastated yang; a suitable formula is Shen Fu Long Mu Tang.

Clause 56

伤寒不大便六七日，头痛有热者，与承气汤。其小便清者，知不在里，仍在表也，当须发汗；若头痛者，必衄，宜桂枝汤。

Shang han with no stool for six or seven days, where there is headache and fever, give Cheng Qi Tang. If the urine is clear, we know it is not in the interior, it is still in the exterior, one must promote sweating; If there is headache, there will be nose bleed, Gui Zhi Tang is appropriate.

DISCUSSION: Shang han disease is a general term for externally contracted febrile disease. During the course of externally contracted disease with fever, if there is no bowel movement for six or seven days and there is also headache and fever, it is essential to determine whether it is in fact an exterior or an interior pattern in order to choose the correct treatment strategy. If the exterior pathogen transforms into interior heat affecting the Yang Ming, there will be constipation. In such a case, headache is a result of the interior heat flaring upwards. The presence of interior heat would be confirmed by scant, dark yellow urination, and the correct strategy would be to use Cheng Qi Tang to purge the interior excess heat. In the clinical situation where one encounters constipation associated with an exterior pattern which is incompletely resolved, Da Chai Hu Tang or a formula such as Chai Hu Jie Re Tang (Chai Hu, Huang Qin, Ban Xia, Zhi Gan Cao, Sheng Jiang, Da Zao, Niu Bang Zi, Lu Gen, Mao Gen) can be used.

However, if the urine is clear, there is no interior heat and this indicates it is a Tai Yang exterior pattern where the headache is a result of pathogenic constraint in the Tai Yang channel. The constipation in this case is due to exterior heat generated by the pathogenic constraint in the muscle layer, and the correct treatment is to release the exterior by promoting sweat. The headache is caused by pathogenic constraint in the channel generating heat, which harasses the yang network vessels; it can therefore be followed by a nosebleed. The appropriate formula is Gui Zhi Tang.

There is further differentiation in regard to the fever that presents in a Tai Yang exterior and a Yang Ming interior pattern: Yang Ming fever is described as steaming fever, whereas in a Tai Yang pattern, there will be a mild rise in temperature and the fever is described as a 'feather-warm fever'.

Case Study

Upper Respiratory Tract Infection

Extracted from Gu Jin Yi An An by Zhang Lu Yu

The patient had suffered from shang han disease with aversion to cold for three days and had then taken two doses of a diaphoretic formula. Three days later, he felt irritable and his pulse was hidden in all three positions. When he consulted Dr Zhang, his left cun pulse was slightly moving and he had a tendency to shiver and sweat. He was told not to take any medicinals but merely to use hot ginger water to facilitate the promotion of sweat. He recovered after coming out in a sweat.

Case Study

Lingering and Recurrent Head Colds

Source unknown

A 43-year-old woman had a tendency to catch cold easily and had been treated with several courses of antibiotics which had not been effective in fully eliminating the pathogen or preventing its recurrence. Recently she contracted a cold again and apart from an itchy and sore throat, she was fatigued and her appetite was poor. Her bowel movement and urination were normal, her tongue was pale red with a thin white tongue coat and her pulse was moderate and forceless.

She was precribed Xiao Chai Hu Tang modified (Chai Hu 10g; Huang Qin 10g; Dang Shen 15g; Ban Xia 10g; Ge Gen 15g; Fang Feng 10g; Su Ye 10g; Qian Hu 10g; Niu Bang Zi 10g; Sheng Jiang 3 pieces). After two packs, her cough was substantially relieved and there was little phlegm. The root of her tongue was greasy, her pulse was moderate and forceful. The same formula was repeated for a further seven packs.

Discussion: This case is due to pathogenic wind attacking the lung where the zheng qi is insufficient. The pathogenic cold constrained in the muscle layer results in impaired diffusion of lung qi and hence there is cough with little phlegm. Xiao Chai Hu Tang was used with the addition of herbs which diffuse the lung qi. Herbs such as Qian Hu, Su Ye, Fang Feng and Ge Gen are effective in diffusing lung qi and can be used to substitute Ma Huang.

Order of Treatment for the Root and Branch

Clause 91

伤寒,医下之，续得下利 清谷不止，身疼痛者，急当救里。后身疼痛，清便自调者，急当救表。救里宜四逆汤，救表宜桂枝汤。

Shang han, the treatment is purging, followed by diarrhoea, unremitting with undigested food particles, the body is aching, one must hasten to rescue the interior. Afterwards there is body pain, the watery stool has righted itself, one must hasten to rescue the exterior. Si Ni Tang is appropriate to rescue the interior, Gui Zhi Tang is appropriate to rescue the exterior.

DISCUSSION: The treatment of a shang han exterior pattern by purging is incorrect and will injure the yang qi. Because the exterior pattern has not been treated correctly, it remains unresolved and so there are aches and pains in the body. The damage to the yang qi causes impaired function of the spleen and stomach and results in a watery stool with undigested food particles, which is a manifestation of an interior Shao Yin pattern. In consequence, there is a concurrent exterior–interior pattern of Tai Yang and Shao Yin.

Tai Yang and Shao Yin stand in an exterior–interior relationship. From the pathological perspective, a Tai Yang pattern is associated with excess and represents the branch, whilst a Shao Yin pattern is associated with deficiency and represents the root. It is vital to establish whether a disorder is acute or chronic and to understand which pattern is the root and which the branch, in order to determine the treatment strategy. Watery diarrhoea with food particles reflects a severe deficiency of yang qi in the interior, indicating a Shao Yin pattern with exuberant interior cold; it is this deficiency pattern which is the root. The need to address the root deficiency pattern is urgent and must take priority over the exterior symptom of body aches and pains. If one disregards this and treats the exterior by promoting sweat, the yang qi of the Shao Yin will be further damaged. When the yang of the spleen and stomach is deficient, with a watery stool with undigested food particles, Si Ni Tang is the formula of choice to rescue the deficient yang. Once yang qi is restored and the function of spleen qi is returned, the stool will be normal. If body aches and pains persist after the interior has been treated, Gui Zhi Tang is needed to regulate ying and wei and expel the exterior pathogen. Although the yang qi has returned, it is still in a delicate state and Ma Huang Tang is contraindicated.

Clause 92

病发热头痛，脉反沉，若不差，身体疼痛，当救其里。四逆汤。

The disease has fever and headache, the pulse is submerged, if there is no recovery and there are body aches and pains, one must treat the interior. Si Ni Tang.

DISCUSSION: Fever and headache are generally indicative of a Tai Yang exterior pattern, where there should be a floating pulse. If the pulse is submerged, an interior pattern must be suspected. In Clause 92, the fever and headache are manifestations of the exterior Tai Yang pattern but in this case, the body pain represents an interior disharmony. This is a concurrent pattern of Tai Yang and Shao Yin, and the strategy is to expel the pathogen from the exterior and simultaneously warm the interior. Formulas which fulfil this requirement are Ma Huang Fu Zi Xi Xin Tang and Ma Huang Fu Zi Gan Cao Tang. If, however, despite taking such a formula, the condition persists, it demonstrates that there is a severe deficiency of yang qi in the Shao Yin. Priority is therefore given to warming the yang and preserving the zheng qi, and so Si Ni Tang is indicated to warm the interior in order to preserve the zheng qi, as was described in Clause 91. This clause cites only a submerged pulse as the indication for prescribing Si Ni Tang; naturally the symptom of diarrhoea with undigested food particles must also be present, but it is taken as read because it was described in the previous clause.

Clause 372

下利腹胀满，身体疼痛者，先温其里，乃攻其表；温里宜四逆汤，攻表宜桂枝汤。

Diarrhoea and abdominal fullness, where the body is aching, first warm the interior, then attack the exterior, Si Ni Tang is appropriate to warm the interior, Gui Zhi Tang to attack the exterior.

DISCUSSION: Where diarrhoea is accompanied by abdominal fullness, it is attributed to spleen and kidney yang deficiency with stagnation of the yang qi of the middle jiao and accumulation of cold. The body pain is a reflection of exterior constraint caused by the invasion of wind cold. Clause 372 therefore describes a dual interior and exterior pattern, with exterior constraint and deficiency cold in the middle jiao. In this case, the interior is warmed first before releasing the exterior. The rationale is that the interior condition is chronic, and the exterior pattern is one of exterior deficiency. Therefore, by warming the interior and strengthening the yang qi, the zheng qi will be assisted in its endeavour to expel the pathogen and will not increase the severity of the exterior constraint. Following the use of Si Ni Tang to support the interior yang, Gui Zhi Tang can be used to assist the zheng qi to expel the pathogen from the exterior.

Clauses 91, 92 and 372 describe dual patterns of the exterior and interior, and the correct sequence of treatment for the root and the branch. This is based on the principle of treating the branch in acute conditions and treating the root if the condition is moderate or chronic. This has great clinical significance.

Treatment Principles for Sweating and Purging

Clause 93 discusses the situation of spontaneous recovery following sweating.

Clause 93

太阳病，先下而不愈，因复发汗，以此表里俱虚，其人因致冒。冒家汗出自愈。所以然者，汗出表和故也。里未和，然后复下者。

Tai Yang disease, first there is purging but there is no recovery, and so sweating is then promoted, because of this both exterior and interior are deficient, the person will then feel dizzy. Patients who feel dizzy will sweat and recover spontaneously. The reason for this being, sweating harmonises the exterior. Where the interior is not harmonised, one should purge later.

DISCUSSION: The standard treatment for Tai Yang disease is sweat promotion. Purgation fails to resolve the exterior pathogen and, in addition, it damages the interior. Furthermore, to purge first before promoting sweat runs counter to the standard sequence. This is because when there is interior deficiency, in this case caused by earlier purgation, sweating can damage the exterior. The subsequent injury to wei, qi, ying and blood then gives rise to a pattern of deficiency in both the exterior and the interior. The fainting sensation is a consequence of incorrect purgation, causing the pathogen to be constrained in the interior and obstructing the ascent of clear yang. This is a pattern of deficient zheng qi with pathogenic constraint in the exterior. When a person who feels faint recovers spontaneously after sweating, it shows that the zheng qi was not seriously depleted, allowing sweating to bring about recovery. The final statement, that in cases of interior disharmony purging can be used later, refers to the situation where there is constipation and steaming fever typical of a Yang Ming pattern where, of course, purgation would be an indicated strategy and Tiao Wei Cheng Qi Tang would be an appropriate formula.

Patterns of True and False Heat and Cold

Clause 11

病人身大热，反欲得衣者，热在皮肤，寒在骨髓也；身大寒，反不欲近衣者，寒在皮肤，热在骨髓也。

Where the patient's body has great heat, nevertheless he wants more clothing, the heat is in the skin, the cold is in the bone marrow; where the body has great cold, nevertheless he does not want more clothing, the cold is in the skin, the heat is in the bone marrow.

DISCUSSION: Fever and aversion to cold are commonly encountered symptoms of externally contracted disease, and the identification of simple patterns of heat or cold are straightforward. This clause describes and differentiates patterns of false heat with true cold, and those of false cold with true heat, where the false manifestations are misleading and so a conscientious approach to diagnosis is required.

The first statement describes a patient who, despite exhibiting signs of heat, feels cold and wants to wear warm clothing. This is an indication of false heat presenting in the face of true cold and is a reflection of exuberant yin cold deep in the interior, which has displaced the deficient yang and pushed it outwards to the surface of the body. Zhang Zhong Jing explains that this is heat in the skin, which is the exterior, with cold in the bone marrow, which represents the deepest level of the interior. This pattern of true cold with a false manifestation of heat is referred to as 'exuberant yin repelling yang' and it is associated with Shao Yin cold conversion patterns.

The second statement describes the converse situation where a patient presents with severe cold signs but nonetheless refuses clothing. The cold is said to be in the skin, and the heat in the marrow. It is the cold symptoms in the superficial layer which are false, whilst the unwillingness to wear warm clothing reflects the true nature of the condition, which is pathogenic heat in the interior. This pattern is also encountered when deep-seated pathogenic heat obstructs the normal distribution of yang qi, resulting in what is termed desertion cold, manifesting as cold in the extremities due to the non-distribution of yang qi. This phenomenon is referred to as 'severe heat with severe reversal' (热深厥深), which derives from the fact that the deeper in the body the heat pathogen lies, the more pronounced is the desertion cold of the extremities.

In patterns of false heat and false cold, the true signs manifest in the tongue and pulse, and other signs and symptoms are a mixture of true and false.

- *In true cold with false heat*, the tongue is pale with a slippery, wet coat; the pulse is slow and submerged or faint and thready, bordering on expiry. Other true manifestations of cold are fatigue and somnolence, little or no thirst, a preference for warm drinks, a desire to wear warm clothes, clear copious urination, a stool which can be either watery or normal, cold extremities and cold in the chest and abdomen. The false symptoms are a malar flush, occasional irritability, shallow rapid breathing, and skin which is hot to touch.
- *In a true heat pattern with false cold signs*, the tongue is red or crimson with prickles and a dry, yellow or black tongue coat; the pulse is submerged and forceful or flooding, slippery and rapid. Other true signs are a thirst for cold drinks, a refusal to wear warm clothing, delirious speech, clouded spirit, dark urine, harsh, rapid breathing and a stool which is either dry or is loose and foul. The false sign is skin which is cold to touch.

Treatment for true cold with false heat is based on restoring the yang with such formulas as Si Ni Tang or Tong Mai Si Ni Tang. Treatment for true heat with false cold relies on formulas such as Bai Hu Tang or Cheng Qi Tang.

Spontaneous Recovery

Clause 58

凡病，若发汗、若吐、若下、若亡血、亡津液，阴阳自和者，必自愈。

In any illness, where sweating is promoted, where there is vomiting, where there is purging, where there is devastation of blood or devastation of fluid, if yin and yang harmonise spontaneously, there will be spontaneous recovery.

DISCUSSION: If sweating, vomiting or purging are used to eliminate a pathogen in circumstances where they are appropriate, there will be no damage to the zheng qi. However, the incorrect application of any of these measures has the potential to injure blood, body fluids and zheng qi. Clause 58 describes such an adverse situation. The reasoning behind the possibility of spontaneous harmonisation of yin and yang which then proceeds to recovery is that, if the pathogen is expelled with only mild damage to blood and fluids and with no serious damage to zheng qi, the patient will recover thanks to the body's natural ability to harmonise yin and yang, and the administration of herbs is not needed. What this tells the reader is that following therapy, the disease must still sometimes run its course before the zheng qi can play its part in the recovery process.

The *Huang Di Nei Jing* proposes the idea that health represents a state where the yin and yang of the body are in equilibrium: "If the yin and yang of man is kept in equilibrium, his body will be strong and his spirit sound; conversely, if the yin and yang fail to communicate, then his vital energy will be in decline and eventually exhausted." This is a clear illustration of the ancient concept of illness being the result of an imbalance of yin and yang. Consequently, the objective of treatment was to restore the balance of yin and yang in order to affect recovery. The espousal of this theory in *Shang Han Lun* is demonstrated in forty-two clauses, where it has a broad range of clinical applications.

There are two methods of restoring the balance of yin and yang for the purpose of aiding recovery. The first is to use herbs to augment qi and generate fluid; the second is to support the body's self-regulatory mechanisms without the use of herbs, for instance, by means of dietary therapy, the ingestion of water or bed rest. The method chosen depends on the nature and severity of the disease and the state of the patient's underlying constitution. If, for instance, there has been significant damage to qi and body fluids, then the use of formulas such as Sheng Mai Yin or Zeng Ye Tang may be employed to augment qi and generate fluids. If, on the other hand, damage to the zheng qi is minimal, as evidenced by a normal stool and normal urination, dietary therapy can be considered.

Clause 59

大下之后，复发汗，小便不利者，亡津液故也。勿治之，得小便利，必自愈。

After potent purging, sweating is then promoted, where the urination is not free, it is because body fluids are devastated. Do not treat, once the urination is free, there will be spontaneous recovery.

DISCUSSION: Both Clause 59 and the previous clause emphasise the natural power of the body to recover. Here, an exterior pattern has been given adverse purgative treatment, which is then followed by the promotion of sweat. The clause specifically ascribes the subsequent inhibited urination to the fluid damage caused by the purgation and sweating. It is not a pattern of water accumulation and to treat it as such would be a serious error, because the administration of herbs which promote urination and drain damp would further deplete fluids. For this reason, there is an exhortation not to treat it. This, however, does not imply that other patterns of inhibited urination should be left untreated. The message is simply that, in the absence of other manifestations, the symptom of inhibited urination is transitory, and that urination will return to normal once the body has had an opportunity to replenish fluids by the normal physiological processes. Patients who are dehydrated by severe sweating, vomiting or diarrhoea, will commonly experience reduced urinary output and the consumption of water is required to replenish depleted fluids and also assist in harmonising the stomach qi.

Section Seven

2.7 TRANSMUTED PATTERNS OF TAI YANG

Transmuted patterns of the Tai Yang channel are numerous and varied but fall into two main categories: patterns of excess heat and patterns of deficiency. They are most often the result of incorrect purging or sweating, and the inappropriate use of fire therapy, such as a hot needle or hot compress, tends to produce a transmuted pattern with more serious manifestations. Ben tun or running piglet is a feature of some transmuted Tai Yang patterns.

There are three transmuted patterns associated with heat, each of which is caused by the incorrect use of sweat promotion or purging in a Tai Yang exterior pattern, resulting in the exterior pathogen falling inwards. The pathogen then transforms into heat, harassing the interior. Transmuted patterns are differentiated according to the location of the pathogenic heat and the organs affected:

- Heat constraint in the chest and diaphragm characterised by vexation where the indicated formula is Zhi Zi Chi Tang.
- Heat congestion in the lung characterised by wheezing, sweating and cough where the indicated formula is Ma Xing Shi Gan Tang.
- Heat affecting the intestines in the Yang Ming characterised by fever and diarrhoea where the indicated formula is Ge Gen Qin Lian Tang.

2.7.1 Heat Constraint in the Chest and Diaphragm

Zhi Zi Chi Tang Pattern

Clause 76

发汗吐下后，虚烦不得眠，若剧者，必反覆颠倒，心中懊侬，栀子豉汤主之；若少气者，栀子甘草豉汤主之；若呕者，栀子生姜豉汤主之。

After sweating, vomiting or purging, there is insubstantial vexation and an inability to sleep, if it is severe, there will be tossing and turning, anguish in the heart, Zhi Zi Chi Tang governs; if there is shortness of breath, Zhi Zi Gan Cao Chi Tang governs; if there is retching, Zhi Zi Sheng Jiang Chi Tang governs.

ZHI ZI CHI TANG: Zhi Zi 14 pieces (broken); Xiang Chi (fermented soybean) 4 ge (wrapped in gauze).

DIRECTIONS: First boil the Zhi Zi in 4 sheng of water, reducing to 2½ sheng. Add Xiang Chi and boil till reduced to 1½ sheng. Strain and divide into two doses. Take the first dose warm and if there is vomiting, do not take the second dose.

ZHI ZI GAN CAO CHI TANG: Zhi Zi 14 pieces (broken); Zhi Gan Cao 2 liang; Xiang Chi 4 ge (wrapped in gauze).

DIRECTIONS: First boil the Zhi Zi and Gan Cao in 4 sheng of water, reducing to 2½ sheng. Add Xiang Chi and boil till reduced to 1½ sheng. Strain and divide into two doses. Take the first dose warm and if there is vomiting, do not take the second dose.

ZHI ZI SHENG JIANG CHI TANG: Zhi Zi 14 pieces (broken); Sheng Jiang 5 liang; Xiang Chi 4 ge (wrapped in gauze).

DIRECTIONS: First boil Zhi Zi and Sheng Jiang in 4 sheng of water, reducing to 2½ sheng. Add Xiang Chi and boil till reduced to 1½ sheng. Strain and divide into two doses. Take the first dose warm and if there is vomiting, do not take the second dose.

DISCUSSION: After the promotion of sweating and purging, the exterior pathogen enters the interior, harassing the chest and causing vexation. Vexation can arise from heat which is said to have formed because it has knotted with a substance such as phlegm, water or food. However, in this case, the vexation is a result of heat which has not bound with a substance and is deemed to be formless or intangible; it is therefore described as xu fan (虚烦) or insubstantial vexation.

The manifestation of heat harassing the chest varies depending on its severity, as does the corresponding treatment. Clause 76 describes a milder case of insubstantial vexation causing insomnia, and also a more serious case where there is such disquietude of the spirit that there is a sense of wretchedness, with fretting and anguish accompanied by restless tossing and turning. The degree of vexation of the spirit is described by Liu He Jian in his book *Shang Han Zhi Ge Zhong* as being like "an elephant's restlessness after ingesting Ba Dou or Cao Wu Tou". Because the vexation is caused by heat, Zhi Zi Chi Tang is chosen to clear the constrained heat and vent it outward, thus eliminating vexation.

Zhi Zi is bitter and cold and enters the heart. It can clear and diffuse the constrained heat and at the same time lead the pathogenic fire downward. Xiang Chi has a mild and light flavour. It can release the exterior, vent pathogenic heat outward and harmonise the stomach qi. The combination of Zhi Zi and Xiang Chi effectively clears and diffuses the pathogenic heat and is highly suitable for the treatment of insubstantial vexation. If there is shortness of breath, Zhi Gan Cao is added to augment qi and harmonise the middle. If there is vomiting, Sheng Jiang is added to descend the rebellious stomach qi and stop the vomiting.

The pathogenesis of Zhi Zi Chi Tang is heat constrained in the chest and diaphragm or the stomach. The key symptoms are insubstantial vexation, insomnia and a red tongue body with a pale yellow tongue coat. This pattern is distinct from a Cheng Qi Tang pattern in Yang Ming, where irritability is accompanied by stomach repletion, and also from a Bai Hu Tang pattern where vigorous fever accompanies irritability.

Clause 77

发汗，若下者，而烦热，胸中窒者，栀子豉汤主之。

After sweating, if there is purging, and vexation and fever, a stifled sensation in the chest, Zhi Zi Chi Tang governs.

Clause 78

伤寒五六日，大下之后，身热不去，心中结痛者，未欲解也，栀子豉汤主之。

Shang han for five or six days, after potent purging, the fever does not abate, if there is a knotted pain in the heart, there is no imminent resolution, Zhi Zi Chi Tang governs.

DISCUSSION: Clauses 77 and 78 describe additional manifestations of the Zhi Zi Chi Tang pattern. In Clause 77, following sweating and purging, pathogenic heat is knotted in the chest causing vexation, fever and oppression in the chest. The chest belongs to upper jiao where the heart and lungs reside. The heart governs blood and the lungs govern qi. Pathogenic heat is constrained in the chest where it can remain at the qi level or it can enter the blood aspect. Vexation with fever is a reflection of the constrained pathogenic heat, and the oppressed sensation is evidence that this constrained heat has affected the qi dynamic of the chest. Clause 78 goes on to describe how this may even affect the flow of blood, causing a knotted pain in the heart. This tells us that the condition is far more serious than a simple heat pattern, as the flow of qi and blood has been affected. The aetiology of this pattern is constrained heat and the treatment is Zhi Zi Chi Tang. The constrained heat harasses the chest and manifests with the symptoms of vexation with fever, anguish in the heart, oppression in the chest and knotted pain due to the heat constraint in the chest, all of which form the Zhi Zi Chi Tang pattern. Further differentiation can be made according to severity.

Ancient Application of Zhi Zi Chi Tang

- *Xiao Er Yao Zheng Zhi Jue:* For the treatment of fever with mania or a clouded spirit.
- *Lin Zheng Zhi Nan Yi An:* There are 73 case studies recorded using Zhi Zi Chi Tang for the treatment of upper, middle and lower jiao constrained heat in the qi aspect or for the diffusion of constrained heat in the triple jiao.
- For the treatment of wind warmth harassing the lung, Zhi Zi Chi Tang is modified with

the addition of Jie Geng, Sang Ye, Xing Ren, Yu Jin and Gua Lou Pi.

- For the treatment of autumn dryness with cough, Zhi Zi Chi Tang is used with the addition of Sang Ye, Gua Lou Pi and Yu Jin.
- For the treatment of liver fire harassing the stomach, Zhi Zi Chi Tang is used with Huang Lian, Yu Jin, Sheng Jiang and Ban Xia.
- For the treatment of vertigo due to phlegm fire, Zhi Zi Chi Tang is used with Ling Yang Jiao, Lian Qiao and Ban Xia.
- For the treatment of jaundice, Zhi Zi Chi Tang is used with Lian Qiao, Chi Xiao Dou, Tong Cao and Tian Hua Fen.
- For treatment of constipation due to damp obstruction, Zhi Zi Chi Tang is used with Gua Lou Pi, Zhi Qiao, Pi Pa Ye and Kou Ren.

Modern Application of Zhi Zi Chi Tang

- For the early onset of externally contracted disease, add Chai Hu, Huang Qin, Lu Gen, Mao Gen to release the exterior and clear the heat.
- For stomach ache due to constrained heat manifesting as stomach pain, a parched throat, constipation and a red tongue with a yellow tongue coat, combine Zhi Zi Chi Tang with Xiao Xian Xiong Tang (Ban Xia, Huang Lian, Gua Lou). This may fit the diagnosis of acute or chronic gastritis, or peptic or duodenal ulcers.
- For the treatment of insubstantial vexation manifesting with an oppressed sensation or distension in the chest, irritability, insomnia, a parched throat and mouth, a pulse which is rapid and fine and a tongue with a pale, yellow tongue coat, add Sheng Di, Bai He, Yuan Zhi and Mai Dong.
- For the treatment of constrained lung/stomach heat in a child manifesting with an ulcerated mouth, swollen gums, a dry bowel movement and a red tongue, combine Zhu Ye Shi Gao Tang and Zhi Zi Chi Tang.

Zhi Zi Chi Tang can be combined with Xie Xin Tang for the treatment of chronic gastritis, chronic cholecystitis or hepatitis, when characterised by complex heat and cold. Gua Lou, Xiang Fu and Bai Mei Hua can be added to relieve pain due to constrained qi. *He Bei Zhong Yi* (1985; (2):14) reported a clinical trial where Zhi Zi Chi Tang was used in the treatment of 106 cases of primary neurasthenia in accordance with the following differential patterns and formula modifications.

1. Hyperactive liver yang heat scorching the heart shen: Zhi Zi Chi Tang with the addition of Long Dan Cao, Sheng Di Huang.
2. Heart and spleen deficiency with insufficiency of qi and blood: Zhi Zi Chi Tang with the addition of Ren Shen, Fu Ling, Bai Zhu.
3. Heart and kidney not communicating with harassment of deficient fire: Zhi Zi Chi Tang with the addition of Sheng Di, He Shou Wu, Mu Dan Pi.

The results were: full recovery = 55 cases; effective = 33 cases; slight improvement = 15 cases; not effective = 3 cases.

NOTE: There are varying interpretations as to whether Zhi Zi Chi Tang can induce vomiting. Cheng Wu Ji and Ke Yun Bo regarded it as an emetic, however Chen Xiu Yuan and Zhang Yin An disagreed. The authors do not consider this formula to be an emetic, and where vomiting occurs after the administration of one dose, it can be ascribed to Zhi Zi Chi Tang effectively dispelling the heat which has formed a knot, causing a fixed pain in the chest. In practice, Zhi Zi Chi Tang can sometimes be seen to promote sweating and induce vomiting.

Case Study

Vexation

Extracted from Jiang Xi Yi Yao 1965; (2):663

A 30-year-old man presented with fever which he had had for three to four days, vexation, fullness of the chest, insomnia and thirst for cold drinks. This was mistaken to be an exterior pattern due to cold and the patient had been given an acrid, warm formula to release the exterior which was not effective. He sought a second consultation with another practitioner who diagnosed it as a constrained heat vexation pattern. Examination: his pulse was rapid and forceful and the tongue red with a thin, white, slippery tongue coat. He suffered from restlessness and vomiting, and his urine was scant and dark. Zhi Zi Chi Tang was prescribed: Zhi Zi 15g, Dan Dou Chi 18g. After two packs, his fever receded and the pulse was normal but his appetite was poor. He was prescribed two packs of Bu Zhong Yi Qi Tang to consolidate treatment.

Zhi Zi Hou Po Tang Pattern

Clause 79

伤寒下后，心烦腹满，卧起不安者，栀子厚朴汤主之。

Shang han after purging, there is heart vexation and abdominal fullness, restlessness lying and sitting, Zhi Zi Hou Po Tang governs.

ZHI ZI HOU PO TANG: Zhi Zi 14 pieces (broken); Hou Po (bark removed and fried) 4 liang; Zhi Shi (soaked in water and fried until yellow) 4 pieces.

DIRECTIONS: Boil the ingredients in 3½ sheng of water, reducing to 1½ sheng. Strain and divide into two doses, taking one dose warm. If vomiting occurs, the second dose should not be taken.

DISCUSSION: This formula is based on a combination of Zhi Zi Chi Tang and Xiao Cheng Qi Tang. Because the abdominal fullness is not due to repletion but to qi stagnation, a modification of Xiao Cheng Qi Tang is used. Zhi Zi clears heat from the interior and eliminates vexation. Xiang Chi (Dan Dou Chi) is omitted because the transformed heat is attacking the abdomen; this is because it is cool and acrid, releases the exterior, and does not address abdominal distension. Zhi Shi and Hou Po, from Xiao Cheng Qi Tang, address abdominal fullness. The combined effect of the three herbs is to clear heat, eliminate vexation and alleviate the abdominal fullness.

Where vexation and abdominal fullness are experienced following purging in shang han disease, it is essential to determine whether they are due to cold, heat, deficiency or excess. If, after purging, vexation persists with abdominal pain and distension, and there is an excess pulse and a yellow tongue coat, this is evidence that the excess pathogen has not yet been eliminated and purging can still be used. However, following purging, if the urination and the stool are normal, or if the stool is loose, there is a preference for warmth and pressure, the pulse is moderate and forceless and the tongue is pale with a white tongue coat, then it is a pattern of interior deficiency. This means that despite the symptoms of vexation and abdominal fullness, Li Zhong Tang should be prescribed to warm the interior.

Case Study

Vexation and Epigastric Distension

Extracted from Shang Han Qie Yao

A 37-year-old woman presented with vexation, anguish and a sense of fullness in the epigastrium. She was constipated, had dark urine, the tongue coat was yellow and greasy and her pulse was wiry and rapid. This was diagnosed as heat constrained in the heart and chest. One pack of Zhi Zi Hou Po Tang was prescribed: Zhi Zi 3 qian, Zhi Shi 3 qian, Hou Po 4 qian.

Zhi Zi Gan Jiang Tang Pattern

Clause 80

伤寒，医以丸药大下之，身热不去，微烦者，栀子干姜汤主之。

Shang han, it is treated with a great purging pill, if the fever does not abate, there is slight vexation, Zhi Zi Gan Jiang Tang governs.

ZHI ZI GAN JIANG TANG: Zhi Zi 14 pieces (broken); Gan Jiang 2 liang.

DIRECTIONS: Boil in 2 sheng of water, reducing to 1½ sheng. Strain, divide into two doses and take one warm. If there is vomiting, discontinue.

DISCUSSION: The signs described in Clause 80 are those of heat harassing the chest and diaphragm. However, the nominated formula shows that there is also cold in the middle. This has occurred as a result of the inappropriate administration of a strong purgative. The correct treatment for Tai Yang shang han is to release the exterior, not purge the interior. The purgation has caused the pathogen to fall inwards, damaging the spleen and stomach and resulting in deficiency cold in the middle jiao; the mild fever is attributed to constrained heat in the diaphragm. This is a complex condition of heat in the upper jiao with cold in the middle jiao. 'Slight vexation' refers to the milder condition of vexation described in Clause 76. The patterns described in Clause 77 (vexation and fever with an oppressed sensation in the chest) and Clause 79 (vexation and fever with abdominal fullness and restlessness both lying and sitting) are consistent with heat caused by incorrect purgation, and are not patterns of heat and cold complex. The vexation described in Clause 80 is associated with a complex pattern of heat in the upper jiao and cold in the middle jiao, and so Zhi Zi Chi Tang is modified with the addition of Gan Jiang to warm the interior. The cold in the middle jiao can be the result of severe purging or due to a pre-existing spleen yang deficiency.

Incorrect purging can damage the spleen yang, impairing transformation and transportation, resulting in diarrhoea. Zhi Zi Gan Jiang Tang simultaneously relieves the residual heat in the chest, warms the middle and stops diarrhoea. Zhi Zi is bitter and cold and clears heat from the upper jiao, thus alleviating vexation. Gan Jiang is acrid and hot and warms the middle jiao, dispersing cold and reviving the spleen yang.

In the Han dynasty there were two types of purging pills, one bitter and cold and the other acrid and hot. The pill referred to in Clause 80 is the bitter, cold type which drains heat and therefore damages the spleen yang and impairs its function of transformation and transportation. The pills of the hot acrid type are mentioned in Clauses 104 and 105 (discussed later in Chapter Four, Shao Yang). Ba Dou is the main ingredient and if used inappropriately excessive diarrhoea and delirious speech can result. From the above examples, it is evident that correct diagnosis is essential before a purgative is prescribed.

Ancient Application of Zhi Zi Gan Jiang Tang

- *Sheng Hui Fang:* Cited in the treatment of diarrhoea with pus and blood as was the associated formula, Gan Jiang San, which is Zhi Zi Gan Jiang Tang with the addition of Dou Chi and 7 stems of Xie Bai.

Modern Application of Zhi Zi Gan Jiang Tang

- Zhi Zi Gan Jiang Tang can be combined with Xie Xin Tang for the treatment of heat and cold complex manifesting as chronic gastritis, chronic cholecystitis or hepatitis. For qi stagnation characterised by epigastric fullness, add Gua Lou, Xiang Fu, Bai Mei Hua.

Zhi Zi Chi Tang Contraindications

Clause 81

凡用栀子汤，病人旧微溏者，不可与服之。

Whenever Zhi Zi Tang is used, if the patient has only a sloppy stool, one should not give this formula.

DISCUSSION: The reference to the formula Zhi Zi Tang in this clause is a reference to all Zhi Zi Chi Tang patterns and is inclusive of its modifications. The statement "whenever Zhi Zi Tang is used" means in situations where Zhi Zi Tang is normally indicated. The thrust of this clause is that even where it might otherwise be used, Zhi Zi Chi Tang is contraindicated for patients with a pre-existing pattern of spleen and kidney yang deficiency or yang deficiency of the spleen and stomach, as demonstrated by a sloppy stool.

Summary of Zhi Zi Chi Tang Pattern

A Zhi Zi Chi Tang pattern is attributed to pathogenic heat constrained in the chest and diaphragm, often referred to as 'heat harassing the chest and diaphragm'. There is no excess phlegm or water bind in the interior and the main symptom is vexation due to formless heat, known as 'insubstantial vexation' or 'xu fan'. The key signs and symptoms are: (1) vexation with an inability to sleep, tossing and turning and anguish in the heart; (2) vexation and fever with an oppressed sensation in the chest; and (3) fever with a knotted pain in the heart.

Zhi Zi Chi Tang both clears and vents pathogenic heat. If the person experiences shortness of breath caused by pathogenic heat damaging the middle qi, Gan Cao is added to augment qi and tonify the middle. If there is vomiting due to disharmony of stomach qi, Sheng Jiang is added to descend the counterflow and harmonise the stomach.

There are two sub-categories of the Zhi Zi Tang transmuted pattern otherwise known as heat harassing the chest and diaphragm. The first is a pattern of constrained heat in the chest affecting the stomach; this is characterised by vexation and abdominal distension and accompanied by restlessness both lying and sitting. For this pattern, Zhi Zi Hou Po Tang is indicated to clear heat, alleviate vexation, relax the middle and reduce fullness. The related transmuted pattern is one of heat in the upper jiao with cold in the middle jiao; it is characterised by unresolved fever, slight vexation, abdominal pain and fullness and a sloppy stool. For this pattern, Zhi Zi Gan Jiang Tang is indicated to clear heat from the chest and diaphragm and warm the middle. It must be remembered, however, that Zhi Zi Chi Tang and its modifications are contraindicated in spleen and kidney yang deficiency where there is a sloppy stool.

Modifications of Zhi Zi Chi Tang

- For severe oppression in the chest with a difficult bowel movement, add Yu Jin, Gua Lou Pi, Xing Ren.
- For treatment of wind warmth, add Sang Ye to release the exterior and diffuse lung qi; where there is a parched throat with phlegm, add Pi Pa Ye, Zhu Ru.
- For constipation, add Zi Wan, Xing Ren, Gua Lou Pi to descend the lung qi; where there is phlegm, add Ban Xia Qu, Zhu Ru.
- For the treatment of jaundice, omit Dou Chi and add Huang Bai, Gan Cao. This is called Zhi Zi Bai Pi Tang.
- For the treatment of alcoholic jaundice characterised by vexation, abdominal fullness and yang jaundice, add Da Huang, Zhi Shi. This is Zhi Zi Da Huang Tang (*Jin Gui Yao Lue*).
- For the treatment of vexation and insomnia, add Huang Qin, Gan Cao, Chai Hu, Wu Mei, Zhu Ye. This is Zhi Zi Wu Mei Tang (*Lei Zheng Huo Ren Shu*).

Case Study

Manic Phase in Bipolar Disorder

Extracted from Henan Zhong Yi 1986; 5:8–10

Following a dispute with his family in 1973, a 27-year-old male suffered an acute episode of mania. Episodes subsequently recurred and in 1976 he was diagnosed with bipolar disorder. Western medication gave him moderate relief but two months prior to the consultation, he had suffered from a severe episode with aggressive behaviour. He presented with a parched mouth, thirst, yellow urination, a dry stool, a red tongue with a dry yellow tongue coat and a slippery, rapid pulse. The diagnosis was hyperactive liver fire with phlegm obstructing the orifices and the treatment principle was to clear fire from the heart, scour phlegm, vent constrained heat, sedate liver yang and purge heat from the large intestine. A modification of Zhi Zi Chi Tang was prescribed: Dan Dou Chi 15g, Zhi Zi 10g, Zhi Shi 10g, Dan Nan Xing 9g, Yu Jin 15g, Zhen Zhu Mu 30g, Long Gu 30g, Ju Hong 15g, Da Huang 13g, Hou Po 10g, Dan Zhu Ye 3g, Sheng Gan Cao 20g. After three packs, he passed a foul, frothy stool, his tongue was red with a thin, yellow tongue coat and his pulse was wiry and rapid. The same formula was then repeated with the addition of 15g of Mai Men Dong for three more days. Following that, the pulse was moderate and the formula was modified as follows: Dan Dou Chi 15g, Zhi Zi 10g, Zhi Shi 10g, Shi Chang Pu 15g, Yu Jin 20g, Dan Nan Xing 9g, Chao Zao Ren 30g, Mai Men Dong 15g, Long Chi 30g, Dan Zhu Ye 5g, Sheng Gan Cao 10g (10 packs). There was no recurrence in the following year.

2.7.2 Heat Harassing the Lungs

Ma Huang Xing Ren Gan Cao Shi Gao Tang Pattern

Pathogenic heat can take advantage of the emptiness caused by a loss of fluids following inappropriate or excessive promotion of sweat or purgation in Tai Yang disease. If the yin fluids are depleted, the pathogen has the propensity to fall inwards, filling the void and consequently harassing the lungs. This section discusses a Tai Yang pattern where inappropriate or excessive promotion of sweat has caused the heat pathogen to fall inwards, resulting in heat congestion in the lungs.

Clause 63

发汗后，不可更行桂枝汤，汗出而喘，无大热者，可与麻黄杏仁甘草石膏汤。

After the promotion of sweat, one should not repeat Gui Zhi Tang, if there is sweating and wheezing, no severe fever, one may give Ma Huang Xing Ren Gan Cao Shi Gao Tang.

Clause 162

下后，不可更行桂枝汤，若汗出而喘，无大热者，可与麻黄杏仁甘草石膏汤。

After purgation, one should not repeat Gui Zhi Tang, if there is sweating and wheezing, no severe fever, one may give Ma Huang Xing Ren Gan Cao Shi Gao Tang.

MA HUANG XING REN GAN CAO SHI GAO TANG: Ma Huang (nodes removed) 4 liang; Xing Ren (skin and tips removed) 50 pieces; Zhi Gan Cao 2 liang; Shi Gao ½ jin (crushed and wrapped in gauze). Note the modern dosage: Ma Huang 12g, Xing Ren 9g, Zhi Gan Cao 6g, Sheng Shi Gao 24g.

DIRECTIONS: First boil Ma Huang in 7 sheng of water, reducing by 2 sheng. Then skim the decoction and add the remaining ingredients. Reduce to 2 sheng and take 1 sheng warm.

DISCUSSION: The words 'after promotion of sweat' in Clause 63 and 'after purgation' in Clause 162 refer to inappropriate or excessive promotion of sweat or purging in a Tai Yang pattern. The pathogenic heat subsequently generated then falls inwards causing heat congestion in the lungs. From the perspective of a differential diagnosis, even though there is wheezing, the presence of sweating shows that it is not a Ma Huang Tang pattern, which is characterised by wheezing with no sweat. Nevertheless, despite the absence of sweat, both these clauses stipulate that it is not a Gui Zhi Tang pattern. They also preclude the possibility of Yang Ming interior heat by saying there is no severe fever, which also indicates that there is no significant exterior heat. The clauses in fact describe a pattern of congestion of pathogenic heat in the lungs, and treatment must be based on the diffusion of lung qi and elimination of lung heat, and not on releasing the exterior by the promotion of sweat. Therefore Ma Huang Xing Ren Gan Cao Shi Gao Tang (also known as Ma Xing Shi Gan Tang) is indicated.

Ma Huang Xing Ren Gan Cao Shi Gao Tang is Ma Huang Tang with the omission of Gui Zhi and the addition of Shi Gao. Ma Huang is acrid and warm; it diffuses lung qi and calms wheezing. Shi Gao is sweet and cold and clears interior heat. The combination of Ma Huang and Shi Gao effectively clears the constrained lung heat, diffuses lung qi and calms wheezing. The dose of Shi Gao is double that of Ma Huang, and thus transforms the acrid, warm properties given to the original formula by Ma Huang into a formula which is acrid and cool. It also counters the diaphoretic function of Ma Huang. Xing Ren redirects lung qi downwards and when assisted by Ma Huang is able to further calm the wheeze. Gan Cao is sweet and neutral, and moderates the strong effects of Ma Huang and Shi Gao.

The use of Ma Huang in this formula designed to treat wheeze accompanied by sweating is explained by its combination with the other herbs. In Ma Huang Tang, the function of Ma Huang is to promote diaphoresis. However, if there is no sweat, it can be combined with Shi Gao to treat interior lung heat, where Ma Huang's function is to vent the heat. Shi Gao is very cold. It is used in the absence of exterior heat evidenced by an absence of high fever, and this use is exemplifed in the combination of Shi Gao and Zhi Mu in Bai Hu Tang, which clears heat from the qi level in a Yang Ming heat pattern.

Indications for Ma Huang Xing Ren Gan Cao Shi Gao Tang

The key indications for Ma Huang Xing Ren Gan Cao Shi Gao Tang are: cough, wheezing, rapid breathing, the absence of vigorous fever, thirst, yellow phlegm, a red tongue tip and margin with a pale yellow tongue coat, and a pulse which is rapid and may also be wiry or slippery.

1. Ratio for herbal ingredients:
   - The ratio of Ma Huang to Shi Gao is 1:2. The large dose of Shi Gao counters the acrid and warm properties of Ma Huang. In practice, the ratio can be anything from 1:5 to 1:10.
   - The ratio of Ma Huang to Gan Cao must be 1:1 because if the dosage of Gan Cao is more than Ma Huang, it will counter the diffusing function of Ma Huang and if less, the dispersing action of Ma Huang will not be moderated.
2. The wheezing associated with Ma Huang Xing Ren Gan Cao Shi Gao Tang must be clearly differentiated from that found in Ma Huang Tang, Xiao Qing Long Tang and Gui Zhi jia Hou Po Xing Zi Tang patterns. A Xiao Qing Long Tang pattern is a pattern of pathogenic wind cold constraining the exterior with phlegm fluids accumulating in the interior; it is characterised by fever, aversion to cold, dry retching, wheezing and a wiry and tight pulse. A Gui Zhi jia Hou Po Xing Zi Tang pattern represents a disharmony of ying and wei, where there is non-diffusion of lung qi; it is characterised by fever, aversion to wind, sweating, wheezing and a pulse which is floating and moderate. The wheezing associated with Ma Huang Tang is caused by an acute attack of pathogenic cold which constrains the defence yang and obstructs the dissemination of lung qi.

Ancient Application of Ma Huang Xing Ren Gan Cao Shi Gao Tang

- *Shou Shi Bao Yuan* records Ma Huang Xing Ren Gan Cao Shi Gao Tang combined with Er Chen Tang used in the treatment of lung heat congestion with phlegm.
- *You Ke Fa Hui* records the use of Wu Hu Tang (five tiger soup), which is Ma Xing Shi Gan Tang with the addition of tea leaves, in the treatment of pathogenic cold having entered Fei Shu (UB 13), which is the back shu point of the lungs, subsequently transforming into heat and obstructing the lung channel, resulting in wheezing, panting, rapid breathing and flaring nostrils.

Modern Application of Ma Huang Xing Ren Gan Cao Shi Gao Tang

With appropriate modifications, this formula can be used to treat such biomedical disorders as the common cold, epidemic influenza, bronchitis, broncho-pneumonia, pneumonia, asthma, whooping cough, measles and tonsillitis.

- *Lung heat and wheezing.* The paediatric department of Tian Jin Chinese Medicine Hospital treated 184 cases of infantile pneumonia using Ma Xing Shi Gan Tang with the addition of Zhi Qian Hu, Zhi Bai Shao, Jie Geng, Ban Xia, Zhe Bei Mu, and fresh Bai Mao Gen. There was full recovery in 168 cases.
- *Measles and pneumonia.* If the lung heat is severe, Ling Yang Jiao powder should be added. For exuberant phlegm heat with wheezing and rapid breathing, Dai Ge San and Pi Pa Ye should be added. For wheezing and constipation, Gua Lou Pi and Sang Bai Pi should be added. For a dry and difficult bowel movement, Da Huang should be added to drain the lung heat via the stool. For congested lung qi, Ting Li Zi is added to descend lung qi and purge lung heat.
- *Whooping cough.* Ye Ju Quan said: "Ma Xing Shi Gan Tang can be used to treat infantile whooping cough characterised by spasmodic cough, vomiting and haemoptysis, irrespective of whether there is fever or not. In all cases of haemoptysis, Ma Xing Shi Gan Tang is effective both in stopping the bleeding and in resolving the cough." *Gu Fang Lin Chuang Yin Yong* 古方临床运用 Ye Ju Quan, 20th century. In a clinical trial, 228 cases of infantile whooping cough characterised by spasmodic coughing, nausea and vomiting and coughing of blood, some with fever and some with no fever, were treated with Ma Huang Xing Ren

Gan Cao Shi Gao Tang with the addition of Bai Bu, Ting Li Zi, Da Zao and Yi Tang (malt sugar). There was full recovery in 195 cases, improvement in 25 cases and insignificant or no result in 8 cases (*Shang Han Lun Yu Lin Chuang*).

- *Acute bronchitis.* For a cough with yellow phlegm, a pale yellow tongue coat and a rapid pulse, the core formula is used with the addition of Sang Bai Pi, Bei Mu, Jie Geng and Jin Yin Hua to clear heat, transform phlegm and stop cough. For fever, Sang Ye, Lu Gen and Bai Mao Gen are added to clear heat and release the exterior pathogen.
- *Infantile broncho-pneumonia.* For coughing and wheezing, the core formula is used with the addition of Jin Yin Hua, Ting Li Zi, Jie Geng and Tian Zhu Huang to clear heat, relieve toxicity, transform phlegm and calm wheeze. For vigorous fever, Chai Hu, Huang Qin, Niu Bang Zi and Jin Yin Hua are added. For measles and pneumonia occurring together, Huang Qin, Qian Hu, Chan Yi and Zi Cao are added to clear heat and vent the pathogen.
- *Tonsillitis.* Tonsillitis is due to pathogenic heat knotted in the throat. Ma Huang Xing Ren Gan Cao Shi Gao Tang can be used with the addition of Ban Lan Gen, She Gan, Niu Bang Zi and Jie Geng.

Case Study

Infantile Pneumonia

Extracted from Hu Bei Zhong Yi Za Zhi 1997; 5:53

A young boy aged 3 years and 10 months had been coughing and wheezing for two days. His temperature was 39°C, and he had laboured breathing, flaring nostrils, central cyanosis, and a swollen throat. He had a rapid heart rate of 120 beats per minute and small to medium rales were heard on auscultation. The tongue was red with a yellow coat and the finger examination showed a purplish vein in qi guan or the qi gate. The Western diagnosis was pneumonia. The Chinese medicine diagnosis was wheezing due to phlegm heat obstructing the lungs.

The treatment principle was to clear lung heat, diffuse lung qi, transform phlegm and calm the wheeze. Ma Xing Shi Gan Tang was modified with Lian Qiao 10g, Jin Yin Hua 10g, Qian Hu 10g, Gua Lou Pi 10g, Zhi Qiao 10g, Ge Fen 15g. After one pack, the fever abated and after a further three packs, the cough and wheeze were virtually gone. He was given a further two packs to consolidate the treatment.

Note: When infants and young children contract an exterior pathogen, the wind cold pattern is generally of short duration because it easily transforms into heat. Where the wind heat pattern develops more serious symptoms, Ma Xing Shi Gan Tang, commonly used in the treatment of pneumonia, can be used with appropriate modifications. It must be remembered, however, that it is a potent formula which is acrid and cool and should be discontinued once the condition improves.

Case Study

Bronchial Pneumonia

Extracted from Xin Zhong Yi 1993; (10):56

A three-and-half-year-old boy had suffered from bronchial pneumonia since the age of 6 months and had been hospitalised six times for this condition. He presented with a temperature of 40.2°C, wheezing, coughing, rapid breathing and flaring nostrils. His appetite was poor, he had no thirst, and his bowel movement was difficult. His abdomen was soft on palpation and his urination was scant and dark. His lips were cyanosed and his tongue was red with a thick, white greasy tongue coat. The colour of the finger vein was purplish green. The diagnosis was wind heat constraining the lung and the treatment principle was to diffuse lung qi and calm the wheeze. The formula prescribed was a modification of Ma Xing Shi Gan Tang: Ma Huang 10g, Lian Qiao 10g, Xing Ren 10g, Chao Su Zi 10g, Fa Ban Xia 10g, Chen Pi 10g, Yu Xing Cao 15g, Sheng Shi Gao 30g, Huang Lian 6g, Zhi Gan Cao 6g. He was asked to take two packs per day. After two days, the fever receded, and on the third day, his wheezing subsided. He was then given one pack per day for the next seven days. He recovered. There was no recurrence in the following three months.

2.7.3 Heat in the Large Intestine

Ge Gen Qin Lian Tang Pattern

This is a Tai Yang exterior pattern where incorrect purging has caused the pathogenic heat to fall inward, manifesting as concurrent fever and diarrhoea. The diarrhoea is the result of purging, which has injured the qi of the intestines. In *Shang Han Lun* it is a concurrent pattern of Tai Yang and Yang Ming.

Clause 34

太阳病，桂枝证，医反下之，利遂不止，脉促者，表未解也；喘而汗出者，葛根黄芩黄连汤主之。

Tai Yang disease, Gui Zhi Tang pattern, but the physician has purged, there is incessant diarrhoea, if the pulse is skipping, the exterior is unresolved; if there is wheezing and sweating, Ge Gen Qin Lian Tang governs.

GE GEN QIN LIAN TANG: Ge Gen ½ jin; Zhi Gan Cao 2 liang; Huang Qin 3 liang; Huang Lian 3 liang.

DIRECTIONS: First boil the Ge Gen in 8 sheng of water, reduce by 2 sheng, then add the remaining ingredients and boil until reduced to 2 sheng. Strain and divide into two doses. Take warm twice a day.

DISCUSSION: Clause 34 describes a Gui Zhi Tang pattern in Tai Yang disease which has been incorrectly treated with purging, when the correct treatment is to release the exterior by promoting sweat. The inappropriate use of purgation has resulted in incessant diarrhoea, and it is an example of wrong treatment damaging the stomach and intestines. A skipping pulse represents extreme heat agitating qi, and here, is a reflection of the exuberant yang qi contending with pathogenic qi.

From the reference to the exterior not being resolved, we can infer that since the pathogen has in part lingered in the exterior, then it has not completely transferred to the interior. This therefore is a situation where there is unresolved exterior with concurrent interior heat or concurrent fever and diarrhoea. The lungs are harassed by both exterior and interior heat, which manifests as wheezing; the sweating is a manifestation of the interior heat steaming the body fluids, which percolate through the muscle layer; the diarrhoea is a result of the interior heat which has affected the intestines. The treatment strategy is to simultaneously release the exterior, clear interior heat and stop the diarrhoea. The indicated formula is Ge Gen Qin Lian Tang. Ge Gen is the chief herb because its acrid and cool properties are able to release heat from the muscle layer and treat diarrhoea by raising the clear yang of the stomach and intestines. Huang Qin and Huang Lian are bitter and cold and clear heat from the stomach and intestines to stop the diarrhoea, and Huang Qin also clears heat from the lungs. Gan Cao harmonises the stomach and moderates the actions of the other ingredients. The combined actions of the four herbs release exterior heat and simultaneously clear interior heat. For this reason, the formula is known as a dual exterior and interior heat clearing formula.

Key Points of Diagnosis

The principal diagnostic features are: fever, thirst, foul sticky diarrhoea, a burning anus, a yellow greasy tongue coat and a rapid pulse. The symptoms of wheezing and sweating described in Clause 34 do not have to be present. A Ge Gen Tang pattern is a concurrent Tai Yang and Yang Ming pattern with exterior excess; the determining symptom is absence of sweat. A Ge Gen Qin Lian Tang pattern, on the other hand, is an interior heat pattern and the key point of diagnosis is the presence of sweat. Simply expressed, Ge Gen Tang focuses on releasing the exterior whilst Ge Gen Qin Lian Tang focuses on clearing interior heat.

Ancient Application of Ge Gen Qin Lian Tang

- Ge Gen Qin Lian Tang with the addition of such herbs as Bai Tou Weng and Qin Pi was used in the treatment of *chang pi* (肠澼), a dysenteric disorder characterised by bloody diarrhoea.

- Ge Gen Qin Lian Tang with the addition of Bei Mu, Ju Hong and Pi Pa Ye was used in the treatment of *fei yong* (肺痈) or lung abscess, which in ancient times could include pneumonia.
- *Sha zhen* (痧疹) or sand papules is an externally contracted febrile disease characterised by papules in the skin which resemble sand. *Sha* is a rash in the surface of the skin which relates to the lungs, so the strategy is to use cool herbs to clear heat from the lungs. *Zhen* or papules are related to heat in the blood and are seen to emanate from the stomach because it belongs to Yang Ming and is the source of qi and blood. Therefore, the treatment is based on herbs which clear heat from both the stomach and the lungs; furthermore, in order to vent the rash, herbs which raise qi and release the exterior are needed. Ge Gen Qin Lian Tang can be used with the addition of Zhi Zi. Ge Gen Qin Lian Tang employs herbs which both ascend and descend qi: Ge Gen and Chai Hu raise qi and release the exterior; Huang Qin and Zhi Zi clear heat and descend qi to drain interior heat (*Shang Han Li Xin Zhu*).

Modern Application of Ge Gen Qin Lian Tang

- In acute colitis characterised by fever, thirst, foul diarrhoea, a burning anus, scant urination, a yellow and greasy tongue coat and a pulse which is slippery and rapid, Gen Ge Gen Qin Lian Tang can be used with the addition of Jin Yin Hua, Ma Chi Qian, Huang Qin and Shao Yao to clear heat and disinhibit dampness.
- For dysentery characterised by diarrhoea with blood and pus, tenesmus, fever, abdominal pain, a yellow tongue coat and a rapid pulse, Ge Gen Qin Lian Tang can be used with the addition of Bai Tou Weng, Qin Pi, Huang Bai, Huang Qin and Shao Yao to clear heat, relieve toxicity and stop diarrhoea.
- For infantile diarrhoea characterised by frequent sloppy bowel movements, dark yellow urine, a parched throat, a yellow tongue coat and a purplish finger vein, Ge Gen Qin Lian Tang can be used with the addition of Fu Ling, Bai Zhu and Yi Yi Ren to tonify the spleen and drain damp. If there is food stagnation, add Ji Nei Jin, Jiao Mai Ya, Jiao Shan Zha and Shen Qu to eliminate food accumulation.
- For chronic colitis characterised by the down-pouring of damp heat, Ge Gen Qin Lian Tang can be used with the addition of Jin Yin Hua, Fu Ling, Bai Shao, Yi Yi Ren, Qin Pi and Che Qian Zi to clear heat and drain damp.

Modifications

- If there is abdominal pain, add Bai Shao and Mu Xiang to ease the bowel spasms.
- If the diarrhoea is accompanied by vomiting, add Ban Xia, Chen Pi and Zhu Ru to harmonise the middle and descend stomach qi.
- If there is a disturbed or clouded spirit, combine with An Gong Niu Huang Wan to clear heat and relieve toxicity.

Summary of Ge Gen Qin Lian Tang Pattern

Ge Gen Qin Lian Tang is a dual exterior and interior releasing formula with its main focus being to clear interior heat and stop diarrhoea. For this reason, it is indicated for heat dysentery and all types of heat related diarrhoea, irrespective of the presence of exterior symptoms.

Case Study

Bacillary Dysentery

Extracted from Zhong Guo Ming Lao Zhong Yi Xue Shu Jing Yan Ji

Gui Zhou Ke Ji Publishing 1996

A 12-year-old girl had dysentery with a temperature of 39.5°C. She was delirious and was hospitalised. Two days after admission to hospital, she vomited a significant amount of blood and was diagnosed with bacterial dysentery. Apart from her elevated temperature, she had coarse, rapid breathing, delirious speech, frequent episodes of haemoptysis, a crimson tongue with a yellow coat, and a rapid pulse. The diagnosis was dysentery due to toxic heat. She was prescribed Ge Gen Qin Lian Tang modified: Ge Gen 12g, Huang Lian 6g, Zhi Zi 9g, Chi Shao 9g, Gou Teng 9g, Xi Jiao 5g, Sheng Di 24g, Dan Pi 9g, Bai Mao Gen 30g, Ce Bai Ye 30g. She took two packs per day and after the first dose, there was no more blood in the sputum and she was no longer delirious. The same formula was repeated for two packs, omitting Ge Gen and Gou Teng and with the dosage of Xi Jiao reduced to 2g, and taken with Yin Qiao Jie Du Pian. She recovered fully and was then given Ye Shi Yang Wei Fang modified to consolidate the treatment and prevent relapse.

2.7.4 Spleen Deficient and Cold

Gui Zhi Ren Shen Tang Pattern

This is a Tai Yang exterior pattern where excessive purging has injured the yang of the spleen and resulted in an interior deficiency pattern of the Tai Yin channel, while the exterior pathogen has not yet been cleared from the Tai Yang.

Clause 163

太阳病，外证未除，而数下之，遂协热而利，利下不止，心下痞硬，表里不解者，桂枝人参汤主之。

Tai Yang disease, the exterior pattern is not eliminated, and there has been multiple purging, pursuant to this a complex of fever and diarrhoea, the diarrhoea is incessant, there is hard glomus below the heart, if the exterior and interior are not resolved, Gui Zhi Ren Shen Tang governs.

GUI ZHI REN SHEN TANG: Gui Zhi (bark removed but not cut) 4 liang; Zhi Gan Cao 4 liang; Bai Zhu 3 liang; Ren Shen 3 liang; Gan Jiang 2 liang.

DIRECTIONS: All ingredients with the exception of Gui Zhi are first boiled in 9 sheng of water until reduced to 5 sheng. Gui Zhi is then added and the decoction is boiled until reduced to 3 sheng, then strained. A dose of 1 sheng is administered warm, once in the day and again at night.

DISCUSSION: A complex of fever and diarrhoea describes fever resulting from an unresolved exterior pattern and diarrhoea due to interior cold. There is reference in Clause 163 to repeated purging despite the presence of an unresolved exterior pathogen. It is adverse treatment which has resulted in a pattern of complex heat and diarrhoea, with the further manifestation of hard glomus in the area below the heart, which refers to the epigastric area. The inappropriate and excessive purgation has damaged the spleen yang, manifesting as diarrhoea, and the unresolved exterior manifests as fever, where, because there is an exterior pattern, there would also be aversion to cold.

The damage to yang qi has impaired the spleen's transformation function, and the failure to separate the clear from the turbid results in stagnation which obstructs the qi dynamic. The subsequent accumulation of turbid damp in the middle jiao manifests as 'hard glomus below the heart' or focal distension in the epigastrium. The failure of the spleen to raise clear yang is reflected in the incessant diarrhoea.

Gui Zhi Ren Shen Tang is Li Zhong Tang with the addition of Gui Zhi. Gan Jiang and Bai Zhu warm the middle to disperse the congealed cold and damp; Gui Zhi releases the exterior pathogen from Tai Yang; Ren Shen and Gan Cao tonify the middle and augment qi, thus assisting deficient spleen yang. The method of first decocting the four ingredients of Li Zhong Tang, which warm the middle and disperse cold, and adding Gui Zhi later, is to preserve the volatile oils of Gui Zhi, thus capturing its pungent and aromatic properties which could be lost by over-boiling. Gui Zhi's function of releasing the exterior is then uncompromised and the exterior pathogen is not constrained by Ren Shen and Gan Jiang.

The pathogenesis of a Gui Zhi Ren Shen Tang pattern is pathogenic wind cold in the exterior in the presence of pre-existing insufficiency of spleen yang. Thus there is cold in both the exterior and interior. Implicit in this pattern are the symptoms of fever and aversion to cold, hard glomus in the epigastrium, persistent diarrhoea, abdominal pain which is eased by warmth and pressure, cold hands and feet, a pale tongue with a white tongue coat, and a pulse that is floating and moderate.

Comparison of Ge Gen Qin Lian Tang and Gui Zhi Ren Shen Tang

The key feature of a Gui Zhi Ren Shen Tang pattern is a complex of fever and diarrhoea due to interior cold accompanied by focal distension in the epigastrium. Ge Gen Qin Lian Tang and Gui Zhi Ren Shen Tang patterns are both transmuted patterns caused by inappropriate purging, and both patterns represent unresolved exterior patterns where inappropriate purging has caused diarrhoea. However, they differ in several important aspects.

- The Ge Gen Qin Lian Tang pattern is a heat pattern characterised by both exterior and interior heat. It manifests with fever, wheezing and foul diarrhoea due to heat in the large intestine. The fever is significant due to the vigorous struggle between the exterior pathogenic heat and the internal defensive yang.
- The Gui Zhi Ren Shen Tang pattern, on the other hand, is a cold pattern characterised by both exterior and interior cold. It manifests with fever, aversion to cold, diarrhoea and focal epigastric distension, and is a result of more extreme purging which has damaged the spleen yang. There remains an unresolved pathogen in the exterior; the fever is milder and may be accompanied by chills.

Modern Application of Gui Zhi Ren Shen Tang

- For upper respiratory tract infections such as the common cold or epidemic influenza characterised by fever, aversion to wind and cold, headache, watery diarrhoea and a floating and weak pulse, Gui Zhi Ren Shen Tang can be used with the addition of Su Ye.
- For colitis characterised by diarrhoea, abdominal pain, aversion to cold, preference for warmth, cold extremities, a pulse that is submerged and weak, and a thin, white tongue coat, whether there are exterior symptoms or not, Gui Zhi Ren Shen Tang can be used with the addition of Fu Ling and Shan Yao to tonify the spleen and drain damp.
- For chronic gastritis characterised by epigastric distension and glomus below the heart, occasional stomach pain, aversion to cold, preference for warmth, a sloppy stool, a submerged, moderate and weak pulse and a thin, white tongue coat, Gui Zhi Ren Shen Tang can be used with the addition of Fu Ling, Yuan Hu and Xiang Fu to warm the middle, regulate qi and stop pain.

Case Study

Gastroenteritis

Extracted from Guo Yi Lun Tan 1997; (2):17

A 46-year-old female presented with an acute bout of gastroenteritis. Four days previously, after washing her hair, she took a nap in the afternoon before her hair was thoroughly dry. She woke with nausea and epigastirc discomfort and in the evening she suffered from diarrhoea. Other symptoms were fever, aversion to wind, a dry throat, preference for warm drinks, glomus below the heart which was eased by pressure, and a poor appetite. She had been given Huo Xiang Zheng Qi San but it was not effective. At the time of consultation, her complexion was pale and she spoke with a low-pitched voice. Her tongue was pale and swollen and her pulse was thready and weak. The treatment principle was to warm and tonify the spleen and release the exterior. A modifed version of Gui Zhi Ren Shen Tang was prescribed: Gui Zhi 10g, Tai Zi Shen 15g, Chao Bai Zhu 10g, Pao Jiang 10g, Zhi Gan Cao 10g, Huang Lian 3g. After four packs, the fever abated and her diarrhoea stopped. She was then given the same formula with a reduction in Pao Jiang to 5g for another four packs, after which she recovered.

2.7.5 Heart Yang Deficiency

There are four variations of a Tai Yang transmuted pattern where there is damage to the yang qi of the heart.

1. *Gui Zhi Gan Cao Tang* pattern is a Tai Yang pattern where excessive promotion of sweat has damaged the heart yang. Gui Zhi Gan Cao Tang is the core formula for the treatment of heart yang deficiency characterised by palpitations.
2. *Gui Zhi Gan Cao Long Gu Mu Li Tang* is the representative formula for vexation caused by depletion of heart yang by incorrect or

excessive use of hot needling. Because the heart yang is deficient, it is unable to contain the heart shen, which then floats upwards, manifesting as vexation.

3. *Gui Zhi Qu Shao Yao jia Shu Qi Long Gu Jiu Ni Tang* is indicated for a transmuted pattern of Tai Yang where fire therapy has damaged the heart yang causing restlessness and fright with a potential for yang desertion.
4. *Gui Zhi jia Gui Tang* pattern is where fire therapy has damaged the heart yang and cold qi rushes to the chest to fill the emptiness. This upsurge of qi is known as *ben tun* or running piglet. Fu Ling Gui Zhi Gan Cao Da Zao Tang pattern is an associated but milder pattern where ben tun does not manifest fully. This is demonstrated by the fact that there is no upsurge of qi, but just a tremor in the periumbilical region which heralds the manifestation of ben tun.

Gui Zhi Gan Cao Tang Pattern

Gui Zhi Gan Cao Tang pattern represents injury to the heart yang which is caused by excessive sweating and manifests with palpitations.

> **Clause 64**
>
> 发汗过多，其人叉手自冒心，心下悸，欲得按者，桂枝甘草汤主之。
>
> After promoting sweat excessively, if the person clasps their hands to their heart, there are palpitations below the heart, a desire for pressure, Gui Zhi Gan Cao Tang governs.

GUI ZHI GAN CAO TANG: Gui Zhi (bark removed) 4 liang; honey-fried Gan Cao 2 liang.

DIRECTIONS: Boil both ingredients together in 3 sheng of water, reducing to 1 sheng. Strain and drink in a single dose.

DISCUSSION: Sweat is the fluid of the heart and it is produced from the steaming of body fluids by yang qi. Excessive promotion of sweat can cause the yang qi to leak out with the sweat, depleting the heart yang, and resulting in palpitations and restlessness, which can be eased by the pressure of the hands on the chest.

Palpitations and restlessness due to heart yang deficiency are indications for Gui Zhi Gan Cao Tang. Gui Zhi is acrid and sweet to warm and unblock the channels. It enters the heart to assist and warm the heart yang. Gan Cao is sweet and warm. It augments heart qi and tonifies heart blood. The combination of these two herbs fulfils the principle of using acrid and sweet flavours to tonify qi and supplement yang, thus restoring the yang of the heart, enabling it to rule the vessels and regulate the pulse. When the heart functions normally, the pulse will be regular and there will be no palpitations.

The focus of this formula is restoration of yang. The pathogenesis is depletion of heart yang from excessive sweating. The heart yang deficiency is characterised by palpitations under the heart with restlessness and a sense of emptiness. The pulse is faint, moderate or intermittent and there is a white tongue coat. The patient may be of thin build and suffer from fatigue, shortness of breath and a sensation of oppression in the chest.

Gui Zhi and Gan Cao were commonly used by Zhong Jing to augment the heart yang in the treatment of heart yang deficiency. Other principal formulas for the treatment of heart disorders associated with heart yang deficiency are Gui Zhi Gan Cao Long Gu Mu Li Tang and Gui Zhi Qu Shao Yao jia Shu Qi Long Gu Mu Li Jiu Ni Tang, both of which are discussed below.

Ancient Application of Gui Zhi Gan Cao Tang

- *Qian Jin Yao Fang:* For the treatment of foul breath, using an equal dose of Gui Zhi and Gan Cao ground into a powder, a large pinch being taken with wine before retiring to bed.
- *Zheng Zhi Da Huan*: In the treatment of difficult child birth or missed abortion, it is recommended to take a decoction of a small bunch of Gui Zhi and 3 qian of Gan Cao.

Modern Application of Gui Zhi Gan Cao Tang

Gui Zhi Gan Cao Tang can be used to treat cardiac disorders characterised by palpitations due to a deficiency of qi, yin or yang, such as coronary heart disease or rheumatic heart disease. It can also be used in the treatment of cardio-pulmonary asthma or asthma where there is an intermittent pulse. With the addition of Rou Gui, it can be used for hypotension: Liu Zheng Cai and his team used Gui Zhi Gan Cao Tang modified with Rou Gui infused in tea in the treatment of 83 cases of hypotension due to heart qi deficiency. The course of treatment ranged from 3 to 12 doses. Blood pressure before treatment ranged from 90-75/67-45 mmHg and the average blood pressure after treatment was 110/70 mmHg (*Xin Yi Yao Xue Za Zhi* 1975; 2:29).

Case Study

Palpitations and Chest Pain

Extracted from Fu Jian Zhong Yi Yao 1964 Vol 5

A 39-year-old male patient had chest pain and palpitations which were relieved with pressure on the chest. He had taken analgesics for a few days to no avail. He experienced occasional spontaneous sweating and his stool and urination were normal. The pulse was soft and moderate and the tongue coat white and slippery. Gui Zhi Gan Cao Tang (Gui Zhi 18g, Gan Cao 9g) was prescribed and the chest pain eased after one pack.

Gui Zhi Gan Cao Long Gu Mu Li Tang Pattern

Gui Zhi Gan Cao Long Gu Mu Li Tang pattern represents the inappropriate use of fire therapy which has injured the heart yang and resulted in vexation.

Clause 118

火逆下之，因烧针烦躁者，桂枝甘草龙骨牡蛎汤主之。

Adverse fire therapy and purgation, if, due to hot needling, there is vexation and agitation, Gui Zhi Gan Cao Long Gu Mu Li Tang governs.

GUI ZHI GAN CAO LONG GU MU LI TANG: Gui Zhi (bark removed) 1 liang; Zhi Gan Cao 2 liang; Mu Li (dry-fried) 2 liang; Long Gu 2 liang.

DIRECTIONS: Boil the above four ingredients in 5 sheng of water until reduced to 2 ½ sheng then strain. Take 8 ge (160 mL) warm three times a day.

DISCUSSION: Excessive sweating caused by the inappropriate use of fire therapy can damage the heart yang and purgative treatment will cause further damage. The depleted heart yang is unable to contain the heart spirit, and so the heart shen is unsettled and there is restlessness and agitation.

Gui Zhi and Gan Cao augment the heart yang. Long Gu and Mu Li sedate and astringe the heart shen to address the vexation. The combined effect of the four herbs is to restore the heart yang and settle the restless heart shen.

Both Gui Zhi Gan Cao Tang and Gui Zhi Gan Cao Long Gu Mu Li Tang can be used to treat heart palpitations. The difference is that the former is suitable for a relatively mild condition caused simply by the excessive promotion of sweat; the latter, on the other hand, is indicated in the treatment of palpitations of a more serious nature which are accompanied by vexation and are the result of inappropriate fire therapy and purging. The key differential symptom in the diagnosis of Gui Zhi Gan Cao Long Gu Mu Li Tang pattern is vexation. Gui Zhi Gan Cao Long Gu Mu Li Tang can be applied where there are palpitations, nocturnal sweating, seminal emission and enuresis due to heart yang deficiency accompanied by vexation and insomnia.

Gui Zhi qu Shao Yao jia Shu Qi Mu Li Long Gu Jiu Ni Tang Pattern

Gui Zhi qu Shao Yao jia Mu Li Jiu Ni Tang pattern represents the inappropriate use of fire therapy which has resulted in yang desertion with manic behaviour. The translation of this formula is: Gui Zhi minus Shao Yao plus Shu Qi, Mu Li, Ling Gu Rescue Reversal Decoction.

Clause 112

伤寒脉浮，医以火迫劫之，亡阳必惊狂、卧起不安者，桂枝去芍药加蜀漆牡蛎龙骨救逆汤主之。

Shang han with a floating pulse, because the physician has used fire to force, if there is devastation of yang there will be manic behaviour, and restlessness both lying down or getting up, Gui Zhi qu Shao Yao jia Shu Qi Mu Li Long Gu Jiu Ni Tang governs.

GUI ZHI QU SHAO YAO JIA SHU QI MU LI LONG GU JIU NI TANG: Gui Zhi (bark removed) 3 liang; Zhi Gan Cao 2 liang; Sheng Jiang (sliced) 3 liang; Da Zao 12 pieces (broken); Mu Li (dry-fried) 5 liang; Shu Qi (washed to remove fishy smell) 3 liang; Long Gu 4 liang.

DIRECTIONS: First boil Shu Qi in 1 dou 2 sheng of water, reducing by 2 sheng. Add the other herbs and boil until reduced to 3 sheng. Strain and take 1 sheng warm.

DISCUSSION: The allusion to shang han with a floating pulse shows clearly that this is an exterior pattern. Fire therapy was used to force sweat to issue beyond the resources of the patient and the excessive and inappropriate sweating devastated yang, which in Clause 112 refers specifically to heart yang. Sweat is the humour of the heart, and yang is the spirit of the heart; therefore excessive sweating has the potential not only to injure the heart yang but it may also result in the non-containment of the heart shen, hence the restlessness, vexation and manic behaviour.

The desertion of heart yang in this pattern is to be differentiated from desertion of kidney yang or defence yang. Kidney yang desertion is characterised by a throbbing heart, which differs from palpitations in that the throbbing is not only palpable, as with palpitations, but it is actually visible, causing detectable movement of the chest. Other symptoms are dizziness, *jue ni* (a sudden loss of consciousness due to yin and yang not communicating, and where the extremities are cold), diarrhoea, muscle twitching and a pulse that is faint and thready. The treatment principle is to revive kidney yang and restore consciousness; appropriate formulas are Zhen Wu Tang and Si Ni Tang. Desertion of defence yang is characterised by excessive leaking sweat, aversion to wind cold, inhibited urination and slight tension in the limbs. The treatment principle is to secure the exterior and resuscitate the yang and the indicated formula is Gui Zhi jia Fu Zi Tang.

This is a modified version of Gui Zhi Tang, in which the ingredients Gui Zhi and Gan Cao have the function of warming and restoring the heart yang. A yang desertion pattern is often accompanied by the accumulation of phlegm turbidity, which obstructs the ascent of clear yang, blocking the orifices and affecting the heart shen. For this reason, Shu Qi (the sprout of Chang Shan) is added to eliminate phlegm. The heavy sedative herbs, Long Gu and Mu Li, settle and anchor the upcast heart shen and calm the spirit. There are various interpretations regarding the omission of Shao Yao, as follows.

1. Cheng Wu Ji suggests that Shao Yao is not indicated for desertion of heart yang.
2. *Yi Zong Jin Jian* comments that Shao Yao has an emolliating effect which will retard the restoration of heart yang.
3. Ke Yun Bo comments that since desertion of yin has already occurred, Shao Yao is of no avail in its function of astringing fluids and is therefore not needed.
4. Cheng Dan An comments in *Shang Han Lun Xin Zhu* that Shao Yao is sour and astringent and is inappropriate in the treatment of phlegm turbidity.
5. The authors feel that the first two explanations most closely concord with the meaning and purpose of the clause.

Modern Application of Gui Zhi qu Shao Yao jia Mu Li Jiu Ni Tang

This formula augments the heart yang, eliminates turbid phlegm and sedates and calms the heart shen. It can be used in the treatment of bipolar disorder characterised by a pale tongue with a moist and slippery tongue coat.

Case Study

Insomnia Due to Fright

Extracted from Shang Han Lun Fang Yi An

Since having an anxiety attack some time previously, a 36-year-old male patient suffered from insomnia and was in need of constant company even during the daytime. He had urinary frequency and a reduced appetite. The palms of his hands and soles of his feet were clammy, his tongue was pale with a thin, white coat and his pulse was wiry. A modified version of Gui Zhi Jiu Ni Tang was prescribed: Gui Zhi 12g, Zhi Gan Cao 24g, Sheng Jiang 9g, Da Zao 6 pieces, Sheng Long Gu 50g, Sheng Mu Li 50g, Yuan Zhi 9g, Gui Yuan Rou 100g, Fu Xiao Mai 100g. After the three packs his condition improved. The formula was repeated for four days with a reduction in the dose of Long Gu and Mu Li to 25g and Gui Yuan Rou to 30g.

Gui Zhi jia Gui Tang Pattern

Gui Zhi jia Gui Tang is the representative formula for heart yang deficiency which has resulted in *ben tun* or running piglet. *Ben tun* is the result of heart yang deficiency where the heart is unable to warm the kidneys in the lower jiao and the resulting accumulation of water leads to an upsurge of water qi.

Clause 117

烧针令其汗，针处被寒，核起而赤者，必发奔豚。气从少腹上冲心者， 灸其核上各一壮，与桂枝加桂汤，更加桂二两也。

Hot needling caused sweating, the needle site is attacked by cold, if a nodule erupts which is red, there will be running piglet. If qi from the lesser abdomen surges upward to the heart, place one cone of moxa on each nodule, give Gui Zhi jia Gui Tang, with the addition of 2 liang of Gui Zhi.

GUI ZHI JIA GUI TANG: Gui Zhi (bark removed) 5 liang; Shao Yao 3 liang; Sheng Jiang (sliced) 3 liang; Zhi Gan Cao 3 liang; Da Zao 12 pieces (broken).

DIRECTIONS: Boil the ingredients in 7 sheng of water until reduced to 3 sheng. Strain and take 1 sheng warm. This is Gui Zhi Tang with the dose of Gui Zhi increased to 5 liang. The purpose of the increased dose is to disperse the upsurge and redirect the counterflow of qi rising from the lower jiao.

DISCUSSION: The use of hot needling to promote sweating has resulted in the opening of the skin pores and interstices with subsequent invasion by pathogenic cold, giving rise to the red nodule. Copious sweating has damaged the heart yang and the running piglet phenomenon arises. This is because qi has taken advantage of the emptiness in the chest and manifests as a sensation of qi surging upwards from the lower abdomen. The appropriate treatment is the application of a cone of moxa on each red nodule to warm the yang and disperse the cold. This is then followed by Gui Zhi jia Gui Tang, which, by supporting the deficient heart yang, discharges the rebellious upsurge of qi.

There are numerous interpretations as to the pathogenesis of ben tun or running piglet. Zhang Xu Gu and Wang Hu suggest that the inappropriate treatment of a Tai Yang exterior pattern has caused the cold pathogen to fall inwards. Since Tai Yang and Shao Yin have an exterior–interior relationship, the pathogen has caused cold from the Shao Yin to surge up, creating the phenomenon of ben tun. Ke Yun Bo suggests that the inappropriate treatment of hot needling to promote sweating has damaged the heart yang and this, together with an attack of pathogenic cold, has caused kidney water to counterflow and manifest as ben tun. *Yi Zong Jin Jian* suggests that hot needling has over-stimulated the heart shen resulting in fright, whilst the kidney water has exploited the deficiency in the upper jiao and surged upwards, manifesting as ben tun. Huang Yuan Yu suggests that the loss of sweat has caused a yang deficiency of the spleen and kidney, which, in turn, has caused wood to be constrained; the exterior cold pathogen causes further constraint, affecting the wood and giving rise to wind qi manifesting as ben tun. Cheng Wu Ji suggests that hot needling damages the yin blood which in turn causes the kidney qi to stir and manifest as ben tun.

In brief, there are two possible causes of ben tun. The first explanation, according to *Jin Gui Yao Lue:* "Ben tun disease emanates from the lesser abdomen with its upsurge of qi reaching all the way to the throat. During an attack, the patient has a desire to die". The second explanation is that found in Clause 117, where a loss of sweat caused by hot needling has injured the yang. The yang deficiency in the upper jiao allows yin to exploit the emptiness, which results in the subjective sensation of qi surging upwards from the lesser abdomen to the throat. A tremor in the umbilical region can presage this sense of upsurging qi. If the qi upsurge assails the stomach, the patient may experience fullness and distension in the epigastrium and abdomen; if the qi assails the chest, there can be an oppressed sensation in the chest accompanied by palpitations; if the qi assails the throat, there can be a stifling sensation or a sense of asphyxiation.

There is a controversial debate as to whether the intention was to use Gui Zhi or Rou Gui. Chen Xiu Yuan and Huang Yuan Yu suggest Gui Zhi is the chief herb; Fang You Zhi and Xu Ling Tai suggest the use of Rou Gui; Zhang Xu Gu suggests that Rou Gui is more appropriate to treat the kidneys. The authors see that Rou Gui is a sound clinical choice to treat ben tun, but in consideration of the dose of 5 liang, it would appear that Gui Zhi is the intended herb, because this dose is too high for Rou Gui.

Functions and Applications of Gui Zhi

Shen Nong Ben Cao states: "Gui Zhi is indicated for counterflow lung qi and cough: it relieves knotted qi in the throat and augments the middle qi", hence the saying that Gui Zhi has the function of addressing the three qi. The first of the three qi is counterflow: Gui Zhi is used as the essential herb in discharging the upsurge of qi in the formulas Ling Gui Zhu Gan Tang, Ling Gui Zao Gan Tang, Ling Gui Wei Gan Tang and Gui Zhi jia Gui Tang. The second is knotted qi: Gui Zhi is used to free knotted qi by invigorating qi and transforming stasis in the formulas Zhi Shi Xie Bai Gui Zhi Tang and Gui Zhi Fu Ling Wan. The third qi is deficient middle qi, and Gui Zhi's function of augmenting middle qi is seen in the formulas Xiao Jian Zhong Tang and Huang Qi Jian Zhong Tang.

The function of Gui Zhi when combined with Shao Yao varies depending on the ratio. When the dosage is equal, such as in Gui Zhi Tang, the focus is on regulating ying and wei. When Shao Yao is double the dose of Gui Zhi, as in Gui Zhi jia Shao Yao Tang, the focus is on moderating pain and harmonising the middle. When the dosage of Gui Zhi is greater than that of Shao Yao, as in Gui Zhi jia Gui Tang, the focus is on redirecting counterflow qi. The clinical applications of Gui Zhi jia Gui Tang include: an exterior pattern, headache, vertigo, gastritis, neurosis, menopausal syndrome, chronic colitis and cardiac disorders with a subjective feeling of qi upsurge.

Ancient Application of Gui Zhi jia Gui Tang

Lei Ju Fang Guang Yi advocated the use of Gui Zhi jia Gui Tang where there was acute qi upsurge in a Gui Zhi Tang pattern.

Modern Application of Gui Zhi jia Gui Tang

Gui Zhi jia Gui Tang is used to treat externally contracted disease, headache, vertigo, gastritis, neurosis, menopausal syndrome and chronic colitis, when characterised by discomfort in the chest with a subjective feeling of upsurging qi. It is also suitable in the treatment of cardiac disease with upsurging qi, arrhythmia or palpitations with a stifling sensation in the chest.

Modifications of Gui Zhi jia Gui Tang

- For scleroderma, Raynauld's disease or frostbite, add Rou Gui.
- If there is qi deficiency with blood stasis, add Huang Qi, Dang Gui, Chuan Xiong, Hong Hua and Tao Ren to augment qi and nourish and invigorate blood.
- If there is severe pathogenic cold, add Gao Liang Jiang.
- If the qi counterflow is severe, add Chen Xiang.

Case Study

Hiccough

Extracted from Liao Ning Zhong Yi Za Zhi; 1980 (5):35

A 70-year-old male patient presented with frequent episodes of hiccoughing, each episode comprising some 20 hiccoughs. Based on the symptom of qi surging upwards, the disorder was diagnosed as ben tun and Gui Zhi jia Gui Tang was prescribed: Gui Zhi 25g, Bai Shao 15g, Gan Jiang 10g, Gan Cao 15g, Da Zao 7 pieces, Chen Pi 10g, Hou

Po 10g. One pack was given, to be taken in two doses. He recovered after a repeat of the same formula the next day.

Note: The high dose of Gui Zhi was prescribed to address the upsurging kidney qi. Hou Po and Chen Pi were added to harmonise stomach qi and redirect counterflow, and Shao Yao and Gan Cao to harmonise the stomach qi.

Fu Ling Gui Zhi Gan Cao Da Zao Tang

Fu Ling Gui Zhi Gan Cao Da Zao Tang is an associated formula indicated where there is heart yang deficiency with symptoms suggesting the imminent manifestation of ben tun. Ben tun stems from heart yang deficiency where the heart is unable to warm the kidneys in the lower jiao; the resulting accumulation of water causes a sensation of tremor or palpitation in the lower jiao which has the potential to surge upwards, manifesting as ben tun.

Clause 65

发汗后，其人脐下悸者，欲作奔豚，茯苓桂枝甘草大枣汤主之。

After the promotion of sweat, the person feels palpitations below the umbilicus, this is about to manifest as ben tun, Fu Ling Gui Zhi Gan Cao Da Zao Tang governs.

FU LING GUI ZHI GAN CAO DA ZAO TANG: Fu Ling ½ jin; Gui Zhi (bark removed) 4 liang; Zhi Gan Cao 3 liang; Da Zao 15 pieces (broken).

DIRECTIONS: Decoct Fu Ling first in 1 dou of gan lan water until reduced by 2 sheng, then add the other ingredients until reduced to 3 sheng. Strain and take 1 sheng warm three times a day.

NOTE: *Gan lan shui* (甘澜水) is water which has been 'worked' by stirring 2 dou of water repeatedly in a large pan until thousands of water bubbles appear. The rationale of using *gan lan* water is to render the water (which is salty in nature) sweet, thus benefiting the spleen.

DISCUSSION: The heart governs fire; it is located in the upper jiao, and interacts with the kidney water in the lower jiao, inhibiting excessive cold or the flooding of the kidney water. When heart yang is damaged by loss of fluids due to sweating, the weakened heart fire can not control the kidney water and cold qi surges from the lesser abdomen up to the chest and throat, in the phenomenon known as ben tun. The characteristic tremor below the umbilicus is the aura heralding the actual manifestation of ben tun and is caused by water and qi knotted in the umbilical region, which has an upward momentum and the potential to surge upwards. Fu Ling Gui Zhi Gan Cao Da Zao Tang is prescribed to warm the yang and suppress the counterflow of water. The purpose of using such a large dose of Fu Ling and decocting it first is to calm the heart shen, tonify the spleen and drain damp. Gui Zhi reinforces the heart yang and redirects the counterflow. Da Zao tonifies the spleen and benefits the middle, and Zhi Gan Cao warms the middle and supplements deficiency. Together, these two herbs prevent the upsurge of water qi by warming and strengthening the middle. The combined effect of the four herbs supports the spleen earth to bank water and also warms the heart yang.

Both the potential to manifest as ben tun and the actual manifestation of ben tun arise as a result of deficient heart yang failing to control water. The difference is in the symptoms and the treatment. The potential for ben tun is characterised by a tremor below the umbilicus, reflecting the stirring of knotted water; the treatment is focused on transforming qi and draining damp. In the actual manifestation of ben tun, the water qi does not remain contained in the abdomen but surges up to the chest and throat. The treatment principle is to quell the stirring of water qi and suppress counterflow.

Ben tun can be differentiated into ben tun qi disorder, ben tun due to cold in the kidney, and ben tun due to cold accumulation, also known as *han shan* (寒疝) or hernial disorder. The pathomechanism of ben tun is related to the dynamic of the ascent and descent of qi. Differential patterns and their treatment are as follows.

1. For knotted cold water qi obstructing qi transformation in the Tai Yang channel, the indicated formula is Fu Ling Gui Zhi Gan Cao Da Zao Tang, otherwise known as Ling Gui Gan Zao Tang.
2. For yang deficiency caused by the the use of hot needling to promote sweat, manifesting as red nodules at the needling site caused by pathogenic cold, the indicated formula is Gui Zhi jia Gui Tang.
3. For damage to yang caused by emotional upset or fright, Ben Tun Tang is the appropriate formula.

Case Study

Ben Tun Qi

Extracted from Xin Pian Shang Han Lun Lei Fang 1984

A 54-year-old male patient complained of a tremor below the umbilicus, restlessness, difficult urination and a sensation of qi surging upwards from the lower abdomen to his chest, which gave him a sense of panic and caused a stifling sensation in the chest as if he could not breathe. The attacks occurred several times per day and were worse in the afternoon. His pulse was submerged, wiry and slightly slippery and his tongue was pale with a thin, white watery tongue coat.

There are two formulas in Shang Han Lun which deal with this disorder. Gui Zhi jia Gui Tang is indicated for qi upsurge with no urinary symptoms and Fu Ling Gui Zhi Gan Cao Da Zao Tang is indicated when there is qi upsurge with inhibited urination. In this instance, the patient suffered from umbilical tremor and difficult urination indicating water accumulation in the lower jiao and Fu Ling Gui Zhi Gan Cao Da Zao Tang was the formula chosen: Fu Ling 30g, Gui Zhi 10g, Rou Gui 6g, Zhi Gan Cao 6g, Da Zao 15 pieces, to be decocted in gan lan water (worked water). He was prescribed three packs.

Summary of Heart Yang Deficiency Patterns

Clauses 64, 118, 112, 117 and 65 all relate to heart yang deficiency patterns. Clauses 64, 118 and 112 are focused on heart yang deficiency patterns which differ only in severity. Clause 64 relates to Gui Zhi Gan Cao Tang: the damage to heart yang is relatively mild and the key symptoms are palpitations with a preference for pressure in the chest area. Clause 118 relates to Gui Zhi Gan Cao Long Gu Mu Li Tang: the damage to heart yang is more serious and the key symptoms are floating heart shen and heart vexation. Clause 112 relates to Gui Zhi Qu Shao Yao jia Shu Chi Mu Li Long Gu jiu Ni Tang where damage to heart yang is the most severe of the three Gui Zhi patterns and is close to yang desertion. The key symptoms are fright, manic behaviour and restlessness. Clauses 117 and 65 are associated with heart yang deficiency affecting the spleen and kidney yang and manifesting as ben tun, or the upsurge of water qi. Clause 117 describes a ben tun pattern where the upsurge of cold water qi from the lower jiao reaches the chest and throat whilst Clause 65 describes a pattern where ben tun is about to manifest but has not actually done so.

2.7.6 Heart Yin and Yang Deficiency

Zhi Gan Cao Tang Pattern

A Zhi Gan Cao Tang pattern represents injury to both the yin and yang of the heart.

Clause 177

伤寒脉结代，心动悸，炙甘草汤主之。

Shang han, the pulse is knotted and intermittent, there are throbbing palpitations, Zhi Gan Cao Tang governs.

ZHI GAN CAO TANG: Zhi Gan Cao 4 liang; Sheng Jiang (sliced) 3 liang; Ren Shen 2 liang; Sheng Di Huang 1 jin; Gui Zhi (bark removed) 3 liang; E Jiao 2 liang; Mai Dong (core removed) ½ jin; Ma Ren ½ jin; Da Zao 30 pieces (broken).

NOTE: Ma Ren refers to Huo Ma Ren. Its main function is to moisten the intestines. In *Shang Han Lun* it is called 'Ma Zi Ren' and in *Shen Nong Ben Cao Jing* it is called 'Ma Zi'. The name 'Huo Ma Ren' comes from *Ri Yong Ben Cao*.

DIRECTIONS: Decoct all ingredients with the exception of E Jiao in 7 sheng of aged rice wine and 8 sheng of water. Reduce to 3 sheng then strain and add the melted E Jiao. Take 1 sheng warm three times a day.

DISCUSSION: In the course of externally contracted disease, symptoms of a knotted and intermittent pulse combined with palpitations indicate that both the yin and yang of the heart are deficient, depriving the heart of nourishment. The "throbbing palpitations" indicate that the condition is serious, and that the kidney yang is also affected. There are several possible causes of a knotted or intermittent pulse: blood stasis, phlegm obstruction, water constraint or qi and blood deficiency. In the pattern described above, the knotted and intermittent pulse is the manifestation of qi and blood being insufficient and unable to fill the vessels and move the blood; therefore the pulse is not smooth and regular, but stops intermittently.

Su Wen: Ling Lan Mi Dian Lun (Chapter 8: Confidential Discourse of the Mystical Orchid) states: "The heart holds the office of the monarch, whence the life spirit emanates." It further states: "The wise monarch ensures peace and order, ensuring health and long life". In this way, it explains that if the heart's function is good, the twelve zang fu will function, thus implying that the function of all the zang fu is dependent on the healthy function of the heart. If heart blood is deficient and the heart yang devitalised, then heart function will be weakened. Zhi Gan Cao Tang nourishes heart blood and bolsters the heart yang, thus restoring the pulse. For this reason, it is also known as Fu Mai Tang or Restore the Pulse Decoction.

Zhi Gan Cao is the chief herb; it tonifies the middle and augments qi, thus strengthening the source of qi and blood, which is the basis of restoring the pulse. Ren Shen and Da Zao tonify qi and generate fluids and, when combined with Sheng Di, Mai Dong, E Jiao and Ma Ren, are able to nourish heart blood and replenish heart fluid to fill the blood vessels. Gui Zhi bolsters heart yang and its function of warming and unblocking is enhanced by Sheng Jiang. The aged rice wine used to decoct the herbs is acrid, sweet and warm, thus promoting the flow of blood and facilitating the unblocking of heart yang.

The pathogenesis of this pattern is deficiency of the vital substance of the heart: yin, yang, qi and blood. The heart lacks nourishment and is unable to govern the blood vessels and regulate the flow of blood. The symptoms arising from this are a knotted and intermittent pulse, palpitations, shortness of breath, fatigue, dizziness, a pale complexion and a pale tongue.

Ancient Application of Zhi Gan Cao Tang

- *Qian Jin Yao Fang* cites Zhi Gan Cao Tang in the treatment of deficient detriment disorder characterised by sweating, an intermittent pulse and palpitations in response to normal daily activities; the condition tends to deteriorate and lapse into a serious disorder within 100 days.
- Ye Tian Shi used this formula in the treatment of febrile disease attributed more to weakness of zheng qi than to the strength of the pathogen; this may be extended to miscellaneous disease, including post-partum disorders.
- Wu Ju Tong modified Zhi Gan Cao Tang, creating the formulas Jia Jian Fu Mai Tang, Yi Jia Fu Mai Tang, Er Jia Fu Mai Tang, San Jia Fu Mai Tang and Da Ding Feng Zhu Tang. These were recommended for the later stages of wen bing characterised by kidney and liver yin deficiency.

Modern Application of Zhi Gan Cao Tang

- Zhi Gan Cao Tang is suitable for the treatment of cardiac disease associated with arrhythmia, atrio-ventricular block and also autonomic nervous system dysfunction characterised by palpitations, an oppressed sensation in the chest, shortness of breath and an intermittent pulse.
- Zhi Gan Cao Tang is indicated in the treatment of palpitations and insomnia due to yin blood deficiency.

Modifications:

- For qi deficiency, add Huang Qi.
- For yin deficiency with hyperactive fire, reduce the dosage of Gui Zhi, add Yu Zhu, Huang Lian, Wu Wei Zi and Gou Qi Zi.

- For residual toxins characterised by low grade fever, add Xuan Shen, Bie Jia, Qing Hao and Ren Dong Teng.
- For heart yang desertion characterised by sweating and cold limbs and a faint and weak pulse, add Fu Zi, Long Gu, Mu Li and Wu Wei Zi.
- For blood stasis characterised by a sharp pain in the chest, a tongue which is purple or has stasis spots, and a choppy pulse, add San Qi, Tao Ren and Hong Hua.
- For phlegm damp characterised by a white, slippery, greasy tongue coat, add Gua Lou and Ban Xia.
- Where there is oedema, omit Gan Cao.
- Where there is a sloppy stool, omit Ma Ren.

Case Study

Palpitations

Extracted from Shang Han Shi Jian Lun

A 16-year-old female patient presented with palpitations, anxiety and jumpiness, an oppressed sensation in the chest, shortness of breath, fitful sleep, fatigue and a reduced appetite. Her bowel movement and urination were normal. The ECG indicated that she had sinus arrhythmia. Her pulse was moderate, forceless and irregular and her tongue was pale with a thin, white moist tongue coat. She was prescribed a modification of Zhi Gan Cao Tang: Zhi Gan Cao 10g, Gui Zhi 10g, Dang Shen 15g, E Jiao 15g, Sheng Di 10g, Mai Dong 10g, Huo Ma Ren 15g, Sheng Huang Qi 15g, Sheng Jiang 3 pieces, Da Zao 3 pieces. One dose was to be taken each day with a small amount of rice wine. After seven packs, the palpitations and anxiety decreased, the shortness of breath was much improved; she felt more energetic and she was sleeping more deeply. Her pulse was moderate and forceful with occasional irregularity. Her tongue was pale and moist with a thin, white tongue coat. The original formula was repeated with the addition of Bai Zi Ren 10g to be taken in one dose each day.

Discussion: This case is characterised by a deficiency of yang and qi. Zhi Gan Cao Tang is used to support yang and nourish yin in order to restore the pulse. Huang Qi is added to further benefit the qi. Coronary heart disease, emphysema and myocarditis can all be treated with Zhi Gan Cao Tang where there is a yin and yang deficiency and an intermittent pulse.

Note: Zhi Gan Cao is indicated for the treatment of ectopic heartbeat and has been proven highly effective. The pathogenesis is a deficiency in both yin and yang, however, this formula is contraindicated in yin deficiency with a red tongue and a scant coat and in interior heat with a yellow tongue coat. If administered in error, there will be insomnia, vexation and a parched throat and mouth. In such a case the formula must be discontinued immediately.

Prognosis of a Knotted and Intermittent Pulse

Clause 178

脉按之来缓，时一止复来者，名曰结。又脉来动而中止，更来小数，中有还者反动，名曰结，阴也；脉来动而中止，不能自还，因而复动者，名日代，阴也。得此脉，必难治。

If the pulse is moderate on palpation, occasionally stopping and then starting again, it is called knotted. Also, a pulse which is stirring but is interrupted, then on returning is small and rapid, occasionally returning to normal but stirring again, it is called knotted, this is yin; a pulse which is stirring but is interrupted, if unable to return, it is because when it returns it is stirring, it is called intermittent, this is yin. If this is the pulse, it will be difficult to treat.

DISCUSSION: Clause 178 is a supplement to Clause 177 which describes a knotted and intermittent (结代脉) pulse. The peculiarity of the knotted pulse or jie mai (结脉) is that it is a slow or moderate pulse which occasionally stops and then starts again. The interruption is ascribed to obstruction of the vessels due to qi stagnation. Bin Hu Mai Xue 濒湖脉学 states: "The knotted pulse is moderate with occasional interruption. This is due to exuberance of yin with desertion of yang". The knotted pulse can also be attributed to an insufficiency of zheng qi where deficient yang fails to promote the flow of qi, and exuberance of yin cold congeals the blood. For this reason it is deemed to be a yin pulse.

The intermittent pulse or dai mai (代脉) is described as a pulse which is regularly interrupted and fails to return to a normal rhythm. This implies that the interruption is of significant duration and the cause is deeply entrenched. *Bin Hu Mai Xue* states: "An intermittent pulse is ascribed to weakness of source qi characterised by abdominal pain and diarrhoea". This mirrors the explanation ascribing an intermittent pulse to an insufficiency of zheng qi, resulting from impaired zang fu function and inadequate source qi. An intermittent pulse is deemed to be a yin pulse on the basis of the deficiency. If the zheng qi is damaged to the point of exhaustion, the condition is serious and so will be difficult to treat.

In short, the identifying feature of the knotted and intermittent pulse is that it is moderate or slow and interrupted or irregular, whilst the skipping or hasty pulse (促脉) is rapid and irregular. In the clinical situation, pulses can be either knotted or intermittent or both. Both pulse images are a reflection of qi and blood deficiency caused by emotional disturbance, congealed stasis obstructing the vessels, or may indicate a severe loss of fluids due to incessant vomiting, diarrhoea or severe haemorrhage following trauma.

2.7.7 Spleen Deficiency

There are two variations of Tai Yang transmuted pattern where there is damage to the spleen.

1. Fu Ling Gui Zhi Bai Zhu Gan Cao Tang pattern is a pattern of spleen deficiency with damage to spleen yang.
2. Hou Po Sheng Jiang Ban Xia Gan Cao Ren Shen Tang pattern is one where damage to spleen qi has resulted in abdominal fullness.

Fu Ling Gui Zhi Bai Zhu Gan Cao Tang Pattern

Fu Ling Gui Zhi Bai Zhu Gan Cao Tang pattern is a result of incorrect purging or inducing vomiting in shang han disease which has injured the spleen yang and resulted in the accumulation of water in the middle jiao. It is also known as Ling Gui Zhu Gan Tang.

Clause 67

伤寒若吐、若下后，心下逆满，气上冲胸，起则头眩，脉沉紧，发汗则动经，身为振振摇者，茯苓桂枝白术甘草汤主之。

If there is vomiting in shang han, and if after purging there is fullness below the heart due to reversal, an upsurge of qi to the chest, on standing there is dizziness, the pulse is submerged and tight, and if the promotion of sweat causes stirring in the channels, with the body quivering and trembling, Fu Ling Gui Zhi Bai Zhu Gan Cao Tang governs.

FU LING GUI ZHI BAI ZHU GAN CAO TANG: Fu Ling 4 liang; Gui Zhi (bark removed) 3 liang; Bai Zhu 2 liang; Zhi Gan Cao 2 liang.

DIRECTIONS: Boil the ingredients in 6 sheng of water, reducing to 3 sheng. Strain and take the decoction warm three times a day.

DISCUSSION: The use of purgatives and emetics constitutes incorrect treatment in shang han disease because it has the potential to damage the yang qi, in particular, the yang qi of the spleen and stomach. This emptiness in the middle jiao may result in the accumulation of water qi, which surges upwards to the heart. Because the spleen yang is deficient, it is unable to raise the clear yang, so the orifices are misted by the water qi which has risen to the upper jiao, causing dizziness or a sense of faintness. The water qi represents a preponderance of yin and is reflected in the submerged pulse, whilst the tightness of the pulse is a reflection of excess cold. Fullness below the heart due to reversal refers to epigastric fullness resulting from disturbance of the qi dynamic. Dizziness can be interpreted as a sense of faintness or as dizziness in response to movement.

The reference in Clause 67 to the promotion of sweat causing quivering and trembling illustrates the fact that any further fluid loss through incorrect treatment will cause adverse outcomes, and serves as a warning that the promotion of sweat is contraindicated. The correct treatment for yang deficiency with water retention is to warm the channels, restore the yang and drain damp by promoting urination. The promotion of sweat would have the opposite effect, damaging the yang qi and depriving the channels of warmth, subsequently giving rise to the adverse outcome of quivering or trembling. This is explained by the fact that the sweating comes in the wake of the earlier adverse treatments of vomiting and purgation, and the loss of sweat exacerbates the drain on the yang and the qi, which are already deficient. The channel qi is already depleted and so the channels are easily destabilised when assailed by the water qi, resulting in quivering and trembling. The stirring of the channels cited in Clause 67 is a reference to this harassment of qi.

Fu Ling is the chief herb and is used for its function of draining damp and promoting urination. Gui Zhi warms the yang, redirects the counterflow qi and, when combined with Fu Ling, transforms qi, unblocks the yang and disinhibits water. Bai Zhu tonifies the spleen and dries damp, with these functions enhanced by Gui Zhi. Gan Cao harmonises the middle.

The pathogenesis of a Fu Ling Gui Zhi Bai Zhu Gan Cao Tang pattern is spleen yang deficiency with water qi counterflow. This manifests as fullness below the heart due to rebellious qi, qi upsurge, palpitations, dizziness and the rumbling of water in the abdomen. The patient can present with water marks, or dark discolouration of the forehead, cheeks, nose and corners of the mouth, and will have a white, watery tongue coat and a submerged, wiry and tight pulse.

The patterns described in Clause 65 (Fu Ling Gui Zhi Gan Cao Da Zao Tang, also known as Ling Gui Zao Gan Tang) and Clause 67 (Fu Ling Gui Zhi Bai Zhu Gan Cao Tang, also known as Ling Gui Zhu Gan Tang) bear many similarities, as do the formulas representing them. Both relate to water qi harassment and their respective formulas both have Fu Ling as the chief herb, to disinhibit water and drain damp, combined with Gui Zhi and Gan Cao. One, however, contains Da Zao and the other Bai Zhu. The first, containing Da Zao, and described in Clause 65, is used for water retention in the lower jiao characterised by tremor beneath the umbilicus whilst the second, containing Bai Zhu, and described in Clause 67, is indicated for water accumulation in the middle jiao with counterflow fullness beneath the heart.

Ancient Application of Ling Gui Zhu Gan Tang

- *Jin Gui Yao Lue:* For the treatment of phlegm fluids below the heart characterised by such symptoms as fullness in the chest and vertigo.
- *Ji Sheng Fang:* Omitting Gui Zhi and adding Ren Shen and Ban Xia for the treatment of deficiency cold with water accumulation in the spleen and stomach manifesting with vomiting and a reduced appetite.
- *Huang Han Yi Xue*: *Yan Ke Jin Nang:* For the treatment of fullness in the chest with water qi upsurge characterised by dizziness and water swelling of the eyelids.

Modern Application of Ling Gui Zhu Gan Tang

Ling Gui Zhu Gan Tang can be used to treat patterns where there is an accumulation of phlegm fluids such as chronic bronchitis, bronchial asthma and oedema, including that associated with impaired cardiac or renal function as may be found in congestive heart failure, chronic nephritis or hydronephrosis. Other disorders for which it is suitable include vertigo, palpitations, gastritis, duodenal ulcer, colitis, leucorrhoea and bi syndrome.

Modifications

- For chronic bronchitis characterised by clear, watery sputum, a pale tongue with a thin, white coat and a slippery pulse, add Chuan Bei Mu and Zi Wan to transform phlegm. For phlegm damp, combine with Er Chen Tang.
- For vertigo related to spleen yang deficiency with phlegm damp obstruction and counterflow fullness below the heart characterised by vertigo, nausea and tinnitus, add Ban Xia, Yi Ren and Ge Gen. If the vertigo is severe, add Ze Xie.

- For heart failure associated with qi deficiency of the heart and spleen with water accumulation, add Ren Shen, Mai Dong, Wu Wei Zi and Dan Shen. Where there is severe oedema, add Ze Xie, Zhu Ling and Ze Lan Ye to strengthen the heart and drain damp.
- For wheezing characterised by a submerged and wiry pulse and a watery tongue, add Su Zi, Yi Yi Ren, Kuan Dong Hua and Bai Guo to transform phlegm and calm wheeze.
- For chronic mature onset bronchitis characterised by cough and copious watery phlegm, add Dang Shen, Ban Xia and Chen Pi.
- For chronic colitis associated with spleen deficiency and diarrhoea, increase the dosage of Bai Zhu and Fu Ling and add Yi Yi Ren and Shan Yao to tonify the spleen and drain damp. If there is yang deficiency with exuberant cold, add Gan Jiang and Fu Zi to warm the middle and disperse cold. If accompanied by abdominal pain, add Wei Mu Xiang and Bai Shao.
- For leucorrhoea associated with spleen deficiency and cold, add Shan Yao, Pao Jiang and Qian Shi to tonify the spleen, drain damp and disperse cold.
- For stomach pain associated with spleen deficiency and damp, add Yuan Hu, Xiang Fu and Gao Liang Jiang to disperse cold and ease pain. If there is counterflow and nausea, add Fa Ban Xia, Sheng Jiang, Chen Pi and Zhu Ru to descend qi and relieve vomiting. If spleen qi is deficient, add Dang Shen and Huang Qi to augment qi and tonify the spleen.
- For stomach prolapse characterised by counterflow fullness below the heart with the sound of rumbling water, add Sheng Ma, Chai Hu and Zhi Qiao to raise the yang and augment the stomach qi.
- If there is hypertension, add Niu Xi, Hong Hua and Qian Cao. If there is an intermittent pulse, omit Bai Zhu and add Wu Wei Zi. If there is a flushed face with heat and vexation due to water qi with deficient heat, add Bai Wei.

NOTE: This formula is acrid and warm and indicated for the accumulation of phlegm fluids due to yang deficiency. If there is yin deficiency with hyperactive fire, it must be used with caution. If there is fullness in the middle characterised by a greasy tongue coat and water swelling, the dose of Gan Cao should be reduced or omitted entirely.

Case Study

Chronic Gastritis

Extracted from Jiang Su Zhong Yi, 1996

A 42-year-old male patient had suffered for more than ten years from pain and distension in the epigastrium, with bloating and discomfort after meals. Other symptoms were aversion to cold, a preference for warmth and pressure on the stomach, reflux of thin fluids, and a sloppy stool. His tongue was pale with a thin, white and greasy tongue coat and the pulse was soggy. He had been diagnosed as having chronic gastritis and the Chinese medical diagnosis was spleen and stomach yang deficiency with water accumulation. The treatment principle was to warm the yang and tonify the spleen, redirect counterflow and harmonise the stomach. A modifed version of Ling Gui Zhu Gan Tang was prescribed: Fu Ling 20g, Zhi Gui Zhi 8g, Chao Bai Zhu 10g, Fa Ban Xia 10g, Fo Shou Hua 6g, Gao Liang Jiang 3g, Jiu Xiang Chong 10g, Chao Mai Ya 15g. After ten packs, the stomach pain had eased and the reflux reduced. The same formula was continued with slight modifications for several months, after which his condition remained good with no relapse over the following two years.

Hou Po Sheng Jiang Ban Xia Gan Cao Ren Shen Tang Pattern

Hou Po Sheng Jiang Ban Xia Gan Cao Ren Shen Tang pattern is representative of the inappropriate promotion of sweat having damaged spleen qi and resulted in abdominal fullness.

Clause 66

发汗后，腹胀者，厚朴生姜甘草人参汤主之.

After promoting sweat, the abdomen is distended, Hou Po Sheng Jiang Ban Xia Gan Cao Ren Shen Tang governs.

HOU PO SHENG JIANG BAN XIA GAN CAO REN SHEN TANG: Hou Po (bark removed and dry-fried) ½ jin; Sheng Jiang ½ jin (sliced); Ban Xia ½ jin (soaked); Gan Cao 2 liang; Ren Shen 1 liang.

DIRECTIONS: Boil the ingredients in 1 dou of water, reducing to 3 sheng. Strain and take 1 sheng warm three times a day.

DISCUSSION: The incorrect promotion of heavy sweating has damaged spleen qi, impairing its transformation function and generating phlegm damp; this impedes the qi dynamic, causing abdominal distension. This clause describes a complex pattern of excess on deficiency, and the treatment strategy is to simultaneously supplement the deficiency and reduce the excess with the formula Hou Po Sheng Jiang Ban Xia Gan Cao Ren Shen Tang.

Hou Po loosens the chest and descends qi; Sheng Jiang harmonises the stomach and dissipates the fullness; Ban Xia dries damp and eliminates phlegm, thus dispersing constraint. These three herbs have the combined effect of eliminating the knotted phlegm and restoring the qi dynamic of the middle jiao. The remaining two herbs, Ren Shen and Gan Cao, strengthen the spleen and augment qi. The pathogenesis of this pattern is spleen deficiency with stagnation of qi resulting in the accumulation of phlegm damp. This is characterised by abdominal distension with no pain on palpation.

Ancient Application of Hou Po Sheng Jiang Ban Xia Gan Cao Ren Shen Tang

- *Zhang Shi Yi Tong:* For the treatment of stomach deficiency characterised by vomiting, glomus and poor appetite.
- *Lei Ju Fang Guang Yi:* For the treatment of *huo luan* (acute gastritis) characterised by vomiting, diarrhoea and abdominal distension due to deficiency.

Modern Application of Hou Po Sheng Jiang Ban Xia Gan Cao Ren Shen Tang

It is commonly used in the treatment of vomiting and diarrhoea with abdominal distension as found in chronic gastritis or stomach ulcers associated with spleen deficiency with bloating.

The authors consider Hou Po Sheng Jiang Ban Xia Gan Cao Ren Shen Tang pattern to be a complex pattern of excess on deficiency, where there is more excess than deficiency. For this reason, the dosage of Hou Po and Sheng Jiang is larger than Ren Shen and Gan Cao in order to alleviate the abdominal distension, and the dosage of Ban Xia should be 10g. For more significant qi deficiency, Bai Zhu and Fu Ling are added to assist Ren Shen and Gan Cao in their function of reinforcing the spleen and augmenting qi, whilst enhancing the formula's action of resolving damp. If damp is a predominating factor, Cang Zhu, Chen Pi and Fu Ling can be added to strengthen the spleen's function of transforming water.

Case Study

Gastritis

Extracted from Xin Zhong Yi 2005 August Vol 37 No. 8

A 46-year-old female patient complained of chronic abdominal fullness which had started five months previously. The epigastric distension worsened after meals, there was no nausea or vomiting, her stool and urination were normal, and she had no menstrual problems. The examination revealed a distended epigastrium which was relieved by warmth and pressure. Her tongue was pale with a thin, white greasy coat, and her pulse was moderate and weak. Liu Jun Zi Tang and Ban Xia Xie Xin Tang had previously been prescribed but without effect. An endoscopy had resulted in the diagnosis of atrophic gastritis. The Chinese medicine diagnosis was epigastric pain. She was prescribed Hou Po Sheng Jiang Ban Xia Gan Cao Ren Shen Tang: Fa Ban Xia 15g, Hou Po 15g, Sheng Jiang 15g, Zhi Gan Cao 6g, Dang Shen 5g. After three packs, the abdominal distension eased and a further fifteen packs of the same formula was prescribed to consolidate the treatment.

> **Case Study**
>
> **Diabetes with Abdominal Distension**
>
> ***Extracted from Guo Yi Lun Tan 1997; (3):19***
>
> A 65-year-old male patient had suffered from diabetes for five years and was insulin dependent. During the previous year, his stool alternated between diarrhoea and constipation. Ever since over-eating one week earlier, he had suffered from epigastric and abdominal distension, belching and nausea. He felt fatigued and had a bland taste in the mouth. His tongue coat was white and his pulse was wiry and thready. His blood sugar was 10.2 mmol/L. The Western diagnosis was lowered gastric motility due to diabetes. The Chinese medical diagnosis was spleen deficiency with qi stagnation. The treatment principle was to strengthen the spleen and to alleviate abdominal fullness. Three packs of Hou Po Sheng Jiang Ban Xia Gan Cao Ren Shen Tang were prescribed: Hou Po 15g, Sheng Jiang 12g, Ban Xia 12g, Dang Shen 10g, Gan Cao 10g. After the first pack, the abdominal fullness was reduced and the nausea eased. After the further two packs, there were no more symptoms.

2.7.8 Spleen and Heart Deficiency

Xiao Jian Zhong Tang Pattern

Xiao Jian Zhong Tang pattern is a shang han pattern where there is interior deficiency, with insufficiency of the heart and spleen manifesting as palpitations and vexation.

> **Clause 102**
>
> 伤寒二三日，心中悸而烦者，小建中汤主之。
>
> *Shang han for two or three days, if there are palpitations in the heart and vexation, Xiao Jian Zhong Tang governs.*

XIAO JIAN ZHONG TANG: Gui Zhi (bark removed) 3 liang; Zhi Gan Cao 2 liang; Da Zao (broken) 12 pieces; Shao Yao 6 liang; Sheng Jiang (sliced) 3 liang; Yi Tang 1 sheng.

DIRECTIONS: Decoct the first four ingredients in 7 sheng of water and reduce to 3 sheng. Then strain the decoction and add Yi Tang, reducing the flame to allow it to melt without caramelising. Take 1 sheng three times a day. Because of its sweet flavour, Xiao Jian Zhong Tang is not suitable for patients who suffer from nausea or vomiting.

DISCUSSION: Clause 102 describes the situation where the patient has contracted shang han two or three days earlier. Neither diaphoretic nor purgative treatment was given and the patient now has palpitations and vexation. The palpitations are associated with yang deficiency whilst the vexation is associated with yin deficiency, and so we can understand that the disorder is a pattern of dual deficiency of yin and yang, where there is also an insufficiency of qi and blood.

The objective of Xiao Jian Zhong Tang is to warm and nourish the middle qi in order to resolve the pathogen, a strategy demonstrative of the adage: 'In deficiency, one must reinforce the middle'. Xiao Jian Zhong Tang is a variation of Gui Zhi Tang where the dosage of Shao Yao is doubled and Yi Tang is added. Gui Zhi regulates the spleen and stomach and harmonises yin and yang; Shao Yao nourishes the ying blood; Yi Tang warms and nourishes the spleen and stomach and, combined with Shao Yao, is able to supplement yin. The pathogenesis of the Xiao Jian Zhong Tang pattern can be attributed to either of the following: (1) deficiency cold of the spleen and stomach, resulting in an insufficiency of qi and blood which is characterised by occasional abdominal pain relieved by warmth and pressure; or (2) deficiency detriment disorder characterised by palpitations and vexation, where the vexation is due to insufficient qi and blood failing to nourish the heart, combined with pathogenic harassment. The formula Jian Zhong Tang or 'Strengthen the Middle Decoction' is named for its function of supplementing the spleen in order to bolster the source of qi and blood.

NOTE: Deficiency detriment disorder or *xu lao* (虚劳) was first mentioned in *Jin Gui Yao Lue* and was discussed by many authors in the Ming dynasty. In simple terms it refers to deficiency of both yin and yang. Because yang deficiency is characterised by cold and yin deficiency can lead to heat, a patient suffering from deficiency detriment often presents with a complex pattern of heat and cold.

Ancient Application of Xiao Jian Zhong Tang

- *Qian Jin Yao Fang:* For the treatment of deficiency due to taxation fatigue or late-stage febrile disease manifesting with heaviness in the limbs, aching muscles, shortness of breath, wheezing, a sensation of fullness in the chest, rapid breathing lower back ache, palpitations, a parched throat and lips, a lack-lustre complexion, poor appetite, pain in the hypochondrium, abdominal distension, heaviness in the head or progressive weight loss.

Modern Application of Xiao Jian Zhong Tang

Used in the treatment of stomach disorders, which may include gastritis, duodenal ulcer, stomach prolapse, chronic hepatitis, low grade fever, night sweats, post-partum deficiency and abdominal pain.

Modifications

- For spontaneous sweating, add Huang Qi.
- For night sweats, add Fu Xiao Mai, Mu Li.
- For palpitations and fright, add Long Gu, Mu Li.
- For poor appetite, add Ji Nei Jin, Shen Qu, Shan Zha.
- For pain in the hypochondrium, add Chai Hu, Yu Jin, Chuan Lian Zi, Yuan Hu.
- For qi deficiency, add Dang Shen, Huang Qi.
- For deficient detriment disorder with cough, add Wu Wei Zi, Bai Bu.
- For chronic constipation in the elderly, add Bai Shao 30g, Huang Qi, Rou Cong Rong, Suo Yang.

Case Study

Palpitations and Anaemia

Extracted from Si Chuan Zhong Yi 1987; 12:22

A 35-year-old female patient had suffered palpitations for over three months. Even slight exertion could cause coughing or wheezing, vertigo, dizziness or tinnitus. She had a poor appetite, a pale complexion and also suffered with a plum-stone throat or globus hystericus. Her tongue was pale with a thin, white tongue coat and her pulse was thready and moderate. Her haemoglobin reading was 80 g/L (N=119–160). The principle of treatment was to tonify the middle and generate blood. Xiao Jian Zhong Tang was prescribed with the addition of Ban Xia 18g, Jie Geng 20g and Ju Hong 30g. After three days, she improved and was given another twelve packs to consolidate the treatment.

2.7.9 Kidney Yang Deficiency

There are two transmuted patterns associated with damage to kidney yang, both characterised by vexation. The first is a Gan Jiang Fu Zi Tang pattern, where the yang has been damaged by inappropriate purgation, and the second is a Fu Ling Si Ni Tang pattern, where both yin and yang have been damaged by inappropriate diaphoresis and purgation. Whilst bearing many similarities, in the Gan Jiang Fu Zi Tang pattern, the pathogen has completely transmitted to the interior and no exterior symptoms remain. The Tai Yang and Shao Yin channels stand in an exterior–interior relationship and any incorrect treatment of Tai Yang disease has the potential to injure Shao Yin. Because Shao Yin is related to the heart and kidneys, it is associated with fire and water, representing the root of yin and yang. If both yin and yang are damaged, this will result in the non-interaction of yin and yang and may manifest as vexation. Fu Ling Si Ni Tang principally addresses Shao Yin yang deficiency characterised by aversion to cold, cold extremities due to devastation of yang, and a faint and thready pulse. Fu Ling Si Ni Tang restores yang whilst supporting yin.

Gan Jiang Fu Zi Tang Pattern

Gan Jiang Fu Zi Tang pattern represents the situation where, after the promotion of sweating, Tai Yang disease has been treated improperly with purging and the damage to yang qi has resulted in vexation.

Clause 61

下之后，复发汗，昼日烦躁不得眠，夜而安静，不呕不渴，无表证，脉沉微，身无大热者，干姜附子汤主之。

After purging, sweating is again promoted, in the daytime the patient is vexed, agitated and unable to sleep, in the night-time, however, quiet and peaceful, there is no vomiting and no thirst, an absence of exterior symptoms, a pulse which is submerged and faint, if no vigorous fever, Gan Jiang Fu Zi Tang governs.

GAN JIANG FU ZI TANG: Gan Jiang 1 liang; Fu Zi 1 piece (raw with skin removed and cut into eight slices).

DIRECTIONS: Boil the ingredients in 3 sheng of water and reduce to 1 sheng. Strain and take in a single dose.

DISCUSSION: When the sequence of treatments is incorrect and purging therapy is administered before the promotion of sweat in Tai Yang disease, the yang qi is damaged and the patient will exhibit symptoms of yang deficiency. Yang is the energy which prevails in the day and yin is the energy of the night, and so, in the daytime, the depleted yang qi manages to resist the interior yin cold, but struggles to do so, and the struggle results in vexation. At night, the impaired yang is insufficient to contend with the prevailing yin and so the patient is sedated and quiet. This is to be distinguished from normal restful sleep because the patient's qi is flagging and their spirit is depressed. The submerged, faint pulse denotes yang deficiency with exuberant yin; the absence of exterior symptoms confirms that it is an interior pattern; the statement that there is an absence of a vigorous or high fever implies that the patient does have a slight fever. However, when taking into account the submerged, faint pulse, it is clear that the slight fever is a false sign, and the pattern is one of true cold and false heat, where the true yang is being displaced to the exterior by the exuberant yin. The absence of vomiting shows that the stomach qi is not too badly damaged, and the absence of thirst indicates that it is a pattern of interior cold. The treatment principle therefore is to disperse cold and warm the interior and Gan Jiang Fu Zi Tang is appropriate. Fu Zi resuscitates devastated yang and in its raw state this function is more potent. Its combination with Gan Jiang not only increases the warming function of the formula but also moderates the toxic properties of the unprepared Fu Zi. The direction to take the decoction in one single dose relates to the urgency of the condition.

Ancient Application of Gan Jiang Fu Zi Tang

- *San Yin Fang:* Used for the treatment of cold strike with sudden syncope characterised by nausea and copious salivation.
- *Wei Sheng Bao Jian:* With the addition of Ren Shen ½ liang for the treatment of yin exuberance repelling yang, characterised by generalised coldness, a submerged and faint pulse, vexation and no thirst.

Modern Application of Gan Jiang Fu Zi Tang

This formula is indicated in the case of severe yang desertion because of its capacity to resuscitate yang and warm the kidneys and spleen. It can be used in the treatment of congestive heart disease with oedema, liver cirrhosis with ascites, stomach pain due to cold, nephritis with oedema, hypovolaemic shock due to infection, dizziness due to low blood sugar, hypotension and Meniere's syndrome when due to yang deficiency. For treatment of hypovolaemic shock with low blood pressure, this formula should be combined with Sheng Mai San.

Fu Ling Si Ni Tang Pattern

Clause 69

发汗，若下之， 病仍不解，烦躁者，茯苓四逆汤主之。

Having promoted sweat, where there was purging, if the disease is still not resolved, and there is vexation, Fu Ling Si Ni Tang governs.

FU LING SI NI TANG: Fu Ling 4 liang; Ren Shen 1 liang; Fu Zi 1 piece (raw with skin removed and cut into eight slices); Zhi Gan Cao 2 liang; Gan Jiang 1½ liang.

DIRECTIONS: Boil the ingredients in 5 sheng of water, reducing to 3 sheng. Take 7 ge warm three times a day.

DISCUSSION: Inappropriate promotion of sweat in the treatment of Tai Yang disease will injure yang, and incorrect purging will cause damage to yin. If, after the promotion of sweat and subsequent purging, the disease is not resolved, then there will be transmutation. The Tai Yang channel has an exterior–interior relationship with the Shao Yin, so incorrect treatment of Tai Yang disease may have an adverse effect on the Shao Yin. The Shao Yin division comprises the heart and kidney, the organs of water and fire, representing true yin and true yang, with the kidneys seen as the source of prenatal yin and yang. Damage to the Shao Yin can disturb the interaction of fire and water, resulting in non-communication of the heart and kidney, and manifesting as restlessness and vexation. The underlying disorder is yang deficiency in the Shao Yin. The symptoms include aversion to cold, cold limbs due to devastation of yang, and a pulse that is faint and thready. Fu Ling Si Ni Tang supports the yang and nourishes the yin which was damaged by the purgation.

Gan Jiang and Fu Zi rescue devastated yang; Ren Shen augments qi and benefits the source, generates fluids, calms the spirit and eases the palpitations. The combination of Gan Jiang, Ren Shen and Fu Zi not only restores the yang but also augments the yin. Fu Ling tonifies the spleen and calms the spirit. Gan Cao tonifies qi, harmonises the middle and moderates the action of the other herbs.

The pathogenesis of this pattern is deficiency of both yin and yang. Yang deficiency is predominant and so there are cold extremities, a faint and thready pulse verging on expiry, cold diarrhoea and a pale tongue with a slippery white tongue coat. In modern clinical practice, Fu Ling Si Ni Tang is used in the the treatment of disorders arising from spleen and kidney yang deficiency which include abdominal distension and diarrhoea with vexation, as can be found in chronic gastritis and colitis, and also for the fluid retention of congestive heart failure.

Summary of Fu Ling Si Ni Tang Pattern

Fu Ling Si Ni Tang is a shang han pattern where there is a pre-existing deficiency of both yin and yang, although yang deficiency predominates. Incorrect sweat promotion causes a further deterioration of yin and yang and the indicated treatment is to support the yang first before supplementing the yin. This is based on the theory of tonifying yang in order to generate yin.

Comparison of Gan Jiang Fu Zi Tang and Fu Ling Si Ni Tang Patterns

Both Fu Ling Si Ni Tang and Gan Jiang Fu Zi Tang patterns are transmuted patterns of Tai Yang which are characterised by vexation. Although tthe formulas for both are based on Si Ni Tang and its modifications, there are significant differences. Gan Jiang Fu Zi Tang is indicated for yang deficiency with exuberant yin cold. In the daytime, the patient is vexed and agitated and can not sleep, but is very quiet and restful at night; there is a mild fever, no vomiting, no thirst, no exterior symptoms, and the pulse is submerged and faint. The daytime vexation represents the struggle of weak yang, assisted by environmental yang qi, in its attempt to prevail over the exuberant yin; and the nighttime restfulness is a reflection of the complete predominance of yin over yang. The treatment is based on the urgent resuscitation of yang. In a Fu Ling Si Ni Tang pattern, yang is deficient, but there is also damage to yin, and vexation is apparent day and night; the accompanying symptoms are aversion to cold, cold extremities, diarrhoea, and pulse which is faint and thready. The treatment strategy is to resuscitate yang and augment yin.

Case Study

Vexation

Extracted from Zhong Yi Za Zhi 1965; 1:28

The patient had a weak constitution and was very thin. He presented with extreme vexation and had suicidal thoughts. Previous to the consultation, he had suffered from headache and slight vexation and had undergone treatment using cold herbs to clear heat. The medication was not effective and the condition had worsened. His complexion was grey and he felt tired and also had a wheeze, shortness of breath, oily sweat, cold extremities and a submerged and thready pulse. He was given a formula based on Fu Ling Si Ni Tang: Fu Ling 30g; Korean Ginseng 30g; Pao Fu Zi 30g; Pao Gan Jiang 30g; Gan Cao 30g. The herbs were to be decocted and taken in a single dose. After the medication, his irritability eased considerably and the same formula was repeated in a reduced dosage for a further ten packs.

Zhen Wu Tang Pattern

Clause 82

太阳病发汗，汗出不解，其人仍发热，心下悸、头眩、身瞤动，振振欲擗地者，真武汤主之。

Tai Yang disease, sweat is promoted, there is sweating with no resolution, if the person still has fever, palpitations below the heart, dizziness, the body is twitching, trembling and about to fall down, Zhen Wu Tang governs.

ZHEN WU TANG: Fu Ling 3 liang; Shao Yao 3 liang; Bai Zhu 2 liang; Sheng Jiang (sliced) 3 liang; Fu Zi (skin removed, broken into 8 and dry-fried) 1 piece.

DIRECTIONS: Boil all five ingredients in 8 sheng of water, reducing to 3 sheng. Strain and take 7 ge warm three times a day. If there is a cough, add Wu Wei Zi ½ sheng, Xi Xin 1 liang, Gan Jiang 1 liang; if urination is uninhibited, omit Fu Ling; if there is diarrhoea, omit Shao Yao and add Gan Jiang 2 liang; if there is vomiting, omit Fu Zi and add Sheng Jiang to give a total of ½ jin.

DISCUSSION: Although the promotion of sweat is a standard strategy in the treatment of Tai Yang exterior excess, strong promotion of sweat in Tai Yang exterior deficiency is contraindicated. If inappropriate sweating is promoted in a deficient patient, the interior will be damaged and a transmuted pattern is likely to develop. Clause 82 describes a situation where even after sweating, the exterior pathogen remains unresolved. The loss of sweat has damaged the yang qi of the Shao Yin and a transmuted pattern has arisen. The deficent kidney yang is unable to transform qi and control yin, and this is a pattern of deficient yang with exuberant yin and water qi. The fever is a manifestation of upcast yang; the palpitations below the heart are a result of water qi harassing the heart. The upper body is yang and the head is the focus of yang qi, with all yang channels meeting at the vertex. The water qi follows the movement of yang qi and causes vertigo or dizziness. The insufficiency of yang qi throughout the body, combined with the agitation of the water qi, results in muscle twitching and body tremor, to the point where the equilibrium is unstable and the person almost loses balance and falls to the ground.

Fu Zi is acrid and hot and its function is to fortify kidney yang, tonify the fire of ming men (the life gate) and support the kidney function of transforming water. In *Ben Cao Zheng Yi* 本草正义 (*Rectification of the Meaning of the Materia Medica Zhang Shan Lei*, 1914): "Fu Zi is a pure yang herb which penetrates the twelve channels, reaching the exterior to expel exterior cold, and reaching the interior to warm the true yang." Bai Zhu is bitter and warm. It strengthens the spleen's function of transforming and transporting, dries damp and promotes urination. Fu Ling is sweet and bland and so drains damp by promoting urination. The combination of these two herbs enhances the formula's function of draining damp. Sheng Jiang is acrid and warm, it disperses the water qi, warms and harmonises the stomach and assists Fu Zi to warm the yang and transform qi. Shao Yao is sour and cold. It eases spasm and nourishes yin, thus counteracting the harsh properties of Fu Zi and protecting the yin. When Shao Yao is combined with Fu Zi, the Fu Zi exerts a warming effect to counter the coldness of Shao Yao, and when combined with Shao Yao, it resuscitates the devasted yang without being too hot. Clause 82 lists additional symptoms for which modifications must be made. For cough, add Gan Jiang to warm the lungs and transform phlegm, Xi Xin to disperse cold, warm the lung and dry phlegm, and Wu Wei Zi to astringe the lung qi. Where there is copious or frequent urination, omit Fu Ling. Where there is diarrhoea, omit Shao Yao and add Gan Jiang. Where there is vomiting, omit Fu Zi and add Sheng Jiang to harmonise the stomach and redirect qi downward.

2.7.10 Dual Deficiency of Yin and Yang

The two patterns representing dual deficiency of yin and yang are:

1. Gan Cao Gan Jiang Tang and Shao Yao Gan Cao Tang represent yin, yang, interior and exterior deficiency.
2. Shao Yao Gan Cao Fu Zi Tang pattern is a pattern of yin and yang deficiency after sweat promotion.

Clause 60

下之后，复发汗，必振寒，脉微细。所以然者，以内外俱虚故也。

After purgation, sweat is again promoted, there will be shivering cold, the pulse is faint and thready. The reason for this being, the interior and exterior are both deficient.

DISCUSSION: Incorrect purgation will damage the interior yin fluids and sweat promotion will damage the exterior yang. This clause describes a situation where, contrary to fundamental treatment protocols, purging was carried out ahead of sweat promotion. Although the exterior pathogen has been resolved by the sweating, the interior zheng qi has been damaged by the purgation, giving rise to a transmuted pattern. Insufficient yang is unable to warm the body and secure the exterior, and so the body shivers with cold. A faint pulse is one which lacks force under the pressure of the fingers, and is verging on expiry; a thready pulse is one which under the fingers feels thin and fine like a thread. The faint and thready pulse is testament to a dual deficiency of yin and yang, with the faint pulse reflecting a deficiency of wei qi and yang, and the thready pulse indicating a deficiency of ying blood and yin. Thus the faint and thready pulse reflects not only a deficiency of the exterior and interior, but also a dual deficiency of yin and yang, and so Zhong Jing used the term interior and exterior deficiency to refer to both conditions.

In treating the above pattern, it must be remembered that it is a dual pattern of devastated yang and exhausted yin. The practitioner, therefore, must not only address those deficiencies, but also assess their relative severity and tailor the treatment accordingly. Because incorrect purgation and sweating are the cause of the pattern, and in view of the symptom of shivering cold, more emphasis should be placed on fortifying yang. Gan Jiang and Fu Zi fortify yang, Ren Shen augments qi and yin; appropriate formulas are Zhen Wu Tang or Fu Zi Tang.

Gan Cao Gan Jiang Tang and Shao Yao Gan Cao Tang Patterns

These patterns represent yin, yang, interior and exterior deficiency and as such, the treatment strategy is first to warm and restore the yang and then to nourish the yin.

Clause 29

（一）伤寒脉浮，自汗出，小便数，心烦，微恶寒、脚挛急，反与桂枝欲攻其表，此误也。得之便厥、咽中干、烦躁吐逆者，作甘草干姜汤与之，以复其阳。（二）若厥愈足温者，更作芍药甘草汤与之，其脚即伸。（三）若胃气不和 谵语者，少与调胃承气汤。（四）若重发汗，复加烧针者，四逆汤主之。

(1) Shang han the pulse is floating, there is spontaneous sweating, frequent urination, there will be heart vexation, a slight aversion to cold, and cramps in the feet, but Gui Zhi Tang is given to attack the exterior, this is a mistake. Having given it, there is jue, the throat is dry, and if there is vexation and agitation with vomiting due to reversal, administer Gan Cao Gan Jiang Tang to restore the yang. (2) If the jue recovers and the feet become warm, then after administering Shao Yao Gan Cao Tang, the feet will then stretch. (3) Where the stomach qi is disharmonious, if the

speech is delirious, give a little Tiao Wei Cheng Qi Tang. (4) Where heavy sweating was promoted, if then there is repeated hot needling, Si Ni Tang governs.

GAN CAO GAN JIANG TANG: Zhi Gan Cao 4 liang; Gan Jiang 2 liang.

DIRECTIONS: Boil the ingredients in 3 sheng of water, reduce to 1 sheng 5 ge (1½ sheng), then strain. Divide into two doses to be taken warm twice in the one day.

SHAO YAO GAN CAO TANG: Bai Shao 4 liang; Zhi Gan Cao 4 liang.

DIRECTIONS: Boil the ingredients in 3 sheng of water, reducing to 1 sheng 5 ge (1½ sheng), strain and take warm twice a day.

DISCUSSION: The first sentence in Clause 29 describes a situation where incorrect treatment has resulted in a transmuted pattern and the next four sentences particularise four situations, each requiring a different formula.

1. The pattern described in the first sentence is not a Gui Zhi Tang pattern. Although the floating pulse, spontaneous sweating and slight aversion to cold are all representative of a Tai Yang exterior deficiency pattern, there are manifestations of an interior pattern: frequent urination indicates that yang qi is deficient and unable to control the gates; the vexation and foot cramps are symptoms of yin deficiency, where yin can not nourish the sinews. In this pattern, an exterior cold pathogen was contracted on a background of a pre-existing deficiency of both yin and yang. The appropriate strategy is to release the exterior whilst simultaneously supporting the yang. The administration of Gui Zhi Tang was a critical error, because by releasing the exterior through diaphoresis, there was further depletion of yin as shown by the dry throat; desertion of yang has caused coldness in the four limbs, termed jue; because yin is deficient, the heart shen is not nourished and there is vexation; deficient yang can not control yin, and the yin pathogen harasses the stomach causing vomiting. This pattern represents a dual deficiency of yin and yang, but the correct treatment is to give priority to the restoration of yang, and so Gan Cao Gan Jiang Tang is indicated.
2. Once the yang is restored, as evidenced by the feet being warm, the second stage of treatment is the administration of Shao Yao Gan Cao Tang. Where yin is deficient the sinews are not nourished, and so Shao Yan Gan Cao Tang is chosen to nourish the yin and relax the sinews, thus allowing them to stretch.
3. The root of this disorder, namely a dual deficiency of both yin and yang, has allowed the pathogen to transform into dryness. This is because the administration of herbs to restore yang tend to consume yin. The depleted yin is unable to control yang and there is dryness in the stomach, affecting the Yang Ming. The dryness can generate heat causing stomach disharmony characterised by delirious speech. Because the onset of the condition is recent, a small dose of Tiao Wei Cheng Qi Tang will be effective in draining the heat so as to relieve the dryness.
4. Further promotion of sweat would repeat the original error and the use of hot needling would compound the adverse treatment. Devastation of yang would undoubtedly result and so Si Ni Tang is required to resuscitate the yang.

Gan Cao Gan Jiang Tang warms the middle, disperses cold and restores the yang qi of the middle jiao. The objective of Gan Cao and Gan Jiang in this formula is the same as in Li Zhong Wan; however, in this formula, the dosage of Gan Cao is double that of Gan Jiang in order to tonify and harmonise the qi of the middle jiao, and to moderate the drying properties of Gan Jiang. Together, they disperse cold, rescue yang, and restore the proper function of the spleen and stomach qi. Shao Yao Gan Cao Tang augments yin, nourishes blood and softens the liver and is thus able to nourish the sinews and relieve the spasms and leg cramps.

Ancient Application of Gan Cao Gan Jiang Tang

- *Wai Tai Mi Yao*: For the treatment of vomiting.

- *Zhi Zhi Fang*: For the treatment of haemorrhage due to stomach coldness.
- *Zhu Shi Ji Yan Fang*: Nominates Er Shen Tang (an alternative name for Gan Cao Gan Jiang Tang) for the treatment of haemoptysis.

Modern Application of Gan Cao Gan Jiang Tang

Gan Cao Gan Jiang Tang can be used to treat a variety of cold patterns, including cough or asthma, vertigo, acid reflux, chest or epigastric pain, diarrhoea, enuresis and dysmenorrhoea, provided they are characterised by symptoms for which Gan Cao Gan Jiang Tang is indicated. For effective outcomes, appropriate modifications are essential and the dosage of Gan Jiang can be varied from 15–20g with no adverse effects. (Tang Zhu Xuan et al *Zhejiang Zhong Yi Za Zhi* 1:40, 1982).

Modifications

- For haemoptysis, add Wu Wei Zi.
- For blood in the stool add Qing Bai Ye, Ban Xia and Zao Xin Tu.
- Where there is spleen deficiency, the dosage of Gan Jiang can be increased.

NOTES: (1) This formula is contraindicated where there is a rapid pulse and a crimson tongue with a dry, yellow tongue coat. (2) It was reported that too large a dose of Gan Jiang can cause facial swelling and scant urination, however the symptoms resolve when the medication is stopped.

In *Shang Han Lun Yu Lin Chuang,* Prof Nie Hui Ming reported using Gan Cao Gan Jiang Tang for the treatment of abdominal pain due to stomach cold with the following modifications.

- If the abdominal pain is characterised by a preference for pressure, Dang Shen, Gui Zhi, Xiang Fu and Yan Hu should be added.
- If there is intestinal rumbling and diarrhoea, Fu Ling, Chao Yi Ren, Chao Bai Zhu and Dang Shen should be added.
- For the treatment of haemoptysis and blood in the stool due to spleen and stomach deficiency, Fu Long Gan can be used with the addition of Xian He Cao and Bai Ji. Fu Long Gan (伏龙肝) is an alternative name for Zao Xin Tu (灶心土), which is the yellow roasted earth taken from the ashes of an oven. It enters the spleen and stomach channels and warms the middle. If Zao Xin Tu is required in a formula, it must be wrapped in gauze and decocted first. It is then removed and the other herbs cooked in the decoction.

Ancient Application of Shao Yao Gan Cao Tang

- *Gu Jin Yi Tong:* For the treatment of abdominal pain.
- *Huo Ren Shi Zheng Fang:* Shen Gong San (an alternative name for Shao Yao Gan Cao Tang) was cited in the treatment of diabetes.
- *Zhu Shi Ji Yan Fang:* To treat weakness in the legs and difficulty in walking.
- *Yi Xue Xin Wu:* This formula was used with the addition of Gan Jiang to treat abdominal pain due to cold and characterised by moderate pulse. If there is heat, characterised by a flooding pulse, then Huang Lian should be added.

Modern Application of Shao Yao Gan Cao Tang

Modern research has shown that Shao Yao Gan Cao Tang has a moderating effect on both skeletal and smooth muscle and is therefore able to relieve cramps. It can be used extensively in the treatment of gastro-intestinal disease, upper respiratory tract disease, urinary tract disorders and gallbladder disease. In addition, it can be used to treat headache, sciatic pain, intercostal neuralgia, leg cramps and dysmenorrhoea. It also has an anti-inflammatory action and can inhibit the production of stomach acid.

Professor Nie Hui Ming used this formula to treat stomach pain associated with disharmony of the liver and stomach, modifying it with the addition of Chai Hu, Zhi Shi, Yu Jin to regulate qi and ease pain. Further modifications are as follows.

- For cholelithiasis, add Jin Qian Cao, Chai Hu, Ji Nei Jin.
- For headache, add Dang Gui, Bai Zhi, Gao Ben.
- For leg cramps, add Niu Xi, Mu Gua, Yi Ren.

- For pain associated with qi stagnation, add Xiang Fu, Wu Yao, Chai Hu.
- For pain with blood stasis, add Hong Hua, Dan Shen, Yan Hu.

Shao Yao Gan Cao Fu Zi Tang Pattern

This is a pattern of yin and yang deficiency following inappropriate promotion of sweat.

> **Clause 68**
>
> 发汗，病不解，反恶寒者，虚故也，芍药甘草附子汤主之。
>
> *After promoting sweat, if the disease is not resolved, instead there is aversion to cold, it is due to deficiency, Shao Yao Gan Cao Fu Zi Tang governs.*

SHAO YAO GAN CAO FU ZI TANG: Shao Yao 3 liang; Zhi Gan Cao 3 liang; Fu Zi 1 piece (blast roasted, skin removed and cut into eight slices).

DIRECTIONS: Boil the ingredients in 5 sheng of water, reducing to 1½ sheng. Strain and divide into three doses to be taken warm three times in the one day.

DISCUSSION: Clause 68 describes what started as a Tai Yang exterior pattern. The promotion of sweat should resolve the pathogen, and if resolved, there would no longer be aversion to cold. However, in this case, the aversion to cold remains after the promotion of sweat, and this is ascribed to deficiency. The deficiency is of yin and yang. This can be surmised from the formula, which supplements both yin and yang, and it must also be surmised that the sweating was excessive, and it is the inappropriate sweating which has depleted the yin fluids and the yang qi. Shao Yao Gan Cao Fu Zi Tang, which is Shao Yao Gan Cao Tang with the addition of Fu Zi, fortifies yang and augments yin, and so is the indicated formula. Fu Zi is acrid and hot; it warms the channels and by restoring yang, reinforces the defensive qi. Shao Yao is cool and sour; it conserves yin and nourishes blood. Gan Cao is sweet and warm; it tonifies the middle qi and supplements blood. The combined effect of the three herbs is to tonify yin and yang.

> **Case Study**
>
> **Abdominal Pain**
>
> ***Extracted from Shang Han Lun Chan Shi***
>
> The patient presented with severe abdominal pain and a generalised cold sweat. For the previous eight years he had suffered from extreme sensitivity to cold and had been given such potent herbs as Ren Shen and Lu Rong, and also the formula Si Jun Zi Tang using a large dose of Ren Shen, but these treatments were not effective. His pulse was thready and choppy and his tongue coat was white and greasy. He was given Shao Yao Gan Cao Fu Zi Tang. After the initial dose, the patient had intestinal rumbling and diarrhoea and felt irritable. This was followed by an attack of cold sweat, after which the abdominal pain eased considerably. The same formula was repeated for two more days and he recovered fully.
>
> **Discussion:** The potent tonic herbs were not effective because they did not address the key point of the patient's pattern, which was yang deficiency, not qi deficiency. The aversion to cold, the white greasy tongue coat and the thready, choppy pulse show interior cold congealed in the channels. The cold sweat is a sign of devastated yang. Fu Zi is required to rescue yang, warm the interior and dispel cold from the channels, eliminating the congealed cold and thus promoting the flow of qi and blood to ease the pain. Gan Cao and Shao Yao relax spasms to ease pain, and together supplement qi and preserve yin, thus countering the harsh properties of Fu Zi. The return of the yang qi is shown by the movement of qi in the abdomen and the irritability. The diarrhoea and cold sweat are a means of expelling the pathogenic cold.

Section Eight

2.8 TRANSMUTED PATTERNS FOLLOWING INAPPROPRIATE THERAPY

2.8.1 Transmuted Patterns Caused by Fire Therapy

Incorrect or inappropriate fire therapy can result in the conversion of physiological fire to pathological fire. The pathogen is fuelled by the fire therapy and this results in a transmuted pattern where fire harasses the mind causing vexation, and scorches the vessels causing bleeding. This phenomenon is known as fire counterflow. There are three transmuted patterns arising from inappropriate fire therapy. These are fire harassment due to (1) fire fuming therapy (Clause 114); (2) Incorrect moxibustion (Clauses 115 and 116); and (3) Inappropriate administration of a hot compress (Clause 110). In this section, the prognosis of transmuted patterns associated with fire counterflow (Clause 111) and fire therapy used in warm disease are also discussed (Clause 113).

Fire Harassment Following Fuming Therapy

An ancient method of promoting sweating in the treatment of exterior disorders was fire fuming therapy. This is inappropriate in the treatment of Tai Yang disease and could give rise to the transmuted pattern of fire counterflow with blood in the stool. The term fire counterflow (火逆) refers to the situation where there is a patient with a constitutional yin deficiency who suffers an attack by an exterior pathogen, and is then treated inappropriately with fire therapy to promote sweating. Because the fire therapy has been used inappropriately and excessively, it transforms into interior pathogenic fire, which exacerbates the pre-existing yin deficiency and fuels the existing empty fire. The fire obstructs the proper dispersal of yin and results in impediment from the waist down, causing a sensation of heaviness. The frenetic flow of blood is due to the fire depleting the yin, harassing blood and scorching the vessels.

Clause 114

太阳病，以火熏之，不得汗，其人必躁；到经不解，必清血，名为火邪。

Tai Yang disease, because of fuming by fire, sweating is not obtained, the person will be agitated; if it reaches the channel and does not resolve, there will be blood in the stool, it is called fire evil.

DISCUSSION: The correct treatment for a Tai Yang exterior pattern is to use herbs to release the exterior and promote sweat. The use of fire fuming therapy is inappropriate because it can fail to promote sweat and instead result in the introduction of fire to the interior. The resulting harassment of the heart shen causes vexation, and if the fire enters the blood, it will flow recklessly and leave the channels, so there will be qing xue (清血) or blood in the stool. As stated in *Shang Han Lun Tiao Bian*: "If pathogenic fire harasses the blood and infiltrates the intestines, there will be blood in the stool".

The reference to agitation in the above clause has been subject to various interpretations by ancient scholars. Zhang Yin An suggested that the fire fuming therapy damages the heart shen; Wang Hu suggests the ensuing heat pathogen may damage the stomach; Cheng Wu Ji suggests that the fire and heat cause the yin deficiency. Based on the vexation resulting from fire fuming therapy, Zhang Yin An's interpretation is more appropriate. The incorrect use of fire therapy harasses the ying blood causing the heart shen to be disturbed. In regard to the statement: "if it reaches the channel and does not resolve", Cheng Wu Ji's annotation in *Zhu Jie Shang Han Lun* explains that after six days, the pathogen has completed its passage through the channels and on the seventh day returned to Tai Yang. The significance of this is twofold: if on completing its passage through the six channels, there is headache on the seventh day, then there will be spontaneous recovery. However, as in this case, if the pathogen is not resolved, there will be exuberant heat which falls deep into the interior, harassing the blood and causing bleeding.

Zhang Zhong Jing describes the condition without suggesting treatment. Guo Yong, in his book *Shang Han Bu Wang Lun*, suggested the appropriate treatment is to nourish yin and cool blood and recommended the formula Xi Jiao Di Huang Tang (Sheng Di 12g, Dang Gui 9g, Gan Cao 4.5g, Huang Lian 6g, Chao Zhi Zi 3g, Xuan Shen 9g and Huang Qin 6g). An alternative formula is Liang Xue Di Huang Tang from *Xue Zheng Lun* (Sheng Di 4 qian, Dang Gui 3 qian, Gan Cao 1.5 qian, Huang Lian 2 qian, Chao Zhi Zi 1 qian, Xuan Shen 3 qian, Huang Qin 2 qian).

The purpose of Clause 114 is to heighten the practitioner's awareness of the risks of fire therapy and its potential to injure blood, so that adverse outcomes can be avoided. A parallel of this pathogenesis of 'fire evil' can be seen in the contemporary use of radiotherapy, which can cause nosebleed or blood in the stool.

Fire Harassment Following Moxibustion

Clause 115

脉浮、热甚，而反灸之，此为实。实以虚治，因火而动，必咽燥、吐血。

The pulse is floating, the fever is extreme, despite this moxibustion is used, this is excess. Excess has been treated as deficiency, because of the fire there is activity, the throat will be parched, and there will be vomiting of blood.

DISCUSSION: A floating pulse with a high fever indicates an exterior excess yang pattern. The correct treatment is to release the exterior using acrid cooling herbs. The phrase, 'excess has been treated as deficiency', alludes to the fact that moxibustion is used for deficiency or yin patterns and its use in a yang pattern has the adverse effect of exacerbating the pathogenic heat. Fire scorches the network vessels causing the blood to move recklessly and leave the vessels, resulting in the vomiting of blood; the fire also injures the body fluids, causing the throat to feel parched. This is referred to as fire counterflow.

Both Clause 114 and Clause 115 describe the adverse outcomes of inappropriate fire therapy. Clause 114 describes the consequences of fire fuming therapy and Clause 115 describes a similarly adverse outcome after inappropriate moxibustion. Both treatments cause bleeding due to the frenetic movement of blood, the former resulting in the passing of blood in the stool and the latter in the vomiting of blood. Both clauses are therefore associated with the transmission of the pathogen from the qi level to blood level. The Qing dynasty scholar Ye Tian Shi summarised this in his statement: "If the condition has entered the blood level and it is feared that there will be a frenetic flow of blood, one must cool and disperse blood". Under such circumstances, blood cooling formulas such as Xi Jiao Di Huang Tang can be used to cool the blood or, alternatively, Zhu Ye Shi Gao Tang modified with Shi Hu, Sha Shen and Lu Gen can be used to clear heat and nourish yin.

Clause 116 elaborates on the incorrect application of moxibustion where there is pre-existing yin deficiency with heat signs, and describes its prognosis. The correct treatment for a patient with empty heat characterised by a faint and rapid pulse is to nourish yin and clear heat.

Clause 116

（一）微数之脉，慎不可灸。因火为邪，则为烦逆，追虚逐实，血散脉中，火气虽微，内攻有力，焦骨伤筋，血难复也。（二）脉浮，宜以汗解，用火灸之，邪无从出，因火而盛；病从腰以下，必重而痹，名火逆也。（三）欲自解者，必当先烦，烦乃有汗而解，何以知之？脉浮，故知汗出解。

(1) A faint and rapid pulse, be warned one should not use moxibustion. Because fire is an evil, it will cause vexation and counterflow, by targeting deficiency and pursuing excess, blood will be dissipated in the vessels, even if the fire evil is mild, it will attack the interior vigorously, scorching the bones and injuring the sinews, the blood

will be difficult to restore. (2) If the pulse is floating, it is appropriate to resolve with sweating, using fire or moxibustion, the evil has no place to exit, because the fire is superabundant; the disease is from the waist down, there will be heaviness and impediment, this is called fire counterflow. (3) If there is about to be spontaneous resolution, there must first be vexation, only after vexation will there be sweating and resolution, how does one know this? The pulse is floating, so it is known that sweating brings resolution.

DISCUSSION: Clause 116 is better analysed in three sections.

1. Caution must always be exercised when using moxibustion in a pattern of yin deficiency, and the first section warns that it is not to be used at all when there are signs of heat. A pulse which is faint and rapid is indicative of deficiency heat, where the treatment principle is to nourish yin and clear heat. Vexation and counterflow (烦逆) refer to the phenomenon of fire counterflow, where vexation and other adverse symptoms are the result of exacerbation of heat caused by moxibustion or other fire therapies, which are in diametric opposition to the correct strategy of clearing heat and nourishing yin. The ultimate outcome is generation of excess heat or fire.

   The phrase 'targeting deficiency and pursuing excess' is applied to this situation because the faint pulse is rightly assumed to indicate a deficiency pattern, and the mistaken objective of using moxibustion was to target this deficiency. However, attention was not given to the speed of the pulse, which indicates the presence of heat, where moxa is contraindicated. The phrase 'pursuing excess' refers to the outcome of inappropriate fire therapy, which transforms deficiency heat into excess heat. Moxibustion not only directly exacerbates the heat by introducing fire, but also aggravates internal heat indirectly by further consuming yin, thus generating excess heat, referred to in the clause as 'pursuing excess'. The fire pathogen dissipates the blood, harasses the heart, giving rise to vexation, and scorches the tissues normally nourished by blood. This represents severe injury to blood, which is difficult to restore, and implies that once moxibustion has been incorrectly used in this way, full recovery is difficult even with the adoption of yin and blood nourishing herbs.
2. The second section confirms that a floating pulse indicates an exterior pattern and reminds the practitioner that the appropriate treatment is sweat promotion. The statement that the fire is superabundant and so has no place to exit explains the transformation of deficiency heat into excess heat, which is constrained within the body. The transmutation manifests not only with vexation, but also with a sensation of heaviness and impediment in movement. This is because exuberant yang heat has scorched the yin blood, the kidney and liver yin can not nourish the sinews, and so there is heaviness and impediment in the lower part of the body. There are several interpretations of the heaviness and obstruction experienced from the waist down. Cheng Wu Ji suggests that the yin qi is exuberant in the lower half of the body. Cheng Jiao Qian proposes that the ying qi in the lower jiao is stagnant and exhausted. However, this is a pattern of severely depleted yin, and the authors feel that the most logical explanation is the failure of deficient yin blood to nourish the sinews.
3. For the fire pathogen to be resolved and expelled from the interior, there must first be a return of zheng qi. The vexation which precedes the sweating described in the third section, heralds the uprising of zheng qi as it contends with the pathogen. When it prevails, there is resolution by sweating, because it is an exterior disorder, as evidenced by the floating pulse.

This is a transmuted pattern arising from incorrect treatment, with a pathogenesis of hyperactive yang consuming yin. The vexation followed by sweating when the pulse is floating is a sign of imminent spontaneous recovery. Zhang Zhong Jing did not nominate any treatment but the appropriate strategy is to tonify the liver and kidneys by nourishing yin and blood. Herbs which clear heat and generate fluids should also be used. Of note, Ke Yun Bo suggested that sedating and calming herbs should not be used as they may prevent sweat promotion and thus prevent resolution.

Fire Harassment Following a Hot Compress

Clause 110 describes the application of a hot compress, which is one kind of fire therapy used to promote sweating in the treatment of Tai Yang zhong feng, and also outlines the subsequent transmuted pattern and its prognosis.

Clause 110

（一）太阳病二日，反躁，凡熨其背而大汗出，大热入胃，胃中水竭，躁烦必发谵语。十余日振栗自下利者，此为欲解也。（二）故其汗从腰以下不得汗，欲小便不得，反呕、欲失溲、足下恶风、大便硬、小便当数，而反不数及不多；大便已，头卓然而痛，其人足心必热，谷气下流故也。

(1) Tai Yang disease for two days, but there is agitation, whenever a hot poultice is applied to the back and there is profuse sweating, severe heat will enter the stomach, exhausting the stomach fluids, there will be agitation and vexation with delirious speech. If more than ten days have passed and there is shivering and spontaneous diarrhoea, this means it is about to resolve. (2) And so the sweat will not issue from the waist down, the patient tries to pass urine but can not, instead there is vomiting and almost a loss of continence, the bottoms of the feet are averse to wind, the stool is hard and, although urination should be frequent, it is infrequent and scant; once a stool is passed, there is an extraordinary headache, and the soles of the patient's feet will be hot, this being due to the downward flow of the grain qi.

DISCUSSION: Clause 110 should be read in two parts. The first part describes the incorrect treatment of Tai Yang disease, the adverse effects of that treatment and the mechanism of recovery. Tai Yang disease is an exterior pattern and if treated correctly by promoting sweat to resolve the exterior, there should be no vexation. If, after two days, the Tai Yang pattern remains unresolved and vexation arises, this is indicative of interior heat, similar to that found in a Da Qing Long pattern. At this point, the correct treatment strategy is to release the exterior and clear interior heat. The application of a hot poultice contravenes that principle by introducing excess heat. This exacerbates the existing interior heat and consumes stomach fluids, giving rise to agitated behaviour and delirious speech, which are manifestations of fire counterflow. If, after the passage of ten days, there is shivering and sweating, it is a sign of the zheng qi expelling the exterior pathogen, whilst the diarrhoea is a sign of the expulsion of interior heat. This is because during the ten days, the fire has abated sufficiently for stomach fluids to replenish, facilitating sweating to release the exterior, and the proper descent of stomach qi is restored, facilitating the expulsion of heat via the stool. Therefore the two signs of shivering sweat and diarrhoea demonstrate that the transmuted pattern has reached a turning point and recovery is imminent.

The second section of Clause 110 describes additional symptoms which can occur as a result of adverse fire therapy. Exuberant yang affects the upper half of the body causing sweating in the upper part, and also causes the stomach qi to rebel, manifesting as vomiting. Yang qi does not flow to the lower half of the body, and there is also fluid deprivation because of the heat. Because yang qi fails to transform and descend fluids to the lower half of the body, there is no sweat from the waist down, and although the person feels like passing urine, they are not able to because of the non-descent of fluids. Although urination is difficult, there is a paradoxical tendency to incontinence due to deficient yang being unable to control the lower orifices; because fluids are not descending, the stool is hard; because deficient yang fails to warm the extremities, the lower limbs will be averse to wind.

Patterns of yang deficiency are characterised by frequent copious urination, but here the urination is scant. This is not because it is a heat pattern, but because yang qi is not descending fluids and not supporting the transformation of qi. The absence of sweat in the lower half of the body, the dry stool and the inability to pass urine are all due to deficient yang, not to heat, and the clause goes to some length to be clear that the scant and infrequent urination and dry stool do not represent a Yang Ming pattern. In a Yang Ming excess pattern, consumption of yin by heat produces a dry stool, and in a Tai Yang Yang Ming pattern, the excess stomach heat can inhibit the spleen's transportation of fluids, diverting them from the large intestine to the urinary bladder, which results in a dry stool and frequent urination (see Clause 247 in Chapter Three, describing a Ma Zi Ren Wan pattern).

Further to the symptoms discussed above, is the unexpected phenomenon of severe pain in the head experienced on defaecation and accompanied by a sensation of heat in the soles of the feet. This is the result of the sudden descent of yang qi which causes the stool to descend; this departure of yang qi from the upper jiao suddenly deprives the head of yang, causing pain, and the descent of the yang qi warms the soles of the feet. It is this descent of yang which is described as "the downward movement of grain qi". A converse development is where the yang qi remains constrained in the upper jiao leaving a sensation of cold in the lower jiao.

Various complex patterns are recognised in Chinese medicine. A heat and cold complex where there is heat in the upper jiao and cold in the lower jiao is principally attributed to exuberant yang obstructing the normal ascent and descent of qi. As such, it bears comparison to the Si Ni San pattern, where cold extremities are ascribed to the constraint of yang. The phenomenon of severe headache being experienced on bowel movement is open to numerous interpretations. Cheng Wu Ji suggested that the descent of yang qi to the lower jiao results in inadequate ascent of clear yang to the head. Huang Yuan Yu proposed that the bowel movement drained fire from the head. Cheng Jiao Qian maintained that once the stool was passed, qi in the upper part of the body descended and that of the lower part of the body ascended. These various interpretations are not mutually exclusive but differ as to whether the focus is on the zheng qi or the pathogen.

Whilst the objective of this Clause 110 is to define and describe the outcomes of adverse fire therapy, it also carries significance for diagnosis and treatment in miscellaneous diseases. A cursory reading of the symptoms could lead one to misdiagnose this pattern as one of deficiency cold in the lower jiao, resulting in incorrect tonification and warming strategies. In general terms, the correct treatment strategy is to clear heat and nourish yin, whilst also regulating qi to guide the yang downwards, where it has failed to flow. If clearing heat is a priority, Tiao Wei Cheng Qi Tang can be used; if the focus is on nourishing yin and clearing empty heat, Zhu Ye Shi Gao Tang is a suitable formula. Irrespective of specific strategies employed in particular circumstances, the golden rule of treating in accordance with the pattern identification remains.

Case Study

Chronic Aversion to Cold

Source unknown

A 38-year-old female patient of average constitution regarded herself as being weak and deficient. Her chief complaint was constant aversion to cold and wind, even in the summer months. Other symptoms were an oppressed sensation in the chest, shortness of breath, cool extremities, a submerged and wiry pulse and a red tongue tip with the root being slightly yellow. She had previously been prescribed Bu Zhong Yi Qi Tang and also a formula to tonify the kidney yang to no avail. However, at the consultation she was diagnosed with yang constraint and Si Ni San was given to disperse constraint and free the yang. The result was satisfactory.

Prognosis of Fire Counterflow Patterns

Clause 111

太阳病中风，以火劫发汗。邪风被火热，血气流溢，失其常度，两阳相熏灼，其身发黄。阳盛则欲衄，阴虚小便难。阴阳皆虚竭，身体则枯燥，但头汗出，剂颈而还。腹满、微喘、口干、咽烂，或不大便，久则谵语，甚者至哕、手足躁扰、捻衣摸床。小便利者，其人可治。

Tai Yang zhong feng, fire was used to force sweating. Evil wind was fuelled by the fire, blood and qi flow and spill over, losing normality, these two yang fume and scorch each other, the body turns yellow. Yang exuberance results in a tendency to nosebleed, yin deficiency and inhibited urination. Both yin and yang are deficient and exhausted and the body is withered and dried, sweat pours from the head alone, stopping at the neck. There is abdominal distension, slight wheezing, a dry mouth, ulceration of the throat, or there is no stool, if it persists there will be delirious speech, even to the point of vomiting, the arms and legs are agitated and restless, the patient twists their clothing and plucks at the bedding. If urination is free, the patient can be treated.

DISCUSSION: The recommended treatment for Tai Yang zhong feng is Gui Zhi Tang, to promote a mild sweat and release the exterior pathogen via the muscle layer. The use of fire therapy to promote sweat is excessive; it not only fails to resolve the external pathogen but, by introducing fire into the interior, aggravates the condition, with fire harassing the interior and injuring qi and blood. The fuming and scorching of the two yang, which are the wind and fire, obstruct qi flow of the liver and gallbladder, and result in the chaotic flow of bile, causing jaundice. The flaring of hyperactive fire scorches the yang network vessels, which can refer either to the collaterals in the superficial layers of the body, or to those ascending to the upper jiao. The scorching of the vessels results in nosebleed; if the fire pathogen descends to the lower jiao and injures yin, there will be inhibited urination. If both yin and yang are depleted and there is exhaustion of qi, the sinews will not be warmed and nourished and the body will become dried up and withered. If the fire is not expelled and there is constrained heat in the interior, it manifests as sweating from the head only, because of the insufficiency of yin fluids. Where fire blazes upwards and damages fluids in the upper jiao, there may be a dry mouth or even an ulcerated throat. If the heat pathogen is knotted in the interior, there will be constipation with mild abdominal pain due to the obstruction of qi. Heat knotted in the interior can also obstruct the dissemination of lung qi causing a slight wheeze. If the condition is protracted, fire will harass the heart shen and there may be delirious speech, and further deterioration may damage the stomach qi and cause vomiting. The restlessness of the arms and legs and the fingers plucking at the bedclothes are the unconscious actions of a semi-comatose patient and are attributed to the exhaustion of fluids by excess heat. Yang is not anchored and there is a potential for yang desertion. A key indicator in prognosis is the amount of fluid remaining as evidenced by urination. Even though severe heat has consumed fluids and urination is scant, if urination is uninhibited, it demonstrates that the function of qi transformation is unimpaired, which, in turn, demonstrates the physiological health of the zang fu. If there is no significant dysfunction of the zang fu, then prognosis is good.

Jaundice with sweating from the head is the result of pathogenic heat attacking the interior, scorching the liver and gallbladder and causing the flow of bile to be chaotic. This must be differentiated from yellowing due to damp heat in the Yang Ming. Clause 111 is a discussion of exuberant fire damaging yin and causing blood to flow recklessly, giving rise to nosebleed.

This clause gives an understanding of how the use of fire or warmth in a pattern of yin deficiency can cause bleeding, because of the further depletion of yin and the exacerbation of interior heat. The theory of preserving yin by the avoidance of fire therapy inspired the wen bing (warm disease) specialists of later centuries to advocate the preservation of yin and to avoid the indiscriminate use of acrid warm herbs in the treatment of disease caused by pathogenic warmth. The principle was transcribed to the treatment of warm diseases, where such formulas as Ma Huang Tang and Gui Zhi Tang are inappropriate.

There is no formula recommended by Zhang Zhong Jing, however, *Shang Han Lun Ji Zhu* suggests the formula: Ren Shen Di Huang Mu Li Fu Ling Tang (Ren Shen 3 liang; Gan Di Huang ½ jin; Long Gu 3 liang; Mu Li 4 liang; Fu Ling 4 liang). The ingredients are boiled in 1 dou of water, reduced to 3 sheng. The decoction is taken warm three times a day.

Inappropriate Fire Therapy in a Wen Bing Pattern

Clause 113

形作伤寒，其脉不弦紧而弱，弱者必渴，被火必谵语，弱者发热，脉浮，解之当汗出愈。

Resembling shang han, the pulse is not wiry or taut but weak, if weak there will be thirst, if treated with fire there will be delirious speech, if with the weakness there is fever, the pulse is floating, resolution by sweating should bring recovery.

DISCUSSION: The condition described in Clause 113 bears resemblance to a shang han pattern, whereby it is presumed to manifest with the symptoms of fever, aversion to cold, headache and body aches and pains. However, the pulse is neither wiry nor taut, but weak. The allusion to the weak pulse differentiates this pattern from a typical shang han pattern, as does the presence of thirst, by which it may be inferred there is also fever. The presence of thirst and fever are symptoms of warm disease. Clause 6 states clearly: "Tai Yang disease, there is fever and thirst, with no aversion to cold, it is wen bing (warm disease)." The strategy of treatment in warm disease at the defensive level is to administer cool acrid herbs to release the exterior. If fire therapy is used, not only will fluids be depleted but there is potential for interior pathogenic heat to be exacerbated, giving rise to a transmuted pattern with clouded spirit and delirious speech. Therefore, Zhang Zhong Jing proposes that resolution should be obtained by the promotion of sweat.

There have been numerous interpretations of Clause 113. (1) Cheng Wu Ji suggested it represents a pattern of interior heat; (2) Qian Huang suggested it was a warm disease pattern; (3) You Zai Jing suggested yin deficiency with a concurrent exterior pattern; (4) Ke Yun Bo suggested internal injury due to over-exertion or taxation fatigue combined with exterior wind cold. Based on the pulse and symptoms, Qian Huang's interpretation is the most appropriate.

There are two key points to be gleaned from this clause. (1) The differentiation between warm disease and shang han can be made on the basis of the pulse and the presence or absence of thirst: if the pulse is taut but there is no thirst, it is shang han and if the pulse is floating and weak and there is thirst, it is warm disease. (2) Although warm disease is included in the broad definition of shang han, diagnosis and treatment must be differentiated according to the narrow concept.

Summary of Transmuted Patterns caused by Fire Therapy

Fire counterflow is a transmuted pattern which occurs as a result of the inappropriate use of fire therapy. During the Han dynasty, fire therapy was a popular form of treatment for many diseases. It included the use of warm needling, where moxa is placed on the handle of the needle; hot needling, where a red-hot needle is inserted; fuming, where the patient is subjected to steam; warm compresses and direct or indirect moxibustion. The chief objectives of fire therapy were to promote sweating, disperse cold, warm the channels, resuscitate and assist yang. These functions enabled it to promote the flow of yang qi, unblock obstruction and vanquish yin. It was applied in such conditions as abdominal cold, bi syndrome due to wind-cold damp and diarrhoea due to cold and deficient yang. It was also used in the treatment of swellings and flat abscess, and hot needling was commonly used to cauterise boils and abscesses. Fire therapy is contraindicated for heat patterns both of the empty and full type.

There are two categories of fire counterflow patterns. The first is where excessive or inappropriate loss of sweat damages the heart yang, causing the heart shen to float upwards, manifesting with vexation, and where the harassment of the fire pathogen causes manic behaviour. The second category is where the fire pathogen falls inward and injures ying yin causing haemoptysis and blood in the stool. Parallels can be drawn between the fire counterflow in *Shang Han Lun* and modern radiotherapy, which also results in injury to yin and blood. In contemporary times, the more moderate forms of fire therapy are still in common use. Warm compresses, moxibustion and warm needling are effective means of warming the channels, dispersing cold and invigorating the network vessels to unblock obstruction.

2.8.2 Transmuted Patterns Caused by Emetic Therapy

Incorrect use of emetics may result in the transmuted patterns of cold in the stomach with false heat signs, or dry heat in the stomach.

True Cold False Heat

Excessive or inappropriate use of emetics can damage the yang qi of the stomach, resulting in a pattern of deficiency and cold in the stomach with accompanying manifestations of false heat.

Clause 120

太阳病，当恶寒、发热，今自汗出，反不恶寒、发热、关上脉细数者，以医吐之过也。一二日吐之者，腹中饥、口不能食；三四日吐之者，不喜糜粥，欲食冷食，朝食暮吐，以医吐之所致也，此为小逆。

Tai Yang disease, there should be aversion to cold and fever, now there is spontaneous sweating, but if there is no aversion to cold or fever and the guan pulse is thready and rapid, it is because the physician has wrongly induced vomiting. If there is vomiting for one or two days, there is hunger in the abdomen but the mouth is unable to eat; if there is vomiting for three or four days, the patient doesn't want gruel, he wants to eat cold food, food eaten in the morning is vomited in the evening, it is because of the physician inducing vomiting, this is a minor adverse treatment.

DISCUSSION: Tai Yang disease is characterised by aversion to cold and fever and, as an exterior pattern, it is treated by promoting sweat in order to release the exterior. Diaphoresis harmonises the exterior and resolves the fever and the aversion to cold. In Clause 120, the patient has spontaneous sweating with no fever or aversion to cold, which indicates that the exterior pathogen is already resolved. The rapid and thready guan pulse shows that although the exterior pattern has been resolved, there is an interior disharmony, indicating that there has been transmutation. The guan pulse represents the spleen and stomach, and a rapid thready pulse in the guan position is a sign of the damage to stomach qi caused by incorrect emetic therapy.

The reference to one or two days, and to three or four days of emetic treatment is not precise and merely illustrates that a longer period of incorrect emetic treatment will result in more serious symptoms. The relatively short duration of one or two days is indicative of a relatively mild transmutation, with mild symptoms of a sense of hunger in the stomach, but no appetite and an inability to eat. However, when emesis has been carried out for a longer period, nominated in the clause as three or four days, the damage to stomach qi is significant, and the symptoms more serious. The patient does not want to eat hot gruel, but only cold foods, and anything eaten in the morning is vomited later in the day, showing it has remained in the stomach and not been digested for the whole of that time.

Clause 120 describes the damage done to stomach qi by incorrect emesis, which robs the stomach of yang qi and steals its fluids. Yang qi is debilitated, fluids are depleted, and so there is yang deficiency combined with dryness, manifesting as false heat. The underlying pattern is one of cold and deficiency; the yang qi is inadequate and unable to decompose and transform water and grain. The resulting accumulation of stagnant food in the stomach results in the reversal of stomach qi, and so the food taken earlier in the day, which remains unprocessed and undigested, is vomited later in the day. Although more serious than the simple loss of appetite which follows a shorter period of emetic therapy, it is still not considered to be severe or irreversible and such emetic therapy is therefore described as minor adverse treatment, indicating a relatively mild transmutation.

The preference for cold food, accompanied as it is by fever and a pulse which is thready and rapid in the guan position, could seem to be at odds with the symptom of vomiting food taken earlier in the day. The presence of fever, the desire for cold food and the pulse concord with a heat pattern. However, vomiting due to stomach heat typically occurs immediately after eating because it is caused by the obstruction of heat, resulting in immediate ejection. The failure of the stomach to digest the food, leading to its regurgitation much later in the day, is attributed to stomach deficiency with cold, where there is insufficient yang qi to fuel the digestive process. Despite the fever and the desire for cold food, it is this pattern of cold and deficiency which is the true pattern. The fever and the desire for cold food are false heat signs, as is the rapid pulse image.

The emphasis of this clause is on the identification of the transmuted pattern and no guiding formula is proposed. However, suitable formulas for the milder of the two patterns are Xiao Ban Xia Tang combined with Fu Ling Tang, or Xiang Sha Liu Jun Zi Tang and for the more serious pattern of vomiting food taken earlier in the day, Ju Pi Zhu Ru Tang or Xuan Fu Dai Zhe Tang with the addition of Hou Po. For severe cold, Gan Jiang instead of Sheng Jiang can be used.

Dry Heat in the Stomach

Inappropriate emetic therapy can give rise to dry heat in the stomach, where the pathognomonic sign is vexation.

Clause 121

太阳病，吐之，但太阳病当恶寒，今反不恶寒，不欲近衣，此为吐之内烦也。

Tai Yang disease, there is vomiting, but Tai Yang disease should have aversion to cold, now however there is no aversion to cold, no desire to wear more clothing, this means the vomiting has caused interior vexation.

DISCUSSION: Clause 121 describes the incorrect use of emetic therapy in a Tai Yang exterior pattern. In Tai Yang disease the patient exhibits aversion to cold because of the pathogen constrained in the muscle layer, and for this reason, the prescribed treatment is the promotion of sweat. Here, vomiting has been wrongly used; the cold signs disappear, and there is vexation. The vexation has arisen for two reasons: first, because emesis can easily damage the stomach fluids and the subsequent dryness generates heat; second, because the emetic treatment has caused the exterior pathogen to fall inward, the Yang Ming is affected, and so a pattern of heat and interior vexation arises. The fact that there is no aversion to cold and no wish to wear additional clothing shows that the pathogen is no longer in the exterior.

Heat in the Interior

Clause 123

（一）太阳病，过经十余日，心下温温欲吐而胸中痛，大便反溏，腹微满，郁郁微烦。（二）先此时自极吐下者，与调胃承气汤；若不尔者，不可与。（三）但欲呕、胸中痛、微溏者，此非柴胡证，以呕故知极吐下也。调胃承气汤。

(1) Tai Yang disease, having passed through the channel for ten days or more, there is discomfort below the heart with a desire to vomit and pain in the chest, the stool however is loose, the abdomen slightly full, there is constraint with mild vexation. (2) If, prior to this time, there was severe emesis and purgation, give Tiao Wei Cheng Qi Tang; if it is not so, it should not be given. (3) But even if there is a desire to vomit,

> pain in the chest and slight looseness, this is not a Xiao Chai Hu Tang pattern, because the vomiting is known to be due to severe emesis and purgation.

DISCUSSION: Clause 123 is best read in three sections.

1. The pathogen has passed through the Tai Yang channel and is no longer in the exterior. The discomfort under the heart shows that it has fallen inward. Because the chest lies adjacent to the foot Tai Yang channel, the pathogenic qi will first attack the chest; if it lodges between the chest and epigastrium, there will be a knotted sensation below the heart and a desire to vomit, which is a reflection of qi constraint in the chest. The pathogenic qi harasses the chest and diaphragm, affecting the qi dynamic and giving rise to chest pain; the heat pathogen enters the interior, causing disharmony which manifests as slight abdominal fullness and a sense of constraint with slight vexation. Knotting of heat in the intestines would normally cause constipation but there is 'slight looseness' of the stool, as can be found in a Shao Yang pattern. The abdominal fullness, on the other hand, is reminiscent of a Yang Ming pattern. The information given is inconclusive, and further investigation and analysis is needed to identify the pattern and understand the aetiology.
2. The second section describes how the incorrect use of harsh emetics and purgatives has resulted in disharmony of stomach qi. If emesis and purgation were induced prior to the pathogen leaving the Tai Yang channel, then this constitutes adverse purgation of an exterior pattern, damaging fluids and causing stomach dryness to transform into an excess pattern of stomach heat. Although the indicated treatment for excess stomach heat is purging, because this disorder is the result of incorrect emesis which has already damaged the stomach qi, there is concern that a strong purgative will do further damage. So it is suggested to give the patient Tiao Wei Cheng Qi Tang, which mildly purges heat and also moistens dryness. However, if the sloppy stool is not the result of purging and is accompanied by abdominal fullness, then the pattern is one of yang deficiency, not heat, and so Tiao Wei Cheng Qi Tang should then not be given, because if the vomiting has not been caused by emetics, it could be a Shao Yang pattern.
3. The last sentence considers the possibility that the symptoms of nausea, chest pain and a loose stool are an indication of a Xiao Chai Hu Tang pattern. However, based on the history of emetic therapy, the pathogenesis is different and so we know it is not this pattern. The nausea and vomiting, the pain in the chest and the sloppy stool of Shao Yang disease are the result of heat affecting the qi dynamic of the Shao Yang, and not, as here, the result of previous emetic therapy which has damaged the stomach qi.

Summary of Transmuted Patterns caused by Emetic Therapy

Incorrect emetic therapy may result in a transmuted Tai Yang exterior pattern. On the basis of differences in the yin and yang of the zang fu, and the different properties of herbs used in the emetic medication, there are two developments. (1) Damage to yang qi causing stomach deficiency with cold accumulation characterised by the vomiting of food which has been eaten much earlier in the day (Clause 120). (2) Damage to stomach fluids with subsequent dryness transforming to stomach heat, giving rise to vexation (Clause 121).

Treatment for variations of this pattern is also cited in Clauses 70 and 207: if there is abdominal fullness and constipation, Tiao Wei Cheng Qi Tang can be used; if there is fever accompanied by vexation, with no aversion to cold and no desire to wear more clothing, one must understand the pathogenesis and observe the pulse sign in order to select an appropriate formula. Formulas such as Bai Hu Tang or Zhu Ye Shi Gao Tang may be considered.

2.8.3 Transmuted Patterns caused by Sweating

In Clause 70 the inappropriate promotion of sweat can lead to two patterns. One is associated with deficiency and the second with excess, and each is treated differently.

Clause 70

发汗后,恶寒者,虚故也；不恶寒,但热者,实也，当和胃气，与调胃承气汤。

Following the promotion of sweat, if there is aversion to cold, it is due to deficiency; if there is no aversion to cold but there is heat, it is due to excess, one must harmonise the stomach qi, give Tiao Wei Cheng Qi Tang.

DISCUSSION: Although the promotion of sweat is the correct strategy in the treatment of a Tai Yang exterior pattern, sweating which is inappropriate may fail to resolve the exterior pathogen and may cause it to fall inward. This transmutation can manifest as a pattern of cold and deficiency or one of heat and excess. If there is pre-existing yang deficiency, the loss of sweat can further damage the yang qi, giving rise to patterns of deficiency cold and their possible transmission into the yin channels. The key diagnostic features of a cold pattern are aversion to cold, the absence of heat signs, a submerged, faint or faint and thready pulse, the absence of any strange taste in the mouth and no thirst. No formula is specified, but consideration can be given to the use of Shao Yao Gan Cao Fu Zi Tang, as cited in Clause 68 for deficiency cold following inappropriate diaphoresis. Alternatively, if the person has a pre-existing pattern of yang excess, then the loss of sweat could lead to fluid damage transforming to dryness, exacerbating the heat, and increasing the possibility of transmission to a Yang Ming or other heat excess pattern. A Yang Ming excess heat pattern can be diagnosed on fever, a big pulse, a dry throat and thirst, with no aversion to cold. The appropriate formula is Tiao Wei Cheng Qi Tang to clear internal heat and harmonise the stomach qi.

2.8.4 Transmuted Patterns caused by Purgation

In the case of a person with an accumulation of phlegm fluids who contracts Tai Yang disease, if an inappropriate treatment such as purgation is used, it can lead to a transmuted pattern such as chest bind or concurrent fever and diarrhoea.

Clause 139

太阳病，二三日，不能卧，但欲起，心下必结，脉微弱者，此本有寒分也。反下之，若利止，必作结胸；未止者，四日复下之，此作协热利也。

Tai Yang disease, on the second or third day, the person can not lie down, but wants to get up, there will be knotting below the heart, if the pulse is faint and weak, there was originally coldness. Nevertheless, purgation is used, when the diarrhoea stops, there will be knotting in the chest; if there is no cessation, on the fourth day there is again purgation, this will cause a complex of fever and diarrhoea.

DISCUSSION: Clause 139 describes a situation where Tai Yang disease is contracted by a person who has an accumulation of phlegm fluids. In such a case, inappropriate purgation can lead to transmutation. One would expect that Tai Yang disease which has lasted two or three days is still mild; however, the symptoms of difficulty sleeping (inability to lie down), restlessness (desire to get up) and a knotted bind below the heart all indicate a complex pattern where the exterior Tai Yang pathogen was unresolved at the time of purging, and has combined with a pre-existing accumulation of water in the interior, giving rise to knotted bind below the heart. If the practitioner mistakes this for an excess pattern and employs purging, the pathogen will enter the interior. There are two scenarios associated with this transmutation. The first is where, after purgation, the diarrhoea stops and the pathogenic heat forms a knot with the retained water in the upper jiao, manifesting as chest bind; the second is where the diarrhoea persists, purging is used again on the fourth day, causing the pathogen to descend, resulting in concurrent fever and diarrhoea.

So what precisely is the pattern which preceded the adverse treatment? Ke Yun Bo suggested an externally contracted pattern where there was an accumulation of phlegm fluids similar to a Xiao Qing Long Tang pattern; Qian Tian Lai, however, suggested that the purgation gave rise to heat constrained in the diaphragm, which is a Zhi Zi Chi Tang pattern. The authors believe that Ke Yun Bo's interpretation is the more logical, because the knotting below the heart and the faint, weak pulse indicating deficiency cold, according to the clause, were present before the purgation; furthermore, there is no evidence of simple heat constraint in the interior.

There are two possible interpretations as to the nature of the chest bind which occurs after the purgation. Some suggest it is due to excess heat and others attribute it to excess cold. Based on the pathogenesis of deficiency cold, as indicated by the faint and weak pulse, and the pre-existing condition of yin accumulation as suggested by Ke Yun Bo, excess cold due to the yang deficiency and the accumulation of phlegm fluids is more likely. For this, a suitable formula is San Wu Bai San. The concurrent fever and diarrhoea is a result of yang deficiency of the spleen and stomach, with the deficiency cold diarrhoea resembling that of a Gui Zhi Ren Shen Tang pattern.

Clause 140 specifies pulse signs for the differentiation of various transmutations of Tai Yang disease following adverse purgative treatment.

Clause 140

太阳病，下之，其脉促，不结胸者，此为欲解也；脉浮者，必结胸；脉紧者，必咽痛；脉弦者，必两胁拘急；脉细数者，头痛未止；脉沉紧者，必欲呕；脉沉滑者，协热利；脉浮滑者，必下血。

Tai Yang disease, after purgation, if the pulse is skipping, and there is no chest bind, this means recovery is imminent; if the pulse is floating, there will be chest bind; if the pulse is taut, the throat will be sore; if the pulse is wiry, there will be constrained tightness in both sides of the chest; if the pulse is thready and rapid, there will be constant headache; if the pulse is submerged and taut, there will be nausea; if the pulse is submerged and slippery, there will be a complex of fever and diarrhoea; if the pulse is floating and slippery, blood will descend.

DISCUSSION: Diaphoresis is the standard treatment for Tai Yang exterior disease. Purgation is not only incorrect, but has the adverse effect of causing transmutation. In this clause, Zhang Zhong Jing cites the pulse signs of the various transmuted patterns and their corresponding manifestations.

1. The interpretation of the skipping pulse with no chest bind is that recovery is imminent. This is based on a skipping pulse being rapid and pertaining to yang, and indicates that yang qi flourishes and is able to dispel the pathogen. Thus it signals recovery.
2. The significance of a floating pulse in predicting chest bind after purgation resides in the relative strength of the exterior pathogen, which is reflected in a floating pulse. A strong exterior pathogen has a greater potential to exploit the interior emptiness by falling inward. When the pathogen falls inward, it combines with the water and phlegm in the chest, causing chest bind.
3. A taut or tight pulse governs cold, stagnation and pain. Following purgation, the exterior pathogenic cold falls inward and lodges in the Shao Yin channel, from where it ascends to the throat. Thus, if the pulse is taut, the throat will be sore.
4. A wiry pulse is associated with the liver and gallbladder. If, after purgation, the pathogen enters the Shao Yang channel, it will result in tightness and pain in the sides of the chest.
5. A thready, rapid pulse associated with unresolved headache is explained by the fact that a thready pulse governs deficiency and a rapid pulse governs heat. This means that an upsurge of deficiency heat can cause headache.
6. A submerged and taut pulse is associated with vomiting and nausea because a submerged pulse denotes an interior disharmony caused by the pathogen falling inwards, and a taut pulse indicates cold, which is the result of purgation having damaged the yang qi. The taut or tight pulse also reflects the accumulation of yin fluids and cold which results in rebellious qi, manifesting as vomiting.
7. A submerged pulse indicates interior disharmony, whilst a slippery pulse is a yang

pulse and indicates damp. In this case, the damp has combined with heat, because when the exterior pathogen falls inward, it transforms into heat. Heat then harasses the intestines and manifests as concurrent fever and diarrhoea.

8. Where a floating pulse is also slippery, the floating nature indicates an unresolved exterior pathogen whilst the slippery nature pertains to yang, and in this instance denotes the interior heat, which is the result of purgation having caused the exterior pathogen to fall inward, where it transformed into heat. Heat injures the yin blood causing blood to be chaotic, and blood appears in the stool.

From the above, it can be seen that each transmutation has its corresponding pulse sign. Nevertheless, this clause by no means suggests that diagnosis can be made on the basis of the pulse signs alone, and as implied by the above explanations, accurate diagnosis relies on all four examinations.

Clause 140 does not nominate a specific formula for any of the transmuted patterns, however suitable formulas have been recommended by the Ming dynasty practitioner Wang Ri Xiu. His suggestions are as follows: for a floating pulse with chest bind, Gui Zhi Qu Shao Yao Tang; for a tight pulse with a sore throat, Xiao Chai Hu Tang with the addition of Gui Zhi; for a thready, rapid pulse with an unresolved headache, Dang Gui Si Ni Tang; for a submerged, tight pulse with vomiting, Gan Cao Gan Jiang Tang; for a submerged, slippery pulse with concurrent fever and diarrhoea, Bai Tou Weng Tang; and for a floating, slippery pulse with bleeding, Shao Yao Gan Cao Tang with the addition of Qin Pi (*Shang Han Lun Yu Lin Chuang* by Nie Hui Ming).

2.8.5 Summary of Transmuted Patterns Following Inappropriate Therapy

Transmuted patterns arising from adverse treatment of Tai Yang disease and their prognosis are summarised in Clause 153.

Clause 153

太阳病，医发汗，遂发热、恶寒；因复下之，心下痞。表里俱虚，阴阳气并竭，无阳则阴独。复加烧针，因胸烦、面色青黄、肤瞤者，难治；今色微黄，手足温者，易愈。

Tai Yang disease, the physician has promoted sweat, it is followed by fever and aversion to cold; because purgation was repeated, there is glomus below the heart. The exterior and interior are both deficient, yin, yang and qi are also exhausted, there is no yang but yin alone. Hot needling is then used, causing chest vexation, if the facial complexion is greenish yellow, and the skin twitches, it is difficult to treat; now the complexion is slightly yellow, if the hands and feet are warm, recovery is easy.

DISCUSSION: The correct treatment for a Tai Yang exterior pattern is the promotion of sweat. However, if fever and aversion to cold persist after the promotion of sweat, then this shows that the sweating was inadequate. If the physician then uses purging to resolve the exterior pattern, the original error of inadequate diaphoresis is compounded. The reason inadequate sweating can lead to a transmuted pattern is that, although it is insufficient to achieve its purpose of releasing the exterior, nevertheless, it has still injured the exterior wei yang, which is left in a depleted state to try and contend with the pathogen. This, together with the damage to the interior by the incorrect purgation, then results in deficiency of both the exterior and the interior, and of yin, yang and qi. Although the exterior pathogen has fallen inward and there is no longer a pathogen in the exterior, the adverse treatments have resulted in a transmuted pattern of glomus below the heart. The indicated treatment for this transmuted pattern is Xie Xin Tang, however in Clause 153 the physician again uses incorrect treatment, this time in the form of a fire needle. The fire therapy gives rise to heat, which harasses the heart, manifesting as vexation.

This series of errors has damaged both the exterior and the interior and yin and yang, thus giving rise to a transmuted pattern or huai bing (坏病). The glomus below the heart described in this clause is characteristic of many transmuted patterns, and here the glomus is due to deficiency. The exhaustion of yin, yang and qi is related to the depletion of interior yin, exterior yang and damage sustained by zheng qi. From this it can be understood that the interior deficiency affects blood as well as qi. The statement, "there is no yang but yin alone", alludes to the fact that there is no longer an exterior pattern but only an interior disharmony. Based on five phase theory, green is associated with the liver and yellow with the spleen, and a greenish-yellow complexion is indicative of the liver qi harassing the spleen. The lungs govern the skin and the spleen governs the muscles. If the lung and spleen qi are deficient, there will be emptiness in the skin and muscle layer, which can give rise to muscle twitching. Cold limbs indicate damage to the qi of the internal zang, which is why Zhang Zhong Jing pronounced that such a condition was difficult to treat. A return of the complexion to a slightly yellow colour indicates that the stomach qi is not devastated and can still transform qi and generate blood. If the limbs are warm then the yang deficiency is still mild, and so the prognosis is good and recovery can be expected. Whether the limbs are warm or cold is an important clinical predictor as to the strength or weakness of the zheng qi.

Clause 160 describes the adverse treatment of shang han disease with emetics, purgation and inappropriate sweat promotion. These damage the yang qi, impairing the function of controlling water. If allowed to persist, this condition can develop into a flaccidity pattern known as *wei zheng* (痿证).

Clause 160

伤寒吐下后，发汗、虚烦，脉甚微，八九日心下痞硬，协下痛、气上冲咽喉、眩冒、经脉动惕者，久而成痿。

Shang han after emetics and purgation, there is sweat promotion insubstantial vexation, the pulse is extremely faint, after eight or nine days there is a hard glomus below the heart, if there is pain under the ribs, an upsurge of qi to the throat, dizziness and twitchiness in the channel vessels, if it persists, there will be flaccidity.

DISCUSSION: Clause 160 details the damage to qi and body fluids, caused by emetics and purgatives in a Shang Han disorder. The zheng qi also sustains injury. Damage to the yang qi facilitates pathogenic exploitation of the interior, which manifests as insubstantial vexation. Insubstantial vexation is the result of unformed heat, which refers to heat which has not combined or knotted with a tangible substance such as water, phlegm or blood stasis. Therefore, because it is without substance, it is referred to as insubstantial vexation. This term is also used in discussions on Zhi Zi Chi Tang patterns in Section 2.7.1; formless heat causes insubstantial vexation.

Insufficiency of yang qi is characterised by a faint pulse. If zheng qi is still not restored after eight or nine days, the depleted yang may proceed to a level of greater yang deficiency, where it fails to control water and results in flooding. Manifestations of pathogenic water vary according to the movement of the water qi: if water qi surges upward, harassing the chest and epigastrium, a hard glomus may form below the heart or in the upper epigastrium; if it is located in the sides of the ribs, pain will be felt in that region; if it surges upwards, there may be throat impediment; if it harasses and obstructs the clear yang, there may be dizziness. These symptoms are all associated with the flooding of water due to yang deficiency. A further development arises when body fluids are damaged in the presence of a deficiency of yang qi, which is unable to transform and transport fluids. In this case, deficient yang qi not only fails to warm the muscles but also fails to nourish the sinews, with the result that there is twitching. If the condition persists and yang qi further declines, there will be weakness of the limbs and limitation of movement and agility, referred to in the clause as flaccidity, and known as wei zheng (痿证).

Clause 160 can be compared with Clause 67, which is also associated with the harassment of water qi and describes a Fu Ling, Gui Zhi Bai

Zhu Gan Cao pattern, where it says: "If there is vomiting in shang han, and if after purging there is fullness below the heart due to reversal, an upsurge of qi to the chest, on standing there is dizziness, the pulse is submerged and tight, and if the promotion of sweat causes stirring in the channels, with the body quivering and trembling, Fu Ling Gui Zhi Bai Zhu Gan Cao Tang governs". There is a strong similarity between Clause 67 and Clause 160. Clause 67 describes the manifestations of water qi and advocates the administration of Fu Ling Gui Zhi Bai Zhu Gan Cao Tang; Clause 160 gives greater emphasis to the severe deficiency of yang qi which is the underlying cause of the water qi harassment, and which is evidenced by the extremely faint pulse. No formula is suggested in Clause 160, but the appropriate strategy is to warm yang in order to control water. Fu Ling Gui Zhi Bai Zhu Gan Cao Tang combined with Zhen Wu Tang is suitable, or alternatively, a large dose of Fu Ling Gui Zhi Bai Zhu Gan Cao Tang may be used with the addition of Fu Zi to warm the yang and control water.

Clause 122

病人脉数，数为热，当消谷引食。而反吐者，此以发汗，令阳气微，膈气虚，脉乃数也。数为客热，不能消谷；以胃中虚冷，故吐也。

The patient's pulse is rapid, rapid relates to heat, and there should be insatiable hunger with huge consumption. If instead there is vomiting, this is due to the promotion of sweat, causing yang qi to be faint, diaphragm qi is deficient, the pulse is still rapid. Rapid relates to visitant heat, an inability to digest food; because there is deficiency cold in the stomach and so there is vomiting.

DISCUSSION: A rapid pulse denotes heat and is associated with excessive hunger and a large intake of food. This is because stomach heat accelerates the decomposition of food. In Clause 122, however, the opposite situation obtains: instead of an increased appetite due to heat, we find vomiting due to yang deficiency, which has been brought about by inappropriate diaphoresis. With the passage of time, the yang qi of the chest and diaphragm are also affected. A yang deficient pulse should be moderate and weak but, paradoxically, it is rapid. A rapid pulse indicates heat, but a rapid pulse must be differentiated as to whether it is rapid and forceful, in which case it denotes excess heat, or rapid and forceless, denoting deficiency, and this information is not given. Lu Jiu Zhi said: "A rapid pulse is associated either with exuberant heat or with severe deficiency". The reference to visitant heat in this clause is therefore significant, because although this term can refer generally to the invasion of pathogenic heat, here, it refers to the transient, evanescent heat of a deficiency pattern, which can be deficient qi or deficient yang, and not only deficient yin.

Thus we know the pattern is one of deficiency, and so the rapid pulse must be forceless. We are told that there is an inability to digest food, and in the last line of the clause, this is attributed to deficiency cold in the stomach. Stomach cold must be differentiated from stomach heat. In stomach cold there will be a poor appetite, an absence of thirst, the vomiting of clear watery fluid, a slippery white tongue coat and a pulse which is rapid and forceless. In stomach heat there is insatiable hunger, thirst, the vomiting of a putrid substance soon after eating, a dry, yellow tongue coat and a pulse which is rapid and strong.

Clause 122 emphasises the absence of stomach heat symptoms and states clearly that the rapid pulse is not due to heat but due to deficiency of yang. The recommended formula for stomach cold is Xiao Jian Zhong Tang with the addition of Ding Xiang and Wu Zhu Yu to warm the stomach and disperse cold, redirect counterflow and stop vomiting. This pattern complex of cold with deficiency heat is commonly seen in chronic gastritis, stomach or duodenal ulcers, chronic liver and gallbladder diseases and chronic colitis.

Section Nine

2.9 ZANG BIND, CHEST BIND & GLOMUS

Glomus is the common translation for *pi* (痞) which refers to accumulation and the associated sense of distension. When the accumulation is of qi alone, it has no form because it has not knotted with a substantial pathogen such as water, phlegm or food. It is then described as 'formless' and, having no form or substance, is soft on palpation. It is not tangible, there is no pain on pressure and it is regarded as a subjective sensation of blockage. When an accumulation is the result of the knotting of pathogenic qi with a substance such as water or phlegm, then it is referred to as a 'formed' knotted bind or 'hard glomus', which is a symptom of various patterns, including chest bind. Because it has form, it manifests as a tangible mass, which on palpation is firm or even hard, and there is pain on pressure.

A distinction needs to be made between the presence of water or phlegm which knots together with heat to form the knotted bind of chest bind, and water, food or phlegm which can stagnate qi, giving rise to qi glomus. Qi glomus is soft because there is no knotting of water or phlegm with the heat. Where glomus combines with a substantial pathogen such as phlegm, water or food, a hard glomus is formed.

The disease location and symptoms of chest bind, glomus and zang bind bear similarities but the patterns differ in their pathogenesis. Chest bind is the result of incorrect purging in Tai Yang, causing the pathogen to fall inward, transforming into pathogenic heat which becomes knotted with any pre-existing phlegm or water accumulation in the chest. Glomus is a disorder which is a direct consequence of incorrect purgation, which damages the spleen and stomach, and is characterised by a blocked sensation in the middle jiao. Zang bind is a serious condition where the pathogenesis is not incorrect treatment but zang dysfunction leading to the congestion of pathogenic qi in the zang organs. It is generally the result of deficient yang unable to support the spleen's function of transformation and transportation.

Comparison of Chest Bind and Zang Bind

Clause 128

问曰：病有结胸、有脏结，其状何如？

答曰：按之痛，寸脉浮，关脉沉，名曰结胸也。

Question: A disease with chest bind and zang bind, what are the symptoms?
Answer: Pain on pressure, the cun pulse is floating, guan pulse is submerged, it is called chest bind.

Clause 129

何谓脏结？

答曰：如结胸状，饮食如故、时时下利，寸脉浮、关脉小细沉紧，名曰脏结。舌上白胎滑者，难治。

Question: What is zang bind?
Answer: It is like chest bind, the intake of food and drink are as usual, there is frequent diarrhoea, the cun pulse is floating, the guan pulse is small, fine, submerged and tight, it is called zang bind. If the tongue coat is white and slippery, it is difficult to treat.

DISCUSSION: Clauses 128 and 129 describe chest bind and zang bind, respectively. Chest bind and zang bind are ancient names of diseases which are compared here to elucidate the differences. Chest bind is characterised by hard glomus below the heart. Zang bind has similar symptoms and disease location, but is due to congestion of yin cold in the zang organs and is discussed later in the section. The fundamental difference is one of aetiology: chest bind is the result of incorrect purging and zang bind is the result of spleen yang deficiency.

In chest bind, the exterior pathogen has fallen inward as a consequence of incorrect purgation in the treatment of Tai Yang disease.

The subsequent binding of pathogenic heat with water or phlegm in the chest is what causes the symptoms of chest bind. The pattern is a yang excess pattern characterised by pain aggravated by pressure. Both its categorisation as yang excess and the disease location are demonstrated by the pulse: the cun pulse relates to the upper jiao, indicating the disease location, and the floating pulse, which is a yang pulse, is a reflection of the heat which has formed in the chest; the submerged guan pulse relates to the middle jiao and is a reflection of the water accumulation 'below the heart', which refers to the upper epigastric region.

The sensation of pain when pressure is applied is a key symptom of chest bind. Citations from clauses which relate to chest bind and which describe this symptom of pain on the application of pressure are: "there is pain in the diaphragm which resists pressure" (Clause 134); "if there is pain below the heart, stone-hard upon palpation" (Clause 135); "if from below the heart to the lesser abdomen there is hard distension and pain such that the patient will not allow anyone near" (Clause 137); "Minor chest bind disease, just below the heart, if there is pain on palpation" (Clause 138); "If there is fullness with hard pain below the heart, it is chest bind" (Clause 149). Nevertheless, diagnosis must not be made on the basis of pain alone but on a full assessment of all signs and symptoms, including the pulse. The pattern often corresponds to the biomedical diagnosis of acute pancreatitis or intestinal obstruction.

Whilst chest bind is caused by incorrect purgation, zang bind is attributed to the congestion of pathogenic qi in the spleen zang arising from spleen yang deficiency and the subsequent congelation of yin cold. Although the spleen is affected, there is no excess pathogen in the stomach, and so the appetite is normal; however, the accumulation of yin cold damages spleen yang and impairs its function of transformation and transportation, giving rise to frequent diarrhoea.

In zang bind, the cun pulse is floating and the guan pulse is small, thready, submerged and tight. The floating cun pulse relates to the upper jiao and is associated with yang. The guan pulse is small and fine, representing the qi and blood deficiency inherent in zang bind; the submerged and tight pulse is a reflection of the interior cold; the white and slippery tongue coat is a sign of yang deficiency with yin cold accumulation. The conclusion to be drawn is that this is a deep-seated pattern, where the accumulated yin cold is an interior excess and is the result of long-term yang deficiency. It would be a mistake to assume that purgation should be used on the basis that this is a pattern of interior excess. The interior excess is yin and the underlying pattern is deficiency cold, and so purgation is contraindicated because it would further damage the yang and deplete zheng qi. For this reason, Zhang Zhong Jing stated that this disorder is difficult to treat.

Clauses 128 and 129 both describe a floating pulse which in *Shang Han Lun* has two possible interpretations. A floating pulse which is also forceful is associated with pathogenic heat falling inward and knotting with phlegm fluids in the chest and diaphragm; the cun pulse relates to the location, and the floating, forceful pulse is a reflection of the accumulation of phlegm fluids. If the floating pulse is forceless, it relates to zang deficiency with congealed yin cold; here its forceless nature represents the yin cold and the floating nature is a reflection of deficient yang being displaced and outcast by exuberant yin. Cheng Wu Ji said: "A floating cun pulse with a guan pulse which is submerged relates to pathogenic bind in the yang; a floating cun pulse with a guan pulse which is thready, small, submerged and tight, relates to pathogenic bind in the yin" (*Zhu Jie Shang Han Lun*).

Chest bind is caused by the knotting of pathogenic heat and water. The key symptom is pain aggravated by pressure; there is no appetite, due to the interior excess; the stool is dry and the tongue has a dry, yellow coat, indicating yang excess. The guiding formula for chest bind is Da Xian Xiong Tang. In zang bind, the appetite is normal but there is frequent diarrhoea due to the underlying yang deficiency. The treatment must therefore address the principle of warming yang and dissipating cold accumulation. An appropriate formula is Si Ni Tang or Li Zhong Wan to warm the yang with the addition of Zhi Shi to dissipate accumulation.

Comparison of Chest Bind and Glomus

Clause 131A

病发于阳，而反下之，热入因作结胸；病发于阴，而反下之，因作痞也。所以成结胸者，以下之太早故也。

In disease stemming from yang, there is adverse purgation, heat enters and so chest bind forms; in disease stemming from yin, there is adverse purgation, and so glomus forms. The reason for chest bind is that purgation was used too early.

DISCUSSION: Clause 131A explains the difference between chest bind and glomus on the basis of aetiology. Both are the result of incorrect purgation, but they are differentiated here as either stemming from yang or stemming from yin. The concept of disease as stemming either from yang or from yin can be interpreted from two different perspectives. The first is the concept of yin and yang as representing interior and exterior, and the second relates to yin and yang in relation to the relative strength of the constitution and pre-existing disease, which in this case is the presence of water retention, phlegm or food stagnation. In referring to a disease which stems from yang, Clause 131A is describing an exterior excess pattern and, because of the later development of chest bind, it is understood that there is a pre-existing accumulation of water and phlegm; incorrect purgation causes the exterior pathogen to fall inward and transform into heat where it combines with the water and phlegm to cause chest bind. Disease stemming from yin refers to a pattern of interior deficiency, where incorrect purgation further damages the spleen and stomach, the qi dynamic is impaired and qi accumulates in the middle, manifesting as glomus.

The statement that "purgation was used too early" refers to the fact that purgation was used too early in the course of shang han exterior disease, thus giving rise to chest bind. By "too early" it means when the exterior pathogen is not fully resolved, and thus the clause reinforces the principle of not purging in the presence of an exterior pathogen, even where there are some symptoms indicating purgation. This is because, as explained earlier, purgation can cause the exterior pathogen to fall inward.

In chest bind, there is a pre-exisitng accumulation of water or phlegm fluids in the chest; purgation causes the pathogen to enter the chest, transform to heat and knot with the fluids to form chest bind. Glomus is not associated with interior excess; it is due to pre-existing stomach qi deficiency exacerbated by purgation. Glomus in this clause refers to qi glomus. It is formless and is ascribed to stagnant qi, not to the knotting of heat and fluids as in chest bind. The word glomus is generally defined as a subjective sensation of blockage. It is not related to an exterior pathogen falling inward, and so the timing of purgation does not apply.

Although both chest bind and glomus are the result of incorrect purgation, they differ in their aetiology and pathomechanism. Chest bind is caused by purgation in the course of Tai Yang disease, which causes the heat pathogen to fall inward, whilst glomus is the result of spleen deficiency, exacerbated by purging, which impairs the qi dynamic.

2.9.1 Zang Bind

Zang bind results from devastation of yang qi with yin cold congealing in the zang fu. It differs from chest bind in that chest bind is caused by excess heat, whereas the pathogenesis of zang bind is deficiency cold.

Clause 130

脏结无阳证，不往来寒热，其人反静，舌上胎滑者，不可攻也。

Zang bind, with no yang pattern, no alternating chills and fever, if the person is nonetheless calm, and the tongue coat is slippery, one should not attack.

DISCUSSION: Zang bind refers to a condition where there is severe depletion of zang qi and congealed yin cold, so the main feature is yin excess, and there are no yang signs such as fever, a floating pulse or alternating chills and fever. Although the zang bind manifests with hard glomus and fullness below the heart, there is no alternation of chills and fever, and so it is not a half exterior and half interior Shao Yang pattern. The reference to the person being calm demonstrates the absence of vexation associated with Yang Ming interior heat, thus confirming that it is not a yang pattern and not a disease of the three yang channels. This is a pattern of yin cold with no yang symptoms, which is a key point of diagnosis for zang bind. The slippery tongue coat is characteristic of the congelation of yin cold where yang qi is deficient and unable to transform fluid and, as such, further testifies to zang bind being a pure yin cold pattern with no sign of yang. Clause 130 is better read in combination with Clause 129, discussed at the start of section 2.9, which describes zang bind in great detail. When these two clauses are read together, the secret to understanding the true nature of zang bind is unlocked. The statement in Clause 129 that zang bind is difficult to treat is based on the fact that it is a pattern of devastated zang qi with devitalised yang. Having grasped that, the assertion in Clause 130, that one should not attack is easily understood. *Shang Han Bu Wang Lun* recommends that Guan Yuan (Ren 4) should be needled; *Shang Han Yun Yao* suggests the use of moxibustion on Qi Hai (Ren 6) and Guan Yuan (Ren 4), and the administration of Ren Shen San Bai Tang with the addition of Gan Jiang, and if there is severe cold, to add Fu Zi; *Shang Han Quan Sheng Ji* advises: "It is appropriate to use moxa on Guan Yuan and then give Wu Zhu Yu Si Ni Tang to warm the cold".

In regard to translation of the word zang (脏) in this clause as 'zang organ', it should be noted that the original text used the character of classical Chinese, written 藏. The flesh radical 月 was added later, giving the modern traditional character臟, which is now commonly written 臓, the simplified counterpart being 脏. The character 藏 also has the meaning 'repository' or 'storehouse' and is also pronounced 'zang'; however, although there is a semantic correspondence, there should be no confusion that in *Shang Han Lun*, and in this clause, the character 藏 refers to 'zang organ'.

Clause 167

病胁下素有痞，连在脐旁，痛引少腹入阴筋者，此名脏结，死。

The disease normally has glomus under the ribs, extending to the side of the umbilicus, if the pain goes to the lesser abdomen and enters the yin tendon, it is called zang bind, the person will die.

DISCUSSION: Clause 167 raises the issue of prognosis in zang bind. The condition described is critical and is attributed to a long-term deficiency of the zang qi and subsequent congelation of yin cold, which has been characterised by glomus in the hypochondrium. The sensation of distension associated with glomus is a result of the stagnation of qi and blood. The channels and network vessels are obstructed, causing discomfort. The fact that pain extends to the level of the umbilicus and from there to the lesser abdomen shows involvement of the spleen and liver, and is testament to just how pervasive the disease is. Here, the term shao fu is used in its broader application, referring to the whole of the lower abdomen, thus also involving the kidneys, and from there, it travels to the yin tendon or penis, which not only follows the path of the liver channel, but has a relationship with the kidneys as the ruler of life, death and reproduction. The implication of the deep-seated bind in these three zang, representing accumulation and concretion in the liver, spleen and kidneys, bodes poorly, and the likely outcome is death. A parallel can be drawn with benign and malignant tumour.

2.9.2 Chest Bind with Heat Excess

Da Xian Xiong Tang Pattern

Clause 134

（一）太阳病，脉浮而动数，浮则为风，数则为热，动则为痛，数则为虚。头痛、发热、微盗汗出，而反恶寒者，表未解也。（二）医反下之，动数变迟，膈内拒痛，胃中空虚，客气动膈，短气躁烦，心中懊侬，阳气内陷，心下因硬，则为结胸，大陷胸汤主之。

（三）若不结胸，但头汗出，余处无汗，剂颈而还，小便不利，身必发黄。大陷胸汤方。

(1) Tai Yang disease, the pulse is floating but stirring and rapid, floating indicates wind, rapid indicates heat, stirring indicates pain, rapid indicates deficiency. There is headache, fever and mild night sweats, but if there is aversion to cold, the exterior is not resolved. (2) However, the physician uses adverse purgation, stirring and rapid change to slow, there is pain in the diaphragm which resists pressure, emptiness and deficiency in the stomach, the visitant qi stirs the diaphragm, there is shortness of breath, agitation and vexation, anguish in the heart, yang qi fills the interior, causing hardness below the heart, which is chest bind, Da Xian Xiong Tang governs. (3) If there is no chest bind, but sweat issues from the head, there is no sweat elsewhere, it stops at the neck, the urination is not free, the body will turn yellow. Da Xian Xiong Tang formula.

DA XIAN XIONG TANG: Da Huang (skin removed) 6 liang; Mang Xiao 1 sheng; Gan Sui 1 qian bi (= 1 small teaspoon).

DIRECTIONS: First decoct Ma Huang in 6 sheng of water, reducing to 2 sheng. Strain, add Mang Xiao and bring to the boil again before adding powdered Gan Sui. Take 1 sheng warm. Discontinue medication once there is a loose stool.

DISCUSSION: Clause 134 is better read in three sections, as marked (1), (2) and (3) in the translation.

The first section is an analysis of an unresolved Tai Yang pattern which is based on the pulse sign, specifying that the floating pulse relates to the exterior pattern, the rapid pulse to heat and the spinning pulse, which refers to a pulse that is rapid, slippery and tight, is a reflection of pain caused by the constrained pathogenic qi. Taken together, these three pulse images (seen here in the rapid, floating and stirring pulse) indicate pathogenic cold invading the exterior and obstructing the flow of qi in the Tai Yang channel, thus giving rise to body aches and pains, and also confirm that the pathogenic cold has subsequently transformed into heat.

The statement "rapid indicates deficiency" alludes to the fact that the heat pathogen has not as yet knotted with phlegm or fluids in the interior, which would constitute an excess. The heat is formless and the term 'deficiency' describes the absence of knotted excess; it does not imply deficiency of zheng qi. The headache and fever represent the exterior pattern and the mild night sweats are representative of the exuberant yang heat which is tending to fall inward and damage the yin. However, if the heat pathogen had indeed fallen inwards, there would be no aversion to cold, and the aversion to cold is affirmation that the exterior pathogen is unresolved.

In the second section (2), adverse purgation refers to purgation in the presence of an unresolved exterior pattern. Even if there is interior excess, purging is contraindicated until the exterior is fully resolved. The adverse consequences of inappropriate purgation are then described, which are the symptoms of chest bind. Whilst not stated explicitly, it is understood that this occurs when there is an underlying condition of phlegm or water accumulation.

The change in the pulse sign from spinning and rapid to slow indicates a change from a yang pattern to a yin pattern. Yu Jia Yan explains that a slow pulse is a sign of knotted bind which fails to dissipate. Here, the slow pulse is a reflection of congealed qi obstructing dispersion and it should also be forceful. The emptiness and deficiency of the stomach are the result of purgation; 'visitant qi' is a reference to exogenous qi, migrating like a visitor from another country and entering the interior; this pathogenic invasion disrupts the qi of the chest and diaphragm and knots in the chest, causing shortness of breath. The chest is yang and houses the heart; the pathogenic heat in the chest harasses the heart, giving rise to vexation, agitation and anguish.

When purgation causes heat to fall inward, it knots with the pre-existing phlegm and water in the chest and creates chest bind; because the heat has knotted with form and substance, there is hardness below the heart, characterising chest bind. The treatment strategy is to purge heat and expel water, and the indicated formula is Da Xian Xiong Tang.

The third section (3) describes the development of yellowing following incorrect purgation in an unresolved exterior pattern. In this case, the pathogenic heat falls inward and combines with pre-existing damp, manifesting as a transmuted pattern of damp heat jaundice or yellowing. The damp locks-in the heat and obstructs its dispersion, so sweating is limited to the head. The combined heat and damp obstruct the waterways, giving rise to inhibited urination; thus the damp heat has no exit and its retention results in jaundice and yellowing of the skin.

Da Xian Xiong Tang is a potent formula that purges heat and expels water. Gan Sui is acrid, bitter and cold; it not only purges heat but also dispels water and is specifically indicated for water accumulation in the chest and abdomen. *Ben Cao Feng Yuan* states: "If the passage of water is uninhibited, water qi can be dispersed; if the passage of grain is uninhibited, food accumulation can be eliminated." Gan Sui drains and expels water and eliminates food stagnation, thus benefiting the passage of water and grain. Da Huang is bitter and cold; it purges heat and eliminates excess. Mang Xiao softens hardness and thus dissipates the knotted heat and water. The combination of Da Huang and Gan Sui clears heat and dispels phlegm fluids; Mang Xiao enhances Gan Sui's function of eliminating water and clearing pathogenic heat. The combined effect of the three herbs results in a potent formula to clear heat and drain accumulated water. Gan Sui is toxic and should be discontinued as soon as the condition is resolved.

Clause 134 describes two consequences of incorrect purgation in Tai Yang disease where there is a pre-existing accumulation of water or damp. The first is chest bind and the second is jaundice or yellowing. The nature and severity of the transmuted pattern arising from this is dependent on the patient's constitution and any pre-existing condition.

A Da Xian Xiong Tang pattern must be differentiated from a Zhi Zi Chi Tang pattern. The former represents a knotted bind of heat and water caused by the earlier invasion of a pathogen. It is characterised by vexation, anxiety and hard glomus below the heart. The latter is a glomus pattern where formless heat is constrained in the chest and diaphragm and the glomus is soft. Whilst it is similarly characterised by vexation and anguish, there is no hard glomus and, on palpation, the physician can only find softness.

The application Da Xian Xiong Tang and Da Cheng Qi Tang must also be clearly differentiated. Each contains Da Huang and Mang Xiao and is a bitter, cold formula with potent purging properties; however, the aetiology and disease location of their associated patterns differ, as do their ingredients. Da Cheng Qi Tang is indicated for stomach and bowel excess. Its chief herbs are Da Huang and Mang Xiao to purge the excess heat and Zhi Shi and Hou Po to descend qi and eliminate stagnation. Da Xian Xiong Tang on the other hand, is indicated for the congestion of heat and water in the chest and abdomen and uses Gan Sui as the chief herb to drain the pathogenic water downward and to free the waterways. Da Huang is the deputy and is decocted first in order to moderate its effect on the large intestine.

There are three key points to bear in mind when using Da Xian Xiong Tang. (1) The directions must be strictly adhered to: Da Huang is decocted first; the decoction is then strained before Mang Xiao is added, then it is brought to the boil again before finally adding Gan Sui powder, after which it is not strained again. The decoction is taken warm. (2) Gan Sui is the chief herb and should be taken in either powder or pill form as it is not water soluble. The instruction for the dosage of Gan Sui is 1.7 qian which is approximately 1 gram. (3) Da Xian Xiong Tang is a potent formula which purges and expels water. It is indicated only for patients with a strong constitution. Once the condition is resolved, it should be stopped.

Clause 135

伤寒六七日，结胸热实，脉沉而紧，心下痛，按之石硬者，大陷胸汤主之。

Shan han for six or seven days, chest bind with heat excess, the pulse is submerged and tight, if there is pain below the heart, stone-hard upon palpation, Da Xian Xiong Tang governs.

DISCUSSION: If shang han disease has persisted for six or seven days, there is a possibility of chest bind. Even where there has been no purging, the exterior pathogenic heat can fall inward and knot with water in the chest. Chest bind is caused by excess heat in the interior and the reference to excess heat is a reference to the exterior pathogen having penetrated the interior.

The three key symptoms are a submerged and tight pulse, pain below the heart and glomus which, on palpation, is found to be stone-hard. The submerged pulse relates to the interior and here, it is a reflection of the retained water qi. A tight pulse is associated with an excess pattern characterised by pain, thus a submerged and tight pulse is a reflection of the excess pathogenic heat being knotted in the chest and causing pain. The expression "pain below the heart" refers to pain caused by the obstruction of the knotted heat and water below the diaphragm. The description of the glomus as hard and stone-like characterises its excess nature, manifesting as fullness, tightness and pain. The treatment strategy is to drain heat and dissipate knotted bind and the indicated formula is Da Xian Xiong Tang.

A pulse which is submerged and tight can be characteristic of either a Da Xian Xiong Tang pattern, where chest bind represents the knotting of heat and water, or a yin cold pattern with water accumulation. Cheng Jiao Qian clarified this apparent ambiguity by stating: "The tight pulse associated with the chest bind pattern is pain and should not be interpreted as coldness". Chest bind with a submerged, tight pulse associated with yin cold and water accumulation is addressed in Clause 67 and the indicated formula is Fu Ling Gui Zhi Bai Zhu Gan Cao Tang.

From the modern perspective, parallels can be drawn between chest bind and inflammatory conditions of the smooth muscle, exhibiting cramp or spasm, such as acute cholecystitis with signs of infection, cholelithiasis, pancreatitis and intestinal obstruction characterised by acute abdomen with rebound pain.

Ancient Application of Da Xian Xiong Tang

Yi Xue Zhong Zhong Can Xi Lu advocated Zhe Sui Gong Jie Tang (赭遂攻结汤) (Sheng Zhe Shi 2 liang; Po Xiao 5 qian; Gan Jiang 2 qian; Gan Sui 1 qian 5 fen) for intestinal obstruction with mild heat.

Modern Application of Da Xian Xiong Tang

- *Acute pancreatitis.* Da Xian Xiong Tang with the addition of Chai Hu, Huang Qin, Mu Xiang, Yan Hu Suo was used in the treatment of 1000 cases of acute pancreatitis and combined with acupuncture treatment (Zheng Xian Li et al: *Ji Fu Zheng Tong Xun* 1974; 1:14).
- *Intestinal obstruction.* Da Xian Xiong Tang with the addition of Hou Po and Zhi Shi was used to treat acute intestinal obstruction characterised by abdominal pain resistant to pressure, abdominal distension, glomus and fullness and dark yellow urination where the tongue was red with a dry, yellow coat and the pulse was rapid. For excessive water retention in the intestines with intestinal rumbling and obstruction, Gan Sui Tong Jie Tang (Gan Sui, Tao Ren, Chi Shao, Sheng Niu Xi, Hou Po, Mu Xiang, Da Huang) was used. (*Xin Ji Fu Zheng Xue* pp212, People's Publishing Company 1978).

Case Study

Peritonitis

Extracted from Shang Han Qie Yao

A 15-year-old female had suffered from headache and generalised discomfort. After five or six days she had a sudden attack of acute abdominal pain, with her fever worsening in the afternoon, and general malaise. It was diagnosed as peritonitis and the family requested Chinese medicine treatment. Her pulse was tight and forceful, the tongue coat yellow and thick, but not dry. There had been no bowel movement for seven days, there was rebound abdominal pain, her urination was dark and scant, she had no appetite and her speech was delirious. She was prescribed Da Xian Xiong Tang with modifications: Da Huang 2 qian, Mang Xiao 2 qian, Dong Gua Zi 5 qian, Sheng Yi Mi 5 qian, Gan Sui powder 3 fen (wrapped separately).

Da Huang was decocted first, the decoction was then strained before adding Mang Xiao. The decoction was then brought to the boil once or twice and the Gan Sui powder added. One hour after the medication, the patient had a bowel movement but the stool was formed. After a second dose, she passed a loose, watery stool and the fever and abdominal pain receded.

Discussion: The symptoms of constipation, delirious speech and tidal fever are characteristic of a Yang Ming bowel excess pattern where Da Cheng Qi Tang is indicated. However, the symptom of rebound abdominal pain which was resistant to pressure, and a tongue coat which was thick and yellow but not dry, showed it not to be a Cheng Qi Tang pattern. The pattern of abdominal pain mirrored a Da Xian Xiong Tang pattern, supported by the three key diagnostic signs of a tight pulse, pain below the heart (epigastric pain) with hard glomus on palpation. The aetiology was seen to be incorrect treatment of the original exterior disorder which had manifested with tidal fever, headache and general malaise, on a background of pre-existing water accumulation. Since no purgatives had been taken, it can be seen to be a chest bind pattern which has occurred in the absence of purgation.

Comparison of Da Chai Hu Tang and Da Xian Xiong Tang Patterns

Clause 136

伤寒十余日，热结在里，复往来寒热者，与大柴胡汤；但结胸，无大热者，此为水结在胸胁也，但头微汗出者，大陷胸汤主之。

Shang han for more than ten days, if there is heat bind in the interior, with alternating chills and fever, give Da Chai Hu Tang; if there is only chest bind, without vigorous fever, this is water knotted in the chest and ribs, if a slight sweat issues only from the head, Da Xian Xiong Tang governs.

DISCUSSION: When shang han disease has persisted for more than ten days, there is the possibility of the exterior pathogen having transformed into heat and fallen inward. There are two possible developments, one which calls for treatment by Da Chai Hu Tang and the other, where Da Xian Xiong Tang is the indicated formula.

1. A Da Chai Hu Tang pattern represents a semi-interior, semi-exterior pattern with heat bind in the interior. Pathogenic heat knotted in the interior is a manifestation of a Yang Ming pattern where there should be constipation and a dry, yellow tongue coat. However, if the pattern includes the symptoms of alternating chills and fever, then it is understood that the pathogenic qi is harassing the Shao Yang. From this it can be deduced that the pattern is a complex pattern of excess heat in the Yang Ming combined with qi constraint in the Shao Yang, and is also known as a Yang Ming Shao Yang concurrent pattern or bing bing. Further to the symptoms cited above, there is nausea, distension, pain and fullness below the heart or fullness and congestion in the hypochondrium. The indicated formula is Da Chai Hu Tang to address both the Yang Ming and Shao Yang channels.
2. A Da Xian Xiong Tang pattern represents chest bind due to excess heat having fallen inward and knotted with water in the chest. The slight fever which subsequently manifests differs both from the alternating chills and fever of Shao Yang and from the steaming fever of Yang Ming. A chest bind pattern is characterised by glomus below the heart which is both hard and painful, and by slight sweating which comes only from the head. This phenomenon results from the generalised dispersion of heat being blocked

by the bind of heat and water, and the sweat having no escape other than the highest point, the head. Da Xian Xiong Tang is indicated because it addresses the knotting of pathogenic heat with water directly. Ke Yun Bo said: "The aetiology of chest bind is heat falling inward, and the root of chest bind is the knotting of water". If either of these two components is absent, there is no chest bind.

Major Chest Bind with Yang Ming Bowel Excess

Clause 137

太阳病，重发汗而复下之，不大便五六日，舌上燥而渴、日晡所小有潮热，从心下至少腹硬满而痛不可近者，大陷胸汤主之。

TaiYang disease, repeated sweat promotion then purging, no stool for five or six days, the tongue surface is dry and there is thirst, in the late afternoon there is mild tidal fever, if from below the heart to the lesser abdomen there is hard distension and pain such that the patient will not allow anyone near, Da Xian Xiong Tang governs.

DISCUSSION: Sweat promotion is the indicated treatment for Tai Yang disease, but it must be discontinued once the disease is resolved. Continuous or repeated sweating and purging will lead to severe fluid damage, causing the heat pathogen to fall inward, where it can knot with water and form chest bind. The fluid damage also results in stomach dryness, giving rise to constipation, which in Clause 137 has lasted for five or six days; additional symptoms are a dry tongue coat, thirst and tidal fever.

The expression *ri bu* (日晡), translated here as 'late afternoon', in fact refers to the period of time represented by the 9th earthly branch, *shen shi* (申时). This covers the hours between 3 pm and 5 pm, when the large intestine qi of Yang Ming peaks. Tidal fever is a fluctuating fever which comes and goes in waves and, at this time of increased qi in the Yang Ming, it spikes upward, signifying Yang Ming excess. Hard distension in the abdomen is also a feature of a Yang Ming bowel excess pattern; the reluctance to be approached confirms the excess nature of the pain, as it is aggravated by pressure. These symptoms lead to a diagnosis of Yang Ming bowel excess, where there is the additional feature of heat bind in the chest and abdomen. Da Xian Xiong Tang is the appropriate formula to sweep away the water and purge the heat.

Simple Yang Ming bowel excess must be differentiated from chest bind. If there is no water accumulation, then the condition is a simple Yang Ming bowel excess pattern and Cheng Qi Tang is the indicated treatment. If there is an accumulation of interior water which has knotted with heat, then it is a chest bind pattern and the indicated formula is Da Xian Xiong Tang. For optimal analysis and clear differentiation, both similarities and differences must be observed.

The similarities are found in the constipation, the afternoon tidal fever, the dry tongue coat, thirst and abdominal fullness with pain which resists pressure. The differences between simple Yang Ming bowel excess and chest bind are as follows.

Aetiology and pathogenesis. A simple Yang Ming bowel excess pattern with stomach dryness and constipation is caused by interior heat; the complex pattern of Yang Ming bowel excess with chest bind is caused by inappropriate sweating and purging which have damaged fluids, following which exterior heat has fallen inwards and knotted with water.

Distension. The distension of a simple Yang Ming heat excess pattern is located in the stomach and intestines; the distension of chest bind is located in the chest and diaphragm, and is described as 'hard distension'.

Pain. A Yang Ming bowel excess pattern is characterised by periumbilical pain resistant to pressure; chest bind is associated with abdominal pain which extends from the epigastrium to the lesser abdomen.

Fever. In a simple Yang Ming bowel excess pattern, there is significant tidal fever and also delirious speech; in the chest bind pattern there is only slight tidal fever and no delirious speech.

Contraindication of Purgation in Chest Bind with a Floating and Big Pulse

Clause 132

结胸证，其脉浮大者，不可下，下之则死。

Chest bind pattern, if the pulse is floating and big, one should not purge, purging will cause death.

DISCUSSION: When a chest bind pattern is characterised by a pulse which is submerged, excess and forceful, and glomus below the heart which is hard and painful, purgation is permitted. If, however, the pulse is floating and big, purgation is contraindicated. This is because a floating pulse indicates an unresolved exterior pathogen and a big pulse indicates the interior excess is yet to manifest, therefore purging should not be used.

A pulse which is floating and big can either be forceful or forceless. If the pulse is floating, big and forceful, it indicates that the exterior pathogen has only partially fallen inward. The indicated treatment at this juncture is to release the exterior before purging the interior water accumulation. This is because if purgation is used when an exterior pattern is not fully resolved, the exterior pathogen may fall inward causing the condition to deteriorate. A pulse which is floating, big and lacks force indicates interior deficiency, with the excess yet to manifest; the correct strategy is first to support the deficiency before purging the water accumulation; alternatively, the strategy of simultaneous supplementation and purgation may be employed. If one fails to observe the pulse and resorts first to purgation, the exterior pathogen will fall inward and the patient's condition will deteriorate. The significance of Clause 132 is that it cautions practitioners to diagnose correctly, and to use Da Xian Xiong Tang only when there is interior excess and the exterior pathogen is fully resolved.

Prognosis of Chest Bind

Clause 133

结胸证悉俱, 烦躁者亦死。

Chest bind signs are all present, if there is vexation and agitation, the patient will die.

DISCUSSION: The signs of chest bind referred to here are: pain which extends from the area below the heart to the lesser abdomen and which is aggravated by pressure, constipation, a dry tongue coat, thirst, and a submerged and excess pulse. The presence of all of these signs already indicates a critical condition. Vexation and agitation reflect the deep-seated nature of the pathogen and the dissipation of zheng qi, which is evidence of the ever-mounting strength of the pathogenic qi.

The treatment of chest bind must be dictated by its pathogenesis and be in keeping with the course of its development. Clause 133 describes the consequences of not treating chest bind at an early stage: timing of the treatment is the essence and missing the opportunity to purge may have a tragic outcome. Clause 132 describes chest bind which is characterised by a floating, big pulse, where purging is contraindicated. Because purgation was wrongly used, zheng qi was further depleted, providing an opportunity for the pathogen to fall inward. Clause 133, describes a case of inappropriate early purgation and the prognosis is not good. In comparing Clauses 132 and 133 we see that incorrect treatment has been given in both cases. In Clause 132 it is too early, and in Clause 133 it is too late; failing to purge at the correct time has resulted in a disastrous outcome.

The vexation described in Clause 133 and that described in Clause 134 should be contrasted: the vexation of Clause 134 is relatively mild and the symptoms of chest bind are absent; this indicates an excess pattern where the zheng qi is intact. In Clause 133, the vexation is significant, the zheng qi is impaired; thus the prognosis is poor.

Da Xian Xiong Wan Pattern

Clause 131B

结胸者，项亦强，如柔痓状，下之则和，宜大陷胸丸。

If there is chest bind, the neck is stiff, as in soft tetany, purgation will bring harmony, Da Xian Xiong Wan is appropriate.

DA XIAN XIONG WAN: Da Huang ½ jin; Ting Li Zi (dry-fried) ½ jin; Mang Xiao ½ jin; Xing Ren (skin and tips removed, then dry-fried till black) ½ jin.

DIRECTIONS: Pound and sieve the first two ingredients, then add Xing Ren and Mang Xiao to make a paste. Form into large pills, then in a separate bowl, pound 1.7 qian of Gan Sui into powder and combine with 1 ge of honey and 2 sheng of water. Bring to the boil and reduce to 1 sheng. Administer warm with 1 pill as a single dose and the patient will pass a loose stool overnight. If there is no diarrhoea, further doses are taken until there is diarrhoea, which indicates that the medication has taken effect. The instructions must be followed carefully.

DISCUSSION: Chest bind as mentioned in Clause 131B refers to any pattern with the symptoms of chest bind. Tetany is a disorder characterised by a stiff neck which can proceed to full body rigidity. If there is sweating, it is soft tetany; if there is no sweating, it is known as hard tetany. Therefore, the reference to soft tetany is a reference to a stiff neck accompanied by sweating. The significance of the sweating is that in addition to knotting with water in the chest, the pathogenic heat has obstructed the proper distribution of fluids. On the one hand, this results in sweating, on the other, the impaired distribution means that the muscles and sinews are not moistened and nourished, giving rise to a stiff neck.

Da Xian Xiong Wan is Da Xian Xiong Tang with the addition of Xing Ren, Ting Li Zi and honey. Da Huang and Mang Xiao purge heat and dissipate the knotted bind; Gan Sui expels accumulated water and, when combined with Da Huang and Mang Xiao, dissipates the bind of heat and water. Ting Li Zi purges lung heat; Xing Ren descends lung qi, thus facilitating its diffusion and freeing the water passages. Honey is sweet and moistening; it has a moderating effect on the herbs, and thus assists in the expulsion of the pathogen without damaging the zheng qi. Da Xian Xiong Wan represents a potent purging formula which is moderated by the addition of honey.

Da Xian Xiong Wan and Da Xian Xiong Tang are both indicated for chest bind characterised by a hard and painful glomus which is accompanied by tidal fever and constipation and which is a pattern of heat and excess. However, the key diagnostic features for which each is indicated differ. Differentiation must be made according to location, which can be in the middle or lower jiao, not just the upper jiao. If the bind is in the upper jiao, the pathogen is also in the upper jiao; the key diagnostic feature is that the chest bind is accompanied by neck stiffness; the indicated formula is Da Xian Xiong Wan (Clause 131B). If the glomus is in the middle jiao and is characterised by pain below the heart with a knot which is stone-like when palpated, the indicated formula is Da Xian Xiong Tang (Clause 135). Chest bind in the lower jiao represents a more extensive and more serious form of knotting, which involves the Yang Ming, and is characterised by a hard, painful glomus which extends from below the heart to the lesser abdomen and which is aggravated by pressure (Clause 137). Because it involves both the chest and abdomen, it is more serious, but it still is treated with Da Xian Xiong Tang.

Ancient Application of Da Xian Xiong Tang

- *Yi Zong Jin Jian:* In the treatment of the early stage of an excess pattern of diarrhoea.
- *Lei Ju Fang Guang Yi:* In the treatment of phlegm damp characterised by pain in the heart and chest glomus with pain radiating to the neck and arm.

Modern Application of Da Xian Xiong Tang

Modified versions of Da Xian Xiong Tang can be used for chronic bronchitis, asthma, emphysema, pleuritis and pneumothorax when associated with heat and water bind in the upper part of the body.

Xiao Xian Xiong Tang Pattern

Xiao Xian Xiong or minor chest bind pattern is attributed to an exterior pathogen falling inward, which can either be spontaneous or due to incorrect purgation. After sinking inwards, the pathogenic heat then knots with phlegm which has accumulated below the heart, which refers to the epigastric region. Because the phlegm is confined to the epigastrium, so is the manifestation of chest bind, which is characterised by pain upon palpation.

> **Clause 138**
>
> 小结胸病，正在心下，按之则痛，脉浮滑者，小陷胸汤主之。
>
> *Minor chest bind disease, just below the heart, if there is pain on palpation, the pulse is floating and slippery, Xiao Xian Xiong Tang governs.*

XIAO XIAN XIONG TANG: Huang Lian 1 liang; Ban Xia (washed) ½ jin; Gua Lou Shi 1 large piece (equivalent to 30 g).

NOTE: The terms Gua Lou Shi and Quan Gua Lou refer to the whole fruit, incorporating the skin (Gua Lou Pi) and the seed (Gua Lou Ren).

DIRECTIONS: First boil Gua Lou in 6 sheng of water, reducing to 3 sheng. Strain and add the remaining 2 herbs, further reducing to 1 sheng before straining again. Divide into 3 doses and take warm.

DISCUSSION: Minor chest bind or Xiao Xian Xiong Tang pattern is a disorder confined to the epigastrium or 'below the heart'. It is characterised by pain aggravated by pressure and a floating and slippery pulse. A floating pulse is a yang pulse and is associated with heat; a slippery pulse is associated with damp and phlegm. The floating, slippery pulse thus represents a pattern of phlegm and heat and in this instance relates to phlegm heat bind. The indicated formula is Xiao Xian Xiong Tang.

Xiao Xian Xiong Tang is an acrid, bitter formula which transforms phlegm, disperses constraint, drains heat and, by so doing, is able to dissipate chest bind and ease pain. Huang Lian enters the upper and middle jiao and is bitter and cold. Thus it is able to dry damp and drain fire from the epigastrium. Ban Xia is acrid and warm, resolves phlegm and dries damp, thus transforming phlegm damp in the middle jiao. Gua Lou is sweet, cold, moistening and has a descending action. Not only does it assist in the transformation of phlegm heat, but its downward and moistening properties promote the purging of heat bind.

Comparison of Xiao Xian Xiong Tang and Da Xian Xiong Tang Patterns

Xiao Xian Xiong Tang and Da Xian Xiong Tang are patterns of chest bind associated with heat excess but they differ in severity. Xiao Xian Xiong Tang pattern, or minor chest bind pattern, is relatively mild, being characterised by the knotting of heat and phlegm in the epigastrium, with pain elicited by palpation. Da Xian Xiong Tang pattern, or major chest bind pattern, is a more serious condition attributed to the knotting of heat and water; it is characterised by a hard, painful glomus which is aggravated by pressure. Analysis of the herbal ingredients shows that Huang Lian's

Comparison of Da Xian Xiong Tang and Xiao Xian Xiong Tang

	Da Xian Xiong Tang	Xiao Xian Xiong Tang
Aetiology	Heat and water bind	Heat and phlegm bind
Symptoms	Hard glomus and pain from below the heart to the lesser abdomen	Pain below the heart with palpable pain
Pulse Sign	Submerged and tight	Floating and slippery
Treatment	Purge heat, dispel water retention and dissipate bind	Clear heat, transform phlegm, dissipate phlegm bind and loosen the chest

function of clearing heat in Xiao Xian Xiong Tang is far milder than Da Huang's function of purging heat and moving accumulation in Da Xian Xiong Tang. Similarly, Ban Xia's phlegm transforming function in Xiao Xian Xiong Tang is milder than the action of Gan Sui in sweeping phlegm and dispelling water in Da Xian Xiong Tang. Gua Lou's actions of transforming phlegm heat, descending qi, moistening dryness and easing pain is milder than Mang Xiao's action of purging excess and softening hardness.

A parallel can be drawn between some gastroenteric disorders, where epigastric pain is a feature, and a minor chest bind pattern, where epigastric pain is also a feature, and Xiao Xian Xiong Tang can be used for either chronic or acute gastritis characterised by distending pain. The tongue should be red with a yellow, slippery or greasy coat. When serving her internship under Professor Guo Wei Qin of the Cardiac Department of Dong Zhi Men's Hospital in Beijing, the author also observed the use of Xiao Xian Xiong Tang as a base formula in the treatment of chest pain where there was a yellow greasy tongue coat and a slippery pulse.

The purpose of decocting Gua Lou Shi first, is to enhance its function of transforming phlegm and moving accumulation. A sticky yellow discharge from the bowel after administration of the herbs represents elimination of the phlegm, allowing recovery to take place. It should be noted that apart from Gua Lou Shi (Quan Gua Lou), Zhang Zhong Jing sometimes used Gua Lou Gen, also known as Tian Hua Fen, which drains fire, generates fluids and eases thirst. This contrasts with the functions of Gua Lou Shi which are to dissipate knotted bind, transform phlegm and free obstruction in order to ease pain. The application of Gua Lou in this capacity is seen in *Jin Gui Yao Lue,* where Gua Lou Xie Bai Bai Jiu Tang and Gua Lou Xie Bai Ban Xia Tang are indicated to transform stasis and ease chest pain. Gua Lou is also a key herb in the treatment of mammary abscess (*ru yong*) when used with appropriate herbs such as Pu Gong Ying, Ru Xiang and Mo Yao; modern practitioners use Gua Lou, Dang Gui, Sheng Huang Qi to enhance the production and flow of breast milk when obstructed by phlegm stasis.

Ancient Application of Xiao Xian Xiong Tang

- In *Yi Xue Ru Men*, Xiao Tiao Zhong Tang, which is Xiao Xian Xiong Tang with the addition of Gan Cao and Sheng Jiang, is advocated for the treatment of difficult-to-treat disorders associated with phlegm.
- In *Zhang Shi Yi Tong*, Xiao Xian Xiong Tang is cited for the treatment of cough characterised by a flushed face, a greasy, yellow tongue coat and a slippery pulse.
- *Shang Han Lun Lei Fang Hui Can* mentions Xiao Xian Xiong Tang with the addition of Chao Hu for the treatment of fever and tidal heat; where heat is severe, Huang Qin is added; for thirst, Ban Xia is omitted and Tian Hua Fen and Ge Gen are added; for dry retching, Chen Pi is added; for a stifling sensation in the chest, Zhi Qiao and Jie Geng are added; for epigastric pain, Zhi Shi is added; for scant urination, Fu Ling is added; for vexation in the chest, Shan Zhi is added.

Modern Application of Xiao Xian Xiong Tang

- Yue Mei Zhong used Xiao Xian Xiong Tang combined with Da Chai Hu Tang in the treatment of hepatitis. The patient was mildly jaundiced and presented with pain in the ribs and epigastric distension. The left guan pulse was floating and wiry, the right pulse was big and slippery, and the tongue coat was yellow. After 17 days of administration, the condition was resolved. (*Yue Mei Zhong Yi An*, People's Medical Publishing House 1978)
- Xiao Xian Xiong Tang is indicated for chronic gastritis characterised by a dull ache in the stomach area, distension, nausea, constipation, a parched throat and a red tongue with a yellow greasy tongue coat.

Modifications

- For vexation and an oppressed sensation in the chest, add Zhi Zi Chi Tang.
- For acute pain, add Yan Hu Suo, Chuan Lian Zi and Xiang Fu to regulate qi and ease pain.

- For nausea and vomiting, add Chen Pi, Zhu Ru, Sheng Jiang to descend rebellious qi.
- For acid reflux, add Wu Zei Gu to neutralise and restrain acid reflux.
- For chronic hepatitis due to phlegm heat obstruction characterised by epigastric distension, glomus and pain, a yellow greasy tongue coat and a wiry slippery pulse, Xiao Xian Xiong Tang can be combined with Xiao Chai Hu Tang and modified with Yin Chen and Zhi Zi.

Case Study

Recurrent Tonsillitis

Extracted from Greta Young's case studies

A 28-year-old female patient had suffered from chronic tonsillitis for five years, with acute episodes occurring three to four times a year. Her current bout of tonsillitis had persisted for over a month and been triggered by an excessive intake of spicy food and yellow wine. She complained of a subjective feeling of throat obstruction, an oppressed sensation in the chest, glomus, a parched throat with scorching pain, a cough with sticky phlegm, and a dry bowel movement. The throat was inflamed and her tongue was red with a thin yellow tongue coat. Her pulse was floating and slippery. The diagnosis was phlegm heat knotted in the throat and chest and she was prescribed a modified version of Xiao Xian Xiong Tang: Quan Gua Lou 20g, Bei Sha Shen 20g, Ban Xia 10g, Jie Geng 10g, Huang Lian 5g, Xuan Shen 15g, Gan Cao 3g. After five packs, her condition improved and she was given a further five packs to ensure complete recovery.

2.9.3 Chest Bind with Cold Excess

San Wu Bai San Pattern

Clause 141

寒实结胸，无热证者，与三物白散。

Cold excess chest bind, with no heat signs, give San Wu Bai San.

SAN WU BAI SAN: Jie Geng 3 fen; Ba Dou (skin and heart removed, dry-fried and ground to a paste) 1 fen; Bei Mu 3 fen.

DIRECTIONS: Grind Jie Geng and Bei Mu into a powder and pound Ba Dou into a paste. Then blend together and take with white rice water (bai yin). A patient with a strong constitution can take a half qian spoonful but for a patient with a weak constitution, the dose should be reduced. If the disease is above the diaphragm, there will be vomiting and if it is below the diaphragm, there will be diarrhoea. If there is no diarrhoea, drink 1 cup of hot gruel. If there is excessive diarrhoea, drink 1 cup of cold gruel.

DISCUSSION: Cold excess chest bind is due to the knotting of pathogenic cold and water. The are two points to bear in mind in regard to chest bind associated with the knotting of cold and phlegm damp. First, because it is due to knotting in the chest, it resembles other chest bind patterns, in that the glomus is hard and painful and is located in the epigastrium or side of the chest; second, because it is due to the knotting of cold and water, there are no heat signs such as thirst, dryness of the tongue, heart vexation or anguish and no tidal fever in the afternoon. The treatment strategy is to warm the cold, dispel the pathogenic water and eliminate the phlegm bind. The indicated formula is San Wu Bai San.

San Wu Bai San, which translates as 'three ingredients white powder' is made up of the three herbs, Ba Dou, Bei Mu and Jie Geng, each of which are white in colour. Ba Dou is acrid, hot and toxic, drains cold and purges water. Because of its strong action in dispersing cold bind, it is the chief herb. Bei Mu supports Ba Dou by transforming and dissipating stubborn and knotted phlegm. Jie Geng raises and disseminates the lung qi, thus facilitating the dissipation of the knotted bind and also guides the other herbs to the upper jiao. The purpose of taking rice water with the formula is to nourish the stomach and counteract potential damage by the harsh expellant, Ba Dou. The mention of vomiting and diarrhoea is a reference to the after-effect of the herbs: water bind above the diaphragm is expelled through the mechanism of vomiting, and water bind below the diaphragm is expelled via the stool, producing diarrhoea. Diarrhoea is the desired result of the treatment; however, if it is excessive, it shows that the effect of the decoction was too strong and so cold gruel is given to moderate the effect of the acrid hot and warm herbs. If, on the other hand, there is no diarrhoea, warm gruel is given to enhance the effect of the formula. Both white rice water and gruel nourish and protect the stomach and their use here is a good example of the importance given in *Shang Han Lun* to the preservation of the stomach qi.

Chest bind due to the knotting of cold and water in the chest can obstruct the flow of chest yang and disturb the qi dynamic and the subsequent distribution of fluid. Some of the frequently encountered symptoms are aversion to cold, preference for warmth, coughing and wheezing, shortness of breath and, less commonly, constipation. There is no mention of the pulse sign in Clause 141, but based on the fact that it is a pattern of chest bind associated with cold excess, the pulse would be submerged, wiry and forceful.

Modern Application of San Wu Bai San

- Liang et al used San Wu Bai San with the addition of such toxicity relieving herbs as Pu Gong Ying and Jin Yin Hua to treat pulmonary abscess in the ulcerative phase by discharging pus and eliminating toxicity (*Xin Zhong Yi* 4:45, 1981).
- Wang et al used a modified version of San Wu Bai San to treat five cases of pulmonary abscess. They combined San Wu Bai San with Wei Jing Tang and Ting Li Da Zao Tang, Jie Geng Tang and Xie Bai San and also used antibiotic therapy. In the cases where the afternoon dose resulted in several episodes of diarrhoea overnight, cold gruel was given to ease the diarrhoea. The following day, the fever was resolved and the coughing had eased. A formula to transform phlegm and disseminate lung qi was then given (*Zhong Yi Za Zhi* 1955; 4:25).

Summary of Chest Bind Patterns

In *Shang Han Lun*, a chest bind pattern is generally the result of incorrect purging; the pathogenic heat falls inward, where it can knot with accumulated water. Due to differences in constitution and the nature of the pathogen, chest bind is categorised into heat excess chest bind and cold excess chest bind. Heat excess chest bind is further categorised as Da Xian Xiong Tang pattern, Da Xian Xiong Wan pattern and Xiao Xian Xiong Tang pattern, as follows.

- Da Xian Xiong Wan pattern is characterised by the knotting of heat and water in the chest. It tends to be located above the diaphragm, in the upper jiao, and its key features are hard, painful glomus in the chest and stiffness of the neck resembling soft tetany. It is a milder pattern governed by a modified formula and the treatment principle is to drain heat and drive out water from the upper jiao.
- Da Xian Xiong Tang pattern is characterised by the knotting of heat and water below the diaphragm, in the epigastrium or the side of the ribs. Involvement of the abdomen manifests as pain below the heart with a stone-like sensation on palpation, or pain and distension which extends from the epigastric region to the lesser abdomen and which resists pressure. There is a mild tidal fever, constipation and the pulse is submerged and tight. The treatment principle is to purge heat, drive out water and dissipate the knotted bind. However, if the pulse is floating and big, purging is contraindicated and may lead to death.
- Xiao Xian Xiong Tang pattern is ascribed to heat binding with phlegm below the heart and can manifest either with pain on pressure or pain felt without palpation. The pulse is submerged, floating and slippery and the treatment principle is to clear heat, eliminate phlegm and dissipate the phlegm bind.

Cold excess chest bind is due to pathogenic cold binding with water below the heart and is characterised by chest and epigastric pain, the absence of heat signs such as fever or vexation, and less commonly, constipation. The treatment principle is to purge the cold pathogen and expel the water bind. The indicated formula is San Wu Bai San.

2.9.4 Glomus

Glomus or *pi zheng* refers to a localised subjective feeling of fullness and blockage, usually in the epigastric region, described in *Shang Han Lun* as "glomus below the heart". It is attributed to obstruction caused by heat, phlegm water or stagnant qi, which gives rise to blockage and a sense of fullness. The zang fu affected are the spleen and stomach, as is their function in providing the pivotal dynamic of the ascent and descent of qi.

Clause 151

脉浮而紧，而复下之，紧反入里，则作痞，按之自濡，但气痞耳。

The pulse is floating and tight, but again there is purging, the tightness instead enters the interior, causing a glomus, it is soft when pressed, it is only a qi glomus.

DISCUSSION: A floating, tight pulse indicates a shang han exterior excess pattern where Ma Huang Tang is used to promote sweating. If purgation is wrongly used instead, the pathogen falls inward. The tightness which enters the interior refers not to the tight pulse in the opening statement, but to the exterior pathogenic cold which has caused the tight pulse. Because purging damages the qi of the spleen and stomach, their respective functions of ascending and descending are impaired; qi then accumulates, giving rise to a localised sensation of fullness and blockage. There is no formed pathogen and so, because qi glomus is the result of qi stagnation and is a formless qi bind, there is softness on palpation and no sensation of pain.

Reference to the aetiology of glomus being incorrect purging of an exterior pattern, subsequently causing the pathogen to fall inward, is also found in Clause 131 which states: "there is adverse purgation, and so glomus forms". Both Clause 131 and Clause 151 ascribe the aetiology of glomus to incorrect purgation, with subsequent knotting of the pathogen in the epigastrium, giving rise to the clinical feature of blockage below the heart. However, purgation is not the only aetiology and glomus can also arise when the exterior pathogen exploits interior spleen and stomach deficiency.

Comparison of Glomus and Chest Bind

Glomus and chest bind bear certain similarities in that they both share the features of fullness and distension. Differential diagnosis is dependent on understanding the disease mechanism: chest bind is the the result of heat knotting with a formed pathogen in the interior, in this case, with pre-existing water and phlegm. Due to the formed nature of the pathogen, it forms a hard glomus in the chest and is characterised by pain. Qi glomus refers to the stagnation of qi causing disruption to the qi dynamic; because it is formless, there is a subjective sense of blockage below the heart, and softness on palpation which is painless. Although the qi stagnation itself is formless and insubstantial, meaning that it is not knotted with water, food or phlegm, nevertheless any of these substances can be the cause of qi stagnation. Apart from qi glomus, which is soft, there is also hard glomus, which is the result of the knotting of pathogenic heat (Clause 131A) or pathogenic cold (Clause 141) with a substance such as water or phlegm.

2.9.5 Heat Glomus

Da Huang Huang Lian Xie Xin Tang Pattern

Clause 154

心下痞，按之濡，其脉关上浮者，大黄黄连泻心汤主之。

Glomus below the heart, soft upon palpation, the pulse is floating on the guan position, Da Huang Huang Lian Xie Xin Tang governs.

DA HUANG HUANG LIAN XIE XIN TANG: Da Huang 2 liang; Huang Lian 1 liang.

DIRECTIONS: Infuse both ingredients in 2 sheng of boiled water. After a few minutes strain and take warm in two doses.

DISCUSSION: Heat glomus is the result of formless heat knotting below the heart. This stagnates qi and gives rise to glomus. The aetiology can be incorrect purgation causing pathogenic heat to fall inward; pathogenic heat falling inward where there has been no purgation; or non-interaction of the heart and kidney. All can give rise to soft glomus below the heart. "Below the heart" refers to the epigastrium and its description as soft glomus shows that is not due to a formed heat bind. The floating pulse relates to yang heat and the guan position denotes the middle jiao, thus describing the accumulation of pathogenic heat in the middle jiao, for which the indicated treatment is Da Huang Huang Lian Xie Xin Tang. Da Huang is bitter and cold, it purges heat, benefits the stomach and dissipates bind; Huang Lian clears fire from the heart and stomach. The reason for infusing rather than decocting the herbs is because prolonged boiling renders the herbs too concentrated. The infusion is milder and clears the formless heat in the upper jiao without having too strong a descending effect.

There are several interpretations as to the pathogenesis of heat glomus. Among them, Cheng Wu Ji (1066–1156, author of *Zhu Jie Shang Han Lun* and the first to annotate *Shang Han Lun*) suggested that the heat is due to deficiency; You Zai Jing (circa 1749, author of *Shang Han Guan Zhu Ji*) suggests the deficiency relates to the dry bowel but not to general yin or yang deficiency; Wang Ling You, author of *Shang Han Lun Bian Zheng Guang Yi*, said: "This is a pattern of mild pathogenic heat not deficient heat." Modern interpretations generally agree that of these three explanations, the latter two are more apt in describing the pathogenesis of heat glomus accumulation with blockage of the qi dynamic. This is because heat glomus is attributed to the accumulation of formless heat below the heart and not to the formed accumulation of food stagnation. Treatment is therefore focused on clearing heat, not on purging, and for that reason, a stronger formula is not appropriate.

According to Lin Yi, Da Huang Huang Lian Xie Xin Tang comprises only Da Huang and Huang Lian and it is Fu Zi Xie Xin Tang which, apart from Fu Zi, Da Huang and Huang Lian, also contains Huang Qin. However, *Qian Jin Yao Fang* stated that Huang Qin should be included. From the clinical perspective, the addition of Huang Qin increases the efficacy of the formula's heat-clearing function.

NOTE: Lin Yi lived during the Song Dynasty in the 11th century. He and his associates formed a bureau which edited and compiled many medical texts such as *Su Wen, Ling Shu, Shang Han Lun, Qian Jin Yao Fang, Qian Jin Yi Fang, Wai Tai Mi Yao*.

The instructions for administration say that it should be taken as a warm infusion in 2 doses. Contemporary practitioners suggest that it can be taken at frequent intervals during the day like tea, so the herbal effect can be exerted slowly. The Xie Xin Tang of *Jin Gui Yao Lue* is composed of three ingredients, Da Huang, Huang Lian and Huang Qin. These are decocted, reducing the liquid to 1 sheng, then taken warm in one draught. This decoction is indicated for insufficiency of heart qi manifesting with haemoptysis and epistaxis. The stronger effect of the decoction achieves the desired effect of draining heart fire and stopping bleeding.

Ancient Application of Da Huang Huang Lian Xie Xin Tang

- *Qian Jin Fang* used Da Huang Huang Lian Xie Xin Tang in the treatment of heart qi insufficiency manifesting with haemoptysis and nose bleed.
- *Huo Ren Shu* stated that Xie Xin San Huang Tang (which is Da Huang Huang Lian Xie Xin Tang with the addition of Huang Qin) was indicated for women who had had shang han for six or seven days, with dryness and phlegm lodged in the stomach, a difficult bowel movement, vexation, delirious speech, red eyes and toxic qi obstruction.
- *Lin Zheng Zhi Nan* advocated Da Huang Huang Lian Xie Xin Tang in the treatment of severe haemoptysis.

Modern Application of Da Huang Huang Lian Xie Xin Tang

- For epistaxis and haemoptysis.
- For mouth ulcers, modified by adding Zhu Ye, Sheng Di, Zhi Gan Cao, Lian Xin.
- For acute dysentery, combined with Bai Tou Weng Tang and the addition of Mu Xiang and Ju Hua.
- For hypertension characterised by dizziness, a flushed face, a dry throat, a bitter taste in

the mouth, thirst, glomus below the heart, vexation, a dry bowel movement, a strong, wiry pulse and a red tongue with yellow tongue coat, the following modified formula can be used: Da Huang 6g; Huang Lian 5g; Huang Qin 10g. The herbs are infused in boiling water taken strained as a tea.

Case Study

Nose bleed

Extracted from Zhong Guo Yi Yao Xue Bao 1989; (3):9

A 22-year-old male patient had suffered from nose bleeds for two days and was admitted to hospital. He had a dry throat, a bitter taste in the mouth, constipation and dizziness. He was of strong build, had foul breath, his tongue was dull red with a thin tongue coat and his pulse was wiry, rapid and forceful. The diagnosis was exuberant fire in the heart and stomach. The formula used was Da Huang Huang Lian Xie Xin Tang modified: Da Huang 6g, Huang Lian 6g, Huang Qin 9g, Zhi Zi 10g, Bai Mao Gen 15g, Niu Xi 10g. He was given three packs, after which the nose bleed stopped and a follow-up several months later showed there had been no recurrence.

Heat Glomus with an Exterior Pattern

Clause 164

伤寒大下后，复发汗，心下痞、恶寒者，表未解也。不可攻痞，当先解表，表解乃可攻痞。解表宜桂枝汤，攻痞宜大黄黄连泻心汤。

Shang han after severe purgation, sweating is then promoted, if there is glomus below the heart, aversion to cold, the exterior is unresolved. One should not attack the glomus, one must first resolve the exterior, once the exterior is resolved, then one may attack the glomus. To resolve the exterior, Gui Zhi Tang is appropriate, to attack the glomus, Da Huang Huang Lian Xie Xin Tang is appropriate.

DISCUSSION: The indicated treatment for a shang han exterior pattern is to promote sweat in order to release the exterior. Even where there is a concurrent interior pattern, the principle of first releasing the exterior must be adhered to. To purge first constitutes incorrect treatment because purging can damage the stomach qi and cause the pathogenic heat to fall inward, causing obstruction in the middle jiao. Although there is no mention of headache or fever, the presence of aversion to cold signifies that an exterior pattern remains; the glomus demonstrates that there is also an interior pattern. In a pattern which is simultaneously exterior and interior, the exterior must be released first before attacking or clearing the interior. Selection of the most appropriate formula to treat the exterior will depend on the disease condition. Nevertheless, Gui Zhi Tang is the guiding formula nominated for zhong feng exterior deficiency, and Ma Huang Tang is suitable for shang han exterior excess.

The two features which must be present for diagnosis of heat glomus with an exterior pattern are: (1) a floating guan pulse in the guan position; this identifies the nature of the glomus as being caused by yang heat in the middle jiao; and (2) exterior symptoms, such as, but not limited to, aversion to cold, fever and headache. Apart from the floating guan pulse, the pulse should be generally floating in order to confirm the exterior disorder.

The principle of releasing the exterior first before purging the interior comes from the theory propounded in *Huang Di Nei Jing*. If, however, there is an exterior pattern in the presence of acute interior cold due to deficiency, then the principle is to address the interior first by supplementing the deficiency and warming the interior, before addressing the exterior pathogen by releasing the exterior. This situation is discussed in Clause 91, which discusses interior cold treated with Si Ni Tang. However, if the interior deficiency is not severe, then simultaneous treatment of releasing the exterior and warming the interior can be adopted, as in Clause 163, where Ren Shen Gui Zhi Tang is advocated.

Heat Glomus with Exterior Yang Deficiency

Fu Zi Xie Xin Tang Pattern

Clause 155

心下痞，而复恶寒、汗出者，附子泻心汤主之。

There is glomus below the heart, if there is also aversion to cold and sweating, Fu Zi Xie Xin Tang governs.

FU ZI XIE XIN TANG: (Also known as Fu Zi Da Huang Huang Lian Xie Xin Tang.) Da Huang 2 liang; Huang Lian 1 liang; Huang Qin 1 liang; Fu Zi (blast-fried with skin removed, then broken and boiled separately to extract the juice) 1 piece.

DIRECTIONS: Slice the first three ingredients, soak for a while in 2 sheng of boiling hot water, strain, add the Fu Zi juice and take warm in two doses.

DISCUSSION: This is a variant of heat glomus below the heart. The symptoms and signs are similar to the heat glomus discussed in Clause 154 with the additional manifestations of aversion to cold and sweating, which indicate a concurrent exterior yang deficiency. The root of defence yang (wei yang) is the kidney in the lower jiao, and its dispersal is dependent on the lungs in the upper jiao. Exterior yang warms the skin and muscle layer and secures the exterior by governing the interstices (cou li). When weakened defence yang is unable to warm the exterior, there is aversion to cold; when it fails to control the pores, there is sweating.

It is important not to mistake the symptom of aversion to cold as belonging to an exterior pattern. The difference is in the absence of fever and the pulse: the aversion to cold of an exterior pattern is accompanied by fever and a floating pulse whereas the aversion to cold in yang deficiency is accompanied by cold extremities, a pale tongue and a submerged, faint pulse.

Da Huang, Huang Lian and Huang Qin are bitter and cold and clear heat; Fu Zi is acrid and hot, disperses cold, warms the channels, supports the yang and thus secures the exterior. This formula has the dual action of warming the yang and purging interior heat.

In order to retain the light, uplifting and heat-clearing effects of the three bitter, cold herbs, they are not subjected to boiling but are instead steeped in boiling hot water. The juice of Fu Zi is added to warm the yang.

It should be noted here that the descriptions of herbal preparation, decoction methods and administration in *Shang Han Lun* constitute a major contribution and are highly significant in the efficacy of Chinese herbal medicine. The specialist decoction techniques include boiling, reducing, straining and re-boiling to concentrate the liquid and to harmonise the formula, adding additional herbs before re-boiling, using the time required to cook rice as a measure for the decoction time, infusing herbs in hot water instead of boiling, the early or late addition of some herbs to extend or shorten their cooking time, the separate preparation of certain ingredients, the use of specially prepared water and the inclusion of additional ingredients such as honey, wine or vinegar. These are discussed in greater detail in Chapter One.

This glomus pattern is a complex pattern of heat in the upper jiao and cold in the lower jiao. Thus it requires the dual strategy of clearing heat and warming yang. It is this which differentiates a Fu Zi Da Huang Huang Lian Xie Xin Tang pattern from a Da Huang Huang Lian Xie Xin Tang pattern, which represents a simple heat glomus pattern.

Ancient Application of Fu Zi Xie Xin Tang

- *Zhang Shi Yi Tong* cites Fu Zi Xie Xin Tang in the treatment of glomus under the ribs due to heat and cold complex.

Modern Application of Fu Zi Xie Xin Tang

- For chronic colitis characterised by a heat and cold complex, Fu Zi Xie Xin Tang can be used with the addition of Chao Bai Zhu, Mu Xiang, Fu Ling. For spleen deficiency, add Dang Shen, Zhi Gan Cao; for chronic diarrhoea, add Wu Wei Zi.

- For chronic diarrhoea characterised by a heat and cold complex, add Bai Tou Weng, Bai Shao, Ma Chi Xian, Mu Xiang, Zhi Gan Cao.
- For chronic gastritis characterised by glomus and pain below the heart, aversion to cold and a red tongue with a pale yellow tongue coat, omit Da Huang and add Wu Yao and Yuan Hu.

Case Study

Chronic Superficial Gastritis

Extracted from Professor Fu Yanling's Case Study: Pearls Seminar 2007

A 49-year-old male patient had experienced upper abdominal pain for over ten years, following an incident of acute upper abdominal pain following unwise eating. He had sought treatment over the years, but still suffered recurrent pain, which more commonly occurred as a result of excessive cold food or alcohol. He also had occasional acid reflux, nausea, heartburn and alternating dry and loose stools. His pulse was thready and moderate, and his tongue was red with a greasy yellow coat. His complexion was slightly red and his hands and feet were cold. Gastroscopy confirmed a diagnosis of chronic superficial gastritis. The Chinese medicine diagnosis was heat and cold complex with spleen and stomach disharmony. The formula used was a modification of Ban Xia Xie Xin Tang: Ban Xia 12g, Gan Jiang 8g, Huang Qin 10g, Huang Lian 3g, Dang Shen 10g, Zhi Gan Cao 6g, Da Zao 18g, Duan Wa Leng Zi 30g, Gao Liang Jiang 9g, Zhi Xiang Fu 9g. After seven packs there was no more upper abdominal pain, the acid reflux and nausea were substantially reduced, and there was an improvement in his bowel movements The same formula, with appropriate modifications, was repeated for a further 21 packs, after which he enjoyed full recovery.

Discussion: Gastroscopy had shown lesions in the gastric mucosa, some of which were pale, with the majority red, which indicated a predominance of heat. If the majority of lesions is pale and oedematous, then it most likely reflects a pattern of heat and cold complex where cold is the predominant factor. The gastroscopy image in this instance serves as a supplmentary guide for diagnosis.

2.9.6 Glomus Due to Heat and Cold Complex

There are three formulas associated with glomus due to heat and cold complex. They are: Ban Xia Xie Xin Tang, where the focus is on vomiting; Sheng Jiang Xie Xin Tang, where the focus is on undigested food, and the glomus is associated with qi stagnation and characterised by vomiting, foul belching or retching, borborygmi, and diarrhoea; Gan Cao Xie Xin Tang is prescribed where there is severe weakness of the spleen, manifesting with frequent watery diarrhoea with undigested food particles. Its focus is on tonifying the spleen and Gan Cao is the chief herb.

Ban Xia Xie Xin Tang Pattern

Clause 149

（一）伤寒五六日，呕而发热者，柴胡汤证具，而以他药下之，柴胡证仍在者，复与柴胡汤。此虽已下之，不为逆，必蒸蒸而振，却发热汗出而解。（二）若心下满而硬痛者，此为结胸也，大陷胸汤主之。（三）但满而不痛，此为痞，柴胡不中与之，宜半夏泻心汤。

(1) Shang han for five or six days, with vomiting and fever, Xiao Chai Hu Tang signs are present, but other herbs have been used to purge, if the Chai Hu signs are still present, give Xiao Chai Hu Tang again. Even though purgation has been used, it is not adverse, there will be steaming and quivering, followed by fever and sweating and resolution. (2) If there is fullness with hard pain below the heart, it is chest bind, Da Xian Xiong Tang governs. (3) If there is only fullness with no pain, it is glomus, it is not suitable to give Chai Hu, Ban Xia Xie Xin Tang is appropriate.

BAN XIA XIE XIN TANG: Ban Xia (washed) ½ jin; Huang Qin 3 liang; Gan Jiang 3 liang; Ren Shen 3 liang; Zhi Gan Cao 3 liang; Huang Lian 1 liang; Da Zao 13 pieces (broken).

DIRECTIONS: Decoct all ingredients in 1 dou of water, reducing to 6 sheng. Strain and boil again, reducing to 3 sheng. Take 1 sheng warm three times a day.

DISCUSSION: The underlying disorder is a shang han exterior pattern, where, after five or six days, there appear the additional symptoms of vomiting and fever, indicating a change. Fever and vomiting are symptoms associated with Shao Yang and Xiao Chai Hu Tang is the indicated treatment, but purgatives have been given. Following the incorrect purgation, there are three possible developments.

1. The Xiao Chai Hu symptoms of vomiting and fever persist, demonstrating that the person's constitution is relatively strong and was able to withstand the purgation; the pathogen has not fallen inward and so Xiao Chai Hu Tang (referred to simply as Chai Hu) can still be given. The support thus given to the zheng qi enables it to contend with the pathogen; the resulting struggle manifests as steaming and quivering followed by fever and sweating, which leads to resolution. The sweating is likely to be accompanied by shivering, as it is this kind of shivering sweat which represents a vigorous struggle between the zheng qi and the pathogenic qi, with the zheng qi prevailing and driving out the pathogen.
2. After incorrect purgation, the pathogenic heat falls inward, combines with pre-existing water accumulation in the chest and manifests as major chest bind, characterised by hardness and pain below the heart. Da Xian Xiong Tang is the indicated formula.
3. Incorrect purgation damages the spleen and stomach and causes glomus. In this scenario, pathogenic heat exploits the deficiency, giving rise to disharmony of the spleen and stomach. This pattern represents a heat and cold complex due to an impaired qi dynamic and qi obstruction. The fullness and glomus are not in the chest or hypochondrium but below the heart. Therefore, it is not a Shao Yang half-exterior half-interior pattern and Xiao Chai Hu Tang is not indicated. Instead, Ban Xia Xie Xin Tang is used to harmonise the middle and reduce the fullness and glomus.

Ban Xia Xie Xin Tang is Xiao Chai Hu Tang with the omission of Chai Hu, the addition of Huang Lian and with Gan Jiang substituted for Sheng Jiang. Because the glomus pattern is characterised by vomiting, Ban Xia is used to harmonise the stomach, thus averting counterflow, dissipating knotted bind and resolving the glomus. The cause of qi glomus is ascribed to disruption to the qi dynamic, causing counterflow and the manifestation of a heat and cold complex. Huang Qin and Huang Lian are bitter and cold, purge heat and reverse counterflow; Gan Jiang and Ban Xia are acrid and warm, dissipate cold and relieve obstruction. The combined effect of these four herbs harmonises the spleen and stomach and yin and yang. Ren Shen, Zhi Gan Cao, and Da Zao are sweet and warm and supplement the deficiency of the spleen and stomach. By using both hot and cold herbs, this formula regulates yin and yang, revives the qi of the spleen and stomach, and restores the proper ascent and descent of qi. In Ban Xia Xie Xin Tang pattern, it is the impairment of spleen and stomach function and consequent disruption of the qi dynamic which causes the symptoms of glomus and fullness below the heart, nausea, vomiting, poor appetite, intestinal rumbling and diarrhoea. The pulse is submerged and wiry and the tongue coat is thick, greasy and yellow.

The method of decocting Ban Xia Xie Xin Tang is to reboil the strained liquid after the dregs are removed. As with Xiao Chai Hu Tang, the objective is to enhance the harmonising effect. Because of the moderating and harmonising effect of this method of decoction, it is useful in the preparation of paediatric formulas.

Comparison of a Xiao Chai Hu Tang Pattern, Glomus and Chest Bind

The differences between a Xiao Chai Hu Tang pattern, a glomus pattern and chest bind as described in Clause 149 are found in their pathogenesis, in the disease location, and also in the symptoms.

Pathogenesis. A Xiao Chai Hu Tang pattern is attributed to a pathogenic attack on the Shao Yang channel affecting the pivoting mechanism of Shao Yang. A glomus pattern is a heat–cold complex where the focal point is qi stagnation

Comparison of a Xiao Chai Hu Tang pattern, Glomus and Chest Bind			
	Xiao Chai Hu Tang	**Glomus**	**Chest Bind**
Pathogenesis	Attack on Shao Yang affecting pivoting mechanism of qi	Heat–cold complex with stagnation of qi causing obstruction	Pathogenic heat falling inwards and knotting with water
Location	Chest and hypochondrium	Epigastrium	Abdomen from epigastrium to lesser abdomen
Symptoms	Fullness and pain in the hypochondrium	Fullness in the epigastrium with no pain	Fullness and hardness in the epigastrium

and obstruction. Chest bind is the result of pathogenic heat falling inward and knotting with water, causing heat bind.

Disease location. A Xiao Chai Hu Tang pattern is located in the chest and hypochondrium. A glomus pattern is confined to the epigastrium, and chest bind affects an area extending from the epigastrium to the lesser abdomen.

Symptoms. A Xiao Chai Hu Tang pattern is characterised by fullness and pain in the hypochondrium whilst glomus is characterised by epigastric fullness without pain. The key symptom of chest bind is fullness and hardness in the epigastric region.

Ancient Application of Ban Xia Xie Xin Tang

- *Qian Jin Fang* cites Ban Xia Xie Xin Tang in the treatment of diarrhoea characterised by glomus and fullness below the heart, intestinal rumbling and dry retching. Where cold predominates, add Fu Zi; for thirst, add Gua Lou Gen; for severe vomiting, add Ju Pi 1 liang; for pain add Dang Gui 1 liang.
- *San Yin Fang* uses Ban Xia Xie Xin Tang in the treatment of excess heat in the heart characterised by glomus and fullness below the heart, fever, dry retching, vomiting, vexation and a stifling sensation in the chest.

Modern Application of Ban Xia Xie Xin Tang

This formula can be used extensively for acute and chronic gastritis, persistent vomiting, chronic colitis, gastric ulcer, chronic hepatitis and chronic dysentery. It is also indicated in the treatment of stomach pain (including stomach and duodenal ulcers), stomach prolapse and diarrhoea (including chronic colitis), which are characterised by glomus and epigastric fullness, frequent retching, a sloppy stool, intestinal rumbling and discomfort, a white or yellow tongue coat and a submerged, wiry pulse.

Modifications

- For phlegm heat bind, add Quan Gua Lou or combine with Xiao Xian Xiong Tang.
- For bowel excess and interior heat, add Da Huang or combine with Da Huang Huang Lian Xie Xin Tang.
- For qi constraint, add Chai Hu.
- For abdominal fullness, add Zhi Qiao, Shen Qu, Mai Ya.
- For frequent diarrhoea, add Chao Yi Ren, Fu Ling.
- For severe vomiting, add Chen Pi, Zhu Ru.
- For pain, add Yuan Hu, Yu Jin.

Sheng Jiang Xie Xin Tang Pattern

Clause 157

伤寒汗出解之后，胃中不和，心下痞硬，干噫食臭，胁下有水气，腹中雷鸣，下利者，生姜泻心汤主之。

Shang han after resolution by sweating, if there is no harmony in the stomach, there is hard glomus below the heart, dry belching with a foul food odour, water qi under the ribs, intestinal rumbling, diarrhoea, Sheng Jiang Xie Xin Tang governs.

SHENG JIANG XIE XIN TANG: Sheng Jiang (sliced) 4 liang; Zhi Gan Cao 3 liang; Ren Shen 3 liang; Gan Jiang 1 liang; Huang Qin 3 liang; Ban Xia (washed) ½ jin; Huang Lian 1 liang; Da Zao 12 pieces (broken).

DIRECTIONS: Boil the ingredients in 1 dou of water, reducing to 6 sheng. Strain and boil further to get 3 sheng. Take 1 sheng three times a day.

DISCUSSION: Shang han disorder comprises both zhong feng (wind strike) and shang han (cold injury) patterns. This clause describes a situation where sweating has brought resolution; however, after resolution from the exterior pattern, there is middle qi deficiency. The cause can be attributed to excessive diaphoretic therapy which has damaged the spleen and stomach, or to pre-existing weakness of the middle jiao. The exterior pathogen falls inward and exploits the middle jiao deficiency, disrupting the qi dynamic. This, in turn, causes obstruction of qi, giving rise to glomus: "if there is no harmony in the stomach, there is hard glomus below the heart" The exterior pathogen which fell inward has transformed into heat and joined the deficiency cold in the middle jiao. Deficient yang does not support the function of transformation and transportation, and so undigested food remains in the stomach, which is the source of the foul and putrid belching; deficient yang also results in water accumulation, which causes intestinal rumbling and diarrhoea. This complex of heat and cold causes obstruction in the middle jiao and is the basis for the glomus below the heart.

The main characteristic of a glomus pattern is glomus below the heart which is soft on palpation. The glomus described in Clause 157, however, is hard because the pathogenic qi has combined with water and undigested food, both of which have accumulated as a result of spleen and stomach dysfunction.

Sheng Jiang Xie Xin Tang is a modified version of Ban Xia Xie Xin Tang, with a reduction in the dosage of Gan Jiang and the addition of Sheng Jiang. A Sheng Jiang Xie Xin Tang pattern is associated with disharmony of the stomach accompanied by indigestion and retained water. The chief herb is Sheng Jiang, which dissipates water accumulation. Gan Jiang warms the middle and assists Sheng Jiang in dispersing water accumulation. The combination of Sheng Jiang and Ban Xia constitute the small formula Xiao Ban Xia Tang which can discharge counterflow and regulate the stomach. Huang Qin and Huang Lian are bitter and cold, clear heat and also regulate the spleen and stomach. Ren Shen, Da Zao and Gan Cao strengthen the middle to restore the qi dynamic.

Comparison of Ban Xia Xie Xin and Sheng Jiang Xie Xin Tang

Both formulas are indicated for spleen and stomach deficiency characterised by glomus and fullness below the heart, nausea, diarrhoea and intestinal rumbling. However, a Sheng Jiang Xie Xin Tang pattern represents a more serious disorder, where there is food stagnation and water retention, resulting in a hard glomus accompanied by foul belching, severe intestinal rumbling and diarrhoea.

Modern Application of Sheng Jiang Xie Xin Tang

- Chronic digestive disorders characterised by nausea, vomiting and diarrhoea.
- Stomach pain associated with acute and chronic gastritis, stomach and duodenal ulcer or stomach prolapse.
- Chronic hepatitis.

Modifications

- For inhibited urination, add Fu Ling, Zhu Ling, Che Qian Zi.
- For a sluggish digestion, add Shan Zha, Ji Nei Jin and Huo Geng.
- For abdominal fullness and distension, add Hou Po, Da Fu Pi.
- For spleen deficiency accompanied by water retention, add Fu Ling, Gui Zhi.

Case Study

Diarrhoea Due to External Invasion

Extracted from Guo Yi Lun Tan 1987

An 8-year-old girl contracted a cold following a sudden change in the weather. She presented with fever and aversion to cold. She could not eat anything, belched frequently and suffered a putrid reflux of food. She also had borborygmi and diarrhoea up to seven times daily. Her pulse was soggy and her tongue coat was thick and greasy. The treatment principle was to harmonise the stomach and reduce food stagnation. The formula prescribed was based on Sheng Jiang Xie Xin Tang: Sheng Jiang 10g, Dang Shen 3g, Bai Zhu 5g, Fu Ling 10g, Gan Jiang 3g, Huang Qin 5g, Huang Lian 3g, Ban Xia 3g, Hou Po 3g, Da Zao 5 pieces. After two packs, the diarrhoea stopped and her appetite improved but her pulse was floating because the exterior was not fully resolved. The same formula was repeated omitting Hou Po and adding Su Ye 6g, Jin Jie Shui 6g, Huo Xiang 5g. After two packs, there was slight sweating and she recovered.

Note: Research has shown that Sheng Jiang contains a volatile oil which enhances blood circulation, thus promoting sweating, and gingerol, a constituent of ginger, enhances the production of gastric juice and promotes gastric peristalsis, thus assisting the digestive process.

Gan Cao Xie Xin Tang Pattern

Clause 158

(一) 伤寒中风，医反下之，其人下利，日数十行，谷不化，腹中雷鸣，心下痞硬而满，干呕、心烦不得安。(二) 医见心下痞，谓病不尽，复下之，其痞益甚。此非结热，但以胃中虚，客气上逆，故使硬也。甘草泻心汤主之。

(1) Shang han or zhong feng, the physician has nonetheless purged, the person has diarrhoea, ten or more times in one day, with untransformed food, rumbling in the abdomen, hard glomus and fullness below the heart, and dry retching and inconsolable vexation. (2) The physician sees the glomus below the heart, thinking the disease is not ended, again purges, making the glomus more severe. This not knotted heat, but is due to deficiency in the stomach, visitant qi ascends in reverse, thus causing the hardness. Gan Cao Xie Xin Tang governs.

GAN CAO XIE XIN TANG: Zhi Gan Cao 4 liang; Huang Qin 3 liang; Gan Jiang 3 liang; Ban Xia (washed) ½ sheng; Da Zao 12 pieces (broken); Huang Lian 1 liang.

DIRECTIONS: Boil the ingredients in 1 dou of water, reducing to 6 sheng. Strain and boil again until reduced to 3 sheng. Take 1 sheng warm three times a day.

DISCUSSION: Two situations are described in this clause. (1) Both shang han (cold injury) and zhong feng (wind strike) are exterior patterns and the correct treatment is sweat promotion. Purgative treatment is incorrect and can damage the spleen and stomach, causing the exterior pathogen to fall inward. The subsequent heat and cold complex obstructs the flow of qi in the middle jiao, and knots with water, giving rise to hard glomus in the epigastrium. The stomach is in charge of the decomposition of food and grain, and the spleen is in charge of transformation and transportation of water and food essences. Impaired function of the spleen and stomach will result in diarrhoea and, if water accumulates in the intestines, there will be abdominal rumbling. Disharmony of the spleen and stomach will affect the ascent and descent of qi, so that qi accumulates in the middle causing obstruction. It is this obstruction which lodges in the epigastrium and manifests as glomus, characterised by dry retching, vexation and restlessness. The treatment is Gan Cao Xie Xin Tang. (2) The physician observes the signs of glomus below the heart and, mistaking it to be the result of incomplete purging, administers further purgative treatment. Far from reducing the glomus, this causes further damage to the spleen and stomach, exacerbating the glomus and causing the additional symptoms of vomiting and diarrhoea. The cause is not excess of the stomach and intestines, but is the result of spleen and stomach deficiency. The principle of treatment is to harmonise the stomach and reduce the glomus.

Gan Cao Xie Xin Tang is Ban Xia Xie Xin Tang with an increased dose of Gan Cao. Gan Cao and Da Zao augment and tonify the qi of the spleen and stomach and have a moderating effect on the other herbs. Ban Xia is acrid and warm. It warms and harmonises the stomach, and thus stops vomiting. Huang Qin and

Huang Lian are bitter and cold and clear heat, thus relieving vexation. Gan Jiang is acrid and warm, disperses cold and warms the middle.

Comparison of the Three Xie Xin Tang Patterns

Ban Xia Xie Xin Tang addresses glomus associated with heat and cold complex and manifesting with nausea, mild intestinal rumbling and diarrhoea. Sheng Jiang Xie Xin Tang is indicated for stomach deficiency with indigestion, food stagnation and water retention characterised by glomus below the heart, vomiting and dry retching, foul-smelling belching, diarrhoea and severe rumbling in the intestines. Gan Cao Xie Xin Tang is indicated for severe deficiency of stomach qi with nausea and vomiting, vexation and restlessness, and incessant diarrhoea with undigested food particles.

Comparison of Xie Xin Tang Glomus Patterns

Ban Xia Xie Xin Tang	Sheng Jiang Xie Xin Tang	Gan Cao Xie Xin Tang
Nausea Mild borborygmi Diarrhoea	Indigestion Food and water retention Foul-smelling belching Severe borborygmi	Nausea Incessant diarrhoea with undigested food particles Vexation and restlessness

Ancient Application of Xie Xin Tang

- *Jin Gui Yao Lue*: For the treatment of *hu huo* (狐惑), a disorder which parallels Behcet's syndrome.
- *Shang Han Liu Shu*: For the treatment of stirred qi in the upper jiao where after purgation there is abdominal fullness, glomus and dizziness.
- *Zhang Shi Yi Tong*: For the treatment of dysentery with no appetite, also known as *jin kou li* (噤口痢), characterised by headache, vexation, nausea, no appetite, vomiting all food, warm limbs, Gan Cao Xie Xin Tang was used with the omission of Da Zao and the addition of Sheng Jiang.

Modern Application of Xie Xin Tang

- For the treatment of gastritis, colitis, chronic pancreatitis, chronic hepatitis, ulceration of the mouth, Behcet's syndrome.
- Wang Zi He and his team conducted a clinical trial using Gan Cao Xie Xin Tang in the treatment of 60 cases of Behcet's syndrome with satisfactory results (*Zhong Yi Za Zhi* 1963; 1:9).

Note: Behcet's syndrome is a progressive systemic disease of unknown aetiology, involving inflammation of the small blood vessels. Major criteria are recurrent aphthous ulceration of the oral and pharyngeal mucous membranes and the genitalia, and skin lesions. There can also be pain in the eye and blurred vision due to severe uveitis (sometimes with hypopyon), retinal vasculitis, and optic atrophy. Secondary clinical features are arthritis of the large joints, intestinal ulceration, meningoencephalitis, dementia, myelopathy, epididymitis and thrombophlebitis.

Modifications

- For lack of appetite, add Pei Lan.
- For an ulcerated throat, add Sheng Ma, Shui Niu Jiao.
- For thirst, omit Ban Xia and add Tian Hua Fen.
- For inflamed, red eyes, add Chi Shao and Ye Ming Sha.
- For pain in the hypochondrium, add Chai Hu.
- For damp, add Chi Fu Ling.
- For exuberant heat, add Shi Gao, Zhi Mu and substitute Sheng Jiang for Gan Jiang.
- For constipation, add Chuan Jun.

Case Study

Diarrhoea

Extracted from Shang Han Lun Fang Yi An Xuan Pian

A 36-year-old male patient had had diarrhoea after eating contaminated food four years earlier. He recovered after treatment, however, after that he suffered diarrhoea after eating greasy food. There were two or three episodes of diarrhoea a day which were accompanied by abdominal distension, borborygmi and a loose stool with mucus and undigested food particles. Other symptoms were: palpitations, insomnia, dizziness, a submerged, thready pulse and a white, slightly greasy tongue coat. The abdomen was soft with mild pain elicited on palpation of the umbilical region. The formula given was Gan Cao Xie Xin Tang: Zhi Gan Cao 12g, Dang Shen 12g, Huang Lian 3g, Huang Qin 9g, Jiang Ban Xia 9g, Gan Jiang 9g, Hong Zao 6 pieces) + Chao Bai Zhu, Hou Po, Fu Ling, Shu Mi, Jiao San Xian (Shan Zha, Shen Qu and Mai Ya). After three packs, the stool was firm, and his appetite and sleep improved. However, the borborygmi and palpitations persisted. The formula was modified by omitting Hou Po and adding Gui Zhi. He had six packs and then was given Shen Ling Bai Zhu San and Gui Pi Wan to consolidate the treatment.

Summary of Glomus Patterns

Glomus is a subjective sensation of blockage in the epigastric region. The aetiology is largely attributed to incorrect purgation, where the exterior pathogen has fallen inward, and knotted with formless qi in the epigastrium. Another possible cause is a pre-existing stomach deficiency which allows the invasion and exploitation of pathogenic heat. The reason for the softness felt on palpation is that the pathogen is not 'formed'. By this, it is meant that the pathogenic factor is heat, which is not formed, as compared, for instance, with water, damp, phlegm or blood accumulation, all of which are 'formed'. Clause 151 describes this as qi glomus.

The five Xie Xin Tang patterns are differentiated, each according to its respective manifestations. These can be separated into two categories: glomus due to heat and glomus due to heat and cold complex. Heat glomus has a second variant where there is an exterior yang deficiency. Glomus due to heat and cold complex may further be differentiated as water glomus, phlegm glomus, or glomus due to deficiency.

DA HUANG HUANG LIAN XIE XIN TANG is indicated for heat glomus characterised by glomus below the heart, softness on palpation, a floating guan pulse, vexation, and a yellow tongue coat.

FU ZI XIE XIN TANG is indicated for heat glomus with an exterior yang deficiency characterised by glomus below the heart, sweating and aversion to cold. The treatment principle, therefore, is to support the yang and disperse the glomus.

BAN XIA XIE XIN TANG is caused by incorrect purgation in a Shao Yang disorder and manifests as complex heat and cold glomus. It is characterised by the counterflow of phlegm manifesting as nausea and diarrhoea, and the treatment is to harmonise the stomach and discharge counterflow.

SHENG JIANG XIE XIN TANG is indicated for stomach deficiency with food stagnation and water retention characterised by hard glomus below the heart, dry retching, foul belching, rumbling intestines and diarrhoea. The treatment principle is to harmonise the stomach, reduce food stagnation and disperse the glomus.

GAN CAO XIE XIN TANG is indicated where repeated purgation has caused severe deficiency of the stomach characterised by hard glomus with a sense of fullness below the heart, dry retching, incessant diarrhoea and intestinal rumbling, vexation and restlessness. The treatment is to harmonise the stomach and tonify the middle.

First and foremost, however, it must be borne in mind that where there is an unresolved exterior pattern, the exterior must be released prior to attacking the glomus.

2.9.7 Patterns Resembling Glomus

Patterns are said to resemble a glomus pattern when they do not bear all the features of a true glomus pattern. They fall into three categories: Chi Shi Zhi Yu Yu Liang Tang pattern, where hard glomus and incessant diarrhoea are the key features; Xuan Fu Dai Zhe Tang pattern, which is characterised by hard glomus with incessant belching; and Huang Lian Tang pattern, where there is no glomus but where the pattern is said to resemble a glomus pattern because it is a heat and cold complex pattern with nausea, vomiting and abdominal pain.

Chi Shi Zhi Yu Yu Liang Tang

This is a transmuted pattern characterised by glomus and diarrhoea. The aetiology is incorrect purgation in a shang han exterior pattern which has resulted in damage to the spleen and stomach, impairing the proper ascent and descent of qi. In *Shang Han Lun*, the treatment of glomus with diarrhoea is differentiated, with Gan Cao Xie Xin Tang being indicated for diarrhoea due to cold in the middle jiao, Gui Zhi Ren Shen Tang being indicated for diarrhoea associated with an exterior pattern, Li Zhong Tang being indicated for interior cold in the absence of an exterior pattern, and Chi Shi Zhi Yu Yu Liang Tang for uncontrollable diarrhoea due to instability of the kidneys, where the corresponding treatment is to astringe and stop the diarrhoea.

Clause 159

伤寒服汤药，下利不止，心下痞硬。服泻心汤已，复以他药下之，利不止，医以理中与之，利益甚。理中者，理中焦，此利在下焦，赤石脂禹余粮汤主之。复不止者，当利其小便。

(1) Shang han having taken herbs, there is incessant diarrhoea, hard glomus below the heart. (2) Xie Xin Tang was already taken, then because other purgatives were used, the diarrhoea can not be stopped, the physician gives Li Zhong, but the diarrhoea is more severe. Li Zhong is to regulate the middle jiao, but this diarrhoea is in the lower jiao, Chi Shi Zhi Yu Yu Liang Tang governs. If the diarrhoea still persists, one should promote urination.

CHI SHI ZHI YU YU LIANG TANG: Chi Shi Zhi 1 jin (broken); Tai Yi Yu Yu Liang 1 jin (broken).

DIRECTIONS: Boil the ingredients in 6 sheng of water, reducing to 2 sheng. Strain and take warm three times a day.

DISCUSSION: The initial statement explains the cause of the transmuted pattern. Shang han is an exterior pattern and instead of promoting sweat, purgation was used. The consequent damage to the spleen and stomach results in qi obstruction, which manifests as hard glomus in the epigastrium, and in incessant diarrhoea. The correct Xie Xin Tang formula (either Gan Cao Xie Xin Tang or Sheng Jiang Xie Xin Tang) was given in order to regulate the spleen and stomach and restore the proper movement of qi, but was ineffective due to the formula being too mild for such a protracted condition. At this juncture, the right strategy is to persist with the same formula; however, the practitioner mistakes the lack of response as being due to insufficient purging and continues to use other purgatives, which damage the qi, exacerbating the deficiency and resulting in persistent diarrhoea. Believing the diarrhoea to indicate deficiency of the middle jiao, the physician changes his strategy to one of regulating and warming the middle using Li Zhong Wan. The subsequent exacerbation of the diarrhoea despite taking this formula shows that the disorder is no longer a middle jiao problem but has progressed to the lower jiao, because repeated adverse treatment has not only damaged the spleen but has also damaged the securing function of the kidneys. The diarrhoea is therefore best treated with astringent herbs. If this is unsuccessful, then herbs which promote urination must be administered on the basis of the strategy to "promote urination to stop diarrhoea".

Chi Shi Zhi and Yu Yu Liang have descending properties and influence the lower jiao. Chi Shi Zhi is sweet, sour, astringent and warm, its chief function being to astringe diarrhoea. Yu Yu Liang is sweet, astringent and bland and it stops diarrhoea by tonifying the spleen. The combination of these two herbs is effective in treating chronic and persistent diarrhoea.

Differential Treatment of Diarrhoea

There are various diarrhoea patterns which can be differentiated either on the basis of their pathogenesis or on the basis of the six channels. Below are some examples of diarrhoea patterns differentiated according to their pathogenesis, which can be used as a guide for selecting the right treatment.

- For diarrhoea with complex heat and cold glomus, harmonise the stomach and eliminate the glomus with Ban Xia Xie Xin Tang.
- For diarrhoea due to deficiency and cold in the Tai Yin, warm the middle and stop diarrhoea using Li Zhong Wan.
- For chronic, uncontrollable diarrhoea due to insecurity in the lower jiao, astringe the diarrhoea using Chi Shi Zhi Yu Yu Liang Tang.
- For diarrhoea caused by water qi accumulation in the intestines, characterised by inhibited urination and diarrhoea, Wu Ling San is the appropriate formula.

Diarrhoea is a frequently encountered disorder in *Shang Han Lun* and is differentiated according to the six channel patterns, each with its corresponding treatment strategy and formula as shown below.

1. **Tai Yang channel diarrhoea:** Where a Tai Yang exterior pattern is accompanied by diarrhoea, it is also known as a Tai Yang and Yang Ming concurrent pattern; the indicated formula is Ge Gen Tang. This can present as an upper respiratory tract infection combined with a gastro-intestinal disorder. If a Tai Yang pattern has been treated incorrectly with purgation, a pattern of concurrent fever and diarrhoea can result, which may parallel the modern Western diagnosis of acute gastroenteritis. The indicated formula is then Ge Gen Qin Lian Tang. Where there are Tai Yang exterior symptoms accompanied by diarrhoea and abdominal distension similar to dyspepsia, Gui Zhi Ren Shen Tang is suitable.
2. **Yang Ming channel diarrhoea:** This is generally characterised by dryness and a hard stool which is accompanied by the discharge of faecal fluid. Although the stool is hard, the fluid discharge of waste is regarded as a form of excess diarrhoea and the indicated formula is Xiao Cheng Qi Tang. This condition often parallels acute intestinal infection or colitis.
3. **Shao Yang channel diarrhoea:** This is associated with fire harassing the Shao Yang gallbladder channel, causing diarrhoea. The indicated formulas are Huang Qin Tang, Da Chai Hu Tang and Chai Hu Mang Xiao Tang. Similarities can be drawn with acute pancreatitis and cholecystitis.
4. **Tai Yin channel diarrhoea:** This is a manifestation of Tai Yin spleen yang deficiency with cold in the interior and is characterised by abdominal pain, an absence of thirst, and a loose stool. The indicated formula is Li Zhong Wan. A parallel can be drawn with chronic dyspepsia.
5. **Shao Yin channel diarrhoea:** This is a Shao Yin channel disorder characterised by kidney and heart yang deficiency with exuberant yin cold accumulation in the lower jiao, causing diarrhoea with undigested food particles. The indicated formulas for this type of diarrhoea are Si Ni Tang, Tong Mai Si Ni Tang, Bai Tong Tang and Zhen Wu Tang. Parallels can be drawn with diarrhoea associated with chronic enteritis, colitis or renal failure with

Differentiation of Diarrhoea: Pathogenesis and Treatment

	Li Zhong Wan	Chi Shi Zhi Yu Yu Liang Tang	Wu Ling San
Aetiology	Deficiency and cold in the Tai Yin	Insecurity in the lower jiao	Water qi accumulation in the intestines
Treatment	Warm the middle Stop diarrhoea	Astringe intestines Stop diarrhoea	Promote urination Stop diarrhoea

Diarrhoea in the Yang Channels

	Tai Yang	Yang Ming	Shao Yang
Pattern	Tai Tang–Yang Ming concurrent pattern	Yang Ming bowel pattern	Shao Yang diarrhoea
Signs and symptoms	Fever, chills, floating pulse accompanied by diarrhoea	Dryness and constipation, accompanied by the discharge of faecal fluid	Abdominal pain, diarrhoea, fever, bitter taste in the mouth, red tongue, yellow tongue coat and wiry pulse
Patho-mechanism	Exterior pathogen invades the large intestine	Knotting of heat in the stomach and intestines	Shao Yang gallbladder heat descending, causing diarrhoea
Modern disease equivalent	Upper respiratory tract infection combined with gastroenteritis or acute enteritis	Acute intestinal infection or colitis	Acute pancreatitis and cholecystitis
Formulas	1. Ge Gen Tang 2. Huang Qin Ge Gen Tang 3. Gui Zhi Ren Shen Tang	Xiao Cheng Qi Tang	Huang Qin Tang Da Chai Hu Tang Chai Hu Mang Xiao Tang

Diarrhoea in the Yin Channels

	Tai Yin	Shao Yin	Jue Yin
Pattern	Spleen yang deficiency with cold in the interior	Shao Yin pattern	1.Heat and cold complex pattern 2. Damp heat pattern
Signs and symptoms	Abdominal pain, poor appetite, no thirst , bland taste, watery diarrhoea, nausea and a submerged and forceless pulse	Diarrhoea with undigested food particles, cold extremities, clear urination, nausea, aversion to cold and a faint and thready pulse	1. Diarrhoea with undigested food particles 2. Diarrhoea, tenesmus, mucus in the bowel, thirst and a yellow tongue coat
Patho-mechanism and treatment	Spleen and stomach coldness	1. Kidney and heart yang deficiency with exuberant yin cold accumulation in the lower jiao 2. Shao Yin yin deficiency characterised by empty fire and non-communication of the heart and kidney	1.Yang deficiency and exuberant yin in the lower jiao 2. Heat and damp in the lower jiao
Modern disease equivalent	Chronic dyspepsia	1. Chronic enteritis, colitis or renal failure with systemic oedema 2. Chronic bacterial, amoebic dysentery, chronic colitis	Acute bacillary dysentery, chronic gastritis, ulcerated colitis or biliary ascariasis
Formulas	Li Zhong Tang	Si Ni Tang Tong Mai Si Ni Tang Bai Tong Tang and Zhen Wu Tang	1.Wu Mei Wan, Gan Jiang Huang Qin Huang Lian Ren Shen Tang, Ma Huang Sheng Ma Tang 2. Bai Tou Weng Tang 3. Si Ni Tang group of formulas

systemic oedema. Where there is a Shao Yin yin deficiency characterised by empty fire and non-communication of the heart and kidney, Tao Hua Tang is the indicated formula. This pattern largely coincides with chronic bacterial or amoebic dysentery and chronic colitis.

6. **Jue Yin channel diarrhoea:** Jue Yin diarrhoea can be categorised as being due to cold or heat. A diarrhoea pattern associated with cold mirrors a Shao Yin diarrhoea pattern and the treatment is Si Ni Tang, Tong Mai Si Ni Tang, Bai Tong Tang and Zhen Wu Tang. The Jue Yin heat pattern, or Bai Tou Weng Tang pattern, is characterised by diarrhoea, tenesmus, mucus in the bowel and thirst and is treated with that formula. It is equivalent to acute bacillary dysentery with diarrhoea, thirst and a yellow tongue coat due to heat and damp in the lower jiao. Other diarrhoea patterns are Gan Jiang Huang Qin Huang Lian Ren Shen Tang and Wu Mei Tang patterns, which are equivalent to chronic diarrhoea associated with chronic gastritis, ulcerated colitis or biliary ascariasis.

These differential patterns of diarrhoea in the yang and yin channels are summarised in the tables opposite.

Ancient Application of Chi Shi Zhi Yu Yu Liang Tang

- *You Ke Fa Hui:* For diarrhoea characterised by a foul-smelling, watery discharge.
- *Lei Ju Fang Guang Yi:* For the treatment of diarrhoea characterised by a bowel movement with mucus discharge, abdominal pain and dry retching, where the pulse is weak and forceless. If accompanied by abdominal pain and dry retching, Tao Hua Tang is advocated either alone or in combination with Chi Shi Zhi Yu Yu Liang Tang.

Modern Application of Chi Shi Zhi Yu Yu Liang Tang

Chi Shi Zhi Yu Yu Liang Tang is indicated for uncontrollable diarrhoea, rectal prolapse, chronic enteritis and leucorrhoea.

Case Study

Rectal Prolapse

Extracted from Qiu Shou Song: Zhejiang Zhong Yi Za Zhi 1966; 2:22.

Following severe constipation ten years previously, the 56-year-old male patient suffered rectal prolapse with blood in the stool and secondary haemorrhoids. The condition was exacerbated by fatigue, his pulse was deficient and thready, and his tongue was pale. He was of thin build and his complexion was pale and dull. He also suffered from a weak back, poor appetite and a loose stool. The diagnosis was qi sinking due to deficiency of the spleen and kidney. The formula used was Chi Shi Zhi Yu Yu Liang Tang modified: Chi Shi Zhi 15g; Yu Yu Liang 15g, Tu Si Zi 9g, Chao Bai Zhu 9g, Bu Gu Zhi 6g, Zhi Gan Cao 4.5g, Sheng Ma 4.5g and Pao Gan Jiang 4.5g. After three packs, his general sense of wellbeing improved but the stool was still slightly sticky. He was given a further three packs of medication. After that, both stool and appetite were normal.

Xuan Fu Dai Zhe Tang Pattern

Clause 161

伤寒发汗，若吐、若下，解后，心下痞硬，噫气不除者，旋复代赭汤主之。

Shang han there is promotion of sweat, if there is vomiting, if there is purgation, after resolution, there is a hard glomus below the heart, unremitting belching, Xuan Fu Dai Zhe Tang governs.

XUAN FU DAI ZHE TANG: Xuan Fu Hua 3 liang; Ren Shen 2 liang; Sheng Jiang 5 liang; Dai Zhe Shi 1 liang; Zhi Gan Cao 3 liang; Ban Xia (washed) ½ sheng; Da Zao 12 pieces (broken).

DIRECTIONS: Boil the ingredients in 1 dou of water, reducing to 6 sheng. Strain and reboil to get 3 sheng. Take 1 sheng warm three times a day.

DISCUSSION: In shang han, even after resolution of the exterior pattern, if the use of diaphoretic, emetic or purgative therapy has damaged the qi of the spleen and stomach, their impaired function will result in the generation of phlegm in the middle jiao. The phlegm obstruction disturbs the qi dynamic and a hard glomus forms in the epigastric area. The unremitting belching can be interpreted as follows. (1) Continuous and relentless belching indicating the condition is serious; (2) the qi dynamic is untrammelled but the frequent belching does not seem to resolve the hard glomus; (3) this pattern remains despite treatment with Xie Xin Tang and so Xuan Fu Dai Zhe Tang is required to transform phlegm and discharge counterflow.

Xuan Fu Hua is the key herb. Although flowers are attributed with an ascending action, Xuan Fu Hua is exceptional in its ability to descend qi and its ascending function is not as strong. It is bitter and acrid, disperses liver qi and regulates qi, warms and transforms phlegm and softens hardness, and is therefore able to reduce glomus. *Ben Cao Hui Yan* said: "Xuan Fu Hua resolves phlegm and eliminates water, regulates qi and facilitates descent". Dai Zhe Shi descends counterflow qi and these two herbs combined sedate the liver, harmonise the stomach, suppress counterflow qi and transform turbidity. Ban Xia and Sheng Jiang are acrid, warm and dispersing. They transform phlegm, eliminate phlegm fluids and discharge counterflow qi; Ren Shen, Gan Cao and Da Zao warm and tonify the spleen. By regulating the middle, they facilitate the ascent of clear yang and the descent of turbid yin, and thus resolve belching.

Xuan Fu Dai Zhe Tang directly targets persistent, irrepressible belching. The term *yi qi* (噫气) may refer either to belching or to hiccough, both of which are a manifestation of counterflow stomach qi. The pathogenesis for yi qi or belching is disharmony of the spleen and stomach with retained phlegm fluids, which leads to the counterflow of turbid stomach qi causing both the belching or hiccough and hard glomus below the heart. Zhang Lu Yu said: "After sweat promotion, emesis and purgation with resolution of the exterior pattern, there is damage and deficiency of the middle qi with counterflow of turbid qi and phlegm fluids hence the hard glomus." (*Shang Han Lun Yan Jiu Da Ci Dian* p 276). The other identifying symptom is the hard glomus below the heart which elicits no pain when pressure is applied. This is because the glomus is an accumulation of phlegm, disrupting the qi dynamic and obstructing normal qi flow. Secondary symptoms are the vomiting of phlegm, dizziness, poor appetite and a sluggish bowel movement. The pulse is wiry and there is a white tongue coat.

It is essential to differentiate between Xuan Fu Dai Zhe Tang and Sheng Jiang Xie Xin Tang, both of which are associated with a hard glomus below the heart and belching. The aetiology of Sheng Jiang Xie Xin Tang pattern is damage to the spleen and stomach caused by sweating. Its principal features are food stagnation with an accumulation of water, hard glomus below the heart, malodorous belching, intestinal rumbling, and diarrhoea. The aetiology of a Xuan Fu Dai Zhe Tang pattern, on the other hand, is deficiency of the spleen and stomach caused not by sweating but by purgation. The damage to the middle qi caused by the purgation results in turbidity and phlegm accumulation. The accumulation of phlegm obstructs the descent of stomach qi, giving rise to counterflow manifesting as belching, which is the principal clinical feature of this pattern.

Belching and hiccough can be associated either with excess or deficiency. Tang Rong Chuan said: "The treatment of hiccough varies: Fire hiccough is treated with Cheng Qi Tang; cold hiccough is treated with Li Zhong Tang with the addition of Ding Xiang, Shi Ti; blood stasis hiccough is treated with Da Chai Hu Tang with the addition ofTao Ren, Dan Pi, and Xuan Fu Hua Tang is indicated for hiccough due to the obstruction of phlegm fluids". Xuan Fu Dai Zhe Tang can be modified as follows: for heat, add Huang Qin, Huang Lian; for cold, add Ding Xiang, Shi Ti; if there is copious phlegm add Chen Pi, Fu Ling; if there is damp, add Ze Xie, Fu Ling. For stomach deficiency where there is hiccough with a tendency to vomit, it can be combined with Ju Pi Zhu Ru Tang.

The dosage in Xuan Fu Hua Dai Zhe Tang is as follows: Sheng Jiang 5 liang (12–15g) to harmonise the stomach, eliminate phlegm and reduce glomus. Dai Zhe Shi 1 liang (2 to 3g) represents the lowest dosage in this formula. Because Dai Zhe Shi is heavy and cold, a large dose would not only carry its effect to the lower jiao, but could also cause further damage to the stomach and spleen. Some schools of thought suggest that the dosage of Dai Zhe Shi should be two to three times the dosage of Xuan Fu Hua, making it 24–30g. The authors feel the lower dose is more appropriate.

Professor Liu Du Zhou illustrated the application of correct dosage in Xuan Fu Hua Dai Zhe Tang when he was in charge of a group of interns at an outpatient clinic. Xuan Fu Hua Dia Zhe Shi Tang was prescribed for a patient suffering from frequent belching. The dose of Dai Zhe Shi was 30g and there were 3 slices of Sheng Jiang. The result was not satisfactory. Professor Liu reduced the dosage of Dai Zhe Shi from 30g to 6g and increased the dosage of Sheng Jiang to 15g. The rationale was that Sheng Jiang can disperse glomus caused by water qi, whilst the purpose of Dai Zhe Shi, in this case, was being used to address phlegm obstruction due to stomach deficiency and so the dosage needed to be low. The explanation was that the higher dose prescribed by the interns had a sedating effect on the liver, rather than a regulatory effect on the stomach. (*Wang San Hu Shaan Xi Zhong Yi Yao* 1998: 2: 28)

Ancient Application of Xuan Fu Hua Dai Zhe Tang

- *Shang Han Lun San Zhu:* For the treatment of stomach reflux and regurgitation.
- *Yi Xue Gang Mu*. For the treatment of nausea and constipation.
- *Yi Xue Zhong Zhong Can Xi Lu:* Shen Zhe Pei Qi Tang, which is Xuan Fu Hua Dai Zhe Tang with the omission of Sheng Jiang, Gan Cao, Da Zao and the addition of Zhi Mu, Tian Men Dong, Dang Gui, Rou Cong Rong, Shi Shuang (dried persimmon frost) was advocated for the treatment of dysphagia.

Modern Application of Xuan Fu Hua Dai Zhe Tang

- For chronic and acute gastritis, muscle spasm of the diaphragm, dizziness, headache, cough, dyspnoea and haemoptysis.
- Zhang Shu Gui and his team used Xuan Fu Dai Zhe Shi Tang in the treatment of gastric distension which was characterised by glomus, epigastric fullness, nausea, dry retching, and abdominal distension with an intermittent pulse. After the stomach contents were emptied and rinsed with saline solution, the patient still suffered from frequent belching and hiccough with a deficient and slippery pulse and a greasy tongue coat. After two doses of Xuan Fu Hua Dai he Tang, the epigastric and abdominal distension abated and a further two doses resulted in full recovery. (Zhang Shu Gui: Xuan Fu Dai Zhe Shi Tang modification in the treatment of 2 cases of gastric distension, *Shanghai Zhong Yi Yao Za Zhi* 1966; 2:63).
- For chronic gastritis with pain, add Yu Jin, Xiang Fu, Yuan Hu; for severe distension, add Zhi Qiao; for poor appetite, add Shan Zha, Shen Qu, Ji Nei Jin; for copious phlegm, add Fu Ling, Chen Pi, Yi Ren.
- For the treatment of plumstone qi (globus hystericus), add Chai Hu, Hou Po, Su Zi; if accompanied by vexation and an oppressed sensation in the chest, add Zhi Zi, Dou Chi; for insomnia, add Long Gu, Mu Li; for stagnation of qi and blood, add Bai Mei Hua (Mei Gui Hua), Chi Shao, Dang Gui.

Case Study

Two Cases of Belching

Extracted from Xin Yi Yao Xue Za Zhi 1977; (6):35

A 40-year-old female patient had a history of duodenal ulcers for several years. She suffered from glomus with the symptoms of epigastric distension and belching, which was especially bad after eating a meal. Her appetite was poor and her stool was loose. Her tongue was pale and swollen with a white tongue coat and her pulse was wiry and slippery. The formula used was a modification of Xuan Fu Dai Zhe Shi Tang: Xuan Fu Hua 9g, Dang Shen 9g, Fa Ban Xia 9g, Dai Zhe Shi 10g, Zhi Gan Cao 6g, Da Zao 12g, Zhi Qiao 9g, Mu Xiang 6g, Hou Po 9g. After five packs, her appetite improved and there was less bloating after meals. The same formula was repeated for a further five packs, after which there was no more belching. This was followed by Xiang Sha Liu Jun Zi Tang to regulate the spleen and stomach.

A 24-year-old female patient had suffered for two months from painful bloating about two hours after meals, accompanied by acid reflux, nausea and vomiting. Her condition gradually worsened and she often had foul belching and vomited undigested food. She was given atropine to relieve the pain but it had no effect. Her complexion was sallow and she was fatigued and thin. Examination showed her blood pressure to be 160/75 mmHg. There was no swelling of lymph nodes and heart and pulmonary function were normal. Endoscopy revealed that she suffered from superficial gastritis with pyloric stenosis. She was given Western medication but it was not effective. At the time of her consultation, she was suffering from vomiting, belching, epigastric fullness, stomach pain, aversion to cold, with cold extremities and a preference for warmth. She was fatigued, had shortness of breath and her stools were loose. Her pulse was submerged and forceless and the tongue was pale with a thin, white tongue coat. The diagnosis was disharmony of the stomach with counterflow. The treatment principle was to harmonise the stomach, warm the middle, disperse cold, augment qi and tonify the spleen. The formula prescribed was Xuan Fu Hua Dai Zhe Shi Tang combined with Ju Pi Zhu Ru Tang modified. After 30 packs her condition improved. Subsequent endoscopy showed no ulceration or other abnormality.

Huang Lian Tang Pattern

Clause 173

伤寒，胸中有热，胃中有邪气，腹中痛，欲呕吐者，黄连汤主之。

Shang han if there is heat in the chest, evil qi in the stomach, pain in the abdomen and nausea and vomiting, Huang Lian Tang governs.

HUANG LIAN TANG: Huang Lian 3 liang; Zhi Gan Cao 3 liang; Gan Jiang 3 liang; Gui Zhi (skin removed) 3 liang; Ren Shen 2 liang; Ban Xia (washed) ½ sheng; Da Zao 12 pieces (broken).

DIRECTIONS: Boil the ingredients in 1 dou of water, reducing to 6 sheng. Strain and take warm three times during the day and twice at night.

DISCUSSION: The reference to shang han represents exterior disease in general and not Tai Yang shang han specifically. A Huang Lian Tang pattern is one of heat and cold complex, where pathogenic heat from the upper part of the body harasses the stomach causing nausea and vomiting, and pathogenic cold from the lower part of the body harasses the spleen, causing abdominal pain due to the cold congealing and stagnating qi. This pattern represents the failure of the upper jiao yang to communicate with the lower jiao yin, resulting in cold in the lower jiao; because the yin in the lower jiao is unable to interact with the yang, heat arises in the upper jiao. Huang Lian Tang is indicated to clear upper jiao heat and simultaneously warm the cold of the middle jiao, thereby regulating heat and cold and restoring the balance.

Huang Lian clears heat from the upper jiao; Gan Jiang disperses cold in the middle jiao. This combination is a classic example of acrid opening and bitter discharging used to restore the qi dynamic of the middle jiao. Ban Xia harmonises the stomach and discharges counterflow to stop vomiting; Gui Zhi disperses cold and frees yang, thus facilitating the interaction of the upper jiao with the lower jiao; Ren Shen, Gan Cao and Da Zao augment qi and harmonise the middle.

The terms *xiong zhong* (胸中), *wei zhong* (胃中) and *fu zhong* (腹中) refer to different regions of the body, but their terms of reference are broad. *Xiong zhong* refers to the area above the diaphragm. The concept of *wei zhong*, or stomach centre, can also include the intestines, and *fu zhong* refers to the abdomen, and can include the stomach; both refer to the area below the diaphragm. Clause 173 uses these terms to explain that there is heat above the diaphragm, and cold and pain below the diaphragm.

Huang Lian Tang is Ban Xia Xie Xin Tang omitting Huang Qin and adding Gui Zhi. It clears heat from the upper part of the body, and disperses coldness and pain from the lower part. Because of the inclusion of Huang Qin, Ban Xia Xie Xin Tang is more effective at clearing heat, whilst Huang Lian Tang, by its replacement of Huang Qin with Gui Zhi, is better at warming and unblocking the channels and is therefore indicated for heat above the diaphragm, with cold and pain below the diaphragm.

The decoction method for Ban Xia Xin Xin Tang entails further boiling after straining; this strengthens its actions so it can discharge glomus.

By contrast, Huang Lian Tang is boiled once only, as befitting its objective of clearing heat in the upper part and dispersing cold in the lower part. The direction to take several small doses rather than one or two large ones is to avoid vomiting after medication.

Ancient Application of Huang Lian Tang

- *Zhang Shi Yi Tong:* For treatment of heat and cold complex with glomus and fullness below the heart.

Modern Application of Huang Lian Tang

- For the treatment of acute and chronic gastritis.
- For the treatment of peptic ulcers characterised by epigastric and abdominal pain, nausea and vomiting. For more severe vomiting, add Fu Ling and Zhu Ru; for pain add Xiang Fu, Bai Shao, Yuan Hu.

Case Study

Stomach Heat and Intestinal Cold

Extracted from Shang Han Lun Lin Chuang Shi Yan Lu

A 26-year-old male patient suffered from diarrhoea, vexation, nausea, no appetite, dizziness and a frequent watery stool, passed many times a day. His hands were cold and his pulse was submerged and thready. The diagnosis was spleen yang deficiency with diarrhoea. The treatment principle was to clear stomach heat, tonify the spleen yang and stop the diarrhoea. The formula used was Huang Lian Tang modified: Huang Lian 10g, Gan Jiang 10g, Rou Gui 6g, Dang Shen 10g, Ban Xia 10g, Zhi Gan Cao 10g, Da Zao 8 pieces. After three packs, there was no more diarrhoea. A formula to tonify the spleen and stomach was then administered to consolidate treatment.

Summary of Patterns Resembling Glomus

Although a salient feature is glomus below the heart, patterns resembling a glomus pattern are so-called because they do not bear all the features of a typical glomus pattern. Therefore the key to diagnosis is to be focused on the main symptoms. The Chi Shi Zhi Yu Yu Liang Tang pattern is characterised by repetitive and uncontrollable diarrhoea with a hard glomus below the heart following adverse purgation. The Xuan Fu Dai Zhe Tang pattern is characterised by hard glomus below the heart with unremitting belching due to stomach deficiency caused by adverse sweating. The Huang Lian Tang pattern has no glomus but is a pattern of heat and cold complex which bears resemblance to a glomus pattern.

Section Ten

2.10 PATTERNS RESEMBLING TAI YANG

2.10.1 Wind Cold Damp Bi Syndrome

Gui Zhi Fu Zi Tang and Qu Gui jia Bai Zhu Tang Patterns

Clause 174

伤寒八九日，风湿相搏，身体疼烦，不能自转侧，不呕、不渴、脉浮虚而涩者，桂枝附子汤主之。若其人大便硬，小便自利者，去桂加白术汤主之。

Shang han for eight or nine days, the wind and damp vie with each other, the body aches vexatiously, the person can not turn over, if there is neither vomiting nor thirst, the pulse is floating, deficient and choppy, then Gui Zhi Fu Zi Tang governs. If the person has a hard stool, and urination is free, Qu Gui jia Bai Zhu Tang governs.

GUI ZHI FU ZI TANG: Gui Zhi (skin removed) 4 liang; Fu Zi (dry-fried with skin removed) 3 pieces; Sheng Jiang (sliced) 3 liang; Da Zao 12 pieces (broken); Zhi Gan Cao 2 liang.

DIRECTIONS: Boil the ingredients in 6 sheng of water, reducing to 2 sheng. Strain and take warm three times a day.

QU GUI JIA BAI ZHU TANG: Fu Zi (dry-fried with skin removed) 3 pieces; Bai Zhu 4 liang; Sheng Jiang (sliced) 3 liang; Zhi Gan Cao 2 liang; Da Zao 12 pieces (broken).

DIRECTIONS: Boil the ingredients in 6 sheng of water, reducing to 2 sheng. Strain and take warm three times a day. After the first dose, the patient will experience a sensation of painful obstruction. Wait for half a day then continue the medication and when the three doses have been taken, the person will be drenched in sweat. This is to be expected: the reason is that Fu Zi and Bai Zhu have entered the skin to drive out the water which was not previously eliminated. As a rule, 4 liang of Gui Zhi is used. This is one formula with two strategies. When the stool is hard, and the urination is uninhibited, omit Gui Zhi; if the stool is not hard and the urine is inhibited, add Gui Zhi. In some cases, 3 pieces of Fu Zi may be too much. For weak patients and women who have just given birth, a reduced dose is appropriate.

DISCUSSION: When shang han has persisted for eight or nine days without resolution it is attributed to attack by wind, damp and cold, obstructing the exterior and disturbing the harmony of ying and wei. The disharmony of ying and wei affects the circulation of qi and blood, giving rise to aches and pains in the body and stiffness, making it difficult to move or turn over in bed. The statement that there is no vomiting confirms that it is not a Shao Yang pattern and the absence of thirst shows that it is not a Yang Ming pattern. The floating pulse indicates that the wind damp is in the exterior and has not entered the interior; the deficient pulse is a reflection of weak defensive qi, and the choppy pulse is evidence of the stagnation of damp and congelation of cold. This pulse image combined with the symptoms indicates that this is a pattern of wind cold damp bi (painful obstruction) and Gui Zhi Fu Zi Tang is indicated to warm the channels, transform dampness and expel wind cold.

Jin Gui Yao Lue: Chapter 2, Jing Shi Yue (Tetany, Dampness and Summerheat) states that in a damp bi pattern, there is inhibited urination and a loose stool. From that it can be surmised that a Gui Zhi Fu Zi Tang pattern is also characterised by a loose stool and inhibited urination. The comments regarding the stool and urination address variations in outcome. Due to its action of transforming qi, freeing the yang qi and eliminating damp, Gui Zhi Fu Zi Tang can cause the stool to be hard and urination uninhibited. For this reason, rather than using Gui Zhi to free the yang, Bai Zhu is added to parch the damp. The hard stool represents damp obstructing the spleen's transformation function and in such a case, Gui Zhi should be omitted and Bai Zhu added to strengthen the spleen and dry damp.

Gui Zhi Fu Zi Tang is Gui Zhi Tang with the omission of Shao Yao, a slightly larger dose of Gui Zhi, and the addition of Fu Zi; it should not be confused Gui Zhi jia Fu Zi Tang where Shao Yao is not omitted. This formula expels wind and scatters cold from the channels, freeing obstruction. Fu Zi is acrid and hot; it warms the interior yang, scatters cold, expels cold damp from the channels and eases pain. Sheng Jiang is acrid and warm and assists Gui Zhi and Fu Zi in expelling the pathogenic wind cold, and assists Gui Zhi and Fu Zi in their action of warming. Zhi Gan Cao and Da Zao are warm; they benefit zheng qi and moderate the dispersing properties of Gui Zhi and Fu Zi; Gan Cao and Sheng Jiang assist in the transformation of yang and support the generation of yin, thus regulating and harmonising ying and wei, and facilitating the expulsion of the pathogen.

If the stool is hard and urination uninhibited, then Gui Zhi Fu Zi qu Gui Zhi jia Bai Zhu Tang, which is Gui Zhi Fu Zi Tang omitting Gui Zhi and adding Bai Zhu, can be applied in the same circumstances as Gui Zhi Fu Zi Tang; it represesents a situation where qi transformation has been restored but there is residual damp obstructing the spleen. Gui Zhi is omitted since it is a herb used to treat the exterior, and Bai Zhu is used instead to tonify the spleen and eliminate damp.

Wind cold damp bi comes under the scope of miscellaneous disease. The initial stage is characterised by fever, aversion to cold, sweating, body aches and pains and a floating pulse, and thus resembles a Tai Yang exterior pattern. However, the body aches of wind cold damp bi are distinguished by stiffness and difficulty in movement; they both have a floating pulse but whereas a Tai Yang exterior pulse is moderate or tense, the pulse in bi syndrome is deficient and choppy. Because of the superficial similarities with a Tai Yang exterior pattern, bi syndrome is categorised as a pattern resembling Tai Yang.

Although Gui Zhi Fu Zi Tang and Gui Zhi qu Shao Yao jia Fu Zi Tang, cited in Clause 22, are similar formulas which differ only in dosages, their action is quite different. Gui Zhi Fu Zi Tang is indicated for wind cold damp bi syndrome, where there is obstruction in the muscle layer manifesting as body pain and stiffness and difficulty in moving. The dose of Gui Zhi (4 liang) and Fu Zi (3 pieces) is designed to warm the channels, expel cold and ease pain. Gui Zhi qu Shao Yao jia Fu Zi Tang is indicated for a Tai Yang exterior pattern accompanied by fullness in the chest and aversion to cold. The smaller dose of Gui Zhi (3 liang) and Fu Zi (1 piece) is designed to warm the channels and restore yang.

In the original text, the endnote states that individual reactions to Gui Zhi Fu Zi qu Gui jia Bai Zhu Tang may vary and one should not be alarmed if there are such symptoms as impediment or painful obstruction ('bi'), or being drenched in sweat. This is due to the process of Bai Zhu and Fu Zi expelling wind and damp from the skin and muscle layer; once the pathogen is eliminated, the patient's condition will return to normal. There have been various interpretations of this reaction: Ke Yun Bo explained that when the patient suffered from 'bi' or impediment after the initial dose, and then after three doses was drenched in sweat, it was due to Bai Zhu and Fu Zi endeavouring to expel the water which was trapped underneath the skin. Cao Ying Fu's explanation was that the sensation of 'bi' or impediment after the initial dose was due to Fu Zi causing numbness, which is in-line with the modern pharmacological knowledge that Fu Zi contains aconitine which can cause numbness and sweating. Zhang Zhong Jing said the dosage of Fu Zi could be too high and suggested a reduction in dosage for invalids and postpartum women. It is important to follow the precaution of decocting Fu Zi first, keeping the initial dosage low, thereafter only increasing the dosage gradually.

The principal function of Gui Zhi Fu Zi qu Gui jia Bai Zhu Tang is to warm the interior and expel the cold damp pathogen from the exterior. It is indicated in the treatment of fluid accumulation under the skin which has been caused by damp and cold. Bai Zhu is a principal herb used for spleen deficiency and because of its function of drying damp, it is also used in the treatment of bi syndrome. Although Bai Zhu is used to stop diarrhoea, a single large dose of Bai Zhu can also be used to treat constipation due to spleen deficiency. Bai Zhu is the herb of choice for spleen deficiency with impaired transportation of fluids.

Ancient Application of Gui Zhi Fu Zi Tang

- *Tai Ping Hui Min He Ji Ju Fang:* For treatment of the invasion of pathogenic wind characterised by dizziness.
- *Mai Yin Zheng Zhi:* For treatment of cold jue, with acute chest pain and a faint pulse. (Cold jue is a description of yang deficiency characterised by cold extremities due to the non-dispersal of yang qi.)

Modern Application of Gui Zhi Fu Zi Tang

Gui Zhi Fu Zi Tang is indicated in the treatment of an early-stage externally contracted pattern characterised by fever, headache, aversion to cold, sweating, frequent urination, vexation and leg cramps. Qu Gui jia Bai Zhu Tang is indicated in the treatment of arthritis (both cold bi and damp bi patterns) and sciatic pain. If there is damp, Cang Zhu and Yi Yi Ren can be added; if there is acute pain, add Wei Ling Xian; for stiffness in the joints, add such herbs as Ji Xue Teng, Sang Zhi, Xun Gu Feng.

Case Study

Wind Cold Damp Bi

Extracted from Shang Han Lun Fang Yun Yong Fa

After giving birth two weeks earlier, a 34-year-old female patient found she had gained weight. Her complexion was pale, her breast milk was thin. Her appetite normal but she had a loose stool two to three times a day and her urination was scant. She complained of spontaneous sweating and of aching joints and muscles which were worse in wet weather. Her tongue was pale with a white, slippery tongue coat and her pulse was floating and wiry but disappeared under pressure. She was prescribed Gui Zhi Fu Zi Tang: Gui Zhi 12g, Zhi Fu Zi 15g, Zhi Gan Cao 9g, Sheng Jiang 9g, Hong Zao 10g. After two packs, her joint pain was substantially relieved and she was given a further five packs to consolidate the treatment.

Gan Cao Fu Zi Tang Pattern

Clause 175

风湿相搏，骨节疼烦，掣痛不得屈伸，近之则痛剧，汗出短气，小便不利，恶风不欲去衣，或身微肿者，甘草附子汤主之。

The wind and damp vie with each other, there is vexatious joint pain, there is pulling pain and an inability to bend and stretch, the pain is worse with contact, if there is sweating and shortness of breath, urination which is not free, aversion to wind with reluctance to remove clothing, or slight oedema, Gan Cao Fu Zi Tang governs.

GAN CAO FU ZI TANG: Zhi Gan Cao 2 liang; Fu Zi (dry-fried with skin removed) 2 pieces; Bai Zhu 2 liang; Gui Zhi (skin removed) 4 liang.

DIRECTIONS: Boil the ingredients in 6 sheng of water, reducing to 3 sheng. Strain and take 1 sheng warm three times a day. After the initial dose a slight sweat will be raised and resolution will follow. If the appetite returns, and vexation follows the cessation of sweat, then administer a further 5 ge. If there is concern that the initial dose of 1 sheng is too much, then it is appropriate to start with 6 to 7 ge.

DISCUSSION: The struggle between wind and damp obstructs the flow of qi and blood, which is also congealed by cold. The obstruction in the channels results in stiff, painful joints. Damp is heavy and turbid, further impeding the movement of the joints. The pain is described here as a pulling pain, referring to the taut restrictive pain which typifies wind cold damp bi, with its classic symptoms of stiffness and pain and restriction in movement, and the inability to extend or flex the joints.

Damp obstructs, thereby affecting not only the flow of qi but also the transformation of qi, which involves the three jiao. Its affect on the upper jiao is to cause shortness of breath, and its affect on the lower jiao is manifested by inhibited urination. Lodged in the muscle layer, damp manifests as a heavy sensation and there may also be slight swelling or oedema. Gan Cao Fu Zi Tang warms the channels, disperses cold and eliminates damp. It is indicated to eliminate the three pathogenic qi, which are wind, cold and damp, on a background of interior yang deficiency

Fu Zi is acrid and hot; it scatters cold, warms the channels, supports the yang, and eliminates damp. Bai Zhu is bitter and warm; it tonifies the spleen and dries damp. The dosage of Fu Zi in Gan Cao Fu Zi Tang (2 pieces) is less than in Gui Zhi Fu Zi Tang (3 pieces) and Gan Cao is used to moderate the heating and dispersing properties of those two herbs. The dosage of Bai Zhu is only half that in Gui Zhi Fu Zi Tang, the objective of the reduction being to decelerate the action of the formula, thus prolonging its effect, so that it can more effectively eliminate the dampness. This changes the focus of the formula.

Comparison of Wind Cold Damp Patterns and Formulas

The patterns represented by these three formulas are all characterised by aches and pains in the muscles and joints accompanied by aversion to wind and sweating. Gui Zhi Fu Zi Tang is indicated where pathogenic wind damp attacks the most superficial muscle layer; its focus is on the most exterior level. Gui Zhi Fu Zi Qu Gui jia Bai Zhu Tang is indicated where pathogenic wind damp attacks the less superficial muscle layer and its sphere of action is slightly deeper than Gui Zhi Fu Zi Tang. Finally, Gan Cao Fu Zi Tang is indicated where pathogenic wind damp has attacked the joints, representing a deeper level than Gui Zhi Fu Zi Tang. All three formulas can be used in the treatment of arthritis, where joint pain is attributed to wind, cold and damp, but each differs in the level or location of disease that it treats.

Case Study

Wind Cold Damp Bi

Extracted from Shang Han Lun Fang Yun Yong Fa

A 32-year-old male patient worked on a duck farm and spent a lot of time in water. He had suffered from bi syndrome for seven years, with an acute flare-up over the previous seven days. He presented with pain in the shoulder joint, lower back, hip and knee joints, with no redness or swelling. There was limited range of movement in the left hand and leg, and stiffness and pain in the lower back. His throat was swollen and inflamed and he was thirsty, preferring hot drinks. Other symptoms were shortness of breath, scant urination and slight fever of 37.4°C. The tongue coat was thin and white and the pulse was submerged, thready and rapid. The formula prescribed was Gan Cao Fu Zi Tang: Pao Fu Zi 10g, Bai Zhu 6g, Gui Zhi 12g, Zhi Gan Cao 6g. After one pack, the fever had receded and the joint pain was reduced. However, urination was still scant. He was prescribed a further two packs of the same formula. At the third consultation, he presented with generalised joint pain and stiffness, including difficulty in moving his neck. He had a slight fever, sweating and aversion to wind. His tongue coat was white and greasy and the pulse was floating and rapid. He reported that the previous day he had been very thirsty and had drunk some well water, following which he was shivering with cold and suffered joint pain. He was prescribed Gui Zhi jia Ge Gen Tang: Ge Gen 12g, Gui Zhi 10g, Bai Shao 10g, Zhi Gan Cao 6g, Sheng Jiang 10g, Hong Zao 12 pieces. After two packs his general condition improved but he still suffered from joint pain. At the fourth consultation he was again prescribed a modified version of Gan Cao Fu Zi Tang: Pao Fu Zi 20g, Bai Zhu 9g, Gui Zhi 24g, Zhi Gan Cao 12g. After one pack, there was considerable improvement and he was prescribed one more pack to consolidate the treatment.

2.10.2 Suspended Phlegm Fluids

The condition known as *xuan yin* (悬饮), or suspended phlegm fluids, is characterised by the retention of phlegm fluids in the chest with pain in the hypochondrium, described in *Shang Han Lun* as "glomus below the heart which extends under the ribs" and described in *Jin Gui Yao Lue* as water accumulation in the chest and hypochondrium causing localised pain and a productive cough. This is also known as a Shi Zao Tang Pattern.

Shi Zao Tang Pattern

Clause 152

（一）太阳中风，下利呕逆，表解者，乃可攻之。（二）其人漐漐汗出，发作有时，头痛、心下痞硬满、引胁下痛、干呕、短气、汗出不恶寒者，此表解里未和也。十枣汤主之。

(1) Tai Yang zhong feng, there is diarrhoea and counterflow vomiting, if the exterior is resolved, one may still purge. (2) If the person has continuous sweating, occurring at a set time, headache, hard glomus and hard distension below the heart, pain which extends under the ribs, dry retching, shortness of breath, sweating with no aversion to cold, then the exterior is resolved but the interior is not harmonised. Shi Zao Tang governs.

SHI ZAO TANG: Equal parts of Yuan Hua (dry-fried); Gan Sui, Da Ji, Da Zao (10 plump pieces). Note that the name of this formula means 'ten dates soup'.

DIRECTION: Grind the first 2 ingredients into a powder. Then boil Da Zao in 1 sheng of water, reducing to 8 ge, strain and add the ground herbs. The dose for a strong person is 1½ qian and for patients with a weak constitution is ½ qian. It should be taken warm in the early morning, between 5 and 7am (known as ping dan 平旦 or 'morning calm'). If there is only mild diarrhoea, then the disease has not been eliminated and a further dose should be given the next day, with an increase of ½ qian. Once diarrhoea occurs, nourishing gruel should be given.

DISCUSSION: The first statement describes the situation where, in the course of Tai Yang zhong feng, the exterior pattern has proceeded to a secondary pattern of retained phlegm fluids. This accumulation is called suspended phlegm fluids because turbidity is suspended in the chest, and it affects both the interior and the exterior, and also the triple jiao. If the accumulated fluid affects the intestines, there will be diarrhoea and if it harasses the stomach, there will be vomiting. Because the phlegm fluids are lodged deeply under the ribs, formulas commonly used to promote urination will not yield satisfactory results and so, a potent formula which moves and expels water is needed. However, because there is a risk of the exterior pathogen falling inwards following any harsh draining method, harsh expellants can be administered only after complete resolution of the exterior pathogen, otherwise, any of a number of transmuted patterns could arise.

The second statement is a discussion of the clinical features of *xuan yin* or suspended phlegm fluids. Some of the symptoms and signs are similar to that of Tai Yang disease and differentiation between the two is essential. *Xuan yin* is the result of water accumulation in the chest and hypochondrium, obstructing the qi dynamic and manifesting as a hard glomus in the epigastric region. Comparison can also be drawn between *xuan yin* and chest bind, insofar as hard glomus below the heart is a principal feature of both. The differentiation is set out in the table Comparison of Suspended Phlegm Fluids and Major Chest Bind Pattern. Apart from pain in the hypochondrium, there is an inability to turn from one side to the other in bed and there are breathing difficulties and coughing. Rapid breathing and even talking can cause a pulling pain under the ribs. If the retained water pathogen migrates to the zang fu, there will be varying manifestations specific to each zang or fu. For example, if phlegm fluids harass the stomach, there will be stomach qi counterflow with dry retching; harassment of the lung will result in lung qi counterflow with cough and shortness of breath; if retained fluids harass the skin and muscle layer, the harmony of ying and wei will be disturbed and there will be sweating; and phlegm fluids obstructing the clear yang will result in headache. The symptoms of sweating and headache must not be confused with similar symptoms found in a Tai Yang exterior pattern. Differentiation is made on the basis that the headache is not accompanied by aversion to cold and the sweating is intermittent rather than constant.

Shi Zao Tang is a potent water expellant suitable for treating the stubborn nature of suspended fluids. Yuan Hua, Gan Sui and Da Ji (大戟, not to be confused with 大蓟, which stops bleeding) are bitter, cold and toxic and are harsh expellants indicated for driving excess water from the chest and abdomen. They are therefore appropriate to expel retained phlegm fluids from the chest and hypochondrium. However, their coldness, toxicity and very potency all present a potential risk for injury to the spleen and stomach. The ten pieces of Da Zao are included in the formula specifically to moderate the harsh effects of these herbs and offer protection for the spleen and stomach. The reason for not using Ren Shen, Huang Qi, Bai Zhu or Gan Cao is that those herbs tend to cause stagnation which would only impede the draining of the pathogenic fluid.

Comparison of Suspended Phlegm Fluids, Glomus and Chest Bind

The principal clinical features of suspended phlegm fluids or *xuan yin* are hard glomus below the heart and a pulling pain under the ribs. Secondary features are a cough, rapid breathing, headache, dizziness, mild intermittent sweating, no aversion to cold, dry retching, diarrhoea, inhibited urination, a submerged, wiry pulse and a white, slippery tongue coat. The difference between major chest bind and suspended phlegm fluid can be seen in their pathogenesis, the location of the disease, their manifestations and in their treatment principle.

PATHOGENESIS: The pathogenesis of major chest bind is heat and water knotting together. Suspended phlegm fluid, on the other hand, is a result of the retention of phlegm fluids.

LOCATION: In major chest bind, the disorder is located below the chest and diaphragm, principally in the middle jiao, but it can extend lower to include the lesser abdomen. Suspended phlegm fluid is located in the chest and hypochondrium, with associated glomus felt in the epigastric region.

MANIFESTATIONS: Major chest bind is characterised by tidal fever, vexation, thirst and a dry, yellow tongue coat. In contrast, suspended phlegm fluid is characterised by a hard glomus below the heart, a pulling pain in the hypochondrium, headache, sweating, dry retching and cough.

TREATMENT PRINCIPLE: The treatment principle for major chest bind is to purge heat, dispel water and dissipate bind; the indicated formula is Da Xian Xiong Tang. The treatment principle for suspended phlegm fluid is to expel water accumulation; Shi Zao Tang is the guiding formula.

Comparison of Suspended Phlegm Fluids and Major Chest Bind Pattern

	Suspended Phlegm Fluids	Major Chest Bind
Pathogenesis	Retention of phlegm fluids	Knotted heat and water in the chest caused by incorrect purgation of shang han or due to transmission from Tai Yang to Yang Ming
Location	Chest and hypochondrium, with glomus below the heart	Below the diaphragm: stomach and lesser abdomen, with glomus below the heart
Manifestations	Hard glomus with a pulling pain under the ribs; mild sweat, occasional headache, dry retching, shortness of breath, cough and no aversion to cold	Pain below the heart with palpable hard and stone-like glomus, tidal fever, vexation, thirst, dry yellow tongue coat, submerged, tight or submerged moderate and forceful pulse
Treatment principle	Purge and eliminate water retention	Purge heat, dispel water and dissipate bind
Formula	Shi Zao Tang	Da Xian Xiong Tang

NOTE:

- The three chief herbs can be ground into powder, encapsulated and then taken with a decoction of Da Zao.
- The patient's constitution must be taken into consideration and the dosage adjusted accordingly: 1½ qian for patients of strong constitution and ½ qian for weaker patients. Consideration should also be given to individual tolerance and the initial dose should be 1g (0.2 qian) and then increased gradually.
- The time of medication is the early morning on an empty stomach. This can limit the duration of effect of the herbs on the stomach, thus minimising any adverse effects.
- The medication may cause slight nausea, vomiting and dizziness. If such side-effects worsen, the medication should be stopped.
- This formula is contraindicated for pregnant women, for patients suffering from a gastrointestinal disorder where there has been recent haemorrhaging, and for patients with a vigorous fever.

Ancient Application of Shi Zao Tang

- *Wai Tai Mi Yao:* In the treatment of retained fluids in the chest and diaphragm characterised by dizziness, yellowing of the eyes and skin, pulling pain under the ribs.
- *San Yin Fang:* Kong Xian Dan 控涎丹 (Shi Zao Tang with the omission of Da Zao and the addition of Bai Jie Zi) was used in the treatment of phlegm accumulation in the chest and diaphragm.
- *Dan Xi Xin Fa:* Zhou Che Wan 舟车丸 (Shi Zao Tang with the omission of Da Zao and the addition of Qian Niu, Da Huang, Qing Chen Pi, Guang Mu Xiang) in the treatment of a disorder similar to suspended phlegm fluids but milder.

Modern Application of Shi Zao Tang

Shi Zao Tang can be used in the treatment of such diseases as exudative pleurisy, cirrhosis of the liver with ascites, and chronic nephritis. Zhang Zhi Xiong et al used Shi Zao Tang to treat 51 cases of pleural effusion. 96% showed substantial improvement after 11 days and 88.2% showed full recovery after 20 days (*Jie Fang Jun Yi Xue Za Zhi* 1965; 2:150).

Nie Hui Ming used Shi Zao Tang in the treatment of ascites in patients whose waist measured in excess of 100cm. There was initial reduction in abdominal fluid but it recurred and so was not deemed effective. (Nie Hui Ming: *Shang Han Yu Lin Chuang.)*

Case Study

Suspended Phlegm Fluids

Extracted from Xiong et al: Jie Fang Jun Yi Za Zhi 1965; 2:150

The patient was admitted to hospital with severe chest pain on the left side, dyspnoea and alternating chills and fever. Three days after admission, her condition worsened. She complained of fatigue and suffered from breathlessness with rapid and difficult breathing. She had a thick, greasy tongue coat and a slippery, wiry pulse. X-ray confirmed the presence of pleural effusion. Aspirated fluid: 50 mL; ESR 44 mm/hr (Westergren). The diagnosis was suspended phlegm fluids and the formula prescribed was Shi Zao Tang ingredients ground and taken with a decoction of Da Zao. An hour and a half after the medication, there was intestinal gurgling which was followed two hours later, by five episodes of watery diarrhoea. The formula was administered on alternate days and after three doses, the chest pain was substantially reduced and the fever resolved. A further four doses were prescribed to consolidate the treatment and she recovered after 26 days.

2.10.3 Excess Phlegm in the Diaphragm

When excess phlegm lodges in the diaphragm, obstructing the qi dynamic, it manifests as a hard glomus in the chest. This is also known as a Gua Di San pattern.

Gua Di San Pattern

Clause 166

病如桂枝证，头不痛、项不强、寸脉微浮、胸中痞硬、气上冲喉咽不得息者，此为胸有寒也，当吐之，宜瓜蒂散。

The disease resembles a Gui Zhi Tang pattern, there is no headache, no stiffness

> in the neck, the cun pulse is slightly floating, there is hard glomus in the chest, qi surges up to the throat making it difficult to breathe, it is due to cold in the chest, one should induce vomiting, Gua Di San is appropriate.

GUA DI SAN: Gua Di (dry-fried until yellow) 1 fen; Chi Xiao Dou 1 fen.

DIRECTIONS: Grind the ingredients separately and sieve before combining. Take 1 ge of Xiang Chi (Dan Dou Chi) and boil in 7 ge of water, making a thin gruel. Strain and mix with a 1 qian spoonful of the powder and take warm. If there is no vomiting, gradually increase the dosage. As soon as the person vomits, stop the medication. Gua Di San should not be given to patients suffering from haemorrhage or those with a weak constitution or deficiency.

NOTE: Gui Di San is an emetic formula which was used to eliminate phlegm excess. This treatment method is no longer in practice.

> **Clause 355**
>
> 病人手足厥冷，脉乍紧者，邪结在胸中，心下满而烦，饥不能食者，病在胸中、当须吐之，宜瓜蒂散。
>
> The patient suffers from cold in the hands and feet, if the pulse is all of a sudden tight, evil is knotted in the chest, there is fullness below the heart and vexation, hunger with no ability to eat, then the disease is in the chest, one should induce vomiting, Gua Di San is appropriate.

DISCUSSION: Clauses 166 and 355 are both associated with excess phlegm where emesis is induced using the formula Gua Di San. Clause 166 describes a disorder which resembles a Gui Zhi Tang pattern, in that both are characterised by fever, sweating and aversion to cold. In the Gua Di San pattern, however, there is no headache or stiffness of the neck and the pulse is not floating in all three positions as in an exterior pattern. The slightly floating pulse of Gua Di San pattern is in the cun position only, which is a reflection of the phlegm harassing the chest and diaphragm. The resulting disturbance of the qi dynamic in the upper jiao manifests as hard glomus and the obstruction of phlegm, causing counterflow qi, which surges up to the throat affecting the person's breathing. In Clause 166, when Zhong Jing explains that this is due to cold in the chest, he is referring to phlegm cold, and so the treatment strategy is to induce the expectoration of phlegm by emesis.

Clause 355 describes a patient who has already contracted shang han or some miscellaneous disease which has resulted in the accumulation of phlegm damp or, perhaps, food stagnation. Either of these conditions constitutes a formed pathogen which obstructs the chest. The cold phlegm has damaged the chest yang and impaired its distribution, and so, the extremities are not warmed and the limbs are cold. This is known as phlegm jue. The tight pulse indicates the presence of a pathogen which has caused stagnation in the flow of qi and blood. The phlegm not only obstructs the qi of the chest, resulting in epigastric fullness and vexation, but also affects the stomach, so that even when hungry, the person can not eat because of the phlegm obstruction.

Gua Di San is a bitter, cold and slightly toxic herb with a strong emetic action. Chi Xiao Dou is sweet, sour and neutral; it drains damp by promoting urination and is effective in reducing fluid retention; it also moderates the toxicity of Gua Di. When Chi Xiao Dou is combined with Gua Di, it enhances the purging effect while the pungency of Xiang Chi acts as a guide and carries the herbs to the upper jiao.

Special Instructions for Gua Di San

- It must be taken hot in one single dose.
- It is for use in patterns of phlegm excess. If, after administration, there is no vomiting, but instead there is unbearable vexation, vomiting must be induced by inserting a finger down the throat. Once the patient vomits, administration must cease.
- If, once vomiting is induced, it continues uncontrollably, administer Jiang Zhi (ginger juice) or Cong Bai decoction to ease the vomiting.
- This formula is contraindicated for patients suffering from chronic disease, ageing patients and patients with a weak constitution.

Ancient Application of Gua Di San

- *Wai Tai Mi Yao:* Gua Di San with the omission of Dan Dou Chi in the treatment of acute jaundice with hardness below the heart, vexatious thirst with a desire to drink, wheezing and yellowing of the eyes.
- *Wen Bing Tiao Bian:* Gua Di San, omitting Dou Chi and adding Shan Zhi Zi in the treatment of Tai Yin wen bing (Tai Yin febrile disease) when characterised by the accumulation of phlegm damp, vexation, restlessness, nausea and hard glomus in the chest.

Modern Application of Gua Di San

Gua Di San, as an emetic, can be used to eliminate toxic accumulation in the stomach characterised by an oppressed sensation in the chest, nausea and general malaise, such as in food poisoning, particularly when there is an urge to vomit but an inability to do so.

Summary of Patterns Resembling Tai Yang

Patterns resembling Tai Yang disorders share similar clinical features but differ in important detail. In common with Tai Yang patterns, they have such symptoms as fever, aversion to cold and sweating and are therefore known as 'patterns resembling Tai Yang'. This nomenclature makes clear that they are not, in fact, true Tai Yang patterns, and thus also elucidates the need for a different treatment strategy.

Wind cold damp bi syndrome is a disorder characterised by stiffness and pain which is caused by pathogenic wind, cold and damp obstructing the flow of qi and blood in the joints and muscles. Gui Zhi Fu Zi Tang is the indicated formula for a pattern of wind cold; Gui Zhi qu Gui jia Bai Zhu Tang is indicated where cold and damp predominate; and Gan Cao Fu Zi Tang is indicated to eliminate the three pathogenic qi, which are wind, cold and damp, on a background of interior yang deficiency

Suspended phlegm fluid is a disorder of accumulated fluids in the chest and hypochondrium characterised by occasional slight sweating, headache, fullness and hard glomus below the heart, a pulling pain in the hypochondrium, dry retching, shortness of breath, sweating and no aversion to cold. The indicated formula is Shi Zao Tang to expel water.

Phlegm accumulation is associated with phlegm obstruction in the chest and diaphragm, and although it is characterised by fever, sweating and aversion to cold, it is not a Gui Zhi Tang pattern as evidenced by the additional symptoms of hard glomus in the chest, qi upsurge to the throat affecting the person's breathing, cold extremities, a tight pulse, pathogenic bind in the chest manifesting as fullness and vexation, and hunger with no desire to eat. The indicated treatment is to induce vomiting using Gua Di San.

Section Eleven

2.11 HE BING (CONCURRENT PATTERNS) & BING BING (LAGOVER PATTERNS)

He bing or concurrent patterns, and bing bing or lagover patterns, both represent a situation where the pathogen manifests in more than one channel simultaneously; there are, however, important differences. *He bing* is the term used to describe a disorder involving two channels at the same time, which is also referred to as a concurrent pattern. These patterns are named according to the channels affected and include: Tai Yang Yang Ming he bing, Tai Yang Shao Yang he bing and Tai Yang Yang Ming Shao Yang he bing, otherwise called "concurrent pattern of the three Yang channels". Bing bing or lagover patterns, on the other hand, are a reflection of a more serious manifestation of disease, where the original pattern is unresolved, but has passed on to one or more other channels and so, not only affects the new channel or channels, but lags behind, continuing to affect the original channel.

2.11.1 Tai Yang Yang Ming He Bing or Concurrent Pattern

Ge Gen Tang Pattern

Clause 32

太阳与阳明合病者，必自下利，葛根汤主之。

If there is Tai Yang and Yang Ming concurrent disease, there will be diarrhoea, Ge Gen Tang governs.

GE GEN TANG: Ge Gen 4 liang; Ma Huang (nodes removed) 3 liang; Gui Zhi (bark removed) 2 liang; Sheng Jiang (sliced) 3 liang; Zhi Gan Cao 2 liang; Shao Yao 2 liang; Da Zao 12 pieces (broken).

DIRECTIONS: First boil Ma Huang and Ge Gen in 1 dou of water, reducing to 6 sheng. Skim off the foam, add the other ingredients and boil until it is reduced to 3 sheng, then strain and take 1 sheng warm. The instructions and contraindications for the administration of Ge Gen Tang are as per Gui Zhi Tang (see Clause 12).

DISCUSSION: A concurrent pattern of Tai Yang and Yang Ming refers to the invasion of a pathogenic influence which, due to the virulence of the pathogen, has resulted in the presence of that pathogen in both channels simultaneously. It is characterised by fever, aversion to cold, a stiff neck (Tai Yang exterior pattern), and a flushed face, sore eyes, dry nose, frontal headache and restless sleep (Yang Ming exterior pattern). The Yang Ming exterior pattern must not be confused with a Bai Hu Tang pattern. *Shang Han Zong Bing Lun* and *Lei Zheng Huo Ren Shu* both state: "Yang Ming channel disorder is also known as exterior channel pattern". Yi Zong Jin Jian states: "Ge Gen is associated with a Yang Ming exterior pattern where there is a flushed face and forehead, headache, fever with no sweating, aversion to cold, sore eyes, a dry nose and restless sleep", which precisely describes a Yang Ming channel disorder.

When the pathogen attacks the Yang Ming channel it constrains qi, and there is fever and aversion to cold. The subsequent struggle of the Yang Ming channel qi against the exterior pathogen results in disruption of the Yang Ming qi, and causes disharmony of the stomach and large intestine, manifesting as diarrhoea. The attack of the exterior pathogen thus gives rise to a disorder with both exterior and interior symptoms. Ge Gen Tang resolves the exterior and expels the pathogen from the stomach channel, thereby harmonising the interior and resolving diarrhoea.

This disorder is comparable to the contraction of an exterior pathogen where there is pre-existing food stagnation, and where the exterior pathogen has constrained and harassed the intestines, resulting in fever, aversion to cold, nausea and diarrhoea. The treatment principle is to release the exterior, which has the indirect effect of also harmonising the interior.

Modern Application of Ge Gen Tang

Ge Gen Tang can be used in the treatment of the common cold, influenza, pneumonia, meningitis, encephalitis, shoulder pain, chronic neuralgia, skin disorders and acute dysentery.

Ge Gen jia Ban Xia Tang pattern

Clause 33

太阳与阳明合病，不下利，但呕者，葛根加半夏汤主之。

Tai Yang and Yang Ming concurrent disease, there no diarrhoea, there is just vomiting, Ge Gen jia Ban Xia Tang governs.

GE GEN JIA BAN XIA TANG: Ge Gen 4 liang; Ma Huang (nodes removed) 3 liang; Zhi Gan Cao 2 liang; Shao Yao 2 liang; Gui Zhi (bark removed) 2 liang; Sheng Jiang (sliced) 2 liang; Ban Xia (washed) ½ sheng.

DIRECTIONS: First boil Ge Gen and Ma Huang in 1 dou of water, reducing to 2 sheng. Skim the decoction, add the other ingredients and boil until reduced to 3 sheng. Strain and take 1 sheng warm. Cover the patient with a blanket to promote a mild sweat.

DISCUSSION: Clause 33 continues the discussion of a concurrent Tai Yang and Yang Ming pattern described in Clause 32, where there is an unresolved exterior pattern which affects the interior and disturbs the normal qi dynamic. Clause 32 describes an exterior pattern with diarrhoea and Clause 33 goes on to describe an exterior pattern with vomiting, which is a manifestation of stomach disharmony. Ge Gen jia Ban Xia Tang releases the exterior, whilst Ban Xia harmonises the stomach and descends counterflow. In practical terms, this is a frequently encountered disorder found in various forms of gastroenteritis where there is diarrhoea, nausea or vomiting.

Case Study

Exterior Invasion of Wind Cold with Food Stagnation

Extracted from Shang Han Lun Fang Yun Yong Fa

In the evening following overconsumption of watermelon and other food, a 22-year-old male suffered six episodes of watery diarrhoea accompanied by nausea and vomiting. His temperature was 39°C and there was aversion to cold, headache, lower back pain, stiffness of the neck, thirst, an absence of sweat, a thin, yellow tongue coat and a floating, rapid pulse. His abdomen was hard and resisted pressure. The formula prescribed was Ge Gen Tang modified: Ge Gen 15g, Ma Huang 10g, Gui Zhi 6g, Shao Yao 10g, Zhi Gan Cao 10g, Sheng Jiang 10g, Hong Zao 12 pieces, Fa Ban Xia 10g. After two packs, his temperature dropped to 37.5°C and the diarrhoea stopped the next afternoon. There was no thirst but the backache persisted. One further pack of the same formula was given with the dose reduced to one-half and Ban Xia omitted.

Ma Huang Tang Pattern

Clause 36

太阳与阳明合病，喘而胸满者，不可下，宜麻黄汤。

Tai Yang and Yang Ming concurrent disease, if there is wheezing and fullness in the chest, one should not purge, Ma Huang Tang is appropriate.

DISCUSSION: It is essential not only to recognise the severity of the concurrent pattern, but also to determine whether it is the Tai Yang or the Yang Ming channel which requires more focused treatment. Clause 36 focuses on treatment of the Tai Yang channel because the disorder is one of constrained exterior qi. This has resulted in the disordered flow of lung qi, manifesting as wheezing and fullness in the chest. The lungs and large intestine stand in an exterior–interior relationship, and the non-descent of lung qi can lead to stagnation in the large intestine, manifesting as constipation. However, the pattern described in Clause 36 is characterised by fullness in the chest, not abdominal fullness. Therefore purging is inappropriate, and the indicated formula is Ma Huang Tang, which diffuses constrained lung qi and promotes sweating, thus releasing the exterior.

In *Shang Han Lun,* there are many strategies to treat wheezing: for wind cold excess causing wheeze, where there is no sweat, the indicated formula is Ma Huang Tang (Clause 35); for wind cold deficiency, where wheeze is accompanied by sweating, the indicated formula is Gui Zhi jia Hou Po Xing Zi Tang (Clauses 18 and 43); for wheeze due to lung heat with sweating, the indicated formula is Ma Xing Shi Gan Tang (Clauses 63 and 162); and for wheeze due to interior heat where there is sweating, the indicated formula is Ge Gen Qin Lian Tang (Clause 34). It can be said that wheezing is often accompanied by sweating. Clause 36, however, describes a pattern where there is wheezing and fullness in the chest, which is a concurrent pattern of Tai Yang and Yang Ming. The pathogenesis of this pattern is pathogenic qi constraint in the Tai Yang channel which manifests as wheezing with no sweat. The indicated formula therefore is Ma Huang Tang.

2.11.2 Tai Yang Shao Yang He Bing or Concurrent Pattern

Huang Qin Tang and Huang Qin jia Ban Xia Sheng Jiang Tang Patterns

> **Clause 172**
>
> 太阴与少阳合病，自下利者，与黄芩汤；若呕者，黄芩加半夏生姜汤主之。
>
> Tai Yang and Shao Yang concurrent disease, if there is spontaneous diarrhoea, give Huang Qin Tang; if there is vomiting, Huang Qin jia Ban Xia Sheng Jiang Tang governs.

HUANG QIN TANG: Huang Qin 3 liang; Shao Yao 2 liang; Zhi Gan Cao 2 liang; Da Zao 12 pieces (broken).

DIRECTIONS: Boil the four ingredients in 1 dou of water, reducing to 3 sheng. Strain and take 1 sheng warm immediately, then once later in the the day and again at night.

HUANG QIN JIA BAN XIA SHENG JIANG TANG: Huang Qin 3 liang; Shao Yao 2 liang; Zhi Gan Cao 2 liang; Da Zao 12 pieces (broken); Ban Xia (washed) ½ sheng; Sheng Jiang (sliced) 1½ liang or 3 liang. The alternative dose of Sheng Jiang represents the larger dose recorded in some editions of *Shang Han Lun* where various dosages from 1½ to 3 liang are recorded. In the clinical situation, the dosage can be adjusted according to the requirements of the individual patient.

DIRECTIONS: Boil the above six ingredients in 1 one dou of water, reducing to 3 sheng. Strain and take 1 sheng warm, then once again later in the day and again at night.

DISCUSSION: This is a Tai Yang and Shao Yang concurrent pattern where the focus is on Shao Yang. The spontaneous diarrhoea refers not to the result of purging, but to diarrhoea caused by constraint in Shao Yang, where heat has harassed the stomach and intestines. The stool is watery and may contain mucus; there may also be abdominal pain, a burning sensation in the anus, tenesmus and dark urination. Huang Qin Tang clears Shao Yang heat. If there is vomiting, then Huang Qin jia Ban Xia Sheng Jiang Tang can be prescribed to clear heat and descend counterflow. Huang Qin is bitter and cold and clears heat from the liver and gallbladder. Shao Yao is sour and slightly bitter; it astringes yin, harmonises the ying and eases pain. Gan Cao and Da Zao augment qi, tonify the middle and strengthen the zheng qi. The combined effect of the four herbs clears heat, harmonises the middle and stops the diarrhoea. Ban Xia and Sheng Jiang are added to harmonise the stomach and stop the vomiting.

Although Clause 172 is associated with a Tai Yang and Shao Yang concurrent pattern, the symptoms of diarrhoea and vomiting which indicate this formula show that the focus is on constrained heat in the Shao Yang, and it is such key symptoms which must be considered in diagnosis.

In *Shang Han Lun*, there are three clauses discussing diarrhoea in concurrent patterns.

1. Clause 32 describes a Tai Yang and Yang Ming concurrent pattern where the focus is the exterior and the prescribed formula is Ge Gen Tang, to release the exterior and harmonise the interior.
2. Clause 172 describes a Tai Yang and Shao Yang concurrent pattern where the focus is Shao Yang and the formula is Huang Qin Tang, to clear heat and stop the diarrhoea.
3. Clause 256 describes a Yang Ming and Shao Yang concurrent pattern where the focus is Yang Ming, and the diarrhoea is attributed to interior heat and food stagnation, which manifests as a hard stool with a foul watery discharge. The treatment is Da Cheng Qi Tang, which purges heat, frees intestinal obstruction and thus stops the diarrhoea.

Ancient Application of Huang Qin Tang

- Huang Qin Tang is indicated in the treatment of a difficult bowel movement and heat dysentery with tenesmus. *Yi Fang Ji Jie* regarded this as the mother of all formulas in the treatment of dysentery.
- *Lei Zheng Huo Ren Shu:* Huang Qin Tang with the omission Da Zao is advocated in the treatment of epistaxis and dysentery.
- *Wen Bing Tiao Bian:* Si Ling Qin Shao Tang (Huang Qin Tang with the omission of

Da Zao and the addition of Zhu Ling, Fu Ling, Ze Xie, Bai Zhu, Hou Po, Chen Pi, Mu Xiang) is advocated in the treatment of dysentery associated with food stagnation and damp.

Modern Application of Huang Qin Tang

- For acute gastroenteritis with watery diarrhoea and mucus, abdominal pain, a burning sensation in the anus and generalised fever, Huang Qin Tang combined with Ge Gen Qin Lian Tang can be used.
- For acute gastritis with nausea, vomiting and abdominal pain, Huang Qin jia Sheng Jiang Ban Xia Tang with the addition of such herbs as Chen Pi and Zhu Ru may be used.
- For dysentery, Huang Qin Tang may be used combined with Bai Tou Weng Tang.

Case Study

Dysentery

Extracted from Jing Fang Ying Yong Ling Xia

An 18-year-old male had contracted summer diarrhoea. The initial onset was marked by alternating chills and fever, abdominal pain, bloody diarrhoea, a burning anus, tenesmus, thirst, a thin, yellow tongue coat and a slippery, wiry pulse. He was prescribed Huang Qin Tang combined with Bai Tou Weng Tang modified: Huang Qin 9g, Huang Lian 6g, Bai Shao 9g, Mu Xiang 4.5g, Qin Pi 12g, Ma Chi Qian 30g, Huang Bai 9g, Ban Di Jin 斑地锦 30g, Gan Cao 4.5g. After three packs, the diarrhoea and abdominal pain stopped. A further three packs were prescribed to consolidate the treatment.

2.11.3 Concurrent Pattern of the Three Yang Channels

The three yang channels are Tai Yang, Yang Ming and Shao Yang. When disease appears concurrently in all three, the treatment depends on the manifestations, which indicate whether the focus should be on Tai Yang, Yang Ming or Shao Yang.

Clause 268

三阳合病，脉浮大，上关上，但欲眠睡，目合则汗。

Concurrent disease of the three yang, the pulse is floating and big, rising from the guan to the cun position, the person wants only to sleep, when the eyes close there is sweating.

DISCUSSION: In a concurrent pattern of the three yang channels, the floating pulse is a manifestation of a Tai Yang pattern, the big pulse is associated with Yang Ming and the long, forceful pulse which extends from the guan to the cun position represents the wiry pulse of a Shao Yang pattern. The desire to sleep is a reflection of exuberant interior heat harassing the heart shen and resulting in a clouded spirit, which is reminiscent of the somnolence of a Shao Yin pattern. However, Shao Yin somnolence is due to yang deficiency with exuberant yin cold and a faint, thready pulse. The sleepiness of the three yang concurrent pattern, on the other hand, is characterised by a pulse which is floating and big, and is therefore associated with interior heat. Thus we can see that sleepiness can be differentiated as being due to heat, cold, deficiency or excess. Sweating after the eyes close may refer to night sweat, or to exuberant yang heat causing fluids to vent outward, which occurs more easily in sleep when the exterior yang is not guarding the exterior. Shao Yang is half interior and half exterior and governs the pivot of qi between exterior and interior. Therefore, here, the sweat which issues when the eyes close is due to Shao Yang interior heat. No formula is advocated for this pattern but Xiao Chai Hu Tang with the addition of Shi Gao and Zhi Mu would be appropriate. Zhi Zi Chi Tang or San Huang Shi Gao Tang can also be used.

2.11.4 Treatment of Bing Bing or Lagover Patterns

Bing bing or lagover disorder refers to a situation where the pathogen is unresolved, lingering in one channel, whilst having transmitted to another, with manifestations occurring in both channels.

Clause 48

（一）二阳并病，太阳初得病时，发其汗，汗先出不彻，因转属阳明，续自微汗出，不恶寒。（二）若太阳病证不罢者，不可下，下之为逆，如此可小发汗。设面色缘缘正赤者，阳气怫郁在表，当解之、熏之。（三）若发汗不彻，不足言，阳气怫郁不得越，当汗不汗，其人躁烦，不知痛处，乍在腹中，乍在四肢，按之不可得，其人短气但坐，以汗出不彻故也，更发汗则愈。（四）何以知汗出不彻？以脉涩故知也。

(1) Lagover disease of the two yang, when Tai Yang first contracts disease, sweating is promoted, the sweating at first is incomplete, so it will transmit to Yang Ming, there will be continued slight spontaneous sweating, with no aversion to cold. (2) If the Tai Yang disease pattern is not finished, one should not purge, purging is adverse, in this case one may mildly promote sweat. If the facial complexion is constantly really crimson, then yang qi is gloweringly constrained in the exterior, one should resolve it, by fuming. (3) If the promotion of sweat is not complete, then needless to say, the yang qi is gloweringly constrained and unable to escape; when there should be sweat there is none, the person is agitated and vexed, and does not know the location of the pain, whether it is in the abdomen, or in the four limbs, palpation can not find it, the person is short of breath and can only sit, it is because the promotion of sweat was incomplete, further sweat promotion will result in recovery. (4) How can one know if there is incomplete promotion of sweat? It is because the pulse is choppy.

DISCUSSION: The first section of Clause 48 identifies the aetiology of a lagover pattern in the two yang channels, namely Tai Yang and Yang Ming, as being inappropriate diaphoretic therapy. This includes sweat promotion which is too mild for a serious condition and also incorrect medication which simply fails to produce a sweat. Either way, the sweating is inadequate to expel the pathogen and resolve the exterior. When the pathogen is not expelled, it falls inward, transforms into heat and initiates a Yang Ming pattern. This results in heat steaming from the interior, manifesting as a continuous slight sweat with no aversion to cold.

Because the Tai Yang is not fully resolved and the pathogen affects both channels, it is called lagover disease of the two yang, which refers to the Tai Yang and Yang Ming. In other words, the pathogen is still lingering in the Tai Yang whilst proceeding to the Yang Ming. The second section explains that despite evidence of the pathogen having entered the Yang Ming channel, as long as the pathogen is in the exterior, sweating must be promoted. Even if there is severe and constant redness in the face, this is evidence of yang qi constrained in the Yang Ming channel, but it is not evidence of an accumulation of heat in the bowel, and unless there is bowel excess, purgation is contraindicted. In that case, the appropriate treatment is to promote sweat either by the administration of Ge Gen Tang or by the use of herbal fuming therapy whereby, in ancient times, the steam from a herbal decoction would be used to steam or 'fume' the patient in order to raise a sweat. The third section of the clause discusses the pathogenesis and pulse sign of lagover disease of the two yang. It explains how the promotion of sweat was inadequate to release the exterior fully, thus failing to expel the pathogen from the Tai Yang, and resulting instead in further constraint of the yang qi, causing vexation and irritability. Because the constrained yang affects the flow of ying and wei qi, it leads to pain due to qi stagnation, which is of undetermined location, seeming to be neither in the abdomen nor in the limbs and can not even be identified on palpation. If the constrained qi harasses the lungs, there is shortness of breath on exertion, so the person has to sit down. The strategy is to complete the promotion of sweat to achieve recovery. The final section explains that the cause of this pattern is the inadequate promotion of sweat, which can be identified by the choppy pulse. This is because a choppy pulse represents obstruction to the flow of qi and blood, and in this case the obstruction is the pathogenic constraint of yang. The shortness of breath and choppy pulse are both due to constraint of the yang qi by the exterior pathogen. It should be noted that because this is a pattern of excess, the pulse would be choppy and forceful, as opposed to the choppy pulse of a deficiency pattern where there is shortness of breath and where the pulse would be weak.

Although Clause 48 indicates that the correct treatment is to promote mild sweating, it does not recommend a formula. Yu Jia Yan suggests Gui Zhi jia Ge Gen Tang; Zhang Lu Yu proposes Gui Zhi Er Yue Bi Yi Tang; and Cheng Jiao Qian (Cheng Ying Mao) advocates Da Qing Long Tang. The authors believe the most appropriate formula is Gui Zhi Er Yue Bi Yi Tang.

Clause 142

太阳与少阳并病，头项强痛，或眩冒，时如结胸，心下痞硬者，当刺大椎第一间、肺俞、肝俞，慎不可发汗，发汗则谵语，脉弦，五日谵语不止，当刺期门。

In Tai Yang and Shao Yang lagover disease, where there is stiffness and pain of the head and neck, dizziness, and sometimes something which resembles chest bind with hard glomus below the heart; one should needle Da Zhui (Du 14), Fei Shu (UB 13), and Gan Shu (UB 18); caution must be taken not to promote sweat, as sweating will cause delirious speech and a wiry pulse; and if after five days, the delirious speech persists, one should needle Qi Men (Liv 14).

DISCUSSION: Stiffness and pain in the head and neck are key features of a Tai Yang pattern and show that the pathogen is still in the exterior. Dizziness and glomus signal transmission of the pathogen to the Shao Yang, and are a reflection of how it affects the pivoting mechanism, which controls the ascent and descent of qi as well as its movement between the exterior and interior. So it is surmised that the disorder is a Tai Yang and Shao Yang lagover pattern and it is clear that treatment must target both channels. The instruction to needle Da Zhui (Du 14) and Fei Shu (Urinary Bladder 13) has the objective of releasing the Tai Yang exterior pathogen, whilst needling Gan Shu (Urinary Bladder 18) relieves Shao Yang qi constraint.

A Tai Yang disorder is resolved by sweating, but acrid warm herbs are inappropriate in a Shao Yang pattern, and qi constraint in the Shao Yang can not be resolved by sweating, which would damage fluids and only succeed in augmenting the heat. This would in turn give rise to dry heat in the stomach and delirious speech. The wiry pulse is a sign of a Shao Yang pattern; delirious speech persisting after five days is the manifestation of a Yang Ming heat pattern which has not yet developed into a bowel excess pattern, and so purgation is contraindicated on both counts. The suggested alternative is to needle Qi Men (Liver 14), which is the alarm point of the liver channel. This can clear constrained heat in the liver and gallbladder, cool blood and harmonise the ying. Once the Shao Yang heat has been eliminated, the delirious speech will resolve.

Da Zhui (Du 14) is the meeting point of the three yang channels and needling this point is effective in expelling pathogenic wind; Fei Shu (Urinary Bladder 13) can regulate lung qi and disperse pathogens from the exterior. In contemporary acupuncture practice, these two points can be combined with Feng Chi (Gall Bladder 20) and He Gu (Large Intestine 4) as an effective treatment for externally contracted disease. Chai Hu Gui Zhi Tang can be given as adjunctive treatment to support the acupuncture.

Clause 150

太阳、少阳并病，而反下之，成结胸；心下硬、下利不止，水浆不下，其人心烦。

Tai Yang Shao Yang lagover disease, but nonetheless there is purgation, it will turn into chest bind; hardness below the heart, incessant diarrhoea, an inability to get fluid down, the person is vexed.

DISCUSSION: The aetiology of a Tai Yang Shao Yang lagover pattern is incorrect purgation.

Following purgation, the pathogen falls inward, where it knots with phlegm and water already present in the body. This manifests as chest bind characterised by hardness and fullness below the heart. The incessant diarrhoea is the aftermath of the incorrect purgation which has damaged yang and resulted in the sinking of spleen qi. Due to the pathogenic excess in the upper jiao, the person can not keep water down, and when the pathogen harasses the chest, there is vexation. This is a pattern with pathogenic excess in the upper jiao and qi deficiency in the lower jiao. The treatment strategy is first to support the deficiency by using Li Zhong Wan to warm and supplement the spleen and stomach. Ban Xia Xie Xin Tang and Gui Zhi Ren Shen Tang are also appropriate for this condition.

Clause 171

太阳、少阳并病，心下硬、颈项强而眩者，当刺大椎、肺俞、肝俞，慎勿下之。

Tai Yang Shao Yang lagover disease, if there is hardness below the heart, stiffness of the neck and dizziness, one should needle Da Zhui (Du 14), Fei Shu (UB 13) and Gan Shu (UB 18), taking caution not to purge.

DISCUSSION: Stiffness in the neck indicates that the Tai Yang exterior pattern remains unresolved, whilst the hardness below the heart and dizziness show that it has nevertheless proceeded to Shao Yang. Although the exterior pattern is unresolved, the promotion of sweat would damage fluids and result in a transmuted pattern. Similarly, although there is an interior pattern of constraint, demonstrated by the hardness below the heart, purgation is contraindicated in a Shao Yang pattern and can not be used; purgatives would damage the middle qi causing incessant diarrhoea. Since the promotion of sweat and purgation are both contraindicated, acupuncture is used to release the exterior pathogen from Tai Yang by needling Da Zhui (Du 14) and Fei Shu (Urinary Bladder 13) and heat in the Shao Yang can be eliminated by needling Gan Shu (Urinary Bladder 18). Clause 142 explains that sweat promotion is contraindicated in lagover disease of Tai Yang and Shao Yang, whilst Clause 171 states that purgation is also contraindicated.

2.11.5 Summary of He Bing and Bing Bing

Although concurrent patterns (*he bing*), and lagover patterns (*bing bing*) both represent disease simultaneously presenting in more than one channel, there are important differences.

He Bing or Concurrent Patterns

He bing or concurrent patterns are regarded as a primary disease and are differentiated according to the channels affected: Tai Yang Yang Ming he bing, Tai Yang Shao Yang he bing and Three Yang he bing. Each has its differential treatment protocol, as follows.

- **Tai Yang and Yang Ming he bing.** Treatment is based on the key symptoms. If there is wheezing and fullness in the chest, the focus is on Tai Yang and the prescribed formula is Ma Huang Tang. If there is diarrhoea or vomiting, the focus is on Yang Ming and either Ge Gen Tang or Gen Gen jia Ban Xia Tang can be administered.
- **Tai Yang and Shao Yang he bing.** Treatment targets the pathogenic heat harassing the interior, which causes spontaneous diarrhoea or vomiting, and the indicated formula is Huang Qin Tang or Huang Qin jia Ban Xia Sheng Jiang Tang. Sweat promotion is contraindicated.
- **Three Yang he bing.** When the pulse is floating and big, and flows beyond the guan position, and there is a desire to sleep accompanied by sweating, the focus is Shao Yang.

Bing Bing or Lagover Patterns

Lagover disease is where a pathogen affects one channel and, before it is resolved, transmission takes place affecting a second channel whilst the pathogen still lingers in the first one. Lagover disease is regarded as a secondary disease and is differentiated according to the channels involved. The two patterns are Tai Yang and Yang Ming bing bing and Tai Yang and Shao Yang bing bing.

- **Tai Yang and Yang Ming bing bing.** This refers to an exterior pathogen attacking Tai Yang and subsequently transmitting to Yang

Ming without resolution in the original channel. This condition is attributed to the inappropriate promotion of sweat. The key point is to understand whether the Tai Yang pattern is accompanied by a Yang Ming channel disorder or a Yang Ming bowel disorder. The principal treatment for a Yang Ming channel disorder is the promotion of sweat, and the treatment for a Yang Ming bowel disorder is purgation.

- **Tai Yang and Shao Yang bing bing.** This is where the pathogen passes from Tai Yang to Shao Yang, whilst still lingering in the former. Both sweat and purgation are contraindicated: sweating will damage fluids and exacerbate heat, whilst purgation can cause the pathogen to fall inward, giving rise to chest bind with hardness below the heart, and also result in incessant diarrhoea. Zhang Zhong Jing recommended acupuncture treatment.

Section Twelve

2.12 PROGNOSIS & RECOVERY IN TAI YANG DISEASE

Prognosis in Tai Yang Disease

The Tai Yang recovery period has clinical significance in that the positive influence of the environmental yang qi will enhance the chance of recovery in the following situations.

1. If the disease is not of a serious nature, there is a possibility for the disease to resolve during the recovery period.
2. If, after medication, the disease has not fully resolved, there is a greater chance of full recovery during the recovery period.
3. One can choose the recovery period as the optimal time to administer treatment to expedite recovery.

Tai Yang Recovery Period

There is a specific time for the return of yang qi associated with each of the channels. According to the twelve two-hour periods of traditional Chinese time keeping, based on the twelve earthly branches, the Tai Yang recovery period is from si shi, through wu shi to wei shi, which refers approximately to the period from 9am to 3pm.

Clause 9

太阳病欲解时，从巳至未上。

The time that Tai Yang disease is ready to resolve, is from si to wei.

DISCUSSION: The most favourable period for the resolution of Tai Yang disease is from 9am to 3pm. This is based on the theory of man's response to the influence of heaven, and on man's intimate relationship with the environment. Environmental changes, be they seasonal or diurnal, have a significant impact on wellbeing and on response to illness. For this reason, the six environmental evils or excesses are the cause of many diseases, and likewise the yin and yang of the universe can support the yin and yang of man as his zheng qi struggles to combat and expel the pathogen. The period from 9am to 3pm was nominated in *Huang Di Nei Jing* as "yang within yang" because it is the time of the day when the sun reaches its zenith and when cosmic yang energy is at its peak. Therefore, it is the time when the yang qi of the universe can most influence the yang qi of the body and when the environmental yang qi serves as a catalyst to expel the pathogen. Hence, the period for Tai Yang disease to resolve is during those hours.

Recovery Strategies in Tai Yang

Clause 30

（一）问曰：证象阳旦，按法治之而增剧，厥逆，咽中干，两胫拘急而谵语。师曰：言夜半手足当温，两脚当伸，后如师言。何以知此？（二）答曰：寸口脉浮而大，浮为风，大为虚，风则生微热，虚则两胫挛，病形象桂枝，因加附子参其间；增桂令汗出，附子温经，亡阳故也。厥逆，咽中干，烦躁，阳明内结，谵语烦乱；更饮甘草干姜汤。夜半阳气还，两足当热，胫尚微拘急，重与芍药甘草汤，尔乃胫伸。以承气汤微溏，则止其谵语，故知病可愈。

Question: A pattern similar to Yang Dan, treated according to the rule, but it is more severe, there is desertion reversal, dryness in the throat, arresting spasm in both calves and delirious speech. The master said: Now, in the middle of the night the hands and feet will be warm, both feet will stretch, and later it was as the master said. How did he know?

Answer: The cun pulse is floating and big, floating indicates wind, big indicates deficiency, the wind generates a mild fever, the deficiency causes cramps in both calves. The disease resembles Gui Zhi, so Fu Zi should be added in; increasing Gui causes sweating, but Fu Zi warms the channels, this is because there is devastation of yang. Where there is desertion reversal, a dry throat, vexation and agitation, there is Yang Ming interior bind, delirious speech and derangement; it is better to drink Gan Cao Gan Jiang Tang. In the middle of the night, yang qi returns, the two feet must be warm, if the legs have mild cramps, give a large dose of Shao Yao Gan Cao Tang, then the legs will stretch. Because of Cheng Qi Tang there is slight sloppiness, then the delirious speech will stop, so we know the disease is recovering.

DISCUSSION: The first part of Clause 30 compares the pattern to a 'Yang Dan' pattern, an alternative name for a Gui Zhi Tang pattern, which means there was a floating pulse, spontaneous sweating, and a slight aversion to cold. Accordingly, Gui Zhi Tang was prescribed but the condition deteriorated into a transmuted pattern with symptoms of cold extremities due to desertion of yang qi, a dry throat, leg cramps and delirious speech. The implication is that although it resembled a Gui Zhi Tang pattern, it was, in fact, not. The master, having treated the patient, predicts that yang qi will return during the night and the feet would be warm and the cramping resolved; confirmation is given that it was as he predicted.

From the cold extremities due to desertion of yang, it can be understood that there was a pre-existing interior yang deficiency; from the dry throat and leg cramps, it is understood that there was also a milder insufficiency of yin. This is a pattern of dual yin and yang deficiency and the correct treatment is to warm the yang and release the exterior. The conclusion is drawn that the first physician was not aware of the yang deficiency, and so prescribed Gui Zhi Tang with an increased dose of Gui Zhi to promote sweating and release the exterior, instead of Gui Zhi jia Fu Zi Tang, to release the exterior and scatter cold while fortifying the deficient yang. Thus, not only was the yang not supported, leaving the exterior insecure and resulting in excessive sweating, but the promotion of sweat damaged it further, and also injured yin. The failure to use Fu Zi and support yang gave rise to a transmuted pattern of *jue*, which refers to cold extremities resulting from yang desertion and the non-interaction of yin and yang.

The second section of Clause 30 explains the original error and the master's subsequent treatment. First, it describes the pulse, which is floating and big, not floating and moderate as in a true Gui Zhi Tang pattern. The fact that the pulse is floating confirms the presence of an exterior pattern with pathogenic wind attacking the defence yang. The fact that it is big, and by inference, forceless, denotes insufficiency of zheng qi, representing an interior deficiency. This is what is meant by "floating indicates wind, big indicates deficiency". In this way the clause describes a pattern of pathogenic wind attacking the defence yang; the slight fever is a sign of the exterior pattern and the dry throat and leg cramps show that there is also a yin deficiency, where yin fluids fail to moisten the throat and also fail to nourish the sinews.

Gan Cao Gan Jiang Tang is the master's preferred formula to restore the yang, explaining that the yang qi will return that night, and the feet will be warm, thus demonstrating the return of yang. The clause then goes on to say that once the yang returns, if the cramps are not fully relieved, Shao Yao Gan Cao Tang should be given to supplement yin and ease the spasm. In this way, one formula is given to restore yang, and the other to supplement yin in a pattern of dual deficiency of yin and yang. If the vexation and delirious speech are not resolved or, alternatively, if the return of yang qi is excessive, causing further delirious speech and deranged behaviour, then it is suggested that Tiao Wei Cheng Qi Tang can be given, and after passing a sloppy stool, the delirium will be resolved, and there will soon be complete recovery.

Without reading Clause 29, the use of Gui Zhi Tang with the addition of Fu Zi could be understood to refer to the addition of Fu Zi being used by the master to treat the jue of the transmuted pattern, mentioned in the first section, by rescuing the devastated yang. However, as in Clause 29, Gan Cao Gan Jiang Tang is the formula used by 'the master' to warm the interior and restore yang. These two clauses underscore the theory of supporting the yang in order to nourish the yin.

Section Thirteen

2.13 SUMMARY OF THE TAI YANG CHAPTER

Tai Yang Pattern

Tai Yang exterior syndrome is characterised by a floating pulse, headache, stiff neck and aversion to cold. Differences in constitution and in the virulence of the pathogen result in three sub-types.

1. Tai Yang zhong feng (wind strike)
   Manifestations: fever, spontaneous sweating, aversion to wind cold, stiff neck and headache, a floating and moderate pulse.
   Pathogenesis: disharmony of ying and wei with strong wei and weak ying.
2. Tai Yang shang han (cold injury)
   Manifestations: fever, aversion to cold, absence of sweat, dyspnoea, stiff neck and headache, a floating and tight pulse.
   Pathogenesis: blocked wei qi with constrained ying yin.
3. Mild Patterns of Exterior Depression
   Manifestations: fever and aversion to cold, the presence of more heat than cold, headache and a floating pulse.
   Pathogenesis: prolonged unresolved exterior syndrome.

ADDITIONAL SYMPTOMS IN GUI ZHI TANG AND MA HUANG TANG PATTERNS: During the course of Tai Yang disease, concurrent symptoms may appear. For example, a pathogen may have already impeded the channel qi, giving rise to stiffness in the neck; if, in addition to this, the pathogenic constraint in the exterior also affects the diffusion of lung qi, there may be cough and dyspnoea; if the pathogen causes disharmony between the exterior and interior, there may be vomiting and diarrhoea.

TAI YANG FU PATTERN: If the exterior pathogen is not resolved, the pathogenic cold can transmit along the Tai Yang channel and knot with the qi of the urinary bladder. The knotted pathogen then disrupts the transformation function of the bladder and gives rise to a condition known as water amassment or xu shui. Another possibility is for the pathogenic cold to transform into heat and combine with blood in the lower jiao, giving rise to a condition known as blood amassment or xu xue. Both water and blood amassment are associated with the urinary bladder and known as Tai Yang fu patterns.

TAI YANG TRANSMUTED PATTERNS: Transmuted patterns are those where a new pattern emerges manifesting with symptoms which are not characteristic of Tai Yang disease. The underlying cause is inadequate, inappropriate or excessive treatment; there is a greater propensity for transmutation when there is a pre-existing excess or deficiency of the zang fu. Tai Yang transmuted patterns reflect the inter-relationship of yin and yang and the way in which diseases can be affected by constant changes in the balance of yin and yang. There are numerous manifestations associated with transmuted patterns. Where excessive diaphoresis injures the yang qi, there can be heart palpitations due to heart yang deficiency, vexation due to kidney yang deficiency or oedema due to spleen yang deficiency. Where, due to inappropriate treatment, the exterior pathogen falls inward, pathogenic heat will disturb the chest causing insubstantial vexation (xu fan), chest bind (xian xiong) or a glomus pattern (pi zheng). In general, patterns with excess yang affect the three yang channels and their corresponding fu, while patterns with excess yin affect the three yin channels and their corresponding zang.

PATTERNS RESEMBLING TAI YANG: Certain miscellaneous diseases, with manifestations similar to a Tai Yang pattern, are categorised as patterns resembling Tai Yang. These include patterns of wind damp, suspended phlegm fluids (*xuan yin*) and phlegm excess (*tan shi*).

TAI YANG RECOVERY PERIOD: Tai Yang channel qi peaks between the hours of si to wei (9am to 3pm) and so this is the optimal time for recovery.

陽明

Yang Ming 3

Section One

3.1 OUTLINE OF YANG MING

Pathway of the Yang Ming Channel

The Yang Ming channel comprises the foot Yang Ming stomach and hand Yang Ming large intestine channels, which have an exterior–interior relationship with the foot Tai Yin spleen and hand Tai Yin lung channels respectively. Due to the sequential flow of qi in the channels and to their zang fu inter-relationships, the stomach, spleen, large intestine and lungs are intimately related. The external pathway of the foot Yang Ming stomach channel starts at the eye, traverses the cheeks and jaw before descending to the chest and abdomen, and continues down the leg to the second toe. An internal channel encircles the gums and goes to the forehead, and another channel enters the chest and homes to the stomach and spleen. One branch of the luo connecting channel joins with its yin partner, the spleen channel, and another leads to the head and throat. The external pathway of the hand Yang Ming large intestine channel travels from the tip of the index finger across the shoulder to the chin, where it traverses the teeth and gums of the lower jaw. An internal channel intersects the Du meridian, connects and passes through its yin partner, the lungs, before homing to the large intestine. The luo connecting channel leads to the lung and a second branch goes to the ear.

Physiology of the Yang Ming Channel

The overall physiological functions of the Yang Ming channel are to transport vital substances, to supplement qi and blood, and to descend qi. The stomach and the spleen both belong to the middle jiao. The stomach is in charge of the rotting and ripening of water and grain, in other words, the decomposition of food. It has a preference for moisture and loathes dryness. The spleen extracts the essence of grain and water and dispatches the refined essence, or nutrients, to the channels and zang fu, providing them with blood and qi. Ultimately, it reaches all parts of the body, including the zang and fu organs, whereby it nourishes the body and thus is known as the source of transformation and the root of postnatal qi. The function of the large intestine to descend and excrete waste is the end part of the digestive process but, nevertheless, it is dependent on the descending and dispersing function of lung qi, as well as on the spleen's function of transforming and transporting fluids and food essences. It could well be said that the interrelated and concerted actions of the Yang Ming and Tai Yin parallel basic anabolic and catabolic processes, which are the core of human physiological function.

Pathology of the Yang Ming Channel

The Yang Ming channel is the sea of water and grain and as such is rich in qi and blood; it is also characterised by exuberant yang qi, which is an expression of the strength of zheng qi. In a pathogenic attack, there ensues a particularly vigorous struggle which generates heat. For this reason, any pathogenic invasion of the Yang Ming has the potential to transform into heat and dryness. Yang Ming patterns are therefore characterised by high fever, sweating, aversion to heat with no aversion to cold, thirst and a flooding pulse. The basis of Yang Ming pathology is exuberant internal heat, and the subsequent damage to fluids, with transformation to dryness manifesting as fu (bowel) excess. Although both the stomach and large intestine can be affected, stomach excess is the principal feature of Yang Ming patterns, which are as follows.

1. *Severe interior heat with damage to stomach fluids.* Formless heat lodged in the chest characterised by fever, insubstantial vexation and insomnia.
2. *Stomach heat with fluid exhaustion.* Fever, aversion to heat, thirst and sweating.
3. *Severe interior heat with depletion of fluids in the large intestine with food stagnation, manifesting as bowel excess.* Fever, sweating, constipation, abdominal distension, pain aggravated by pressure, delirious speech and a submerged and forceful pulse.
4. *Yang Ming heat combined with damp in the Tai Yin.* Jaundice at the qi level or, if the pathogenic heat harasses the blood, at the blood level.
5. *Complex heat and water bind in the lower jiao.* Inhibited urination, vexation and thirst.

Yang Ming Disease and Its Transmission Pathway

Yang Ming disease is an interior pattern characterised by interior heat and excess. The origin can be the Yang Ming channel itself, or it can be the result of pathogenic transmission from other channels such as Tai Yang or Shao Yang. Disease stemming directly from the Yang Ming channel is known as 'Zheng Yang Yang Ming'; disease transmitted from the Tai Yang channel as a result of incorrect treatment of Tai Yang disease is known as 'Tai Yang Yang Ming'; and if the disease is transmitted from the Shao Yang due to incorrect promotion of sweat in the treatment of Shao Yang disease, it is known as 'Shao Yang Yang Ming'. Similarly, it is possible for diseases of the three yin channels to exit the body via the Yang Ming channel, giving rise to a scenario of transmission from the zang organ to the fu organ; there is then a possibility for the disease to convert from deficiency to excess. In addition, because of the close relationship of Yang Ming and Tai Yin as joint tenants of the middle jiao, any deficiency in the Yang Ming can lead to a disorder of the Tai Yin and, conversely, Tai Yin excess can give rise to Yang Ming disease.

The potential for transmission of an external pathogen to the Yang Ming is dependent on the following three factors.

(a) The nature of the pathogen: its severity and any factors which would activate the transformation of pathogenic wind cold into heat and dryness and potentiate its transmission into the Yang Ming.
(b) The physical constitution of the individual: a person with underlying yang excess, particularly where it is accompanied by food stagnation, is more prone to stomach and intestinal dryness.
(c) Incorrect or inappropriate treatment: inadequate diaphoresis may result in the pathogenic influence not being released, whilst excessive sweating or purging can cause the exterior pathogen to fall inward and transform into heat, damaging fluids and generating dryness.

Key Manifestations of Yang Ming Disease

The key symptoms for diagnosis of Yang Ming disease are the 'four bigs', which comprise a high fever, profuse perspiration, severe thirst and a big pulse. Vexation is a further symptom usually found in a Yang Ming heat pattern. There is no aversion to cold, but aversion to heat.

Classification of Yang Ming Disease

In broad terms, Yang Ming disease is associated with heat and excess, and can be differentiated into two categories: Yang Ming heat excess pattern, and Yang Ming Fu excess pattern.

1. YANG MING HEAT EXCESS PATTERN. This is the result of exuberant dry heat and is characterised by fever, sweating, aversion to heat but not to cold, vexation, thirst and a flooding, big pulse. Bai Hu Tang is the guiding formula. If the heat is lodged in the chest and diaphragm, the pattern manifests with vexation, anguish and insomnia and the indicated formula is Zhi Zi Chi Tang; if there is heat and water knotted in the lower jiao, characterised by fever, thirst for drinks, inhibited urination and a floating pulse, the indicated formula is Zhu Ling Tang.

2. YANG MING FU EXCESS PATTERN. A Yang Ming fu or bowel excess pattern is the result of a dry heat pathogen knotting with food stagnation in the stomach and large intestine, causing stagnation in the large intestine which is characterised by tidal fever, delirious speech, hard distension in the abdomen or pain in the umbilical region, constipation, sweating of the hands and feet, and a submerged, excess and forceful pulse. The indicated formula is one of the three Cheng Qi Tang formulas. A further concept to consider is the spleen: the stomach heat inhibits the spleen's transportation of fluid, resulting in constipation, frequent urination and a floating, choppy pulse at Fu Yang (St 42) on the instep, the strength of which is indicative of the strength of the qi of the spleen and stomach. This is known as *pi yue* (spleen restraint). If the Yang Ming heat is not resolved and combines with the damp of the Tai Yin, there will be jaundice, characterised by yellowing of the skin and eyes, and by fever and inhibited urination. If the heat of the Yang Ming enters the blood level, there will be a parched throat with no thirst, and epistaxis. This is called blood amassment of Yang Ming.

Treatment of Yang Ming Disease

The two key treatment principles of Yang Ming disease are to clear heat and to purge excess. The strategy of clearing heat in Yang Ming heat patterns is exemplified in such formulas as Bai Hu Tang, Bai Hu jia Ren Shen Tang, Zhi Zi Chi Tang and Zhu Ling Tang. Where there is damp heat characterised by jaundice and yellowing, the formula is Yin Chen Hao Tang. The three Cheng Qi Tang formulas are used to purge heat excess from the intestines and Di Dang Tang is used where there is blood amassment in the Yang Ming.

Contraindications in Yang Ming Disease

Although purgation is an indicated treatment in many Yang Ming patterns, there are certain patterns in which it is contraindicated.

Section Two

3.2 PRINCIPAL FEATURES OF YANG MING DISEASE

Clause 180

阳明之为病，胃家实是也。

Yang Ming is diseased, the stomach's domain is excess.

DISCUSSION: The expression 'the stomach's domain' is inclusive of the stomach and the intestines. The *Ling Shu: Ben Shu Pian (Chapter 2: The Root of Transport)* states: "The large and small intestines both pertain to the stomach, which is Yang Ming". The term 'excess' refers to the invasion of an excess pathogen in the presence of zheng qi which is robust and not deficient. *The Su Wen: Tong Ping Xu Shi Lun (Chapter 28)* states: "When evil qi is abundant, it is excess, if essence qi is depleted, it is deficiency". A pattern where there is both pathogenic heat and stagnation will manifest with excessive thirst, excessive sweating, and a flooding and big pulse. Because heat consumes fluids, there will also be symptoms of dryness such as a dry, hard stool, abdominal distension and tidal fever. Thus it can be seen that the expression 'the stomach's domain' is a reference not only to the location of Yang Ming disease, but it is also a reference to the characteristics of a Yang Ming pattern.

The concept of stomach excess is subject to two different interpretations. Some suggest that the excess refers to the concrete manifestations of a dry stool and food accumulation. Others propose that it is a reference to the presence of a hard glomus such as that found in a Da Xian Xiong Tang pattern. This stands in contrast to the epigastric fullness accompanied by insubstantial vexation, which is a feature of a Zhi Zi Chi Tang pattern. However, the excess nature of Yang Ming disease is not in dispute, nor is the indicated treatment of purging the excess and expelling the pathogen. The following is a summary of Zhang Zhong Jing's purging strategies.

1. *Warming and purging.* For chest bind due to cold phlegm and phlegm fluids, using San Wu Bai San as cited in Clause 146.
2. *Purging heat and dispelling water.* For chest bind due to heat excess characterised by pain in the hypochondrium and epigastrium, with pain and distension in the lesser abdomen, constipation, mild tidal fever, a stiff neck, a thick yellow tongue coat and a submerged, tight or submerged, moderate and forceful pulse. The formula used is Da Xian Xiong Tang and Da Xian Xiong Wan.
3. *Purging blood stasis.* For blood amassment characterised by intense pain in the lesser abdomen, glomus which is hard and painful, manic behaviour and uninhibited urination. The indicated formula for milder blood stasis is Tao He Cheng Qi Tang and for more serious stasis, Di Dang Tang or Di Dang Wan may be used.
4. *Purging and draining phlegm fluids.* For water amassment in the chest and hypochondrium caused by the obstruction of chest yang and disruption of the qi dynamic. This is characterised by mild occasional sweating, headache, hard glomus in the epigastrium, dry retching, shortness of breath, a pulling pain in the hypochondrium and no aversion to cold. The formula used is Shi Zao Tang.
5. *Bitter, cold purging strategy.* For Yang Ming pathogenic heat and also where heat has scorched the fluids, affecting the Shao Yin and causing knotted bind, manifesting as a dry stool and obstruction of intestinal qi. This is known as urgent purgation to protect Shao Yin fluids from further damage. This pattern of bowel excess associated with dryness and heat can be further differentiated into three treatment patterns:
   (i) Potently purging: for dryness and excess manifesting as constipation where there may be a foul watery discharge, and where there is periumbilical pain and distension which resists pressure, tidal fever and delirious speech. The indicated formula is Da Cheng Qi Tang.
   (ii) Purging and freeing intestinal obstruction: for hard abdominal distension which resists pressure, with a hard stool where there may also be a foul watery discharge, tidal fever, sweating and delirious speech. The indicated formula is Xiao Cheng Qi Tang to alleviate glomus and distension.
   (iii) Moderately purging and softening hardness: for dry heat affecting the stomach and intestines manifesting with mild abdominal pain which resists pressure, constipation, steaming fever, thirst and vexation. The indicated formula is Tiao Wei Cheng Qi Tang to purge the dry excess and harmonise the stomach qi.
6. *Moistening and purging.* For dry heat in the stomach which obstructs the spleen's transportation of fluids, characterised by constipation, mild or no abdominal pain, frequent urination, a red tongue with a yellow coat and a floating, choppy pulse at Fu Yang (St 42). The indicated formula is Ma Zi Ren Wan to purge the heat and moisten the dryness.
7. *Suppository and enema.* Indicated for fluid damage with constipation, using Mi Jian Dao, Tu Gua Gen or Da Zhu Dan Zhi to induce defaecation.

Apart from the above purging methods, such formulas as Da Chai Hu Tang, Chai Hu Mang Xiao Tang, Yin Chen Hao Tang, although not specific to Yang Ming disease, can be included in the purgation category, because they target bowel excess.

Clause 182

问曰：阳明病外证云何？答曰：身热，汗自出，不恶寒反恶热也。

Question: What are the exterior symptoms of Yang Ming disease? Answer: Fever, spontaneous sweating, no aversion to cold but aversion to heat.

DISCUSSION: Clause 182 outlines the principal features of Yang Ming disease: fever, spontaneous sweating, and no aversion to cold as is found in Tai Yang, but instead, there is aversion to heat. The spontaneous sweating comes from the body fluids being steamed outwards by the interior heat. Aversion to heat with no aversion to cold emphasises that it is an interior pattern with no sign of an external pattern. The subjective sensation of aversion to heat or cold is a key point of differentiation between Yang Ming, Tai Yang and Shao Yang patterns. Wang Ling You said: "No aversion to cold reflects the pathogen is no longer at the exterior; aversion to heat reflects it is due to interior heat" *(Zhong Han Lun Bian Zheng Guang Zhu)*.

Fever is a commonly encountered symptom in disease of the three yang channels; however, it differs in its presentation. The fever of a Tai Yang pattern is mild and is accompanied by an aversion to cold, both manifestations reflecting the presence of an exterior pathogen in the muscle layer. The fever of Shao Yang comes and goes, alternating with chills, reflecting the location of the pathogen midway between the interior and the exterior or 'half interior half exterior'. The fever of Yang Ming is unlike either of these in that it is a highly vigorous fever where there is distinct aversion to heat, no aversion to cold, and no body chills. Yang Ming fever is not resolved by sweating and is usually accompanied by a huge thirst; the pulse is flooding, big and rapid, and not floating or wiry. Bai Hu Tang is the indicated formula for high fever and sweating in a Yang Ming pattern. The fever associated with Yang Ming bowel excess is described as a tidal fever which peaks in the afternoon. The indicated treatment is purgation using one of the Cheng Qi Tang group of formulas. It is important not to confuse a true Bai Hu Tang pattern with any other pattern simply on the basis of a vigorous fever. A pattern where there is unresolved fever, but where the face is pale and the pulse big but empty and forceless, for instance, must be treated by tonification, using a formula such as Dang Gui Bu Xue Tang or Du Shen Tang to tonify qi and blood.

Clause 186

伤寒三日，阳明脉大。

Shang han for three days, the Yang Ming pulse is big.

DISCUSSION: Here, the term shang han is intended in its broader meaning which encompasses all externally contracted febrile disease. The nominated period of three days simply shows that it is no longer in the initial stage; the description of the big pulse is to distinguish the disease clearly from the floating pulse of a Tai Yang pattern, or the wiry pulse of a Shao Yang pattern. A Yang Ming pattern pulse is flooding, big and forceful, and it is this big flooding pulse which reflects so well the abundance of qi and blood of the Yang Ming channel as the zheng qi robustly contends against the pathogen. To correctly identify the pulse as a Yang Ming pulse, it must be not only big, but also forceful and must be distinguished from a big forceless and hollow pulse which can indicate deficiency detriment disorder, as discussed in *Jin Gui Yao Lue* in Chapter 8 on blood impediment and taxation fatigue.

Pathogenesis of Yang Ming Disease

The three Yang Ming patterns of Tai Yang Yang Ming, Zheng Yang Yang Ming and Shao Yang Yang Ming are each differentiated on the basis of aetiology and pathogenesis: Tai Yang Yang Ming refers to Yang Ming disease originating in the Tai Yang; Zheng Yang Yang Ming, refers to a direct attack on Yang Ming; and Shao Yang Yang Ming is where the pathogen has passed into the Yang Ming from the Shao Yang channel.

Clause 179

问曰：病有太阳阳明，有正阳阳明，有少阳阳明，何谓也？答曰：太阳阳明者，脾约是也；正阳阳明者，胃家实是也；少阳阳明者，发汗、利小便已，胃中燥、烦、实、大便难也。

Question: There are the diseases of Tai Yang Yang Ming, Zheng Yang Yang Ming and Shao Yang Yang Ming, what is meant by this? Answer: Tai Yang Yang Ming, is spleen restraint; Zheng Yang Yang Ming is excess in the domain of the stomach; Shao Yang Yang Ming is where, after the promotion of sweat and urination, there is dryness in the stomach, vexation, excess and difficult defaecation.

DISCUSSION: Yang Ming disease is attributed to three causes: (1) The use of incorrect treatment strategies in Tai Yang disease, specifically, excessive sweating, emesis or purging. Fluids are damaged causing dryness and the resulting pattern is known as pi yue or spleen restraint, which is characterised by a dry stool and frequent urination and is attributed to stomach heat inhibiting the spleen's transportation of water. Because the route of transmission is from Tai Yang, it is known as Tai Yang Yang Ming. (2) An exterior pathogen has attacked Yang Ming directly or, alternatively, undigested food has transformed into heat and dryness, obstructing the qi of the large intestine and causing constipation. This is known as Zheng Yang Yang Ming, where 'zheng yang' means 'direct yang', referring to the fact that the pathogen does not come by way of another channel and is associated with the yang properties of heat and dryness. (3) Incorrect treatment in Shao Yang disease by promoting sweat or urination, or by the use of purgatives, leads to fluid damage and constipation. This is known as Shao Yang Yang Ming. The common feature of all these patterns of Yang Ming bowel excess is dryness and heat, which either results from fluid damage caused by incorrect treatment, or from fluid depletion caused by impaired function of the zang and the fu not producing sufficient yin fluids and giving rise to hyperactive yang.

Clause 181

问曰：何缘得阳明病？答曰：太阳病，若发汗、若下、若利小便，此亡津液，胃中干燥，因转属阳明。不更衣，内实大便难者，此名阳明也。

Question: What is the cause of Yang Ming disease? Answer: Tai Yang disease, if there is sweat promotion, if there is purgation, if there is promotion of urination, this devastates fluids, there is dryness in the stomach, and so it transmits to the Yang Ming. If there is no change of clothes, internal excess with a difficult bowel movement, this is Yang Ming.

DISCUSSION: Although sweat promotion is the indicated treatment for Tai Yang disease, any inappropriate or incorrect treatment such as excessive sweating, purgation or the promotion of urination, will not only fail to resolve the disease but, because such treatment causes fluid loss, will result in dryness and heat in the stomach. The reference to a 'change of clothes' is an oblique reference to passing a stool: according to ancient custom, a change of clothes was made after going to the toilet and 'change of clothes' is a euphemistic expression equivalent to the English 'going to the bathroom'. The statement 'no change of clothes' therefore implies constipation and relates directly to the symptom description of 'interior excess with a difficult bowel movement', which are symptoms characteristic of Yang Ming interior excess. From this, it can be inferred that the disease has progressed in severity.

Preservation of stomach qi and body fluids is an important treatment principle in *Shang Han Lun* and is yet another of Zhang Zhong Jing's major contributions to Chinese medicine. The above clause issues the warning that when treating disease which is in the superficial muscle layer, caution must be exercised so as not to cause an excessive loss of fluids through diaphoresis, diuresis or purgation. This is particularly relevant for a patient with a pre-existing yin deficiency.

Clause 185

本太阳初得病时，发其汗，汗先出不彻，因转属阳明也。伤寒发热、无汗、呕不能食，而反汗出濈濈然者，是转属阳明也。

Originally, when Tai Yang first contracted disease, sweating was promoted, sweating at first was incomplete, so it transmitted to Yang Ming. If there is fever in shang han, no sweating, vomiting and an inability to eat, *nonetheless sweat is streaming forth, it has transmitted to Yang Ming.*

DISCUSSION: Clause 185 explains two causes of transmission to Yang Ming: (1) Inadequate promotion of sweat in Tai Yang disease, where the unresolved exterior pathogen falls into the Yang Ming. (2) Failure to treat Tai Yang shang han, or cold injury, where there is fever and an absence of sweat. The unresolved pathogen constrains yang and transforms into heat, causing stomach disharmony characterised by vomiting and an inability to eat. If these symptoms are accompanied by a streaming sweat, describing sweat which flows continuously, then it is a sign of Yang Ming disease.

It must be remembered that diaphoretic treatment is indicated in Tai Yang disease but must be appropriate to the situation because too much will result in fluid damage and too little will fail to resolve the exterior pathogen. Factors to take into consideration are the patient's constitution, the season and the region. Formulas to choose from are Gui Zhi Tang, Ma Huang Tang, Da Qing Long Tang, Xiao Qing Long Tang, Sang Ju Yin and Yin Qiao San. Although there are various aetiologies of Yang Ming, it is principally caused by treatment which is essentially incorrect or is inappropriate for the individual constitution of the patient.

Clause 188

伤寒转系阳明者，其人濈然微汗出也。

If shang han has transferred to Yang Ming, the person will have a slight streaming sweat.

DISCUSSION: The expression in Clause 188, 'zhuan xi yang ming' (转系阳明) translated as 'transfers to Yang Ming', differs significantly in its implication from the expression 'zhuan shu yang ming' (转属阳明) seen earlier in Clauses 181 and 185 and translated as 'transmitted'. The term 'zhuan shu', means 'moves and belongs to' and implies that complete transmission has taken place: the pathogen is now entrenched in the Yang Ming channel. The term 'zhuan xi', seen in Clause 188, means something more like 'moves and attaches to', implying that there has been some transfer, but not complete transmission. It can be applied to a lagover pattern or bing bing, where the pathogen remains in the Tai Yang whilst simultaneously moving into the Yang Ming.

A shang han or cold injury pattern is characterised by an absence of sweat; a Yang Ming pattern is marked by profuse sweat. The sweating mentioned in this clause is therefore a sign that the disease has moved to the Yang Ming. It is useful to read Clauses 185 and 188 together because then the relevance of sweating is brought into focus. Firstly, the presence of sweating is an indicator of the pathogen having transferred to the Yang Ming; secondly, the reference to a slight streaming sweat emphasises the fact that it is not the volume of sweat which is the issue of correct diagnosis. The slight streaming sweat described in Clause 188 can be interpreted as the early stage of an attack on Yang Ming, with a heavier sweat reflecting more exuberant Yang Ming heat. However, diagnosis can not be made on the basis of sweating alone and can only be confirmed in the presence of other Yang Ming symptoms, namely aversion to heat, thirst and a flooding pulse.

Clause 183

问曰：病有得之一日，不发热而恶寒者，何也？答曰：虽得之一日，恶寒将自罢，即汗出而恶热也。

Question: The disease has lasted for one day, if there is no fever but there is aversion to cold, why is this? Answer: Although it has lasted one day, the aversion to cold will cease spontaneously, then there will be sweating and aversion to heat.

DISCUSSION: Clause 182 describes Yang Ming disease as being characterised by aversion to heat with no aversion to cold, so when Clause 183 describes a disease where there is aversion to cold with no fever, it is alluding to pathogenic constraint at the channel level. Because yang qi is constrained and fails to disperse, there are no prominent heat signs and there is aversion to cold, identifying a Yang Ming channel disorder, as opposed to a bowel pattern. However, Yang Ming disease has a tendency for rapid transmission to the interior, hence the warning: "Although the disease has lasted only one day, the aversion to cold will cease spontaneously, and then there will be sweating and aversion to heat". The aversion to cold is thus shown to be self-limiting because of its imminent transformation into an interior heat pattern, with such symptoms as sweating and aversion to heat. This is a description of the external pattern transferring to the Yang Ming.

Aversion to cold is a symptom found in both Tai Yang and Yang Ming channel patterns. In Tai Yang disease, aversion to cold is more pronounced, more prolonged, and is generally accompanied by a stiff neck and headache. As an exterior disorder, the pathogen in Tai Yang is resolved by the promotion of sweat. In a Yang Ming channel disorder, on the other hand, the aversion to cold is a much less pronounced feature – it is mild and fleeting, and can rapidly transform to heat and be replaced by fever with a flushed face and dry nostrils. *Shang Han Lun* makes no recommendation as to a formula appropriate for a Yang Ming channel disorder, however, Ge Gen Tang is suggested in *Yi Zong Jin Jian*, and *Shang Han Da Bai* also suggests that Ge Gen Tang is suitable providing there is no sweating. If sweating is present, Fang Feng Ge Gen Tang or Sheng Ma Ge Gen Tang should be used.

Clause 184

问曰：恶寒　何故自罢？答曰：阳明居中，主土也。万物所归，无所复传，始虽恶寒，二日自上，此为阳明病也。

Question: Why does aversion to cold cease spontaneously? Answer: Yang Ming resides in the middle, it governs earth. A myriad things converge, without passing further, although it starts with aversion to cold, in two days it finishes spontaneously, this is Yang Ming disease.

DISCUSSION: In Clause 184, Zhang Zhong Jing points to the correspondence between five phase theory and the physiology and pathology of the Yang Ming channel. Yang Ming is located in the middle, comprising the stomach, which has an exterior–interior relationship with the spleen. According to early five phase theory, all qi returned to the middle earth before proceeding to the next phase. Furthermore, the stomach receives and ripens water and grain, distributes the refined essences and eliminates the waste. Like the earth to which it belongs, it is seen as the mother of all beings in the universe, and so, on both the physiological plane as an organ, and the metaphysical plane as the earth, it can be seen that all things come to converge in the stomach. If dryness and heat knot together and accumulate in the stomach and intestines, purgation is the most effective method of eliminating the pathogen. The statement, 'a myriad of things converge without passing further' refers to the accumulation of the dry stool. A further connotation of Yang Ming residing in the middle is the role that Yang Ming plays as the source of engendering qi and blood. Because of this, in the eventuality of external invasion or internal injury, the preservation of stomach qi is an essential strategy in *Shang Han Lun* in the prevention and treatment of disease, as follows.

1. Where there is deficiency of the middle jiao with subsequent insufficiency of ying and wei, regardless of whether the disease is at Tai Yang, Yang Ming or Tai Yin, Gui Zhi Tang can be used.
2. In Yang Ming, there can be a pathogenic attack on Yang Ming where formless heat knots with stagnant food and obstructs the large intestine; there is abdominal distension and constipation; or toxic heat scorching fluids and harassing the heart shen. Irrespective of whether the disease is at Yang Ming, Shao Yin or Jue Yin, Bai Hu Tang can be used to clear heat and Cheng Qi Tang can be used for urgent purgation in order to preserve fluids.
3. Deficiency and cold in the spleen and stomach characterised by abdominal pain, diarrhoea and vomiting is treated with Wu Zhu Yu Tang. Where the deficiency is more severe, Li Zhong Wan should be used.
4. For heat and cold complex where there is spleen deficiency and stomach heat, Ren

Shen, Ban Xia, Hong Zao, Sheng Jiang and Gan Cao or the Xie Xin Tang group with the addition of Huang Qin and Huang Lian are suitable.

5. In the aftermath of febrile disease where stomach yin is injured and residual heat not completely resolved, Ren Shen, Mai Dong and Shi Gao should be used in such a formula as Zhu Ye Shi Gao Tang. In regard to the problem of the accumulation in the bowel and its failure to 'pass further', a flexible approach is recommended: if there is excess due to dryness in the large intestine, the correct strategy is to drain heat by purging, thus providing an exit for the pathogen. The guiding formula is Cheng Qi Tang; however, if the dry heat has affected the Shao Yin and Jue Yin, the manifestation of which is delirious speech and clouded spirit, Niu Huang Cheng Qi Tang or Xuan Bai Cheng Qi Tang can be used.

Summary of the Principal Features of Yang Ming Disease

There are three points to remember in understanding the aetiology of Yang Ming disease.

1. *Direct attack by an external pathogen, which enters the Yang Ming and transforms into heat.* This is particularly associated with a pre-existing condition of hyperactive yang, poor digestion with food stagnation or latent heat, any of which can combine with the external pathogen when it enters the interior.
2. *Transmission to Yang Ming from another channel.* This is closely associated with incorrect treatment of Tai Yang disease, where the pathogen is subsequently transmitted to Yang Ming; however, even in the absence of incorrect treatment, it is possible for transmission to occur and manifest as Yang Ming disease.
3. *Constitutional factors.* This was not discussed in *Shang Han Lun* but from the perspective of Yang Ming disease aetiology and the transmission pathway, the constitution plays a significant role. A constitution which tends to be yang, as mentioned in the first point above, will be more prone to attack from a yang pathogen, and one which tends to food stagnation, whether due to spleen deficiency or to latent heat, will succumb more easily to the consequences of an external pathogen falling inwards and causing knotted bind. This is especially true where there are formed accumulations such as latent heat, phlegm or food stagnation, which then knot with the pathogen, exacerbating excess in the form of distension and obstruction.

There are four factors relevant to the pathomechanism in Yang Ming disease.

1. The Yang Ming channel is located in the middle and is the source of engendering qi and blood. Because it is rich in qi and blood, it tends towards excess. Because there is a strong connection between the interior and exterior, Yang Ming disease originating in the exterior can be easily transmitted to the interior and, conversely, disease originating in the yin channels in the interior, can easily make its way to the Yang Ming as part of the recovery process.
2. Yang Ming governs dryness, which refers to the tendency for the heat of Yang Ming disease to consume fluids, transforming into dryness, which further generates heat. This is the basis for the principal features of Yang Ming disease being associated with heat and excess.
3. Irrespective of the origin of Yang Ming disease, whether it is due to a direct attack from the exterior or due to incorrect treatment, the fundamental pathogenesis of Yang Ming disease is fluid damage and subsequent generation of dryness.
4. The location of Yang Ming disease is the stomach and large intestine. References to 'stomach excess' in *Shang Han Lun* are intended to refer to both the stomach and large intestine.

Key Points in the Diagnosis of Yang Ming Disease

1. *Differentiation of heat and cold.* The early stage of Yang Ming disease is sometimes characterised by slight aversion to cold but it is mild and fleeting. Therefore, Yang Ming disease is identified on the basis of aversion to heat with no aversion to cold.
2. *Differentiation of sweat.* The special characteristic of Yang Ming sweat is that it is a continuous stream of light sweat

occurring when fever has not been resolved. It does not represent an exterior pattern and further sweating must not be promoted. This differentiates Yang Ming sweating from Tai Yang sweating, which is sweating accompanied by an aversion to wind cold, and which is resolved by diaphoresis.

3. *Differentiation of constipation.* Constipation must be diagnosed as to whether it is the difficult defaecation associated with pi yue or spleen restraint, or if it is the dry stool associated with a fu excess pattern, which is accompanied by tidal fever, delirious speech and abdominal distension.
4. *Differentiation of the pulse sign.* The characteristic pulse of Yang Ming disease is flooding, big and forceful; the pulse of a fu excess pattern is submerged and forceful.

Section Three

3.3 YANG MING CHANNEL PATTERNS

Yang Ming channel patterns are defined as an attack by an exterior pathogen on the channel, affecting it at the superficial level. Although the principal Yang Ming patterns are broadly categorised as stomach excess, they must be differentiated according to the eight principles. Diagnosis and treatment of Yang Ming channel patterns are based on the signs and symptoms. If there is a slow, moderate pulse and continuous sweating with a slight aversion to cold, then the exterior is not yet resolved, and because of the exterior deficiency demonstrated by the sweating, Gui Zhi Tang is appropriate. However, if the pulse is floating and there is no sweating, then it is an exterior excess pattern and Ma Huang Tang is the appropriate formula to resolve the exterior by promoting sweat. Yang Ming fu patterns are dealt with in Section Four of this chapter.

Clause 231

阳明中风，脉弦浮大，而短气、腹都满，胁下及心痛，久按之气不通，鼻干，不得汗，嗜卧，一身及目悉黄，小便难，有潮热，时时哕，耳前后肿，刺之小差，外不解。病过十日，脉续浮者，与小柴胡汤。

Yang Ming zhong feng, the pulse is wiry, floating and big, and there is shortness of breath, distension throughout the abdomen, pain under the ribs and in the heart, a sense of qi blockage under prolonged pressure, a dry nose, an absence of sweat, a desire to lie down, the body and eyes are all yellow, urination is difficult, there is tidal fever, constant hiccoughing, swelling in front of and behind the ear, needling gives some relief, the exterior is not resolved. The disease has lasted over ten days, if the pulse is still floating, give Xiao Chai Hu Tang.

DISCUSSION: Clause 231 describes a combined pattern of Yang Ming and Shao Yang manifesting as damp heat jaundice. Yang Ming zhong feng or Yang Ming wind strike refers to a direct attack of pathogenic wind on the Yang Ming channel; a pulse which is wiry, floating and big shows that both the Yang Ming and Shao Yang channels are affected; shortness of breath and abdominal fullness are manifestations of constrained heat in the fu of Yang Ming, whilst pain under the ribs and in the heart is a reflection of the involvement of Shao Yang. This is because the Shao Yang channel passes through the side of the chest and the pathogen has impeded the qi dynamic of Shao Yang. Subsequently, there is pain and the stagnant qi is identified as pain elicited by pressure.

The foot Yang Ming stomach channel emerges below the eye, descends the cheek, enters the upper gums, and curves around the mouth before running along the lower jaw and ascending in front of the ear. A divergent channel ascends either side of the nose, and the hand Yang Ming large intestine channel leads to the side of the nostrils, with a connecting channel running to the ear where it joins the stomach and gallbladder channels. The foot Shao Yang gallbladder channel arises at the outer corner of the eye, ascends to the corner of the forehead, then curves down behind the ear. Therefore, pathogenic heat in the Yang Ming and Shao Yang channels can affect the nose causing dryness, and can lodge in the channels that circle the ear causing swelling both in front of and behind the ear. If the heat pathogen is unable to exit from the Yang Ming and Shao Yang, it will obstruct the passages of the triple jiao and, combining with damp, give rise to damp heat constraint. This stagnation of heat and damp can result in a desire to sleep, a jaundiced appearance and tidal fever. The constant hiccoughing is a manifestation of constrained heat in the Yang Ming obstructing the descent of stomach qi.

This is a dual pattern of Yang Ming and Shao Yang where the promotion of sweat and purgation are both contraindicated, and so the recommended strategy is to first use acupuncture to dissipate the constrained heat. Although the acupuncture gives some relief, it has not completely resolved the exterior pathogen and so, even after ten days, the pulse is still floating. This complex exterior and interior pattern must be treated by a harmonising formula, namely Xiao Chai Hu Tang.

Although Clause 231 describes many Yang Ming signs, Xiao Chai Hu Tang, a Shao Yang formula, is used because, by normalising the pivot mechanism of Shao Yang, the interior and exterior are harmonised. It also clears heat from both the exterior and interior and expels the pathogen that is lodged halfway between the exterior and the interior. In addition, it disperses the constrained qi of the liver and gallbladder and resolves the damp heat jaundice, thus addressing the cause of the other manifestations. This is largely achieved by the actions of the two chief herbs: Chai Hu, which releases exterior heat, moves liver qi, raises spleen yang and resolves Shao Yang; and Huang Qin, which clears heat from the gallbladder, dries damp and treats jaundice. Where there are additional symptoms such as headache, dry nose or sore throat, associated with a floating, wiry, rapid pulse and an exterior wind heat pattern, Xiao Chai Hu Tang can be used with the omission of Ren Shen, Gan Cao and Da Zao and the addition of such herbs as Bo He, Jin Yin Hua, Lian Qiao for a sore throat, and in case of headache, Bo He, Chuan Xiong and Man Jing Zi.

The pattern described in Clause 231 is reminiscent of the contemporary diagnosis of parotitis or mumps, characterised by pain and swelling of the parotid glands, which are situated just in front of and below the ear. This clause mentions acupuncture without specifying points to use in treatment. Appropriate local points are: Yi Feng (San Jiao 17), Si Zhu Kong (San Jiao 23), Ting Hui (Gallbladder 2), Ting Gong (Small Intestine 19), Jia Che (Stomach 6); these can be combined with Zhi Gou (San Jiao 6) to clear obstructions from the San Jiao channel, Qu Chi (Large Intestine 11), Shang Yang (Large Intestine 1) and Shao Shang (Lung 11) to clear heat, and Feng Chi (Gall Bladder 20) to expel wind heat and free obstructions form the gallbladder channel. The guiding herbal formula is Li Dong Yuan's Pu Ji Xiao Du Yin, which relieves toxic heat. The ingredients are: Huang Qin, Huang Lian 15g each; Chen Pi, Gan Cao, Xuan Shen 10g each; Lian Qiao, Ban Lan Gen, Ma Bo, Niu Bang Zi 3g each; Bo He, Jiang Chen, Sheng Ma 3g each; Chai Hu, Jie Geng 6g each. The decoction is prepared by first grinding the herbs, then boiling 15g which is strained and taken as a single dose. For residual symptoms of a Tai Yang exterior pattern, indicating the involvement of all three yang channels, add Jing Jie and Fang Feng. For constipation, add Da Huang.

Clause 232

脉但浮，无余证者，与麻黄汤。若不尿，腹满加哕者，不治。

If there is only a floating pulse, no other sign, give Ma Huang Tang. If there is no urination, and abdominal distension with hiccoughing, it is not treatable.

DISCUSSION: By reading Clauses 231 and 232 in sequence, it can be seen that the reference to the pulse only being floating, emphasises the fact that it is neither wiry nor big; the reference to there being no other sign means there is no concurrent interior pattern. This therefore is an unresolved Tai Yang exterior pattern and so Ma Huang Tang is suitable. However, Clause 232 goes on to elaborate that where there are other symptoms such as urinary difficulty, abdominal distension or hiccough, it is not a simple exterior pattern and can not be treated.

Abdominal distension is a sign of qi stagnation in the stomach and large intestine. The descent of qi is obstructed and can result in hiccoughing. The implication of the inhibited urination is that the pathogen, which is constrained in the upper jiao, is unable to exit via urination and the disease is therefore not treatable. This fits into a pattern of *guan ge* (关格), which manifests with vomiting and obstructed urination, indicating failure of qi to descend. This condition is attributed to a dual deficiency of yin and yang, where the disruption to the qi dynamic affects the ascent and descent of qi and results in non-communication between the upper and lower. It is described in the *Nan Jing* as untreatable.

Clause 234

阳明病，脉迟，汗出多，微恶寒者，表未解也，可发汗，宜桂枝汤。

Yang Ming disease, the pulse is slow, there is copious sweating, if there is a mild aversion to cold, the exterior is not resolved, one may promote sweating, Gui Zhi Tang is appropriate.

DISCUSSION: Tai Yang zhong feng or wind strike is characterised by a moderate pulse, sweating and aversion to wind. In contrast to this, Clause 234 describes a Yang Ming disease where there is a slow pulse, copious sweating and a slight aversion to cold. It is not a typical Yang Ming pattern: the slight aversion to cold represents an attack on the Yang Ming channel by pathogenic wind. The copious sweating of Yang Ming disease shows it to be more deeply seated than a Tai Yang zhong feng pattern, where there is only slight sweating, and this is the key point of differentiation. The slight aversion to cold which is common to both patterns is a reflection of their common aetiology, and so Gui Zhi Tang is indicated for both to promote sweating and harmonise ying and wei.

Clause 235

阳明病、脉浮、无汗而喘者，发汗则愈，宜麻黄汤。

Yang Ming disease, the pulse is floating, if there is no sweating but there is wheezing, the promotion of sweating will bring recovery, Ma Huang Tang is appropriate.

DISCUSSION: The floating pulse of Yang Ming disease described in Clause 235 is a sign of an exterior cold invasion of the Yang Ming; the absence of sweat indicates exterior constraint. The exterior attack is explained by the fact that the Yang Ming large intestine channel has an exterior–interior relationship with the lung channel and is therefore linked by the network vessels. Because of this connection, an attack of exterior pathogenic cold on the Yang Ming channel causes constraint in the lung channel which manifests as wheezing. The floating pulse and absence of sweat confirm it as an exterior excess pattern and so Ma Huang Tang is the indicated formula to promote sweating and release the exterior.

Clauses 234 and 235 both describe Yang Ming channel patterns. The first describes exterior deficiency and advocates Gui Zhi Tang; the second describes exterior excess and advocates Ma Huang Tang. Some annotators suggest that these two clauses are actually describing a combined pattern of Tai Yang and Yang Ming with an unresolved exterior.

3.3.1 Yang Ming Heat Patterns

Yang Ming heat patterns fall into the category of excess heat in the qi aspect. They are characterised by exuberant heat and include patterns represented by the formulas Zhi Zi Chi Tang, Bai Hu Tang and Bai Hu jia Ren Shen Tang, where the treatment strategy is to clear heat from the qi aspect and conserve and nourish fluids. The copious sweating of Yang Ming heat patterns injures fluids. If the disease persists, the Yang Ming heat can knot with water in the lower jiao, which is a transmuted pattern characterised by vexation, thirst, insomnia and inhibited urination. The appropriate formula is Zhu Ling Tang, which clears heat, nourishes yin and disinhibits urination.

Zhi Zi Chi Tang Pattern

Clause 221

（一）阳明病，脉浮而紧、咽燥、口苦、腹满而喘、发热汗出、不恶寒反恶热、身重。（二）若发汗则躁，心愦愦，反谵语；若加温针，必怵惕烦躁不得眠；若下之，则胃中空虚，客气动膈，心中懊憹。舌上胎者，栀子豉汤主之。

(1) Yang Ming disease, the pulse is floating and tight, the throat is dry, there is a bitter taste in the mouth, abdominal fullness and wheezing, fever and sweating, no aversion to cold but an aversion to heat, the body feels heavy. (2) If sweating is promoted, there will be agitation, an unsettled heart with delirious speech; if warm needling is added, there will be apprehension, agitation and inability to sleep; if there is purgation, then the stomach will feel empty and hollow, visitant qi will stir the diaphragm, there will be anguish in the heart. If there is a coat on the tongue, Zhi Zi Chi Tang governs.

DISCUSSION: (1) The first part of Clause 221 draws attention to a pulse which is floating and tight but which, whilst being reminiscent of a Tai Yang pulse, is in fact a Yang Ming pulse. This is because the floating tight pulse is accompanied by symptoms indicative of interior heat, such as a dry throat, a bitter taste, and fever and sweating with an aversion to heat, not cold as in a Tai Yang pattern, and is also accompanied by abdominal distension, which is a key manifestation of a Yang Ming pattern. The floating pulse is a reflection not of an exterior pattern, but of the exuberant heat in the Yang Ming channel; the tightness of the pulse is associated with the Yang Ming bowel excess pattern and the subsequent distension and discomfort. The combination of those two qualities therefore indicates heat in the Yang Ming channel, expressed as bowel excess. The bitter taste is a sign of fire and because the exuberant heat has damaged fluids, the throat is dry. The heat obstructs the normal flow of qi in the interior, causing abdominal fullness and wheezing. The fever is a further sign of interior heat and the profuse sweating is a result of that interior heat steaming body fluids and causing them to percolate through the exterior. Heat also obstructs the flow of channel qi, producing a sensation of heaviness. The treatment strategy responding to these symptoms is to use acrid, cold herbs to clear heat and Bai Hu Tang is the appropriate formula. Diaphoretic and purging therapies are contraindicated.

(2) The second part of Clause 221 describes transmutation resulting from inappropriate sweat promotion in a pattern of heat harassing the diaphragm. It is only one of numerous possible transmutations caused by incorrect treatment where the inappropriate use of acrid warm herbs to promote sweating has damaged fluids and consequently exacerbated heat, which then harasses the heart shen causing vexation, restlessness and delirious speech. If warm needling is used in addition to that, not only does it induce further inappropriate sweating, but it also introduces more heat into the body; this further fuels the fire and produces the aggravated symptoms of apprehension and anxiety, nervousness and insomnia. Abdominal fullness must be distinguished from bowel excess, and if the patient had previously exhibited abdominal fullness which was mistaken for bowel excess and was wrongly treated by purgation, then there will be emptiness in the stomach and pathogenic heat will exploit the deficiency. In this clause, the inward-falling heat has been constrained in the diaphragm causing anxiety and restlessness. The clause goes on to specify that if there is a tongue coat, then Zhi Zi Chi Tang is the correct formula. From this it can be inferred that if there is no tongue coat, indicating serious fluid damage, then Zhi Zi Chi Tang should not be used. Where there is indeed a tongue coat, it will be either yellow or yellow and white, and Zhi Zi Chi Tang is indicated to vent the constrained heat from the chest.

Clause 221 describes two different outcomes of incorrect treatment: a) the incorrect treatment of a Tai Yang exterior pattern causing heat to harass the diaphragm and b) the incorrect treatment of a Yang Ming channel pattern where adverse purgation results in emptiness of the stomach and heat harassing the chest. Although these two situations differ in aetiology, the pathogenesis and symptoms are identical and so the same formula is indicated for each.

Clause 228

阳明病下之，其外有热，手足温，不结胸，心中懊侬，饥不能食，但头汗出者，栀子豉汤主之。

Yang Ming disease treated with purgation, there is heat in the exterior, the hands and feet are warm, there is no chest bind, if there is anguish, hunger with no desire to eat, sweating from the head only, Zhi Zi Chi Tang governs.

DISCUSSION: By Yang Ming disease, Clause 228 is referring to a Yang Ming channel heat pattern. Treatment therefore should be aimed at dispersing and venting the constrained heat. If purgation is used, the pathogenic heat tends to fall inward, knot with phlegm and water in the interior, and subsequently manifest as chest bind. Since it is stated that there is no chest bind, it can be surmised that there is no phlegm or water in the interior. In this case, the incorrect purgation and subsequent falling inward of the heat pathogen has resulted not in chest bind but in constrained heat in the chest and diaphragm. The unresolved exterior manifests in the warm extremities, which are a sign of constrained exterior heat. The interior heat disturbs the shen causing anguish; the constrained heat in the diaphragm affects the stomach qi, resulting in hunger with no appetite; it also obstructs the qi dynamic, preventing the normal diffusion of heat so that the body is unable to sweat, and sweat breaks out from the head only. The indicated treatment is Zhi Zi Chi Tang to disperse heat and vent it outward.

There are two possible aetiologies of a Zhi Zi Chi Tang pattern. (1) The treatment of a Yang Ming bowel excess pattern by purgation where heat is not fully resolved and there is residual heat in the chest and diaphragm. (2) The treatment of a Yang Ming channel pattern by purgation, where the heat pathogen falls inwards resulting in constrained heat in the chest and diaphragm.

Bai Hu Tang Pattern

Clause 176

伤寒脉浮滑，此以表有热，里有寒，白虎汤主之。

Shang han, the pulse is floating and slippery, this is heat in the exterior and cold in the interior, and Bai Hu Tang governs.

BAI HU TANG: Zhi Mu 6 liang; Shi Gao (broken) 1 jin; Zhi Gan Cao 2 liang; Jing Mi (non-glutinous rice) 6 ge.

DIRECTIONS: Boil all ingredients in 1 dou of water. When the rice is cooked, the decoction is ready. Strain and take 1 sheng warm three times a day.

DISCUSSION: The annotations of past *Shang Han* specialists provide clarification of the expression 'cold in the interior'. *Yi Zong Jin Jian* explained that the expression 'cold' simply referred to any pathogen; Fang You Zhi explained that in fact it referred to interior heat; Cheng Jiao Qian suggested it should be read as "cold in the exterior and heat in the interior". However, based on the guiding formula Bai Hu Tang, the ingredients of which jointly target both exterior and interior heat, it is clear that the interpretation of interior heat is correct.

The floating slippery pulse is a reflection of exuberant heat in both the exterior and interior: the floating quality is an indication that qi and blood have surged to the surface as a result of exuberant yang qi; a slippery pulse is classed as a yang pulse and here reflects the exuberant interior heat.

The key diagnostic signs of a Bai Hu Tang pattern are fever, sweating, an aversion to heat rather than to cold, a dry tongue coat, vexation and an insatiable thirst. Bai Hu Tang drains heat, alleviates vexation and generates fluids to quench the thirst. Shi Gao is acrid, sweet and cold and so clears lung and stomach heat in the qi level. Zhi Mu is bitter and cold and not only clears heat but also nourishes yin. Zhi Gan Cao and Jing Mi benefit the stomach qi and protect it against the cold herbs.

In *Shang Han Lun* and *Jin Gui Yao Lue* there are 16 formulas using Shi Gao. Their application is as follows. (1) Externally contracted pathogenic wind cold with constrained interior heat, where Shi Gao is combined with Ma Huang and Gui Zhi to disperse pathogenic wind cold. (2) Heat and cold complex, where Shi Gao is combined with Sheng Jiang and Fu Zi as in Yue Bi jia Zhu Tang (1 piece of Fu Zi is added only if there is aversion to wind). (3) The later stage of febrile disease with unresolved residual heat, where Shi Gao is combined with Zhu Ye as in Zhu Ye Shi Gao Tang. In the early republican era, a practitioner known as Zhang Xi Chun prescribed Shi Gao in large doses of up to 80–100g. However, it must be remembered that Shi Gao is a very cold herb and has the potential to damage spleen qi. A large dose should therefore be prescribed with caution, and smaller doses are advised in patients where there is deficiency cold of the spleen and stomach.

The four key symptoms needed to prescribe Bai Hu Tang are a high fever, copious sweating, severe thirst and a big, flooding pulse, often referred to as the 'four bigs'. Of these, it is generally accepted that copious sweating is the primary indicator for Bai Hu Tang, confirmed by the other three, and the tongue coat should be yellow and dry.

Clause 219

三阳合病，腹满、身重，难以转侧，口不仁、面垢、澹语、谵尿。发汗，则谵语；下之则额上生汗、手足逆冷。若自汗出者，白虎汤主之。

Concurrent disease of the three yang, there is abdominal fullness, a sensation of heaviness, difficulty in turning over, the mouth is numb, the face grimy and there is delirious speech and enuresis. If sweat is promoted, there will be delirious speech; if purgation is used, sweat will appear on the forehead, and the hands and feet will be cold. If there is spontaneous sweating, Bai Hu Tang governs.

DISCUSSION: Clause 219 describes concurrent disease of the three yang in terms of the main manifestations of a Yang Ming heat pattern. The obstruction of stomach qi results in abdominal fullness; vigorous heat in the Yang Ming exhausts qi and consumes body fluids, which in turn causes a sensation of heaviness and an inability to turn over in bed; heat in the stomach causes stomach disharmony manifesting as numbness or lack of sensitivity of the mouth, which results in impaired taste and also impaired speech. Because the Yang Ming channels transverse the face, so heat steaming qi and blood in the channels of Yang Ming gives the face a grimy appearance, as if smeared with a layer of dirt mixed with sweat. When heat harasses the heart shen, it causes delirious speech and when it harasses the urinary bladder, it causes enuresis.

This pattern is characterised by Yang Ming heat in the stomach which as yet has not affected the large intestine. Bai Hu Tang is needed to clear Yang Ming heat. If, based on the abdominal fullness and delirious speech, purgation is carried out erroneously, fluids in the lower jiao will be further depleted and, because yang is not anchored, sweat will appear on the forehead. Finally, the exhaustion of yin and the upcasting of yang results in yang not warming the extremities, so the hands and feet are cold. This is why sweating and purgation are contraindicated in a Yang Ming heat pattern.

The use of Bai Hu Tang in the treatment of concurrent disease of the three yang is significant, because in the clinical situation the focus is frequently on the Yang Ming. If acrid warm herbs are used to promote sweating, this will fuel the Yang Ming heat and the use of Chai Hu to harmonise the Shao Yang does not clear heat from the Yang Ming. For this reason, Zhang Zhong Jing advocated the use of Bai Hu Tang, where Shi Gao, which is acrid, sweet and cold, is effective in clearing the interior Yang Ming heat.

Clause 99 in Chapter 4 Shao Yang Disease also describes concurrent disease of the three yang, but the manifestations are quite different from those described in Clause 219, where there is abdominal fullness, heaviness and delirious speech. In Clause 99 there is fever, aversion to wind, stiffness of the neck, distension under the ribs, warm limbs and thirst. The treatment is therefore focused on Shao Yang, and Xiao Chai Hu Tang is the indicated formula.

From the foregoing, it is clear that identification of the salient features of concurrent disease is essential in order to know which of the three yang predominates, so as to choose appropriate treatment. The relative severity of exterior and interior disease must also be determined. The sensation of heaviness referred to in Clause 219 could lead to a diagnosis of Tai Yang exterior constraint, but there is no aversion to wind and no stiffness of the neck. Since exterior symptoms are negligible, the principal feature is interior heat and Bai Hu Tang is appropriate. As a general rule, the key point of diagnosis for concurrent disease of the three yang where the Tai Yang channel predominates is aversion to cold; the key symptom for concurrent disease where the Shao Yang channel predominates is vomiting; and where Yang Ming predominates, the key symptom is copious sweating.

ZHONG JING'S APPLICATIONS OF BAI HU TANG: Zhang Zhong Jing stipulated three main applications of Bai Hu Tang. The first is addressed in Clause 176, on page 199, where he says: "Shang han, the pulse is floating and slippery, this is heat in the exterior and cold in the interior, and Bai Hu Tang governs". The second application is found in Clause 219 (opposite), where he discusses concurrent patterns of the three yang channels and states that if there is spontaneous sweating, Bai Hu Tang governs. The third application is described in Clause 350 in Chapter 7 Jue Yin Disease, where he says: "Shang han, if the pulse is slippery and there is jue, there is heat in the interior, Bai Hu Tang governs".

Ancient Application of Bai Hu Tang

- *Lei Zheng Huo Ren Shu:* Bai Hu Tang with the addition of Cang Zhu was cited for the treatment of damp warmth characterised by copious sweating and cold extremities.
- *Wen Re Jing Wei:* Bai Hu Tang with the addition of Ling Yang Jiao and Xi Jiao was advocated for the treatment of febrile disease characterised by vigorous fever, clouded spirit and spasm due to the scorching of both qi and blood.
- *Chong Ding Tong Shu Shang Han Lun:* Cong Chi Bai Hu Tang, which is Bai Hu Tang with the addition of Cong Bai, Dou Chi and Xi Xin, was mentioned as a suitable formula in the treatment of febrile disease with interior heat and exterior constrained cold. Also mentioned was Bai Hu Cheng Qi Tang (Bai Hu Tang with the addition of Da Huang and Mang Xiao) for the treatment of toxic warmth characterised by macules, vexatious heat, delirious speech and insomnia.

Modern Application of Bai Hu Tang

- *Encephalitis B.* Bai Hu Tang with the omission of Jing Mi and the addition of Shan Yao, Jin Yin Hua and Lian Qiao was used in the treatment of encephalitis B. Of the 36 cases treated, 30 recovered and 6 died *(Zhong Yi Za Zhi* 1958). Guo Zi Hua et al also used Bai Hu Tang to treat epidemic encephalitis B (*Shanghai Zhong Yi Yao Za Zhi* 1955; 11:1). Note: Bai Hu Tang can be used to resolve the high fever of encephalitis, which is generally resolved in three days. Encephalitis B bears many similarities to summerheat warm patterns, with the initial stage characterised by qi aspect symptoms such as copious sweating, vigorous fever, thirst, a big flooding pulse and a dry yellow tongue coat. The key symptom of encephalitis B is fever, which can lead to tetany, delirium and *re jue* which describes cold extremities due to extreme heat obstructing the flow of yang qi. The more severe the heat, the more severe the jue, since it is the heat which is the underlying factor. Therefore every effort should be focused on resolving the fever.
- *Common cold.* Bai Hu Tang, with the addition of Jin Yin Hua, Lian Qiao, Sang Ye, Ju Hua, Bo He, Jie Geng, Xing Ren, Jing Jie, Ge Gen, Huang Qin and Zhi Shi, was used in the treatment of 689 cases of the common cold manifesting with fever. Where there was stomach pain with nausea, Jie Geng was omitted and Hou Po, Sha Ren, Chen Pi and Chao Lai Fu Zi added. For insufficiency of qi and body fluids, Huang Qin was replaced by

Tai Zi Shen. Administration was three times per day and for more serious conditions, every two hours. There was full recovery in 683 cases, improvement in four cases and no effect in two cases (*Zhong Yi Yan Jiu* 1995; 1:23, p580).

- Chai Ge Bai Hu Tang (Chai Hu 9g; Zhi Mu 9g; Gan Cao 9g; Ge Gen 30g; Sheng Shi Gao 30g; Yin Hua 15g; Huang Qin 15g; Qin Jiao 12g; Fang Feng 12g) was used in the treatment of 44 cases of externally contracted disease with high fever. Administration was 1 dose per day. Where there was extreme thirst, Tian Hua Fen was added; for cough with sticky phlegm, Quan Gua Lou and Chuan Bei Mu were added; where there was a dry stool and a dry yellow tongue coat, Da Huang was added; where there was an aversion to cold and an absence of sweat, Huang Qin and Zhi Mu were replaced by Ma Huang. The results were: highly effective, 32 cases; effective, 9 cases; and ineffective, 3 cases (*Jiang Xi Zhong Yi Yao* 1990; 3:25 p580).
- *Ear, eye, nose and throat disease.* Xiao et al used a modified version of Bai Hu Tang (Shi Gao, Zhi Mu, Gan Cao, Huang Qin, Lian Qiao, Yin Hua) in the treatment of four cases of sympathetic ophthalmia and four cases of papillitis. After a treatment course of four weeks, there was substantial improvement of vision (*Zhong Yi Nian Jian,* Ren Mi Wei Sheng Publishing, 1983).
- *Diabetes (xiao ke).* Bai Hu Tang with the addition of Sheng Di, Tian Hua Fen, Sha Shen, Zhi Zi, Mai Dong and Niu Xi was used in the treatment of diabetes characterised by insatiable hunger, thirst, a dry stool, a dry yellow tongue coat and a slippery rapid pulse (*Shang Han Lun Yu Lin Chuang*, 1993).

Case Study

Concurrent Disease of the Three Yang

Extracted from Tianjin Yi Yao (Tianjin Medical Journal) 1979; 8:35

The patient presented with a shang han pattern where there was fever, headache, numbness in the mouth, vexation, delirious speech, abdominal fullness and a sensation of heaviness. These symptoms are the result of heat in both the exterior and interior and Da Chai Hu Tang is indicated. It is said that if the pulse is floating or floating and slippery, it indicates a concurrent disease of the three yang. Bai Hu Tang was prescribed to clear lung and stomach heat. After two doses, the symptoms improved. Hua Fen, Mai Dong and Zhu Ye were added to the repeat prescription to nourish fluids

Bai Hu jia Ren Shen Tang Pattern

Clause 170

伤寒脉浮、发热、无汗，其表不解，不可与白虎汤。渴欲饮水，无表证者，白虎人参汤主之。

Shang han with a floating pulse, there is fever with no sweating, the exterior is not resolved, one should not give Bai Hu Tang. If there is thirst with a desire to drink water, no exterior pattern, Bai Hu jia Ren Shen Tang governs.

BAI HU JIA REN SHEN TANG: Zhi Mu 6 liang; Shi Gao (broken) 1 jin; Zhi Gan Cao 2 liang; Ren Shen 2 liang; Jing Mi 6 ge.

DIRECTIONS: Boil all ingredients in 1 dou of water until the rice is cooked. Strain and take 1 sheng warm three times a day.

DISCUSSION: A floating pulse, fever and an absence of sweat are symptoms associated with a Tai Yang exterior excess pattern or shang han, and the indicated formula is Ma Huang Tang to release the exterior and promote sweat. If Bai Hu Tang is used, the cold herbs fail to expel the exterior pathogen, causing it to be locked in, and the result is a transmuted pattern. For this reason, Bai Hu Tang is contraindicated, as the pre-requisite for the application of Bai Hu Tang is interior heat with a fully resolved exterior, and with severe thirst. Where there is damage to qi and body fluids, there is aversion to wind, a slight sensation of cold in the back and an insatiable thirst for drinks, Bai Hu jia Ren Shen Tang is the indicated formula because it clears heat from the Yang Ming, diffuses interior heat, and the additional use of Ren Shen augments qi and generates fluids.

The application of Bai Hu jia Ren Shen Tang is based on the core Bai Hu Tang pattern with additional symptoms of severe thirst, vexation, a parched mouth, a tongue which is red and lacks moisture, and a hollow, flooding pulse. The severe thirst and the changes in the tongue and pulse form the clinical basis for the addition of Ren Shen. Other symptoms of critical importance are shortness of breath, reluctance to speak and fatigue. Ke Yun Bo said: "The addition of Ren Shen is based on the theory that qi is the mother of water." Deficiency of yin and qi allows the pathogen to exploit the emptiness. Ren Shen tonifies the true yin and, with the return of yin qi, fluids will be generated". Zhang Zhong Jing was quite specific in regard to the combination of Ren Shen with other herbs: for deficiency cold, he added Fu Zi and Gan Jiang; for qi and yin deficiency, he added Mai Dong; where heat damaged yin and qi, he added Shi Gao. The preparation of Ren Shen has significance for its actions: Hong Shen (red ginseng) is warm and is better to augment the source qi; Sheng Shai Shen (sun-dried ginseng) is cooler and tonifies both qi and yin. Dang Shen and Tai Zi Shen are now commonly used instead of Sheng Shai Shen.

Clause 26

服桂枝汤，大汗出后，大烦渴不解，脉洪大者，白虎加人参汤主之。

Having taken Gui Zhi Tang, after profuse sweating, there is severe vexation and unresolved thirst, if the pulse is flooding and big, Bai Hu jia Ren Shen Tang governs.

DISCUSSION: A dose of Gui Zhi Tang should be followed by mild, not copious sweating. Clause 26 describes a situation where inappropriate and excessive sweating has been promoted. Irritability, insatiable thirst and a flooding big pulse are all manifestations of Yang Ming exuberant heat in the interior. By this we can see that although the exterior has been released, the excessive sweating has damaged stomach fluids and resulted in a Yang Ming interior heat pattern. The irritability and vexation are the result of heat harassing the heart, whilst the severe thirst is a reflection of the damage to qi and yin caused by fluid loss due to sweating, and to the consumption of fluids by exuberant heat. The big, flooding pulse is further evidence of excess heat in the Yang Ming. This condition is described in *Shang Han Lun* as shang han which has lasted for three days with a Yang Ming big pulse. The treatment is Bai Hu jia Ren Shen Tang to clear heat and generate fluids.

Clause 26 must be differentiated from Clause 25 which says: "Having taken Gui Zhi Tang, there is copious sweat, if the pulse is flooding and big, give Gui Zhi Tang as before". Although the signs and symptoms are similar, the pathogenesis and treatment are significantly different. Clause 25 describes the situation where, after taking Gui Zhi Tang, there is profuse sweat and the pulse changes from floating and moderate to flooding and big. The copious sweating is attributed to yang qi pushing outward to the surface; however, despite a change in the pulse, the symptoms remain the same. This is because the Tai Yang exterior pattern remains unresolved and there is no interior pattern, as confirmed by the absence of vexation and thirst. Therefore, Gui Zhi Tang is still indicated. Bai Hu Tang can not be justified because there is no thirst and no sign of an interior pattern.

Clause 168

伤寒若吐若下后，七八日不解，热结在里，表里俱热，时时恶风、大渴、舌上干燥而烦、欲饮水数升者，白虎加人参汤主之。

Shang han following vomiting and purgation, is not resolved in seven or eight days, heat is knotted in the interior, if there is heat in both the exterior and interior, with constant aversion to wind, severe thirst, the surface of the tongue is dry, there is agitation and vexation, a desire to drink several sheng of water, Bai Hu jia Ren Shen Tang governs.

DISCUSSION: The situation of dual exterior and interior heat is directly attributable to the incorrect use of emetics and purgatives which, by damaging fluids, causes the exterior pathogen to fall inward, where it transforms into constrained heat. Heat steams fluids outward causing insecurity of the skin interstices or *cou li* and hence there is frequent aversion to wind. If emetics are used there will be fluid depletion in the upper jiao, and where purgation is used there will be fluid depletion in the lower jiao. This causes exuberant dry heat in the interior, hence the dry tongue, vexation, and a thirst so severe that it is quenched only by drinking a whole litre of water. In spite of the dry heat bind, there is as yet no manifestation of a bowel excess pattern, and therefore Bai Hu jia Ren Shen Tang is used to clear heat and generate fluids.

Sweating and Aversion to Wind in the Three Yang Patterns

Aversion to wind and sweating are symptoms associated with Tai Yang, Shao Yang and Yang Ming patterns. Differentiation is made on the basis of their pathogenesis.

A Tai Yang exterior pattern is attributed to pathogenic cold invading the muscle layer. The corresponding treatment strategy is to release the exterior by promoting sweat. Tai Yang exterior patterns are categorised as Tai Yang zhong feng or wind strike, and Tai Yang shang han or cold injury. Both are characterised by aversion to wind, but are differentiated by the presence or absence of sweating. Tai Yang zhong feng or wind strike is categorised as an exterior deficiency pattern based on the presence of sweat; Gui Zhi Tang is the guiding formula. Tai Yang shang han or cold injury is characterised by the absence of sweat and thus categorised as exterior excess; the guiding formula is Ma Huang Tang. If, after promoting sweat in order to release the exterior, the patient suffers from continuous copious sweating with aversion to wind, then the exterior pathogen has not been resolved; rather, the defence yang has been depleted and Xin Jia Tang should be administered.

In a Shao Yang pattern, there is fever, aversion to wind, a stiff neck and a sense of fullness under the ribs, all of which indicate that the exterior pathogen is not fully resolved, and is at the point of entering Shao Yang; the indicated formula is Xiao Chai Hu Tang. Where there is an aversion to wind which accompanies a reluctance to remove clothing, or where there is mild swelling due to fluid retention caused by the invasion of wind damp, then the formula to use is Gan Cao Fu Zi Tang.

Aversion to wind in a Yang Ming pattern is a sign of the exterior pathogen having fallen inward and transformed into interior heat. The interior heat steams outwards, causing sweating. The pathogen is no longer in the exterior and the aversion to wind is a manifestation of the exterior having been made insecure by the profuse sweating which has opened the interstices of the skin. Because of the damage to qi and body fluids, further promotion of sweat is inappropriate and treatment must be directed at clearing interior heat and generating fluids; Bai Hu jia Ren Shen Tang is the indicated formula. In practice, the four examination methods must be employed in order to determine the correct treatment strategy.

Clause 169

伤寒无大热、口燥渴、心烦、背微恶寒者，白虎加人参汤主之。

Shang han without vigorous fever, if there is a parched mouth and thirst, vexation, the back has a slight aversion to cold, Bai Hu jia Ren Shen Tang governs.

DISCUSSION: An absence of a high fever in shang han disease generally indicates that there is little or no heat in the exterior; there is, however, heat in the interior, as evidenced by the parched mouth, thirst and vexation. When heat consumes fluids, there will be thirst and a dry mouth and when it harasses the heart shen there will be vexation. The symptom of the back being averse to cold has a similar pathogenesis to the recurrent aversion to wind cited in the previous clause, Clause 168, insofar as it relates to an insecure exterior. The back is the residence for the yang and the focal point of yang qi. If there is sweating, there is loss not only of body fluids but also of qi. This loss of yang qi deprives the body of the ability to secure the exterior, and it is the back, as the residence of yang, that is most affected. Hence it is the back which is averse to cold; Bai Hu jia Ren Shen Tang is the indicated formula.

This symptom of the back being slightly averse to cold is also found in Shao Yin patterns; however, the aversion to cold of a Shao Yin pattern is more severe, and is also accompanied by additional symptoms such as a desire to sleep, and a submerged faint pulse; the treatment used is Fu Zi Tang and moxibustion. The symptom of the back being slightly averse to cold in a Bai Hu jia Ren Shen Tang pattern, on the other hand, is accompanied by the symptoms reflecting interior heat: thirst, vexation, a dry mouth and a big, flooding pulse, all reflecting a febrile disease pattern with fluid damage. The treatment strategy is to clear heat and replenish fluids, and so Bai Hu jia Ren Shen Tang is the guiding formula.

Clause 222

若渴欲饮水，口干舌燥者，白虎加人参汤主之。

If there is thirst with a desire to drink water, the mouth is dry and the tongue parched, Bai Hu jia Ren Shen Tang governs.

DISCUSSION: Clause 222 follows and contrasts with Clause 221, which describes the adverse effects of purgation in shang han disease, when pathogenic heat lodges in the upper jiao causing insubstantial vexation and where Zhi Zi Chi Tang is the governing formula. If the pathogenic heat is lodged in the middle jiao, as described in Clause 222, there will be thirst, a parched mouth and a dry tongue. These are manifestations of exuberant heat having dried out the fluids and Bai Hu jia Ren Shen Tang is the governing formula.

Modern Application of Bai Hu jia Ren Shen Tang

This formula is frequently used to treat disorders such as summerheat, epidemic influenza, and lobar pneumonia, where there is damage to both qi and yin.

Case Study

Heat Stroke

Extracted from Zhejiang Zhong Yi Za Zhi 1965; 8:7.

During the previous summer, a 38-year-old female patient was found semi-conscious after her afternoon nap. She presented with a clouded spirit, fever, cold extremities, copious sweating, stertorous breathing, wheezing, slight tetany, a dry yellow tongue coat and a big, hollow, flooding pulse. The diagnosis was summerheat stroke with exuberant fire scorching the Yang Ming and the treatment principle was to clear summerheat, augment qi and generate fluids. The formula prescribed was Bai Hu jia Ren Shen Tang: Bai Ren Shen 15g, Zhi Mu 15g, Jing Mi 15g, Sheng Shi Gao 30g, Gan Cao 9g. After one pack, the sweating stopped, her hands were warm, she was lucid and had an insatiable thirst. A second pack of the same formula was given to consolidate the treatment and she recovered completely.

Zhu Ling Tang Pattern

Clause 223

若脉浮、发热、渴欲饮水、小便不利者，猪苓汤主之。

If the pulse is floating, there is fever, thirst with a desire to drink water, and the urination is not free, Zhu Ling Tang governs.

ZHU LING TANG: Zhu Ling (skin removed), Fu Ling, Ze Xie, E Jiao, Hua Shi (broken): 1 liang each.

DIRECTIONS: Boil the first four ingredients in 4 sheng of water, reducing to 2 sheng. Strain and stir in the melted E Jiao. Take 7 ge warm three times a day.

DISCUSSION: Clause 223 describes a transmuted pattern following incorrect purgation, where the pathogen has fallen inward and transformed into heat. Heat is a yang pathogen and its outward steaming action manifests as fever and is reflected in the floating pulse.

When the heat binds with water, it obstructs the movement of fluids, causing thirst. When it binds with water in the lower jiao, which refers here to the kidney and urinary bladder, being the zang and fu of water, the bind of heat and water impairs qi transformation, causing inhibited urination. Zhu Ling Tang is used to clear heat, nourish yin and disinhibit urination. Zhang Zhong Jing pioneered the strategy of simultaneously nourishing yin and disinhibiting water by using E Jiao to tonify the true yin, combined with Zhu Ling, Fu Ling and Ze Xie to drain damp and promote urination; Hua Shi is cold and drains heat downwards through its action of promoting urination.

Clause 223 should also be read in association with Clause 221 as both describe a transmuted Yang Ming heat pattern caused by incorrect purgation. The three differential patterns and their corresponding treatment strategies are as follows.

1. Following incorrect purgation, if the formless heat lodges in the chest and diaphragm and manifests with anxiety, restlessness and a thin, slightly yellow tongue coat, Zhi Zi Chi Tang must be used to vent constrained heat and drain fire from the upper jiao (Clause 221).
2. If there is a parched mouth and dry tongue and severe thirst, then the heat is in the middle jiao. Because there is damage to both qi and yin, the correct formula is Bai Hu jia Ren Shen Tang to clear heat and generate fluid (Clause 222).
3. Where there is fever, a floating pulse, thirst and inhibited urination, then there is heat and water bind in the lower jiao and the formula is Zhu Ling Tang (Clause 223).

These three scenarios represent a sequence in the potential progress of disease; if Zhi Zi Chi Tang is not effective, Bai Hu Tang can be used, and if this is not effective, Zhu Ling Tang can be used. Each of these patterns and their treatments are clinically relevant today, but the aetiology is usually not incorrect purgation and identification is based on the pattern symptoms.

Clause 224

阳明病，汗出多而渴者，不可与猪苓汤。以汗多胃中燥，猪苓汤复利其小便故也。

Yang Ming disease, if there is profuse sweating and thirst, one should not give Zhu Ling Tang. Because of the profuse sweating, there is dryness in the stomach, Zhu Ling Tang will further promote urination.

DISCUSSION: Patterns of thirst vary and so does their treatment. When Zhu Ling Tang is indicated to treat thirst, it is to treat thirst caused by heat and water bind in the lower jiao, which obstructs the proper dispersal of fluids, and there is thirst. When Bai Hu Tang is indicated for thirst, it is because excessive sweating has damaged the body fluids causing dryness in the stomach. However, if thirst is accompanied by copious sweating, as in Clause 224, the indicated treatment is Bai Hu jia Ren Shen Tang, in order to repair the fluid loss. Zhu Ling Tang is contraindicated because by promoting urination, it has the opposite effect of further depleting fluids and it would exacerbate stomach dryness.

Clinical observation has confirmed that a Yang Ming heat pattern characterised by copious sweating with subsequent injury to yin may cause scant or inhibited urination. Zhang Zhong Jing did not elaborate on this point but it is self-evident that where there is profuse sweating and thirst, indicative of heat and dryness, a formula such as Zhu Ling Tang, which drains damp and is therefore drying, is contraindicated.

Ancient Application of Zhu Ling Tang

- *Yi Fang Ji Jie:* In the treatment of damp heat jaundice, where there is thirst and dark and scant urination.
- *Lei Ju Fang Guang Yi:* In the treatment of lin syndrome or difficult urination with scant and dripping urination, swelling and pain of the penis, and pain and distension of the lower abdomen.

Modern Application of Zhu Ling Tang

Zhu Ling Tang can be modified to treat chronic nephritis, urinary tract infection, hydronephritis, renal tuberculosis, kidney stones, chyluria and haematuria when characterised by inhibited urination, a slight or low grade fever and a thready pulse. It should be noted that the tongue sign for Zhu Ling Tang is red with a scant coat, as compared with Wu Ling San, where the tongue is pale with a white coat.

Modifications

- For yin deficiency characterised by lower back pain, tidal fever and a red tongue with a scant coat, combine with Zhi Bai Di Huang Wan.
- For more severe water retention characterised by swelling and distension in the lower abdomen, and where urination is still inhibited even after taking Zhu Ling Tang, add Yi Yi Ren and Che Qian Zi to drain damp more effectively.
- For more severe heat characterised by vexation, insomnia, fever and thirst, combine with Dao Chi San.
- For haematuria, add Han Lian Cao, Xiao Ji, Bai Mao Gen, San Qi Fen.
- Where urine analysis shows white blood cells, add Huang Bai, Zhi Ye and Jin Yin Hua to clear heat and relieve toxicity.
- For renal tuberculosis, add Bai He, Yu Xing Cao, Bai Bu.
- For kidney stones, add Ji Nei Jin, Jin Qian Cao.
- If inhibited urination is accompanied by oedema in the lower limbs, aversion to cold, a pale tongue and a submerged faint pulse, use Zhen Wu Tang.

Case Study

Haematuria

Extracted from Guang Ming Zhong Yi 1988; 3:17

A 53-year-old male patient had suffered from painful urination with occasional haematuria for ten days. He also complained of lower back pain, weakness in the legs, fatigue, thirst, a sensation of heaviness and irritability. His tongue was red with a thin yellow coat and his pulse was wiry and taut. The diagnosis was *xue lin* or haematuria due to kidney yin deficiency with heart and liver fire scorching the vessels in the lower jiao. The treatment principle was to nourish yin, drain fire and cool blood and the formula used was Zhu Ling Tang with the addition of Bai Shao, Qian Cao, Zhi Zi Tan. After three packs, there was full recovery.

Summary of Yang Ming Heat Patterns

The Yang Ming heat pattern in Clause 224 is referring to exuberant heat in the qi aspect of Yang Ming, which is yet to manifest as an excess pattern. Therefore Bai Hu Tang and Bai Hu jia Ren Shen Tang are the indicated formulas; Zhi Zi Chi Tang or Zhu Ling Tang are used for deviations from the standard Yang Ming pattern.

Apart from qi level heat in the Yang Ming, Bai Hu Tang is also indicated for a concurrent pattern of the three yang where there is delirious speech, sweating, abdominal fullness, a sensation of heaviness with inability to turn over, numbness of the mouth, a grimy face and a floating, slippery or flooding and big pulse. When heat affects the three yang channels, the focus is directed to Yang Ming because the symptoms resemble those of a Yang Ming heat pattern, but there is no bowel excess, so Bai Hu Tang is indicated and diaphoresis and purgation contraindicated. If the Yang Ming heat pattern exhibits a deficiency of qi and yin which manifests as insatiable thirst and irritability or, alternatively, if there is heat bind in the interior with a recurrent aversion to wind, thirst and a dry tongue or, as a third possibility, if there is thirst and vexation with the back being mildly averse to cold, then these patterns reflect exuberant heat which has consumed yin and Bai Hu jia Ren Shen Tang is indicated to clear heat, generate fluids and augment qi.

A Zhi Zi Chi Tang pattern is a heat pattern characterised by vexation, which has arisen as a result of incorrect purgation with three possible developments. The first is where insubstantial vexation is caused by heat harassing the chest and diaphragm. The second is where heat has fallen inward, lodging in the chest, due to incorrect purgation. The third is the initial stage of a Yang Ming heat constraint pattern where there is no accumulation of excess heat and where there is emptiness in the stomach, anxiety, heat in the exterior, hunger with no desire to eat, sweating from the head only, a rapid pulse and a yellow tongue coat. Zhi Zi Chi Tang is indicated to diffuse constrained heat.

A Zhu Ling Tang pattern results from incorrect purgation in a Yang Ming heat pattern, where the pathogen knots with water in the lower jiao. The symptoms are a floating pulse, fever, thirst and inhibited urination. If there is profuse sweating, vexation and thirst, it means there is dryness in the stomach and Zhu Ling Tang is contraindicated because by its diuretic action it will cause further damage to fluids.

3.3.2 Yang Ming Cold Patterns

Although most Yang Ming patterns are associated with heat, Yang Ming disease may also manifest as a cold pattern.

> **Clause 190**
>
> 阳明病，若能食，名中风；不能食，名中寒。
>
> *Yang Ming disease, if the person can eat, it is called zhong feng; if the person can not eat, it is called zhong han.*

DISCUSSION: Yang Ming zhong feng (wind strike) refers to an external pathogen which has not affected stomach function. Moreover, wind is a yang pathogen and, because of its dispersing qualities, assists in the processing of grain and water in the stomach. In Yang Ming zhong feng, therefore, the person can take food. In Yang Ming zhong han (cold strike), however, the invasion is one of cold not wind; cold obstructs and congeals, retarding and impairing the decomposition and transportation of water and grain, and so the person has a poor appetite and can not take food. Whilst a pattern of exterior cold is differentiated according to the presence or absence of sweating, the invasion of interior cold is differentiated on the basis of the ability to eat.

Robust stomach qi is a feature of a zhong feng pattern, where neither the qi nor the yang of the stomach is affected by the wind. Wind is yang and tends to heat not cold, and so the stomach yang is not under attack. A zhong han or cold strike pattern, however, is an attack by a yin pathogen, which assails a constitution already deficient in yang and so less able to resist the cold. Zhong han (cold strike), therefore, will succeed in damaging the yang qi further, and result in a pattern of deficiency cold in the Yang Ming channel.

Although Clause 190 only mentions the ability to eat as a means to differentiate between zhong feng (wind strike) and zhong han (cold strike), consideration must, of course, be given to all aspects of the person's health and constitution. Cheng Jiao Qian said: "Zhong feng (wind strike) is attributed to heat and stagnation in the interior, while zhong han (cold strike) is attributed to cold in the stomach". Apart from a reduced appetite and an inability to take food, a pattern of cold in the stomach is characterised by a sensation of cold in the stomach, a preference for warmth, a pale tongue with a wet, white coat, and a pulse which is moderately slow or submerged and slow.

> **Clause 191**
>
> 阳明病，若中寒者，不能食，小便不利，手足濈然汗出，此欲作固瘕，必大便初硬后溏。所以然者，以胃中冷，水谷不别故也。
>
> *Yang Ming disease, if it is zhong han, the person can not eat, the urination is not free, the hands and feet sweat profusely, this means a firm mass is about to form, the stool will be hard at first and sloppy afterwards. The reason for this being, that because of cold in the stomach, there is no separation of water and grain.*

DISCUSSION: Yang Ming zhong han represents a pattern of pathogenic cold attacking where stomach yang is deficient or, where there is a pre-existing pattern of yang deficiency with cold in the middle jiao. If the middle yang is insufficient, the stomach's function of rotting and ripening is impaired; the stomach can not receive more food, and so the person can not eat; the spleen fails to transform and transport, and instead of being transformed into urine in the urinary bladder, water descends to the large intestine, so there is scant urination and a sloppy stool.

There are two explanations of the issue of sweat from the limbs. The first is cold in the stomach combined with insecurity of the defence yang, and the second is the function of the Yang Ming in ruling the limbs. This function is based on the fact that the Yang Ming is the source of qi and blood, providing the limbs with nourishment and warmth. Thus the limbs are dependent on the Yang Ming to supply them with qi and blood and to transport yang qi. The yang qi not only warms the limbs, but also governs the exterior, controlling the pores. When the yang qi fails to close the pores, there is sweating. The sweat tends to be profuse because impaired transformation of water has allowed it to collect beneath the skin.

When Zhong Jing explains that the hard stool followed by a sloppy one is due to cold in the stomach, he is referring not only to empty cold due to yang deficiency, but also to an excess accumulation of cold. The cold accumulation congeals the unripened grain qi into a firm mass, and it is this congealed mass which forms a hard stool. The non-separation of water and grain is a reference to the insufficiency of yang and its inability to separate the food essences into pure and impure, resulting in turbid water flowing downwards from the stomach to the intestines. The congealed mass is followed by the untransformed water, giving rise to the phenomenon of a hard stool followed by diarrhoea.

Sweat streaming from the extremities can be due either to excess heat or to deficiency cold. The excess heat pattern of Yang Ming is characterised by constipation, frequent urination, an inability to eat, and sweat streaming from the extremities; the indicated treatment is purgation. The deficiency cold pattern of Yang Ming is characterised by cold sweat, non-transformation of grain and water, a thin, white, wet tongue coat, and a submerged and slow pulse; the treatment is to warm the middle and tonify the spleen.

Clause 194

阳明病，不能食，攻其热必哕。所以然者，胃中虚冷故也。以其人本虚，攻其热必哕。

Yang Ming disease, the person can not eat, attacking the heat will cause hiccoughs. The reason for this being, there is empty cold in the stomach. Because the person was already deficient, attacking heat will cause hiccoughs.

DISCUSSION: Clause 194 continues the discussion started in Clause 191, and emphasises the importance of differentiating between an inability to eat due to heat, and the same symptom due to cold. If purgation is used as a result of mistaking the inability to eat for a manifestation of an excess bind of heat and dryness, the deficiency will worsen and there will be qi reversal manifesting as hiccoughs. Hiccough is associated with coldness and deficiency of the stomach and is ascribed to three factors. The first is interior cold in the stomach with an underlying yang deficiency; the second is an invasion of exterior cold; and the third possibility is the incorrect or excessive use of cold, bitter purgative herbs. Any of these can damage the stomach yang, causing the improper ascent of stomach qi manifesting as hiccoughing.

The Yang Ming symptom of being unable to eat can be attributed to excess, deficiency, heat or cold. The excess pattern of stomach heat is characterised by abdominal fullness, constipation, tidal fever, sweating, a dry yellow tongue coat and a submerged, excess and forceful pulse. A Yang Ming pattern of deficient heat in the stomach is characterised by a dry mouth, a red tongue with a scant coat, and a rapid, thready pulse. A Yang Ming pattern of deficiency cold in the stomach is characterised by a bland taste in the mouth, excessive salivation, a stool which is loose, or one which is hard at first but sloppy afterwards, a wet, white tongue coat, and a slow and moderate pulse. In the above three patterns, Cheng Qi Tang is the guiding formula for the pattern of excess heat, but purgation is contraindicated for patterns of deficiency heat and deficiency cold.

Clause 195

阳明病，脉迟，食难用饱，饱则微烦头眩，必小便难，此欲作谷瘅，虽下之，腹满如故，所以然者，脉迟故也。

Yang Ming disease, the pulse is slow, it is difficult to eat one's fill, and if full, there is mild vexation and dizziness, urination will be difficult, this means grain jaundice is about to occur, in spite of purging, there is abdominal fullness as before, the reason for this being, that the pulse is slow.

DISCUSSION: A slow pulse in Yang Ming disease indicates a Yang Ming cold pattern. Because there is insufficient yang qi, the stomach function of decomposing food is impaired, affecting the ability to take food. Therefore, if the person eats an immoderate amount, and particularly if there is consumption of cold, raw or greasy foods which are more difficult to digest, there will be food stagnation; qi reversal ensues manifesting as vexation and dizziness. The disruption to the qi dynamic results in the failure of clear yang to ascend and of turbid yin to descend; this leads to abdominal fullness, which is not alleviated by purgation. The obstruction in the middle jiao also inhibits the movement of water and so urination is scant.

If this condition is not treated, there will be grain jaundice. Grain jaundice refers to jaundice caused by food stagnation which can be associated with both damp heat and with damp cold. Clause 195 describes a pattern of yin jaundice, where cold damp, attributed to an immoderate diet and an insufficiency of stomach yang, has obstructed the middle jiao. The strategy is to warm the middle, support the stomach yang, disperse cold and resolve damp. Purgation is contraindicated because it will further damage the yang qi and only serve to exacerbate the condition, and so abdominal distension will not be resolved; it may worsen, and there may also be inhibited or difficult urination. This is explained in the final statement, where Zhong Jing specifies that the reason for the worsening condition and for it manifesting as grain jaundice is the cold pattern, which is represented by the slow pulse.

In regard to proper eating habits and the need for moderation in eating, *Nei Jing* says: "If the intake of food is doubled, the stomach will be damaged." This is because eating immoderate or excessive amounts places too much strain on the stomach, and if the person is deficient, is even more likely to drain the yang qi of the middle jiao, causing digestive problems. It is therefore important to eat easily digestible food and avoid eating large amounts or consume cold substances which are difficult to digest. The abdominal fullness in Clause 195 is due to food stagnation and the accumulation of damp in the stomach; it is not due to the knotting of heat in the large intestine. Because it is due to middle qi deficiency, the strategy is to "fill the filled" (赛因塞用), which refers to the principle of strengthening the earth and its function of decomposition and transportation in order to resolve the fullness. Li Zhong Wan and Xiang Sha Liu Jun Zi Wan are both suitable.

Clause 195 raises three main issues: first, that it is a pattern of yang deficiency and cold, as shown by the slow pulse; second, immoderate eating can cause the condition to deteriorate and give rise to grain jaundice; and third, due to the fact that the pattern is one of cold and deficiency, purgation is not indicated.

Clause 226

若胃中冷，不能食者，饮水则哕。

If the stomach is cold, and the person can not eat, drinking will cause hiccoughs.

DISCUSSION: The stomach is the yang organ pertaining to earth and serves as the receptacle of food. The stomach is dependent on yang qi to perform its function of decomposition; the subsequent transformation of the grain and water into refined food essences is performed by the spleen; distribution of the food essences is a co-ordinated activity of both spleen and stomach. If these functions are impaired there will be food stagnation and qi reversal manifesting as hiccough. The recommended treatment is Li Zhong Wan with the addition of Ding Xiang and Wu Zhu Yu to warm the middle and redirect qi. Clause 226 is better read in conjunction with Clause 194, which describes a pattern of cold and deficiency in the stomach, where the person is unable to eat, and where hiccoughing arises in response to drinking water. In that clause, the yang qi had been damaged by purgation.

Clause 197

阳明病，反无汗而小便利，二三日呕而咳，手足厥者，必苦头痛；若不咳，不呕，手足不厥者，头不痛。

Yang Ming disease, nevertheless there is no sweating and the urination is free, on the second or third day, there is vomiting and cough, there will be a severe headache; if there is no cough, no vomiting, no reversal cold of the hands and feet, then the head will not ache.

DISCUSSION: Sweating is one of the principal signs of a Yang Ming pattern, which is commonly associated with interior heat. The absence of sweating described in Clause 197 suggests that this pattern is not one of heat. The absence of sweat described here is due to an insufficiency of yang qi unable to transform fluids, and so there is no source for sweat. The uninhibited urination is simply a sign that the disorder is not in the lower jiao. The disruption to the transformation function in the middle jiao has also resulted in water being retained in the stomach. After two or three days, it accumulates to the point where it causes qi reversal and vomiting; similarly, where water harasses the lungs, there will be coughing. These symptoms are manifestations of water accumulation resulting in qi reversal, and so there can also be headache. Conversely, when these signs are absent and the yang qi appears intact, the flow of qi and blood will be normal, there will be no coldness of the extremities, and so there will be no headache.

The root of the above pattern is yang deficiency, due to which has arisen the branch disorder of accumulated cold fluids. This would seem to be similar to a Tai Yin pattern of deficiency and cold in the middle jiao, however the difference lies in the zang and fu involved. In Tai Yin it is the spleen which is deficient and cold, whilst in Yang Ming it is the stomach. It is this difference which accounts for the different symptomatology of those two patterns. The Tai Yin spleen governs ascent; therefore the manifestations of the Tai Yin pattern are a reflection of the spleen's failure to raise qi and ascend fluids, and diarrhoea and distension and pain in the abdomen are the result. The Yang Ming stomach, on the other hand, governs descent; the vomiting, cough and headache are a reflection of qi reversal and the non-descent of qi.

Zhong Jing did not nominate a formula for this pattern, but contemporary scholars suggest that Zhen Wu Tang omitting Fu Ling, Xiao Qing Long Tang or Ge Gen Tang are suitable formulas. Xiao Jian Zhong Tang can also be used and, based on the manifestations of this pattern, Wu Zhu Yu Tang to warm the middle and transform turbidity is also appropriate.

Wu Zhu Yu Tang Pattern

Clause 243

食谷欲呕，属阳明也，吴茱萸汤主之；得汤反剧者，属上焦也.

An urge to vomit after eating food pertains to Yang Ming, Wu Zhu Yu Tang governs; if taking the decoction makes the condition worse instead, it pertains to the upper jiao.

WU ZHU YU TANG: Wu Zhu Yu (washed) 1 sheng; Ren Shen 3 liang; Sheng Jiang (sliced) 6 liang; Da Zao (broken) 12 pieces.

DIRECTIONS: Boil the ingredients in 7 sheng of water, reducing to 2 sheng. Strain and take 7 ge warm three times a day.

DISCUSSION: An urge to vomit after eating can be attributed to heat or to cold. A Yang Ming cold pattern is associated with a deficiency of stomach yang and its inability to support the stomach's function of rotting and ripening: food stagnates in the stomach and obstructs the descent of stomach qi. Wu Zhu Yu Tang is indicated to warm the stomach and redirect qi downward to stop vomiting. Vomiting can also be caused by heat in the upper jiao, obstructing lung qi and impairing its function of dispersing and descending body fluids. Damp then accumulates and can result in vomiting after the ingestion of food. Wu Zhu Yu Tang is acrid and warm and is indicated for cold patterns, so if it is used in error, causing the condition to worsen, then it is a sign that the vomiting is due to heat in the upper jiao, not cold in the middle jiao.

Wu Zhu Yu is acrid, bitter and hot; it warms the liver and stomach, redirects qi and helps to lead turbidity downward; Ren Shen and Da Zao are sweet and warm and augment the middle qi; the heavy dosage of Sheng Jiang (6 liang) disperses cold and eases vomiting. Gan Cao is omitted because of the tendency of that herb to cause water to be retained.

Differentiation of Vomiting

Hot and cold patterns associated with vomiting can be differentiated as follows.

- When vomiting is part of a cold pattern, the stomach's function of receiving food is affected and there is a pale tongue with a white coat and a pulse which is moderate, slow and weak; Wu Zhu Yu Tang is the indicated formula.
- When vomiting is caused by heat, there will be a red tongue with a yellow coat and the pulse will be rapid; Ju Pi Zhu Ru Tang (Ju Pi, Zhu Ru, Da Zao, Ren Shen, Sheng Jiang, Gan Cao) is the indicated formula.

Vomiting is a feature of both a Wu Zhu Yu Tang and a Si Ni Tang pattern; however, although both are patterns of interior cold, the manifestations differ. The vomiting in a Wu Zhu Yu Tang pattern is accompanied by headache, diarrhoea is rarely seen and the formula focuses on localised cold in the stomach and liver. In contrast, the vomiting of a Si Ni Tang pattern is accompanied by more serious vomiting and is attributed to generalised yang deficiency which is characterised by aversion to cold and cold extremities.

Ancient Application of Wu Zhu Yu Tang

- *Zhou Hou Bei Ji Fang:* For the treatment of belching.
- *Lan Shi Mi Cang:* For the treatment of Jue Yin headache or vomiting of phlegm and excessive salivation with cold extremities and a floating, moderate pulse.
- *Yi Fang Ji Jie:* Wu Zhu Yu jia Fu Zi Tang for the treatment of pain associated with inguinal hernia or testicular pain due to cold in the liver channel characterised by a submerged and slow pulse.

Modern Application of Wu Zhu Yu Tang

- *Headache and migraine.* Headache or migraine due to cold in the liver channel, including Jue Yin headache located at the vertex, headache associated with hypertension, or associated with neuralgia due to cold in the liver channel. The pain is usually localised and intermittent; it is often accompanied by excessive salivation or vomiting; the tongue is pale with a slippery, white coat and the pulse is submerged and slow. For blood deficiency, add Dang Gui and Chuan Xiong; for excessive salivation add Xuan Fu Hua, Dai Zhe Shi, Jiang Ban Xia; for severe headache, add Xi Xin and Bai Zhi. Zhao et al treated 13 cases of neuralgic headache using Wu Zhu Yu Tang with the addition of Rou Gui, Dang Gui, Chuan Xiong, Ban Xia, Gao Ben and also by adding Quan Xie and Wu Gong. Between 2 to 12 packs were taken effecting full recovery in all 13 cases. A six month follow-up showed no recurrence (*Zhong Yi Yao Za Zhi* 1982; 6:33).
- *Vomiting.* Vomiting and nausea due to cold in the stomach, manifesting as acute or chronic gastritis, peptic ulcers, morning sickness, and vomiting due to neurological disturbance. Accompanying signs and symptoms are fatigue, a pale complexion, aversion to cold, a loose stool, a wet, white tongue coat and a slow, wiry and forceless pulse. For more severe vomiting, add Ding Xiang; for abdominal distension, add Bai Dou Kou and Hou Po; for more pronounced cold in the stomach, add Gao Liang Jiang and Xiang Fu; for acid reflux, add Mu Li, Hai Piao Xiao or Wa Leng Zi.

Case Study

Vertigo

Extracted from the case studies of Professor Zhang Wen Xuan

A 48-year-old woman had suffered from headache at the vertex, vertigo and vomiting for over a month. She had not responded to conventional Chinese medical treatment based on such formulas as Chuan Xiong Cha Tiao Yin etc. Her complexion was pale and she frequently vomited watery fluids. The headache and vertigo were worse in the morning, easing after the intake of food. Her appetite was poor and the stool was loose. She had a thin, white tongue coat and a thready, soft pulse. She was diagnosed with duodenal ulcers following a barium X-ray. The Chinese medicine diagnosis was cold in the liver channel harassing the stomach. The prescription was Wu Zhu Yu Tang modified: Wu Zhu Yu 10g, Dang Shen 15g, Zhi Gan Cao 5g, Sheng Jiang 12g, Da Zao 5 pieces, Ban Xia 10g, Chen Pi 10g. After six packs there was significant relief, but she still had a mild headache. Her tongue coat was white and wet and her pulse was moderate and weak. She was prescribed a modified version of Liu Jun Zi Tang: Dang Shen 15g, Bai Zhu 10g, Fu Ling 15g, Ban Xia 10g, Chen Pi 10g, Mu Xiang 6g, Sheng Huang Qi 15g, Zhi Gan Cao 5g, Sheng Jiang 10g, Da Zao 3 pieces. She took one pack per day for two weeks and recovery was complete.

Discussion: The key symptoms were vertigo and headache. The diagnosis was cold in the liver channel. Wu Zhu Yu Tang was prescribed because of its action of warming the liver channel and harmonising the stomach.

Summary of Yang Ming Cold Patterns

Although Yang Ming disease is principally associated with heat and excess, there are also patterns of cold and deficiency. The Yang Ming pattern of stomach cold complements the Tai Yin pattern of cold in the spleen, thus providing a broader perspective of cold patterns which affect the middle jiao. The chief points of Yang Ming cold patterns are summarised as follows.

PATHOGENESIS: Yang Ming cold patterns arise as a result of incorrect treatment, or because of pre-existing stomach deficiency. The pathomechanism is deficient yang of the stomach failing to support transportation and resulting in retained fluids.

SYMTOMATOLOGY: The key symptoms are an inability to eat, uninhibited urination, a stool which is hard at first but sloppy afterwards, or an urge to vomit after eating, or hiccoughing occurring after the ingestion of water, or abdominal fullness and vomiting, or cold extremities, or vomiting and cough, or headache, or streaming sweat from the extremities. The tongue coat is white and the pulse is slow.

KEY POINTS OF DIAGNOSIS: A pattern of Yang Ming deficiency cold is diagnosed on the following key points.

1. *Intake of food:* the ability to eat indicates heat; the inability to eat indicates cold.
2. *Urination:* uninhibited or profuse urination is associated with cold; scant or inhibited urination is associated with heat.
3. *Stool:* the phenomenon of a stool which is initially hard, but is followed by diarrhoea, is due to cold; a hard and difficult stool is associated with excess heat; a watery stool with undigested food particles characterises Shao Yin yang deficiency.
4. *Response to medication:* if the condition deteriorates after taking Wu Zhu Yu Tang, it means the heat is in the upper jiao; improvement after taking Wu Zhu Yu Tang shows the pattern was one of cold in the middle jiao.

SUPPLEMENTARY CARE: It is essential to take the medication warm and to refrain from eating food which is cold or raw, and also to avoid eating immoderate or excessive amounts to prevent the development of the condition 'grain jaundice'.

3.3.3 Yang Ming Deficiency Patterns

Yang Ming patterns are not limited to patterns of excess, but may also present as deficiency patterns, where the person has a pre-existing deficiency.

Clause 196

阳明病，法多汗，反无汗，其身如虫行皮中状者，此以久虚故也。

Yang Ming disease, the rule is profuse sweat, if however there is no sweat and it is as if worms are crawling beneath the skin, it is due to prolonged deficiency.

DISCUSSION: The copious sweating of Yang Ming disease is the result of interior heat venting the fluids outward. If, instead, there is no sweating, it is because the person is suffering from a chronic long-term deficiency of yang, resulting in insufficient production of blood and body fluids and the consequent depletion of the source of sweat. The qi and blood deficiency also means that the skin is not nourished, giving rise to a crawling sensation in the flesh, which may also be described as itchiness. In *Shang Han Lun*, itching is differentiated according to excess or deficiency and from that perspective, there is a distinction between the symptom of itchiness occurring in Tai Yang and Yang Ming patterns. The itchiness of a Tai Yang pattern is generally associated with excess, specifically, pathogenic wind cold constraining the exterior and depressing the yang qi. This pattern can be accompanied by alternating fever and chills resembling malaria, where fever predominates and where there is a pale red complexion. This describes a Tai Yang disease with an unresolved exterior and the indicated formula is Gui Zhi Ma Huang Ge Ban Tang to promote a mild sweat. Itchiness in a Yang Ming pattern, on the other hand, is due to deficiency of qi, blood and body fluids. Because of injury to fluids, there is no source of sweat and there can be no sweating. Apart from the absence of sweat, the clinical presentation is noteworthy for the absence of exterior symptoms such as fever and aversion to cold. Instead, there are symptoms of empty heat, dry itchy skin and a thready and forceless pulse. The treatment strategy is to nourish fluids and augment qi to support the root. The recommended formulas are Xiao Jian Zhong Tang, Gui Zhi jia Huang Qi Tang or Chai Hu Gui Zhi Tang.

Section Four

3.4 YANG MING FU PATTERNS

A Yang Ming fu or bowel excess pattern is closely associated with a pattern of interior heat knotting with food stagnation; this causes severe fluid depletion and intestinal obstruction. The indicated treatment is the Cheng Qi Tang group of formulas to purge heat and by clearing heat, to conserve fluids.

Tiao Wei Cheng Qi Tang Pattern

Clause 207

阳明病，不吐、不下、心烦者，可与调胃承气汤。

Yang Ming disease, if there is no vomiting, no purgation, and vexation, one may give Tiao Wei Cheng Qi Tang.

TIAO WEI CHENG QI TANG: Zhi Gan Cao 2 liang; Mang Xiao ½ jin; Da Huang (skin removed and washed in clear wine) 4 liang.

DIRECTIONS: Slice Zhi Gan Cao and Da Huang and boil in 3 sheng of water until reduced to 1 sheng. Strain, add Mang Xiao and bring to the boil once or twice on a low flame. Take warm as a single dose to regulate the stomach qi.

DISCUSSION: If the patient is vexed in Yang Ming disease when no emetics or purgatives have been used, then it is known as 'excess vexation'. The heat has not been able to exit either via the upper jiao through vomiting, or via the lower jiao through purgation, and so the heat pathogen remains lodged in the stomach, harassing the heart shen and causing vexation.

Because the heat has combined with food stagnation, it is considered to have substance and is therefore called excess vexation or *shi fan* (实烦). This distinguishes it from empty or insubstantial vexation known as *xu fan* (虚烦) which is associated with the Zhi Zi Chi Tang pattern and is defined as formless heat lodged in the chest. Symptoms associated with excess vexation are steaming fever, delirious speech, abdominal fullness and constipation. Tiao Wei Chang Qi Tang is indicated to purge heat, harmonise the stomach and thus alleviate vexation.

Da Huang is bitter and cold and purges heat; Mang Xiao is salty and cold, moistens dryness and so disperses the knotted heat bind; Zhi Gan Cao moderates the action of Da Huang and Mang Xiao enabling the herbal effect to be focused in the stomach, and at the same time counters the cold and bitter properties of Da Huang and Mang Xiao to prevent damage to the stomach.

The purpose of Tiao Wei Cheng Qi Tang is to address the early stage of Yang Ming heat bind with dry heat in the stomach which has not yet manifested as an intestinal excess pattern. In *Shang Han Lun* there are seven indications for its use: sweating, steaming fever, vexation, restlessness, a dry stool or constipation, abdominal fullness, and delirious speech. It is essential to be able to distinguish between the vexation of a Tiao Wei Cheng Qi Tang pattern and the insubstantial vexation of a Zhi Zi Chi Tang pattern. The aetiology of Zhi Zi Chi Tang insubstantial vexation is incorrect sweat promotion or purgation resulting in formless heat being constrained in the chest, which can manifest as vexation or insomnia.

There are some variations in the instructions given for Tiao Wei Cheng Qi Tang: Clause 29 says that a small dose should be taken warm twice in one day. The purpose of this direction is to moderate the rapid and potent action of Da Huang and Mang Xiao and to regulate the stomach qi. The directions accompanying Clause 70, however, suggest that the decoction should be taken in one single dose in order to target more directly the large intestine, where the disease is located. It is interesting to note that the dose of Mang Xiao in Tiao Wei Cheng Qi Tang is larger than that in Da Cheng Qi Tang. This would seem to contradict the objective of Tiao Wei Cheng Qi Tang to purge moderately, however, the inclusion of Zhi Shi and Hou Po in Da Cheng Qi Tang results in a more potent purgative action. Moreover, the use of Gan Cao in Tiao Wei Cheng Qi Tang serves to moderate the purgative effect.

Clause 248

太阳病三日，发汗不解，蒸蒸发热者，属胃也，调胃承气汤主之。

Tai Yang disease for three days, the promotion of sweat does not resolve it, there is steaming heat, it pertains to the stomach, Tiao Wei Cheng Qi Tang governs.

DISCUSSION: If sweating has failed to resolve a Tai Yang pattern which has endured for three days, it means that the pathogen has passed on to the Yang Ming channel. The steaming fever is a manifestation of the exuberant heat of the Yang Ming percolating outward. From this it is understood that a Yang Ming pattern prevails and the stomach is implicated. Therefore Tiao Wei Cheng Qi Tang is indicated to purge heat and harmonise the stomach.

Clause 249

伤寒吐后，腹胀满者，与调胃承气汤。

Shang han disease after vomiting, if the abdomen is distended and full, give Tiao Wei Cheng Qi Tang.

DISCUSSION: Clause 249 describes the situation where instead of promoting sweat in Tai Yang shang han, emetics are used to induce vomiting. This incorrect treatment will achieve the objective of expelling the pathogen, however, it also results in the loss of qi and body fluids, depleting the qi and fluids of the stomach. The pathogen then exploits the deficiency and falls inwards, giving rise to stomach dryness and qi stagnation which manifests as abdominal fullness. Tiao Wei Cheng Qi Tang is indicated to moisten the intestines, purge heat and harmonise the stomach.

There are two scenarios associated with the incorrect use of emetic treatment in Tai Yang disease. The first is where the pathogen falls inward into Yang Ming causing dryness; this is characterised by abdominal distension, pain aggravated by pressure, fever, sweating, constipation, a dry yellow tongue coat and a submerged and moderate or submerged and forceful pulse; Tiao Wei Cheng Qi Tang is indicated. The second scenario is where emetic treatment damages yang, leading to a Yang Ming deficient cold pattern; this is characterised by abdominal distension which is alleviated by pressure, a thin watery stool, a moist white tongue coat and a moderate weak pulse; either Xiao Jian Zhong Tang or Li Zhong Tang can be used.

Ancient Application of Tiao Wei Cheng Qi Tang

- *Wai Tai Mi Yao:* For the treatment of shang han disease with fever, shortness of breath, fullness below the heart, indigestion and difficult bowel movement, Tiao Wei Cheng Qi Tang was used with the addition of Sheng Di and Da Zao, known as 'Sheng Di Huang Tang'.
- *Tai Ping Hui Min He Ji Ju Fang:* For the treatment of pathogenic heat affecting the upper and middle jiao, or stomach heat manifesting with a macular rash, Tiao Wei Cheng Qi Tang was used with the addition of Huang Qin, Zhi Zi and Bo He, also known as Liang Ge San.
- *Wen Bing Tiao Bian:* For treatment of Yang Ming febrile disease characterised by dark, scant urination, constipation, vexation and thirst, Tiao Wei Cheng Qi Tang was used with the omission of Gan Cao and adding Sheng Di, Chi Shao, Huang Lian, Huang Bai. This is known as Dao Chi Cheng Qi Tang.

Modern Application of Tiao Wei Cheng Qi Tang

Tiao Wei Cheng Qi Tang has broad application in internal medicine, external medicine and ear, eye, nose and throat disease.

- After six years of observation, Zhao et al reported that early purgation could be combined with heat clearing, toxin relieving (anti-bacterial) herbs for the treatment of acute infectious disease such as acute pneumonia, upper respiratory tract infection, acute pancreatitis and urinary tract infection. These patterns are generally associated with yang patterns of excess heat in the interior with the principal symptoms being fever, a parched throat, thirst for cold drinks, a poor appetite, flushed face, vexation, delirious speech or clouded spirit, rapid breathing, hypochondriac distension and pain, wheezing, profuse phlegm, abdominal pain aggravated by pressure, dark scant urination and constipation. The tongue is red or crimson with a thick, dry yellow or thick white tongue coat and the pulse is full and forceful or slippery and rapid. For this kind of acute infectious disease, it was recommended to use a purgative formula of Da Huang 15–30g, Mang Xiao 9g, Xuan Shen 15g and Gan Cao 6g; administering one dose initially and, if after four hours the fever remained, administering one more dose (Zhao Shu Ying: 'Using purgation to treat acute infectious disease', *Zhong Xi Yi Jie He Za Zhi* 1982; 2:90).
- External disorders such as abscess or dermatitis where there is high fever, thirst, constipation, redness or swelling in the skin, or delirious speech can be treated with Tiao Wei Cheng Qi Tang modified by adding heat clearing and toxin relieving herbs, thus facilitating purging of the heat toxin via the bowel movement.
- Ear, nose and throat disease. Liu et al (Liu Du Zhou *Shang Han Shi Si Jiang*) used Tiao Wei Cheng Qi Tang modified with the addition of Huang Lian and Xi Jiao for the treatment of Yang Ming fire blazing upwards and manifesting as inflammation of the gums with foul breath, headache, epistaxis, vexation and constipation.

Case Study

Insomnia and Vexation

Extracted from Shang Han Shi Si Jiang by Liu Du Zhou

The patient presented with vexation and insomnia. His pulse was slippery and rapid and his tongue coat was thick and yellow. The diagnosis was fire harassing the heart shen. Qin Lian Tang was initially prescribed to clear heat but was not effective and the tongue coat was still yellow. Dr. Liu remembered the passage from *Jin Gui Yao Lue* which said: "If the yellow tongue coat remains, use purgation". He then prescribed Tiao Wei Cheng Qi Tang, after which the patient passed a stool. The vexation was relieved and the tongue coat returned to normal.

Xiao Cheng Qi Tang Pattern

Clause 213

阳明病，其人多汗，以津液外出，胃中燥，大便必硬，硬则谵语，小承气汤主之。若一服谵语止者，更莫复服。

Yang Ming disease, the person sweats profusely, due to body fluids exiting, there is dryness in the stomach, the stool will be hard, the hardness causes delirious speech, Xiao Cheng Qi Tang governs. If after one dose the delirious speech stops, no more should be given.

XIAO CHENG QI TANG: Da Huang (washed in wine) 4 liang; Hou Po (bark removed and dried) 2 liang; Zhi Shi (fried) 3 large pieces.

DIRECTIONS: Boil all three ingredients in 4 sheng of water, reducing to 1 sheng 2 ge. Strain, divide into two doses and take warm. There should be a bowel movement after the first dose and if there is none, a second dose must be taken. Once a stool has been passed, the medication should be stopped.

DISCUSSION: Clause 213 represents the normal course of disease in the Yang Ming channel, where heat transforms into dryness and excess. The copious sweating is attributed to Yang Ming exuberant interior heat steaming the body fluids outward. Sweat is derived from the stomach and grain qi, and the excessive sweating leads to stomach dryness. The subsequent fluid depletion then fails to moisten the intestines, resulting in a dry, hard stool; from this turbid accumulation, heat and turbidity flare upward disturbing the heart shen so there is delirious speech. Xiao Cheng Qi Tang is indicated to purge heat and free the stagnant intestinal qi. The cessation of delirious speech is an indication that the medication has achieved the desired effect of draining heat and accumulation from the large intestine and so no further medication is needed.

The word 'xiao' in Xiao Cheng Qi Tang means minor, and the implication of the formula name is that it has a milder action in moving bowel excess than its related formula Da Cheng Qi Tang. The word 'da' means major, and the inclusion of Mang Xiao in that formula clears heat and moistens the stool, softening hardness and resulting in a more potent purgative action. In Xiao Cheng Qi Tang, there is no Mang Xiao and the objective is more focused on mild purging in order to alleviate the abdominal distension. This is achieved by omitting Mang Xiao and using a smaller dose of Hou Po and Zhi Shi than in Da Cheng Qi Tang. In order to achieve an optimum result, Zhang Zhong Jing's instructions should be followed, with strict adherence to the recommended dosage.

Abdominal fullness or distension is a key point of diagnosis for Xiao Cheng Qi Tang, irrespective of whether the constipation is associated with excess heat in the intestines, with food stagnation, or with gallbladder or pancreatic disease; the main signs and symptoms are abdominal distension, constipation, an inability to pass wind, a thick yellow tongue coat and a slippery and forceful pulse.

Clause 214

阳明病，谵语、发潮热、脉滑而疾者，小承气汤主之。因与承气汤一升，腹中转气者，更服一升；若不转气者，勿更与之。明日又不大便，脉反微涩者，里虚也，为难治，不可更与承气汤也。

Yang Ming disease, if there is delirious speech, tidal fever, a pulse which is slippery and swift, Xiao Cheng Qi Tang governs. Because one sheng of Cheng Qi Tang was given, qi moves in the abdomen, then a further one sheng should be taken; if there is no moving of qi, a further dose should not be given. If the next day again there is no stool, moreover the pulse is faint and choppy, the interior is deficient, it is difficult to treat, one should not give any more Cheng Qi Tang.

DISCUSSION: Clause 214 describes a number of manifestations of Yang Ming disease. Delirious speech is the result of the upsurge of turbid stomach heat harassing the heart shen; tidal fever is characteristic of stomach heat excess and describes the regular waxing and waning in temperature which resembles the ebb and flow of the ocean tide; the slippery pulse represents the accumulation of phlegm or food stagnation, whilst the word 'swift' here (疾) implies pathological rapidity, indicating excess heat. The fact that it is not submerged and full is a sign that the bowel excess pattern is still in its initial stage and therefore, Xiao Cheng Qi Tang is the formula used to moderately purge the heat. Rather than the usual 6 ge dose, a larger dose of 1 sheng is recommended in order to achieve an immediate effect. If, following this larger dose, there is a positive response represented by the sensation of qi moving in the abdomen, then the practitioner can be assured that the treatment is correct but the dose is inadequate, so a further dose is required to achieve the full effect. If, however, following the initial 1 sheng dose, there is no movement of qi in the abdomen, then the Yang Ming heat bind is not deep-seated and further medication is not warranted. If the constipation persists to the next day and the pulse is faint and choppy, then qi and blood are deficient. This is difficult to treat because in a Yang Ming deficiency pattern, neither purgation nor tonification can be used, leaving few other options.

This clause depends on the pulse sign as an important tool in identifying the Xiao Cheng Qi Tang pattern. From this, an implied differentiation is made between the slippery and rapid pulse in a Xiao Cheng Qi Tang pattern, and the submerged and forceful pulse of a Da Cheng Qi Tang pattern. After taking Xiao Cheng Qi Tang, the change from a slippery, rapid pulse to one which is faint and choppy indicates a deficiency of qi and blood. Xiao Cheng Qi Tang is unsuitable, but Huang Long Tang or a modified version of Xin Jia Huang Long Tang can be used to drain heat and simultaneously benefit qi.

Clause 250

太阳病，若吐、若下、若发汗后，微烦，小便数、大便因硬者，与小承气汤，和之愈。

Tai Yang disease, after vomiting purgation and sweat promotion, if there is mild vexation, frequent urination, causing the stool to be hard, give Xiao Cheng Qi Tang, to harmonise and bring recovery.

DISCUSSION: Vomiting, purgation and sweating all cause fluid loss. Purgation, in particular, leads to the depletion of fluids in the lower jiao. Sweating injures qi, giving opportunity for the pathogen to fall inward, occupying the Yang Ming, where it will consume fluids and generate dryness. The pathogenic heat drives fluids to the urinary bladder, manifesting as urinary frequency. Where fluids are damaged by purgation, emesis or diaphoresis, or all three, the stool will be dry and hard. Heat flaring in the Yang Ming channel harasses the heart causing vexation. Xiao Cheng Qi Tang treats the cause of all these symptoms by purging heat and harmonising the stomach and intestines.

Both Xiao Cheng Qi Tang and Ma Zi Ren Wan can be used to treat a dry stool with frequent urination which results from fluid damage caused by incorrect treatment of a Tai Yang disorder. In both patterns, incorrect treatment and subsequent loss of fluids results in the pathogen falling inward and transforming into heat. However, each pattern and its formula represent a different pathogenesis, and each represents a different ratio of heat to fluid damage. The focus of Xiao Cheng Qi Tang is clearing heat, whereby it preserves the fluids. It is used where fluid damage is secondary to interior heat. Ma Zi Ren Wan, by contrast, is used where excessive sweating has damaged fluids and where stomach heat has restrained the spleen's function of transporting water. In this situation, fluid damage is the primary concern, with heat taking second place, and the moistening properties of Ma Zi Ren Wan are needed. If the patient presents with abdominal fullness and pain, a hard dry stool, a thick yellow tongue coat, sweating and vexation but no tidal fever, then Ma Zi Ren Wan is the appropriate formula as it contains Ma Ren, Shao Yao, Xing Ren and honey, creating a milder purging formula which is indicated for patients with a weak constitution and in the treatment of postpartum constipation or chronic constipation in the elderly ascribed to yin deficiency.

Ancient Application of Xiao Cheng Qi Tang

- There are eighteen references to the application of Xiao Cheng Qi Tang in *Shang Han Lun*, most of which are used in Yang Ming bowel excess characterised by abdominal fullness, tidal fever, a hard stool, profuse sweating, delirious speech and a slippery and rapid pulse.
- *Su Wen: Bing Ji Qi Yi Bao Ming Ji:* Xiao Cheng Qi Tang with the addition of Qiang Huo for the treatment of an exterior pattern with interior excess and constipation.
- *Yi Xue Gang Mu:* For the treatment of *zhong xiao* or diabetes of the middle jiao characterised by insatiable hunger, stomach heat, dark urination and slight diarrhoea.
- *Yi Xue Ru Men Liang Fang:* For the treatment of the early stage of dysentery characterised by abdominal pain and tenesmus.

Modern Application of Xiao Cheng Qi Tang

- In the treatment of stomach and intestinal excess with constipation, as may be seen in acute pancreatitis, cholecystitis, infectious hepatitis, cholelithiasis or bacterial dysentery attributed to Yang Ming dry heat bind characterised by abdominal fullness and pain, constipation, tenesmus, diarrhoea with blood and mucus, and protracted tidal fever. Zhang Shou Jie et al (*Yun Nan Yi Yao* 2:102 1982) treated 40 cases of viral hepatitis using Xiao Cheng Qi Tang (Zhi Da Huang 10g; Zhi Shi 15g; Hou Po 15g; Gan Cao 3g) with full recovery in 39 cases and no effect in 1 case where the patient suffered from hepatitis B.
- Huang Xiao Gong et al (*Zhong Yi Za Zhi* 4: 31 1983) used Xiao Cheng Qi Tang modified to treat chronic gastric volvulus. (Sheng Da Huang 3g, added at the end; Zhi Qiao 30g; Hou Po 9g; Jiang Ban Xia 9g; Fu Ling 10g; Xu Geng 9g; Bai Kou Ren 6g; Cang Zhu 9g; Chen Pi 9g; Dan Shen 30g). The patient had suffered from upper abdominal distension for six years and had a poor appetite, abdominal bloating after eating, occasional nausea and vomiting, frequent belching, a dry stool, a purplish tongue with stasis spots, a white, slippery, greasy tongue coat and a wiry, slippery pulse. He was given five packs of the above formula after which the abdominal distension and belching eased substantially. The original formula was repeated with the addition of Chen Xiang 2g for nineteen packs. A barium X-ray confirmed that the gastric volvulus had resolved.
- Chai Zhen Xing et al (*Hu Bei Zhong Yi Za Zhi* 1983; 4:31) used Xiao Cheng Qi Tang in the treatment of various paediatric diseases including food stagnation, oedema, jaundice, cough and wheeze, and infantile convulsions. All were diagnosed according to pattern identification with corresponding modifications to the main formula. Dr Chai confirmed that timely treatment and correct pattern diagnosis produced the most effective results. He summed up the function of Xiao Cheng Qi Tang as follows. (1) Xiao Cheng Qi Tang combined with herbs which clear heat and relieve toxicity can be used for a pattern of Yang Ming dry heat characterised by abdominal pain and fullness, a dry, hard stool, vigorous fever, thirst, haemorrhage and a red tongue with a yellow tongue coat. (2) Xiao Cheng Qi Tang combined with herbs which reduce food stagnation can be used in the treatment of infantile food accumulation syndrome or *gan ji* (疳积), which has transformed into heat resulting in a dry, hard stool, abdominal distension, thirst and fever. (3) Xiao Cheng Qi Tang can eliminate phlegm and clear heat and is therefore indicated for interior heat and phlegm turbidity. Where stomach heat obstructs the lung qi causing cough, wheezing, phlegm rale, and a stifling sensation in the chest, Xiao Cheng Qi Tang is used modified with the addition of Ban Xia, Huang Qin, Gua Lou, Jie Geng. (4) Xiao Cheng Qi Tang with the addition of such herbs as Ling Yang Jiao, Gou Teng, Ju Hua, Sang Ye can extinguish wind in

patterns of tetany or convulsions with high fever and a clouded spirit. (5) Xiao Cheng Qi Tang can unblock network vessels and is indicated for heat patterns with intestinal obstruction.

Case Study

Food Poisoning

Extracted from Zhong Yi Za Zhi 1993; (3):145

A five-year-old girl had a fever caused by eating contaminated food three days earlier. Her temperature was above 39°C and she had convulsions. She was hospitalised and given an anti-pyretic drip and an antibiotic but her condition did not improve. The fever persisted and she also had a sore throat. Her breathing was harsh and rapid and her abdomen was hard. Her tongue was red with a dry yellow coat and her pulse was wiry and rapid. The diagnosis was stomach and intestinal heat bind with an unresolved exterior pattern. The formula prescribed was based on Xiao Cheng Qi Tang: Sheng Da Huang 6g, Hou Po 3g, Zhi Shi 5g, Jin Yin Hua 15g, Lian Qiao 12g, Gou Teng 9g, Jiao Zha Qu (Jiao Shan Zha combined with Jiao Shen Qu) 9g. After one dose, she passed a stool three times and the fever receded. The formula was repeated with the omission of Da Huang and Zhi Shi and the addition of Zhi Qiao and Ji Nei Jin. She recovered after two packs.

Da Cheng Qi Tang Pattern

Clause 238

阳明病，下之，心中懊侬而烦，胃中有燥屎者，可攻。腹微满，初头硬，后必溏，不可攻之。若有燥屎者，宜大承气汤。

Yang Ming disease, there is purgation, if there is anguish and vexation, and a dry stool in the stomach, one may attack. There is mild abdominal fullness, the start of the stool is hard, the end will be sloppy, one should not purge. If there is a dry stool, Da Cheng Qi Tang is appropriate.

DA CHENG QI TANG: Da Huang (washed in wine) 4 liang; Hou Po (bark removed) ½ jin; Zhi Shi 5 pieces; Mang Xiao 3 ge.

DIRECTIONS: First boil Hou Po and Zhi Shi in 1 dou of water, reducing to 5 sheng. Strain and add Da Huang, bringing to the boil and reducing to 2 sheng. Strain again and add Mang Xiao, bringing to the boil once or twice on a mild flame. Divide into two and take warm. Once defaecation is achieved, no more should be taken.

DISCUSSION: Clause 238 first describes the situation where Yang Ming disease persists even after purgation. This is seen in the dry stool, which shows that the heat and dryness are still knotted together, giving rise to vexation. This is excess vexation and so it is permitted to 'attack' by purging and Da Cheng Qi Tang is appropriate. However, the abdominal pain and fullness is accompanied by a stool which is hard at the beginning but sloppy towards the end. This is not a manifestation of Yang Ming excess; on the contrary, it is a manifestation of spleen and stomach deficiency, where the transformation and transportation function is impaired and fails to properly separate the clear from the turbid. It stands in sharp contrast to the abdominal fullness described in Clause 255, where the abdominal fullness is not reduced, which is characteristic of a Yang Ming excess pattern. Purgation is normally contraindicated in a pattern of spleen and stomach deficiency, however, if the stool is dry, purgation can be used.

In analysing anguish and vexation occurring in a Yang Ming pattern following purgation, the pathogenesis must first be understood. There are two possibilities. (1) After purgation, the dry stool has been eliminated and the intestinal qi is restored but there is unresolved residual heat. This is also described in Clause 228 where Zhi Zi Chi Tang is the indicated formula; the vexation is insubstantial because there is no abdominal fullness, constipation or tidal fever. It is characterised by anguish, hunger with no desire to eat and sweating from the head only. The tongue coat should be thin and yellow. (2) The anguish and vexation which follow purgation are accompanied by constipation, abdominal fullness which resists pressure, and a thick yellow tongue coat. This is substantial vexation because it is caused by the knotting of pathogenic heat with the stool, and the correct treatment strategy is to eliminate the heat bind and purge the stool in order to alleviate vexation; the Cheng Qi Tang group of formulas is indicated. If there is concern that the purgation may damage the zheng qi, Zeng Ye Cheng Qi Tang (Xuan Shen, Mai Dong, Sheng Di, Da Huang, Mang Xiao) or Xin Jia Huang Long Tang (Xi Sheng Di, Sheng Gan Cao, Ren Shen, Sheng Da Huang, Mang Xiao, Xuan Shen, Mai Dong, Dang Gui, Hai Shen, Jiang Zhi) can be used.

Clause 239

病人不大便五六日，绕脐痛、烦躁、发作有时者，此有燥屎，故使不大便也。

The patient has not passed a stool for five or six days, if there is pain around the umbilicus, vexation and agitation, occurring periodically, this is because there is a dry stool, causing constipation.

DISCUSSION: The absence of a bowel movement for five or six days is not always evidence of a dry stool caused by excess heat and all signs and symptoms must be taken into account before making a diagnosis. Clause 239 explains that the periumbilical pain is a sign of constipation due to a dry stool. This is because the intestinal bind obstructs qi, causing pain in the large intestine, specifically, in the vicinity of the umbilicus. Vexation is a manifestation of heat in the Yang Ming, which not only causes a dry stool, but also surges upwards, harassing the heart shen. The qi of the Yang Ming peaks between the hours of 3pm and 5pm, at which time there is an intense struggle against the pathogen. With this periodic surge of qi in the Yang Ming, the symptoms are also at their peak. The symptoms of vexation and tidal fever confirm a pattern of interior heat in the Yang Ming and it is this heat in the Yang Ming which causes the dry stool and the constipation. The presence of periumbilical pain, however, provides only partial evidence of a dry stool; further evidence is elicited by palpation, when the pain is exacerbated by pressure, demonstrating excess.

Clause 215

阳明病，谵语、有潮热、反不能食者，胃中必有燥屎五六枚也；若能食者，但硬耳。宜大承气汤下之。

Yang Ming disease, if there is delirious speech, tidal fever but an inability to eat, there will be five or six lumps of dry stool in the stomach; where a person is able to eat, it is just hard. Da Cheng Qi Tang is appropriate.

DISCUSSION: Clause 215 decribes the principal manifestations of excess heat in a Yang Ming bowel pattern, namely delirious speech, tidal fever, and a dry stool. Being unable to eat is a secondary symptom caused by the knotting of dryness and heat obstructing the descent of stomach qi. In the classics, the term 'stomach' was often used to refer also to the intestines, which is easily explained by their close anatomical proximity and also their partnership in the Yang Ming channel. The reference to lumps of stool in the stomach here simply refers to their location centrally in the abdomen, coinciding with the location of the transverse colon. The fact that the stool has separated into pieces shows the extent to which it has dried out, and it is the presence of palpable and in all probability impacted faeces, which is the basis for using Da Cheng Qi Tang. The dry stool further obstructs the downward movement of stomach qi, causing food stagnation which results in an inability to eat. Da Cheng Qi Tang is used to eliminate the obstruction and restore the descent of qi.

Although punctuation was not used in the classical Chinese of the original document, it has been added in later versions to assist in interpretation. In Clause 215, the fullstop inserted before the final sentence: "Da Cheng Qi Tang is appropriate" is a guide to interpretation. It shows that the last two statements are not linked and that the last sentence, "Da Cheng Qi Tang is appropriate" does not relate to the statement which precedes it: "where a person is able to eat, it is just hard". This represents a milder condition, mentioned only for contrast, and should be read as if in parentheses. Even where there is delirious speech and tidal fever, the ability to eat shows that the descent of stomach qi has not been seriously affected, and so the practitioner knows that the stool is hard but does not represent a knotted heat bind. Da Cheng Qi Tang is therefore not appropriate and Xiao Cheng Qi Tang should be used instead.

It must be remembered that no single symptom can be relied upon for a diagnosis. All symptoms must be seen in the context of the whole pattern, including its aetiology and pathogenesis. The symptom of being unable to eat is but one example. Based on the pathogenesis, the symptom of being unable to eat found in Clause 215 has different implications from the same symptom mentioned in Clause 190. In Clause 215 the inability to eat is an indication of the obstruction of the descent of stomach qi, indicating that the hard stool is the result of knotted bind. By contrast, the inability to eat in Clause 190 is caused by pathogenic cold which has damaged the stomach yang, resulting in the non-transformation of water and grain.

Clause 241

大下后，六七日不大便，烦不解，腹满痛者，此有燥屎也。所以然者，本有宿食故也。宜大承气汤。

After strong purging, if there is no stool for six or seven days, unresolved vexation, the abdomen is full and painful, this means there is a dry stool. The reason for this being, originally there was accumulated food. Da Cheng Qi Tang is appropriate.

DISCUSSION: After heavy purging, if there is no bowel movement, and there is vexation and abdominal pain and distension, it means that the stool is dry and there is a long-standing accumulation of food in the Yang Ming, generating heat. Da Cheng Qi Tang is indicated to purge the stool and also to purge the bind of food stagnation. Incomplete defaecation can be associated with two situations: (1) bind due to food accumulation which has not been completely purged by the initial medication, and (2) failure of the initial purging to effectively drain heat. In the latter case, because the intestinal fluids are not fully restored, bind results from heat binding with the stagnant, undigested food. In both cases, Da Cheng Qi Tang is indicated to eliminate the intestinal heat bind.

When initial sweat promotion fails to fully expel the exterior in a Tai Yang pattern, sweat can be promoted a second time providing the Tai Yang disease pattern still prevails. Similarly, in Yang Ming disease, if the results of initial purging are incomplete, further purging can be used. In the absence of any sign of deficiency, repeated purging can be used to eliminate any residual pathogenic heat bind. It is essential to observe the pulse and any other subtle changes. If, after one episode of purgation, constipation and abdominal fullness persist, and there is a parched throat, a black tongue coat and a submerged, excess and forceful pulse, instead of Da Cheng Qi Tang, one can give Wu Ju Tong's Hu Wei Cheng Qi Tang (Da Huang, Xuan Shen, Sheng Di, Dan Pi, Zhi Mu, Mai Dong) to purge heat and nourish fluids.

Clause 242

病人小便不利，大便乍难乍易，时有微热，喘冒不能卧者 ，有燥屎也，宜大承气汤。

The patient's urination is not free, passing a stool is sometimes difficult and sometimes easy, with an occasional mild fever, if there is wheeze and dizziness with an inability to sleep, there is a dry stool, Da Cheng Qi Tang is appropriate.

DISCUSSION: The dryness and heat of a Yang Ming bowel pattern represents an obstruction to the qi of the stomach and large intestine, and manifests with constipation; the depleted fluids result in inhibited urination. The mild fever, wheezing and dizziness, and the inability to sleep are caused by the turbid heat surging upwards, harassing the upper jiao. The underlying cause of all these symptoms is pathogenic heat with dry stool bind in the interior. This obstructs the qi dynamic and so impairs the normal function of the zang fu organs. The strategy is to "remove the firewood from under the cauldron", which refers to the strategy of draining heat in order to preserve fluids. This is achieved by draining heat and purging the stool.

The main difficulty is in determining when best to administer Da Cheng Qi Tang. The fundamental rule is that there must be a dry stool, however, there are important principles which apply. The first is that purgation can not be used merely on the basis of a dry stool. This is particularly true in the treatment of febrile disease; in this situation, other symptoms such as the patient's mental state, abdominal symptoms, sweating, the colour and volume of urination, respiration rate and tongue and pulse signs must all be taken into consideration as part of the diagnostic procedure. The second principle is that purgation can be used even in the absence of such characteristic symptoms as tidal fever, delirious speech, or other symptoms cited above such as wheezing and inability to sleep, providing the main symptoms of constipation and abdominal fullness prevail.

There are two scenarios associated with the dry stool of a Da Cheng Qi Tang pattern: (1) in febrile disease a dry stool is one of the key symptoms of a Yang Ming bowel excess pattern and may be accompanied by vexation, tidal fever, sweating, wheezing and delirious speech; (2) the patient exhibits abdominal fullness and constipation but without obvious signs of toxic heat. As described in Clause 255: "Abdominal fullness is not reduced, or reduction is inadequate so to speak, one must purge, Da Cheng Qi Tang is appropriate".

Clause 220

二阳并病，太阳证罢，但发潮热，手足漐漐汗出，大便难而谵语者，下之则愈，宜大承气汤。

Lagover pattern of the two yang, Tai Yang pattern has finished, but there is tidal fever, sweat pouring from the hands and feet, if passing a stool is difficult and there is delirious speech, purging will bring recovery, Da Cheng Qi Tang is appropriate.

DISCUSSION: The two yang referred to are the Tai Yang and Yang Ming. When the Tai Yang pattern is not resolved, and the pathogen proceeds to the Yang Ming, there arises a lagover pattern involving a Tai Yang exterior pattern and a Yang Ming interior pattern, as described earlier in Clause 48 in section 2.7 Tai Yang Transmuted Patterns. In the situation where Tai Yang disease is fully resolved and the pathogenic heat has transferred to the Yang Ming as described here, the characteristic symptoms are tidal fever, sweating from the limbs, a difficult bowel movement and delirious speech. Such manifestations are indicative of a Yang Ming stomach excess pattern, of which tidal fever is a classic feature. In Clause 220 above, the additional symptom of sweat pouring from the limbs is a reflection of exuberant interior heat steaming the body fluids outward; delirious speech is due to stomach heat harassing the heart shen; the excess and dryness in the bowel obstruct intestinal qi, making the bowel movement difficult. Da Cheng Qi Tang purges the dry bind and unblocks the intestinal obstruction.

In considering *Shang Han Lun* lagover patterns, it is essential for the reader to find the central point. Clause 220 focuses on the symptoms of tidal fever and sweating from the limbs, which distinguish it from a Tai Yang zhong feng Gui Zhi Tang pattern and show clearly that the appropriate treatment strategy is to purge Yang Ming interior heat.

A distinction must also be made between Clauses 220 and 219. Clause 219 describes a concurrent pattern of the three yang with the focus on the Yang Ming: the heat affected the stomach but not the large intestine and the strategy was to clear heat without purging. Clause 220 is also a Yang Ming pattern but the focus is on the large intestine: simply clearing heat is inadequate and potent purging is warranted. The treatment is dictated by the pathogenesis.

Urgent Purgation

Clause 252

伤寒六七日，目中不了了，睛不和，无表里证，大便难，身微热者，此为实也。急下之，宜大承气汤。

Shang han for six or seven days, the vision is not clear, there is no harmony in the eyes, there is neither an exterior nor an interior pattern, passing a stool is difficult, the body emits a mild heat, this is excess. Urgent purgation is needed, Da Cheng Qi Tang is appropriate.

DISCUSSION: If the exterior signs of aversion to cold and fever are absent after six or seven days of shang han disease, and there is no evidence of interior excess, such as abdominal fullness, constipation, delirious speech or tidal fever, then why is there the need to purge urgently? *Ling Shu: Da Huo Lun Pian (Chapter 80 Discourse on Great Perplexities)* says: "The essence qi of the five zang and six fu ascends to fill the eyes". If the patient is unable to see clearly and if the eyes lack harmony, by which it is meant that they are dull and not able to move freely, then it can be understood that the dryness and heat of Yang Ming has exhausted the essence of the liver and kidneys. This implies that the condition is critical, with the kidney essence, qi and blood verging on total devastation. The condition must not be misjudged as being mild simply because the heat emitted by the body is mild. On the contrary, the mildness of the fever is a sign of the severe depletion of essence and the exhausted state of zheng qi, which is unable to contend with the pathogen. There is no mention of a faint and choppy pulse as found in Clause 212, however, the reference to it being an excess pattern intimates that in spite of the condition being critical, there is still a chance of survival. Urgent purgation is needed in order to expel the pathogenic heat and restore fluids. The seriousness of the condition is emphasised by the visual manifestations, which testify to the extent that pathogenic heat has damaged yin.

Clause 253

阳明病，发热、汗多者，急下之，宜大承气汤。

Yang Ming disease, if there is fever and copious sweating, for urgent purgation, Da Cheng Qi Tang is appropriate.

DISCUSSION: The Yang Ming disease in Clause 253 refers specifically to a Yang Ming bowel excess pattern where abdominal fullness and constipation are among the identifying clinical features. Whilst not mentioned in this clause, they can be understood from the reading of the foregoing Clause 252. In addition to abdominal symptoms, the constrained Yang Ming heat gives rise to tidal fever, with sweat which streams from the arms and legs. By purging heat, the root is treated and fluids are preserved. Da Cheng Qi Tang preserves the yin fluids by purging the heat which consumes them, and by eliminating the bound stool, which can itself generate more heat. This purging strategy had a significant impact on the later wen bing specialists, who declared: "In warm diseases, it is never too early to purge."

Clause 254

发汗不解，腹满痛者，急下之，宜大承气汤。

Promoting sweat does not bring resolution, if there is abdominal fullness and pain, for urgent purgation, Da Cheng Qi Tang is appropriate.

DISCUSSION: Clause 254 describes a situation where diaphoresis has failed to release the exterior, and is followed by abdominal fullness and pain. These symptoms are a reflection of interior heat, showing that the disease has entered the interior; the pathogenic heat has consumed and scorched fluids, giving rise to obstruction and a dry stool. Da Cheng Qi Tang is indicated as an emergency measure to purge the heat and preserve the yin.

Pain and distension in the abdomen can be attributed to qi stagnation, food stagnation or stasis; the appropriate treatment strategy is chosen according to the differential diagnosis. In *Shang Han Lun*, the strategy of urgent purgation is used as an emergency measure, purging heat so as to prevent the further devastation of yin. This strategy is used in the presence of the following clinical features: severe abdominal fullness and distension, pain which resists pressure, a submerged but forceful pulse and a greasy yellow tongue coat.

In regard to the adoption of urgent purgation in order to preserve the yin, some specialists suggest that all four symptoms of "glomus, fullness, dryness and excess" (痞满燥实) should be present before purging; but not all support that theory. The fact is that this is a Yang Ming pattern with damage to Shao Yin essence means that faithful adherence to all four signs of glomus, fullness, dryness and excess is neither realistic nor necessary. Primarily, the condition must be recognised as being urgent because of the potential for the essence to be scorched and exhausted by the heat.

Urgent purgation is used where the condition is critical due to injury to stomach yin and kidney essence, and as a preventative measure to pre-empt damage to yin where there is severe heat. In the strategy of urgent purgation, the practioner is not limited to Cheng Qi Tang formulas. It is of interest to note that the later development of five additional modifications of Cheng Qi Tang used in the treatment of wen bing or warm diseases were a consequence of this theory.

Clause 255

腹满不减，减不足言，当下之，宜大承气汤。

Abdominal fullness is not reduced, or reduction is inadequate so to speak, one must purge, Da Cheng Qi Tang is appropriate.

DISCUSSION: Pain is differentiated according to whether it is associated with heat or cold, excess or deficiency. The abdominal pain mentioned in Clause 255 states that purging is appropriate if abdominal pain and distension are not substantially reduced, and the implication is that the abdominal symptoms are caused by excess heat.

Although in Yang Ming patterns, abdominal pain is associated with excess heat, abdominal pain can also be associated with deficiency cold, as written in *Jin Gui Yao Lue: On Pulse, Symptom Complex and Treatment of Abdominal Distension and Abdominal Pain caused by Cold and Indigestion*: "Abdominal fullness can occasionally be reduced. This is due to coldness and warm herbs should be used". Abdominal distension associated with deficiency cold is generally accompanied by a loose stool which when passed, offers no relief. The tongue coat is white and greasy, and the pulse is submerged and slow and the appropriate formula is Li Zhong Wan to scatter cold and warm the middle. As a general rule, abdominal pain and distension caused by excess heat are exacerbated by pressure and are accompanied by constipation, rather than a loose stool. Further, the tongue coat is yellow and greasy and there is a submerged, excess and rapid pulse. The appropriate formula is Cheng Qi Tang.

Clause 217

汗出谵语者，以有燥屎在胃中，此为风也。须下者，过经乃可下之。下之若早，语言必乱，以表虚里实故也。下之愈，宜大承气汤。

If there is sweating and delirious speech, it is because of a dry stool in the stomach, this is wind. If one must purge, since it has passed through the channel then one may purge. If one purges early, speech will be deranged, this is because the exterior is deficient and the interior is excess. Purgation will bring recovery, Da Cheng Qi Tang is appropriate.

DISCUSSION: Clause 217 describes a concurrent exterior and interior pattern. The sweating is not the sweating of interior heat, but the sweating of an unresolved exterior Yang Ming pattern and therefore attributed to wind; the delirious speech represents the interior Yang Ming bowel excess pattern and is therefore attributed to the dry stool.

In this clause, as in Clause 215, the term 'stomach' is used in a general sense to indicate the Yang Ming large intestine. The concurrence of sweating, which is an exterior symptom, and delirious speech, which indicates an interior pattern, demonstrates that this is a concurrent channel and fu pattern.

Purgation must not be used when the exterior pathogen is still not resolved; inappropriately early purgation, before the manifestastion of bowel excess, will cause the pathogen to fall inwards and fuel the interior heat, causing deranged speech. The phrase: "the exterior is deficient and the interior is excess" describes this situation, where the pathogen has left the exterior, leaving it 'empty' or deficient, and entered the interior, making it 'full' or excess. Once this interior excess heat has transformed into bowel excess, purgation is the correct treatment to affect recovery.

There are three principles relevant to this situation: the first is the priority of releasing the exterior before treating the interior in a concurrent exterior and interior pattern; the second is the contraindication of purgation in the presence of an unresolved pathogen; the third is the pre-requisite of bowel excess in purgation. However, the order of treatment of concurrent interior and exterior patterns is actually dependent on circumstances: where the exterior pattern is predominant, releasing the exterior is prioritised; where the interior pattern predominates, the exterior and interior are addressed simultaneously. However, regardless of these basic principles, in the case of a critical condition, whichever pattern is the more critical must be given priority.

Clause 256

阳明少阳合病，必下利，其脉不负者，为顺也；负者，失也，互相克贼，名为负也，脉滑而数者，有宿食也，当下之，宜大承气汤。

In a concurrent pattern of Yang Ming and Shao Yang, there will be diarrhoea, if the pulse, has no deficit, it is favourable; if it has a deficit, this is loss, mutual subjugation and plunder, this is deficit, if the pulse is slippery and rapid, there is accumulated food, one must purge, Da Cheng Qi Tang is appropriate.

DISCUSSION: Yang Ming governs the earth and the stomach is its province; Shao Yang governs wood and the gallbladder is its province; the stomach is paired with the spleen and the gallbladder with the liver. Yang Ming and Shao Yang refer to the stomach and spleen, gallbladder and liver and are related to the earth and wood elements respectively. Thus their interrelationship is affected by the restraining sequence in five element theory. The pattern in Clause 256 is a concurrent pattern of Yang Ming and Shao Yang, which is characterised by exuberant excess heat inhibiting the function of the spleen and stomach, causing diarrhoea.

The pulse sign can be used as a prognostic tool and can predict whether the outcome will be adverse or not. The term *fu* (负) refers to loss or deficit. If the pulse suffers no loss or deficit, it means that the stomach qi is intact and it has not been harassed by the gallbladder qi. Earth has not been invaded by wood and so the zheng qi is unaffected. Therefore, as long as the pulse is not adversely affected, the diarrhoea does not represent serious disease and the prognosis is favourable. However, diarrhoea accompanied by a wiry pulse shows that the Shao Yang has the upper hand and is bullying the stomach; the gallbladder fire is harassing the spleen and the stomach qi is devastated; wood is attacking earth and stomach qi suffers a loss, therefore offering a poor prognosis.

'Subjugation' is a reference to the situation of wood invading earth, where the gallbladder has restrained the stomach and spleen, and the term 'plunder' alludes to the collateral damage to zheng qi which is tantamount to theft. The slippery pulse indicates food accumulation and a rapid pulse is a reflection of the heat in the Yang Ming. These combined pulse images are a reflection of the food stagnation in the Yang Ming with heat and dryness knotted in the large intestine. The appropriate formula is Da Cheng Qi Tang.

In *Shang Han Lun* there are three clauses which discuss concurrent patterns with diarrhoea. Clause 32 is associated with a Tai Yang Yang Ming concurrent pattern, where the corresponding formula is Ge Gen Tang, which releases the exterior and stops the diarrhoea; Clause 172 is associated with a Tai Yang Shao Yang concurrent pattern where the corresponding formula is Huang Qin Tang to clear heat and harmonise the interior; and Clause 256 describes a Yang Ming Shao Yang concurrent pattern where the indicated formula is Da Cheng Qi Tang, because the focus is Yang Ming.

The type of diarrhoea described in Clause 256 refers to the discharge of faecal fluid which can leak from around the knotted stool. The knotting of heat and dryness is associated with food stagnation in the stomach and large intestine, which obstructs intestinal qi resulting in a stagnant hard stool, with the heat percolating fluids from the stool which leak out as a foul watery discharge. The failure of stomach qi to descend also impairs its function of receiving food, so there is an inability to eat, and the accompanying symptoms of tidal fever and abdominal fullness complete the picture for a Yang Ming pattern.

Yang Ming Fu Excess and Prognosis

Clause 212

伤寒，若吐、若下后不解，不大便五六日，上至十余日，日晡所发潮热，不恶寒，独语如见鬼状；若剧者，发则不识人，循衣摸床，惕而不安，微喘直视，脉弦者生，涩者死。微者，但发热谵语者，大承气汤主之。若一服利，则止后服。

Shang han, if, after emesis and purgation, there is no resolution, there is no stool for five or six days, even for more than ten days, in the late afternoon there will then be tidal fever, no aversion to cold, the person will talk to themself as if seeing ghosts; if it is serious, then they will not recognise anyone, will pick at their clothes and pat the bedding, be fearful and restless, will pant slightly and stare straight ahead, if the pulse is wiry, the person will live, if choppy they will die. If mild, where there is only fever with delirious speech, Da Cheng Qi Tang governs. If, having taken one dose, there is diarrhoea, then stop subsequent doses.

DISCUSSION: If shang han disease is treated with either vomiting or purgation, there will be damage to fluids and a potential for the pathogen to fall inward causing heat bind in the Yang Ming. The fluid damage will also result in intestinal dryness and constipation. In Clause 212, the tidal fever is interpreted as a manifestation of bowel excess; talking out loud as if suffering hallucinations, and seeing ghosts can be ascribed to exuberant heat harassing the heart shen. In this situation, the role of Da Cheng Qi Tang is to expedite the exit of the pathogenic heat with the objective of preserving fluids and saving them from further damage. If decisive purging is not employed, the heat will scorch the true yin causing the condition to deteriorate. The inability to recognise people, the constant fiddling with their clothing and bedsheets and the sense of fear and restlessness are all consequences of fire flaring upwards and disturbing the heart shen and of severely depleted yin essence; the panting is not to be confused with the gasping associated with wheezing, but is a reflection of the depletion of zheng qi where the lung qi is verging on expiry. The staring gaze is a sign of the exhaustion of liver blood and kidney essence. Prognosis is made on the basis of the pulse sign. A choppy pulse is indicative of exhaustion of qi and blood, and so the prognosis is poor: the condition is not treatable and the person will die. However, a wiry pulse is evidence that yin qi is adequate and zheng qi still intact. If the condition is mild, manifesting only with fever and confused speech as opposed to the more serious condition earlier described, where the patient was talking out loud to himself and had other signs of significant shen disturbance, Da Cheng Qi Tang is indicated to purge the excess heat. However, the caution is issued to discontinue purging as soon as a loose stool is passed and the condition relieved, in order to avoid excessive purging and damage to zheng qi.

The message behind this clause is that purging can be used to treat a condition of severe internal heat in order to prevent the further consumption of yin. Optimum results are obtained by purging at the appropriate time according to an understanding of the pathogenesis.

Ancient Application of Da Cheng Qi Tang

- *Qian Jin Yao Fang:* Da Cheng Qi Tang omitting Hou Po and adding Sheng Di, Shao Yao and Xing Ren was used to treat *guan ge* (关格) which is a severe form of dysphagia characterised by vomiting and a sensation of obstruction in the throat.

- *Wai Tai Mi Yao:* Cui Shi Cheng Qi Tang, which is Da Cheng Qi Tang with Hou Po omitted and with the addition of Xing Ren and Bai Mi (honey), was used to treat severe constipation where a stool had not been passed for more than ten days.
- *Huang Han Yi Xue: Yan Ke Jin Nang:* For the treatment of constipation due to intestinal heat which causes blurred vision.
- *Lei Ju Fang Guang Yi:* Da Cheng Qi Tang was cited in the treatment of measles where there was aversion to heat, abdominal fullness, vexation, delirious speech, a cracked tongue with a black coat, and constipation or foul smelling watery diarrhoea. It was also used for the treatment of dysentery characterised by vigorous fever, abdominal fullness and pain, a parched throat, diarrhoea with more than ten episodes a day, or diarrhoea with blood.
- *Wen Bing Tiao Bian:* Augmented the scope of purgative therapy with additional purging formulas such as Dao Chi Cheng Qi Tang, Niu Huang Cheng Qi Tang, Xuan Bai Cheng Qi Tang, Zeng Ye Cheng Qi Tang and Xin Jia Huang Long Tang.

Modern Application of Da Cheng Qi Tang

- *Haemorrhagic fever.* Li et al used the purging method to treat 29 cases of haemorrhagic fever during the scant urination phase to alleviate emphysema and cerebral oedema, and reduce azotemia to facilitate the recovery of kidney function. To reduce cranial pressure, mannitol 25g was administered first and Da Cheng Qi Tang was administered 30 minutes later (Da Huang 30g, Mang Xiao 15g, Zhi Shi 15g). Where there was no bowel movement after 4 to 6 hours, the medication was repeated up to three times (Li Xun Lan: *Jiang Xi Yi Yao* 1983; 3: 67).
- *Acute bacterial dysentery.* Zhang et al used Da Cheng Qi Tang modified (Da Huang, Zhi Shi, Hou Po, Mang Xiao, Bai Tou Weng, Huang Lian, Huang Bai, Qin Pi) in the treatment of acute bacterial dysentery characterised by a thick yellow tongue coat, a submerged, forceful pulse, and abdominal pain which was aggravated by pressure. After one dose, there was no more pain. Two packs of Bai Tou Weng Tang was then prescribed (*Shang Han Lun Fang Yun Yong Fa*).
- A summary of 13 journal articles reported a total of 14,409 cases of intestinal obstruction treated by using purgation: 9266 cases were significantly relieved and the success rate was 66.7%. Purgative therapy can be used for simple intestinal obstruction due to faecal impaction, ascariasis or adhesions, but it is contraindicated in cases of obstruction caused by malignant tumour or strangulation (*Shaan Xi Xin Yi Yao* 2:23 1973; *Zhi Liao Hui Bian* pp19 1975; *Zhi Liao Hui Bian* pp 86 1973; *Lin Chuan Yu Ke Yan Zhi Liao Hui Bian* 3:46 1976; *Shang Hai Zhong Yi Za Zhi* 12:20 1964; *Xin Yi Xue* 3:118 1977).

Case Study

Constipation with a Foul Discharge

Extracted from Zhong Yi Za Zhi 1990; 3:21

A 70-year-old female patient presented with a foul watery discharge from the bowel without a bowel motion. Her pulse was thready and wiry and she had a thick white tongue coat. A green watery discharge was passed about ten times a day. She also had a sensation of fullness below the heart, abdominal distension and pain which was worse when palpated, belching, the occasional vomiting of a watery fluid, a dry throat, a preference for cold food, and scant dark-coloured urine. She had been given a herbal formula to nourish the fluids but it was not effective. The diagnosis was knotted heat bind manifesting as constipation with the leakage of fluid. The treatment principle was urgent purgation to preserve fluid and the formula prescribed was Da Cheng Qi Tang: Da Huang 9g, Zhi Shi 6g, Mang Xiao 3g, Hou Po 3g. After one pack in the evening, she passed a stool the next morning, but the belching and abdominal fullness persisted. She complained of thirst and slight fullness in the epigastrium, sweating and disturbing dreams. Her pulse was thready and slippery. She was then given Bai Hu jia Ren Shen Tang, adding Mai Dong 15g, Xuan Fu Hua 6g, Dai Zhe Shi 10g. Full recovery resulted.

Comparison of Cheng Qi Tang Patterns

Clause 208

阳明病，脉迟，虽汗出不恶寒者，其身必重，短气、腹满而喘，有潮热者，此外欲解，可攻里也。手足濈然汗出者，此大便已硬也，大承气汤主之；若汗多、微发热恶寒者，外未解也；其热不潮，未可与承气汤；若腹大满不通者，可与小承气汤，微和胃气，勿令至大泄下。

Yang Ming disease, if the pulse is slow, even though there is sweating with no aversion to cold, the body will be heavy, if there is shortness of breath, abdominal fullness and wheezing, with tidal fever, this is because the exterior is about to resolve, one may purge the interior. If there is sweating from the hands and feet, the stool is already hard, Da Cheng Qi Tang governs. If sweating is profuse, there is a slight fever and aversion to cold, the exterior is not resolved; the fever is not tidal, one must not give Cheng Qi Tang; if there is severe abdominal fullness with constipation, one may give Xiao Cheng Qi Tang, to mildly harmonise the stomach qi, do not induce potent purging.

DISCUSSION: There are three purging formulas, Tiao Wei Cheng Qi Tang, Xiao Cheng Qi Tang and Da Cheng Qi Tang, each with a different application. Clause 208 focuses on the two formulas Da Cheng Qi Tang and Xiao Cheng Qi Tang, and also specifies differential criteria for their application. In a Da Cheng Qi Tang pattern, the pulse is moderate and there is no aversion to cold, showing that the exterior is resolved and the pathogen has fallen inward. The symptoms of abdominal fullness, heaviness, shortness of breath and wheezing are all manifestations of the interior excess heat obstructing the qi dynamic, and when heat consumes body fluids causing intestinal dryness, there will be a dry stool. The presence of tidal fever is a sign that the exterior is resolved and purgation can be used for the interior excess. The term 'hands and feet' (手足) in Chinese can refer to the lower part of the arms and legs as well. This symptom of sweating from the extremities, accompanied as it is by a slow pulse, is a reflection of depressed interior heat which is unable to disperse and so seeks an exit in this limited way. Thus Clause 208 describes the signs and symptoms of Da Cheng Qi Tang.

The clause goes on to describe a Xiao Cheng Qi Tang pattern, where aversion to cold and the absence of tidal fever show that the exterior is not resolved. Nevertheless, the main symptom is the intestinal blockage indicated by the abdominal fullness and constipation, and so Xiao Cheng Qi Tang is used to mildly harmonise the stomach qi and moderately purge heat without the harsher effects of a potent purgative such as Da Cheng Qi Tang.

Comparison of Da and Xiao Cheng Qi Tang

The term 'cheng qi' is often translated as 'to order qi' and in this context has the sense of taking charge of qi, referring to its ability to facilitate the proper descent of stomach and intestinal qi in order to expel turbidity and thus support the zheng qi. Mang Xiao softens hardness and clears heat, thus dissipating the knotted bind and moistening the dry stool. Hou Po and Zhi Shi are strong qi regulating herbs which have a descending effect and move qi and disperse stagnation. Da Huang is bitter and cold and drains by purging the stomach and intestines. The combined effect of these four herbs serves to eliminate stagnation, dispel bind and purge the heat pathogen by draining downwards. The key points differentiating the application of Da and Xiao Cheng Qi Tang and their contraindications are as follows.

1. *Aversion to cold.* This indicates an unresolved exterior and purging is contraindicated.
2. *Absence of tidal fever.* This indicates that the excess dryness is not fully formed and any purging must be undertaken with caution.

Ma Zi Ren Wan Pattern

Clause 247

趺阳脉浮而涩，浮则胃气强，涩则小便数；浮涩相搏，大便则硬，其脾为约，麻子仁丸主之。

> The Fu Yang pulse is floating and choppy, floating denotes strong stomach qi and choppy denotes frequent urination; the floating and choppy pulses contend with each other, the stool is hard, this means the spleen is restrained, Ma Zi Ren Wan governs.

MA ZI REN WAN: Ma Zi Ren 2 sheng; Shao Yao ½ jin; Zhi Shi (roasted) ½ jin; Da Huang (skin removed) 1 jin; Hou Po (roasted) 1 chi (approx. 33 cm); Xing Ren (tips removed and dry-fried) 1 sheng.

DIRECTIONS: Grind all six ingredients into a powder, blend with honey and make into pills the size of Wu Tong fruit. Take ten pills three times a day. The dose can be increased gradually if the initial dosage is found to be insufficient. Once a stool is passed, there should be no further medication.

DISCUSSION: Fu Yang is the pulse located at the acupuncture point Chong Yang (St 42) on the instep. It is a stomach channel point and as such is associated with the Yang Ming channel governing the spleen and stomach. A floating pulse in this location relates to yang and indicates heat in the stomach; a choppy pulse relates to yin and indicates an insufficiency of spleen yin. This is because the spleen's function of transformation and transportation is restrained by the stomach heat. Because the movement of fluids is impaired, body fluids are not distributed but drain directly to the urinary bladder. They therefore by-pass the large intestine and a hard dry stool with frequent urination is the result. The indicated formula for this condition is Ma Zi Ren Wan, which softens the stool by moistening the large intestine.

Da Huang, Hou Po and Zhi Shi purge the stomach heat; Xing Ren disseminates lung qi and assists in the downward movement of fluids. Both Xing Ren and Ma Ren moisten the intestines and facilitate the descent of lung qi; Shao Yao harmonises and astringes yin; the honey has a moistening effect on the bowel.

Pi yue or spleen restraint is characterised by a dry hard stool and constipation with no passing of a stool for up to ten days, which is referred to in *Shang Han Lun* by the antiquated expression 'no change of clothes' because of the custom of changing clothes after going to the toilet. This pattern differs from a Cheng Qi Tang pattern in that the constipation is not accompanied by the manifestations of abdominal fullness, pain aggravated by pressure or frequent urination, all of which are characteristic of the Cheng Qi Tang pattern. Although spleen restraint falls into the category of Yang Ming disease, there has been no transformation into dryness and excess and so there is no associated pattern of heat with such symptoms as tidal or steaming fever, vexation, delirious speech, abdominal fullness and pain or, as sometimes occurs, clouded spirit. From this it can be seen that whereas the Cheng Qi Tang pattern is attributed to Yang Ming bowel excess with exuberant heat and dryness, spleen restraint or *pi yue* is attributed to stomach heat restraining the spleen, and it is this which results in stomach dryness and a deficiency of body fluids.

Clause 245

脉阳微而汗出少者，为自和也；汗出多者，为太过。阳脉实，因发其汗，出多者，亦为太过。太过者，为阳绝于里，亡津液，大便因硬也。

> The pulse is yang and faint and there is a mild sweat, this means there is spontaneous harmony; if there is profuse sweating, this is excessive. If the yang pulse is full, because the sweating was profuse, then this is excessive. Excessive means that yang is exhausted in interior, fluids are devastated, hence the stool is hard.

DISCUSSION: Yang Ming disease is normally characterised by copious sweating and a flooding pulse which reflects the exuberance of the yang qi. In Clause 245, the description of the pulse as yang refers to its floating quality; however, it is faint and forceless. This abatement of sweating with a pulse no longer typical of a Yang Ming pulse shows that the heat has dissipated and recovery is taking place spontaneously. However, if the sweating is copious, and fluids are damaged, the pulse will be floating and forceful, showing that the heat has not been cleared, and the bowel movement will be hard.

Clause 246

脉浮而芤，　浮为阳，芤为阴，浮芤相搏，胃气生热，其阳则绝。

The pulse is floating and hollow, floating is yang, hollow is yin, the floating contends with the hollow, the stomach qi generates heat, the yang will be devastated.

DISCUSSION: A floating pulse represents excess yang and a hollow pulse indicates severe depletion of yin. A hollow and floating pulse, therefore, indicates exuberant yang consuming and harassing the already depleted yin, and as such is a reflection of stomach heat with fluid depletion, where yang consumes yin and yin is unable to nurture yang. The depletion of fluids and the heat in the stomach result in a hard stool; insufficient yin failing to nurture yang leads, ultimately, to the devastation of yang.

Clauses 245 and 246 are both associated with a pulse which indicates fluid damage and at the same time indicates exuberant heat. This is associated with a dry, hard stool. Irrespective of whether sweating is spontaneous, nocturnal or the result of diaphoretic therapy, it must be moderate. Excessive sweating leads to fluid depletion and fluid preservation is essential in order to avoid transformation to dryness. If dryness leads to constipation, Ma Zi Ren Wan can be used to moisten dryness and move the stool.

Ancient Application of Ma Zi Ren Wan

- *Lei Zheng Huo Ren Shu:* Ma Yue Wan, an alternative name for Ma Zi Ren Wan, is indicated for the treatment of chronic (long-term) constipation or constipation in the elderly, which is a result of a deficiency of body fluids.
- *Ji Sheng Fang:* Ma Zi Ren Wan under an alternative name is cited in the treatment of impeded fluid transportation causing fluid retention and swelling.
- *Zheng Zhi Zhun Sheng:* Ma Ren Wan, which is Ma Zi Ren Wan with the omission of Shao Yao, Hou Po and Xing Ren, the substitution of Zhi Shi for Zhi Qiao, and the addition of Ren Shen, is advocated for the treatment of post-partum constipation.

Modern Application of Ma Zi Ren Wan

- Ma Zi Ren Wan can be used to treat post-operative and post-partum constipation, or constipation in the elderly due to an insufficiency of yin fluids characterised by an absence of abdominal fullness or pain and accompanied by thirst, a parched throat and mouth, signs of empty heat or tidal fever, emaciation, a red dry tongue and a thready and rapid pulse. Ma Zi Ren Wan can be prepared as a decoction, called Ma Zi Ren Tang. The decocted version has an increased purgative effect, making it stronger than the pill form and also slightly stronger than Xiao Cheng Qi Tang. Ma Zi Ren Tang is indicated for yin deficiency which is characterised by a dry, hard stool.

Case Study

Spleen Restraint (Pi Yue Zheng)

Extracted from Shang Han Shi Si Jiang by Liu Du Zhou

A 29-year-old male suffered from constipation, passing a hard, dry stool once every five or six days. He experienced extreme difficulty each time and the exertion caused him to sweat profusely. His mouth and lips were parched, his pulse was submerged and slippery and his tongue coat was dry and yellow. The diagnosis was spleen restraint with stomach heat and deficient spleen yin. The formula prescribed was Ma Zi Ren Wan. The constipation was relieved after one dose and he was given two more days of medication to consolidate the treatment.

Mi Jian Dao Pattern

Clause 233

阳明病，自汗出，若发汗，小便自利者，此为津液内竭，虽硬不可攻之；当须自欲大便，宜蜜煎导而通之。若土瓜根及大猪胆汁，皆可为导。

Yang Ming disease, there is spontaneous sweating, if sweating is promoted, if the urination is spontaneously free, this is exhaustion of body fluids in the interior, although there is hardness, one should not attack; there must be a natural urge to pass a stool, Mi Jian Dao is appropriate to lead and unblock. If there is Tu Gua Gen and the bile from a large pig, both can lead.

MI JIAN DAO: Honey 7 ge.

DIRECTIONS: Pour the honey into a copper pot and heat over a moderate flame until it is no longer liquid and reaches a thick consistency. Stir continuously to prevent it from burning and sticking to the pot. Take some of the thickened honey while it is warm and mould it to the thickness of a thumb with a length of two inches or so, tapered at one end. Insert the suppository thus made into the rectum and allow it to remain until there is an urge to defaecate, then release it. It is suspected that this does not originate from Zhong Jing but is included because it proves effective.

TU GUA GEN: Tu Gua Gen (Radix ipomoeae hungaiensis) literally means earth melon root. The directions for using the root in a decoction have been lost.

PIG'S BILE: Drain the bile from the gallbladder of a large pig and mix with a small amount of cooking vinegar. Use as a liquid enema by pouring into the rectum and leaving it for 20 to 30 minutes. A stool will be passed which contains undigested food particles. It is very effective.

DISCUSSION: A patient with Yang Ming disease usually suffers from spontaneous sweating. Therefore, any diaphoretic therapy will cause further depletion of body fluids, and if the urination is uninhibited there will be further fluid loss. The subsequent depletion of fluids means that there is insufficient moisture for the large intestine and a hard stool will result. The hard stool in this case is the result of fluid depletion. It is not the same as the hard stool of a Cheng Qi Tang pattern where it is the result of heat and dryness knotting together to form a dry stool bind. For this reason, it is not appropriate to purge strongly or 'attack', but Mi Jian can be used as a mechanical aid to soften the stool and facilitate its passage. Because its action is local, it is effective only if there is a stool in the rectum. When a stool reaches the rectum, there is an urge to defaecate and so it is then that the honey suppository should be used.

Honey is sweet and moistening and when inserted into the rectum and melted by the body heat, it will liquefy and moisten the intestines. This method is relatively gentle and is suitable for a person suffering from deficiency of yin blood. Pig's bile is bitter and cold and not only moistens the intestines but drains heat and relieves toxicity. Tu Gua Gen is bitter and cold and clears heat and moistens dryness. It is indicated for a blockage of any of the six fu organs characterised by constipation.

Ancient Application of Tu Gua Enema

Zhou Hou Bei Ji Fang records the juice of Tu Gua in the treatment of constipation administered per rectum via a tube.

Modern Application of Honey Suppositories

Mi Dao Jian Wan pioneered the way for the use of suppositories in the treatment of constipation and was centuries ahead of the glycerine suppositories later developed in the West. Honey suppositories can still be used for the elderly, for post-partum or post-operative constipation and for paralytic intestinal obstruction (Shang Hai First People's Hospital, *Zhong Yi Za Zhi* 1957; 8:431).

Purgative Therapy in Yang Ming Disease

Clause 209

阳明病， 潮熱，大便微硬者，可与大承气汤，不硬者， 不可与之。若不大便六七日，恐有燥屎，欲知之法，少与小承气汤，汤入腹中，转矢气者，,此有燥屎也， 乃可攻之；若不转矢气者，此但初头硬，后必溏，不可攻之，攻之必肠满不能食也。欲饮水者，与水则哕。其后发熱者，必大便复硬而少也，以小承气汤和之。不转矢气者，慎不可攻也。小承气湯。

Yang Ming disease, there is tidal fever, if the stool is slightly hard, one can give Da Cheng Qi Tang, if the stool is not hard, one should not give it. If no stool is passed for six or seven days, one fears the stool is dry, the way to find out is, give a little Xiao Cheng Qi Tang, once the decoction enters the abdomen, if faecal qi moves, this means there is a dry stool, so one can attack; if faecal qi does not move, it is hard only at the start, afterwards it will be sloppy, one should not attack, attacking will cause abdominal fullness and an inability to eat. If there is a desire to drink water, giving water will cause regurgitation. If after this there is fever, the stool will again be hard and scant, giving Xiao Cheng Qi Tang will harmonise. If faecal qi does not move, beware that one should not attack. Xiao Cheng Qi Tang.

DISCUSSION: Clause 209 describes the four criteria applied in determining whether or not to 'attack' by purging strongly.

1. *Identification of the stool.* When Yang Ming disease has been confirmed by the presence of tidal fever, a hard stool means that there is heat excess and purgation can be used. If, however, the stool is not hard, it means that the pattern is not associated with heat excess and purgation should not be used.
2. *Identification of the movement of abdominal qi.* If no stool has been passed for six or seven days, then it is most likely because the stool is dry. To confirm that supposition, before administering a strong purgative, a small dose of the milder formula Xiao Cheng Qi Tang should be given first, to determine whether this is in fact the correct strategy. The passing of faecal qi or abdominal gas can be a sign of the presence of a dry stool. Because the action of Xiao Cheng Qi Tang is more focused on moving qi than on softening the stool, a small dose will cause the qi to move, thus confirming that a dry stool is present. However, if there is no sense of qi movement or flatulence and instead, a stool is passed which is hard at the beginning but then loose, this is a sign of cold and deficiency of the spleen and stomach. Purgation is therefore contraindicated and, if used, will result in abdominal fullness and a loss of appetite.
3. *Identification of 'water regurgitation'.* Water regurgitation refers to the regurgitation of any water swallowed. When this occurs in a Yang Ming pattern, it is a sign of yang deficiency, which has resulted in stomach qi counterflow due to water retained in the interior. Purgation should not be used.
4. *Identification of heat accumulation.* Further purgation can only be administered if fever persists and there is a scant hard stool, both of which indicate the accumulation of pathogenic heat. In this case, Xiao Cheng Qi Tang can be given; however, it is subject to the passing of faecal qi. If no gas is passed, purgation should not be used.

Application of Da Cheng Qi Tang and Xiao Cheng Qi Tang

Clause 251

得病二三日，脉弱，无太阳、柴胡证，烦躁、心下硬；至四五日，虽能食，以小承气汤，少少与，微和之，令小安；至六日，与承气汤一升。若不大便六七日，小便少者，虽不受食，但初头硬，后必溏，未定成硬，攻之必溏；须小便利，屎定硬，乃可攻之，宜大承气汤。

Sickness for two or three days, the pulse is weak, there is no sign of a Tai Yang or Chai Hu pattern, there is vexation and agitation, hardness below the heart; on the fourth or fifth day, even if able to eat, give a very small dose of Xiao Cheng Qi Tang to mildly harmonise, and calm a little; on the sixth day, give one sheng of Cheng Qi Tang. Where there is no stool for six or seven days, if the urination is scant, even if there is an inability to eat, the stool is hard only at the start, afterwards it will be sloppy, there is no formation of hardness, attacking will cause sloppiness; the urination must be free, the stool formed hard, then one may attack, Da Cheng Qi Tang is appropriate.

DISCUSSION: If the patient has been sick for two or three days, and it is neither a Tai Yang exterior pattern nor a Shao Yang half exterior half interior pattern, but there is vexation and hardness in the epigastrium, then it is due to Yang Ming interior heat. If after another day or so the person still has a good appetite, then this shows that the Yang Ming interior excess pattern has not yet developed into Yang Ming intestinal dryness. Because the pulse is weak, harsh treatment must be avoided and so a small dose of Xiao Cheng Qi Tang is given to harmonise the stomach and quell the vexation by freeing the intestinal obstruction. If, after six days, the patient is still vexed and still suffers hardness in the epigastrium and there has been no bowel movement, a larger dose of one sheng of Xiao Cheng Qi Tang can be given. Caution must be exercised in the administration of this formula because, although the symptoms indicate an excess pattern, the pulse is a deficient pulse. Therefore, there is a possibility that purging will damage the zheng qi and lead to a transmuted pattern.

If, however, there is no bowel movement at the end of six or seven days, and there is a loss of appetite, then this seems to resemble the bowel excess of a Da Cheng Qi Tang pattern. However, the scant urination shows that fluids are still being transported to the stomach and intestines; only the first part of the stool is dry, and once that is passed, the rest is sloppy. Strong purgation in this situation can injure the spleen yang and cause the stool to be loose. A Da Cheng Qi Tang pattern is characterised by urination which is uninhibited. The fact that it is not scant shows that fluids are being sent from the large intestine to the urinary bladder; therefore, there is reduced moisture in the large intestine and the stool is dry and hard; this is bowel excess and so it is appropriate to purge strongly using Da Cheng Qi Tang.

Significance of the Ability or Inability to Eat

The question of appetite, and the ability or inability to eat, is a recurring issue in *Shang Han Lun*. Clause 190 states: "Yang Ming disease, if the person can eat, it is called zhong feng; if the person can not eat, it is called zhong han"; Clause 215 states: "Yang Ming disease, if there is delirious speech, tidal fever but an inability to eat, there will be five or six lumps of dry stool in the stomach; where a person is able to eat, it is just hard. Da Cheng Qi Tang is appropriate". Clause 251 states: "even if there is an inability to eat, the stool is hard only at the start, afterwards it will be sloppy". Examination of these three clauses shows that the inability to eat is a symptom used to identify certain Yang Ming patterns, for example, in Clause 190 it differentiates Yang Ming zhong feng from Yang Ming zhong han, which is a pattern of deficiency cold; in Clause 215 the inability to eat is a manifestation of the more serious condition of heat and dryness knotting in the large intestine, manifesting as dry constipation and accompanied by delirious speech and tidal fever. This contrasts with the milder condition of heat in the stomach, where there is a dry stool but no other symptoms. Clause 251 shows that the inability to eat is not always indicative of heat and dryness knotting in the intestines. The above analysis is a clear example of how diagnosis can not be made on one sign or symptom alone.

Urination and bowel movement are diagnostically significant and Clause 251 makes multiple references to them: "Where there is no stool for six or seven days"; "if the urination is scant"; "the stool is hard only at the start, afterwards it will be sloppy"; "there is no formation of hardness"; and "the urination must be free, the stool formed hard". In the last instance, the hardness of the stool can be determined by urinary volume. Although the urination is scant and urinary output decreased, fluids are still being transported to the stomach and large intestine. Therefore, the stool is hard initially, due to some depletion of fluids but the rest is sloppy. This shows that the excess of knotted dryness has not formed and that purgation is therefore not indicated. Copious urination is a sign that the fluids are all directed to the bladder and are not retained in the stomach and large intestine. With the large intestine thus deprived of proper moisture, the stool is dry and hard and so purgation is appropriate. However, as with the symptom of being unable to eat, which was discussed above, a single symptom can not be relied upon in isolation. Nevertheless, frequent urination is often associated with a hard stool and where there is a pattern of excess heat, Cheng Qi Tang can be used. Where there is scant urination due to fluid deficiency, then Ma Zi Ren Wan is the formula. Where the stool is only hard at first and then sloppy, it is a Yang Ming deficiency cold pattern of the spleen and stomach and the strategy is to warm the middle and strengthen the transportation function of the spleen. The principle of treating diarrhoea by promoting urination to drain damp is based on the same rationale, and it is on this basis that Wu Ling San can be used in the treatment of watery diarrhoea.

Differentiation of Purgation on the Basis of Urinary Frequency

Clause 203

(一) 阳明病，本自汗出。医更重发汗，病已差，尚微烦不了了者，此必大便硬故也。(二)以亡津液，胃中干燥，故令大便硬。(三) 当问其小便 日几行，若本小便日三四行，今日再行，故知大便不久出。今为小便数少，以津液当还入胃中，故知不久必大便也。

(1) Yang Ming disease, there was originally spontaneous sweating. The physician promoted further sweating, the disease was already despatched, if there is still mild vexation that is not cleared, this means the stool will be hard. (2) Because of devastated body fluids, dryness in the stomach, making the stool hard. (3) One must ask about the urination, how many times a day it is passed. If urination was being passed three or four times a day, now it is twice a day, then you know a stool will be passed before long. If the urination is currently frequent and scant, it is because the body fluids are returning to the stomach, hence you know before long a stool will be passed.

DISCUSSION: Profuse sweating is a feature of Yang Ming disease, and so if the practitioner causes the patient to sweat further, although the pathogenic heat will be eliminated, complete recovery does not take place. This is because the sweating is excessive and whilst it succeeds in resolving the Yang Ming heat, the subsequent damage to fluids results in dryness of the stomach and in mild vexation. The dry bowel movement caused by the depletion of body fluids does not require purgation, because the distribution of fluids to the stomach and intestines will soon resume and the stool will then be normal again. In this situation, purgation is inappropriate and the principle of moistening the intestines should be adopted in order to soften the stool.

Assessing urinary output is one way of determining whether the stomach has harmonised and if proper fluid distribution has returned. This can be measured either by frequency or by amount. If there is a noticeable reduction in urinary frequency, for instance from three or four times a day to only two, or if, on the other hand, frequency remains unchanged but there is a decrease in the amount of urine passed, then we know that the body fluids are not all being sent to the urinary bladder for excretion, and that some are being redistributed and circulated in the body. Therefore, the stomach and intestines will receive moisture and the stool will be softened and normalised.

Differentiation of Purgation on the Basis of Sweating and the Pulse

Clause 240

病人烦热，汗出则解；又如疟状，日晡所发热者，属阳明也。脉实者，宜下之；脉浮虚者，宜发汗。下之与大承气汤，发汗宜桂枝汤。

The patient is vexed and has a fever, sweating brings resolution; then there are malaria-like symptoms, if in the late afternoon there is tidal fever, this pertains to Yang Ming. If the pulse is excess, purgation is appropriate; if the pulse is floating and deficient, sweat promotion is appropriate. For purgation give Da Cheng Qi Tang, to promote sweating Gui Zhi Tang is appropriate.

DISCUSSION: The fever and vexation indicate exterior constraint, so the promotion of sweat should resolve the condition. If, however, after sweating, there are malaria-like symptoms with tidal fever in the afternoon, then it means that the pathogen has entered the interior to form a Yang Ming interior excess pattern. Pulse diagnosis can be used to determine whether the exterior has been fully resolved or not. If it is excess and forceful, then the exterior pathogen is resolved and it is appropriate to purge using use Da Cheng Qi Tang. If, however, the pulse is floating and forceless, even if there is an afternoon tidal fever, then the exterior is not fully resolved and Gui Zhi Tang must be used to promote sweating and release the exterior.

Contraindications in Yang Ming Disease

Clause 204

伤寒呕多，虽有阳明证，不可攻之。

Shang han with frequent vomiting, although it is a Yang Ming pattern, one should not attack.

DISCUSSION: Vomiting in shang han or cold damage can be associated with any of the six channels and the treatment varies accordingly. Clause 204 describes a Yang Ming pattern where vomiting is a manifestation of the counterflow of stomach qi, which has been caused by heat in the chest and diaphragm. In this case, the Yang Ming heat has not knotted in the abdomen, but in the chest, and so heat must be cleared not from the lower jiao, but from the upper and middle jiao. 'Attacking' or purging the stool in the lower jiao would cause a transmuted pattern; the appropriate herbs to use are Shi Gao, Zhi Mu and Lu Gen, which enter the stomach and the lungs.

Shang Han Da Bai states: "If there is aversion to cold and fever, with the initial stage characterised by fullness of the chest and vomiting, it is a pattern of Tai Yang externally contracted pathogenic wind cold with retention of phlegm fluids in the stomach … If chills and fever come and go, and there is vomiting, a bitter taste in the mouth and a wiry, rapid pulse, it is a Shao Yang channel disorder … If there is sweating and vomiting, and the pulse is rapid, it is a vomiting pattern associated with dryness and heat, and Shi Gao Zhi Mu Tang with Zhu Li and Lu Gen juice is indicated. Vomiting associated with the yin channels is due to stomach cold and the indicated formula is Li Zhong Wan to warm the middle". From this passage it can be surmised that vomiting associated with the three yang channels is principally due to heat, and vomiting associated with the three yin channels is generally associated with a cold pattern. This, however, is not absolute. A Yang Ming pattern with vomiting can be differentially diagnosed as excess heat or deficient cold. The distinguishing feature of vomiting in a pattern of Yang Ming deficiency cold is vomitus which is watery; there is stomach pain and a moist white tongue coat. The recommended formula is Wu Zhu Yu Tang.

A concurrent pattern of Shao Yang and Yang Ming is characterised by the vomiting of bitter fluid, pain in the hypochondrium, alternating chills and fever, constipation, a greasy yellow tongue coat and a rapid, wiry pulse; the formula is Da Chai Hu Tang. Clause 204 describes vomiting due to the accumulation of heat in the chest and diaphragm. Because the heat is located in the upper jiao, the appropriate strategy is to clear heat, not to purge.

Clause 205

阳明病，心下硬满者，不可攻之。攻之，利遂不止者死；利止者愈。

Yang Ming disease, if there is hardness and fullness below the heart, one should not attack. Attacking, if followed by incessant diarrhoea the person will die; if the diarrhoea stops, the person will recover.

DISCUSSION: A Yang Ming bowel excess pattern is characterised by hardness and distension in the abdomen resistant to pressure and there may also be periumbilical pain. Purgation is the recommended treatment. If, however, the hardness and distension are in the epigastric area, which relates to the stomach, rather than the abdominal cavity, and the pain or discomfort are not exacerbated by pressure, then it is due to the congestion of unformed or insubstantial heat. Because it is not associated with formed heat, which is the knotting of heat with an excess such as phlegm or food stagnation, purgation is incorrect. Furthermore, if purgation is used, the damage to middle qi may cause diarrhoea. If the diarrhoea is incessant, it is an indication of devastated spleen and stomach qi and so the prognosis is poor and death may ensue.

A clear distinction must be made between the pattern described in Clause 205 and a chest bind pattern. The nature of the bind and its location are the key differentiating factors. Chest bind is attributed to heat and water knotting in the chest and diaphragm, and is characterised by epigastric pain which may extend to the lesser abdomen and a palpable stone-like hardness which resists pressure. It is thus associated with excess and the treatment strategy is to drain and expel water. By comparison, the pattern described in Clause 205 is not caused by the knotting of heat and water in the chest and diaphragm, but by a knotting of insubstantial heat in the epigastric area, and although there is hardness and distension, the pain is not exacerbated by pressure. By this it can be seen that there is no pathogenic excess and so purging is contraindicated. A glomus pattern associated with a heat and cold complex is also characterised by hardness and fullness below the heart and the indicated treatment is Xie Xin Tang, where the main focus is on draining heat rather than purging.

Clause 206

阳明病，面合色赤，不可攻也。必发热，色黄者，小便不利也。

Yang Ming disease, the whole face is crimson, one should not attack. Then there will be fever, yellowing, the urination will not be free.

DISCUSSION: If there is a flushed face in a Yang Ming pattern, it is an indication of pathogenic constraint in the channel and a formula such as Ge Gen Tang is indicated to promote sweat and release the exterior constraint. The incorrect use of purgation would damage the stomach qi and exhaust fluids, and thus facilitate the exploitation of the channel by the pathogen. If, on this background of middle qi deficiency, the pathogen falls inward, it will manifest as an accumulation of spleen damp and there will be inhibited urination, unsurfaced fever or unresolved tidal fever, which gives rise to constrained heat of the gallbladder and liver, manifesting as yellowing. This is described as yang jaundice with a bright yellow complexion accompanied by fever.

Clause 189

阳明中风，口苦、咽干、腹满、微喘、发热、恶寒、脉浮而紧，若下之，则腹满小便难也。

Yang Ming zhong feng, a bitter taste in the mouth, a parched throat, abdominal fullness, slight panting, fever, aversion to cold, and a pulse that is floating and tight, if there is purgation, then the abdomen will be full and urination difficult.

DISCUSSION: Clause 189 describes a complex of symptoms: a bitter taste in the mouth and a parched throat are associated with a Shao Yang pattern; abdominal fullness and panting are symptoms of Yang Ming disease; fever and aversion to cold are signs of Tai Yang. The pulse also has a complex presentation: it is both floating, indicative of an exterior pattern, and tight, which indicates interior cold. The concurrent pattern of the three yang channels is described as 'Yang Ming zhong feng' because the symptoms of Yang Ming are more pronounced than those of Tai Yang and Shao Yang. This is a Yang Ming disease with interior heat which has as yet not developed into a Yang Ming excess pattern; purgation is therefore contraindicated. If purgation were to be used, the damage to fluids would result in dryness, characterised by abdominal fullness, constipation and difficult or inhibited urination. There is an old saying which epitomises this situation: "In shang han disease, the sweating must be promoted early, but purgation should never be used early".

Summary of Yang Ming Fu Patterns

A Tiao Wei Cheng Qi Tang pattern represents the early stage of a Yang Ming dry heat pattern. At this stage, the heat is in the stomach and has not yet manifested as intestinal dryness, which would be characterised by the absence of a bowel movement, vexation, restlessness, steaming fever, and possibly accompanied by abdominal fullness or delirious speech.

A Xiao Cheng Qi Tang pattern is a further development of Yang Ming dry heat where there is a hard stool, abdominal fullness, vexation and delirious speech, and the pulse is slippery and rapid. The purgative effect of Xiao Cheng Qi Tang is comparatively stronger than that of Tiao Wei Cheng Qi Tang but is still more moderate than that of Da Cheng Qi Tang.

A Da Cheng Qi Tang pattern is a pattern of Yang Ming bowel excess where the pathogenic heat and dryness is deeply entrenched, obstructing the intestinal qi. It is characterised by the absence of a bowel movement for five or six days, or even considerably longer, and there is pain and distension in the abdomen, or periumbilical pain, sweating, tidal fever, delirious speech, no appetite, and the patient may also speak aloud to himself, as if delusional or seeing ghosts. There is also agitation demonstrated by unconsciously picking at clothing or twisting the blankets. In addition, there can be inhibited urination and the evacuation of a foul smelling liquid, or there might be a slight fever or wheezing. Da Cheng Qi Tang purges the heat, softens and expels the hard bind and eliminates intestinal stagnation. The name Da Cheng Qi Tang or 'Great Order the Qi Formula' is a reflection of its potency.

The three Cheng Qi Tang have the function of purgation in common, with each being suitable for a different stage of a Yang Ming bowel excess pattern. Tiao Wei Cheng Qi Tang targets the heat of the stomach when the stool is not yet hard; Xiao Cheng Qi Tang is indicated where there is fluid damage and the knotted heat and hard stool obstruct the intestinal qi; Da Cheng Qi Tang is indicated where heat and dryness have formed a hard stool bind and constipation.

Key Points

1. **Differentiation of treatment for a dry stool.** Clauses 208, 209, 215, 217, 239, 241, 242, 248 and 249 all describe various situations associated with a dry stool and the corresponding treatment.
   (i) Sweating: sweat streaming from the extremities (Clauses 208, 217).
   (ii) Mental condition: vexation, delirious speech (Clauses 215, 217, 239, 374).
   (iii) Abdominal condition: abdominal fullness or pain around the umbilicus (Clauses 208, 209, 239).
   (iv) Fever: tidal fever between the hours of 3pm and 5pm or interior heat constraint with slight fever (Clauses 208, 215, 242, 209).
   (v) Ability to eat: the inability to eat is associated with a dry, hard stool; the ability to eat is associated with a stool which is hard but not dry (Clauses 215, 209).
   (vi) Passing of wind from the abdomen: the passing of wind after taking Xiao Cheng Qi Tang indicates the presence of a dry stool; if no wind is passed, the stool is not dry (Clauses 209, 217).
   (vii) The state of urination and stool: frequent urination with no bowel movement indicates the presence of a dry stool (Clause 242). It is also possible to have a dry stool accompanied by inhibited urination and watery diarrhoea with undigested food particles or the evacuation of a foul malodorous fluid.
2. **Contraindications for purgation.** Contraindications for purgation based on the original *Shang Han Lun* text can be summarised as follows.
   (i) Exterior not fully resolved or heat constraint in the Yang Ming channel.
   (ii) Heat that is located in the upper jiao.
   (iii) Deficiency of the middle yang with a stool that is hard at the beginning and sloppy afterwards.
   (iv) Deficiency of ying blood, copious sweating with fluid damage (purgation is contraindicated even if there is bowel excess).
   (v) Xiao Cheng Qi Tang can be given in the absence of a dry stool (abdominal wind is passed after administration).
   (vi) Depletion of qi and body fluids and a slightly choppy pulse (purgation is

contraindicated even if there is bowel excess).

The key criterion for purging is the relative strength of zheng qi and pathogenic qi. However, where there is deficiency, one can purge providing the zheng qi is simultaneously supported.

3. **Methods of decoction and administration.**
   (i) For the treatment of stomach dryness and fire flaring upward, characterised by a flushed face or swollen, inflamed gums, mouth ulcers, vexation or insomnia, Tiao Wei Cheng Qi Tang can be given in repeated small doses to eliminate the heat.
   (ii) If there is a dry hard stool, Da Cheng Qi Tang can be given as a single dose on an empty stomach and repeated until a stool is passed.
   (iii) The administration of Da Cheng Qi Tang must be in strict accordance with Zhang Zhong Jing's instructions. No deviation is permitted.

Section Five

3.5 TRANSMUTED PATTERNS OF YANG MING

The transmuted patterns of Yang Ming disease fall into two categories: a) Yellowing due to damp heat; and b) Blood aspect patterns.

3.5.1 Yellowing Due to Damp Heat

Yellowing due to damp heat is classified as follows: a) Yin Chen Hao Tang pattern, where there is equal heat and damp; b) Zhi Zi Bai Pi Tang pattern, where heat predominates; and c) Ma Huang Lian Qiao Chi Xiao Dou Tang, where the stagnation of damp heat is accompanied by an exterior pattern. Their common pathogenesis is damp heat due to stasis heat which has caused constraint of the gallbladder and liver qi.

Clause 199

阳明病，无汗，小便不利，心中懊侬者，身必发黄。

Yang Ming disease, there is no sweating, if the urination is not free, and there is anguish in the heart, the body will turn yellow.

DISCUSSION: Copious sweating is a characteristic feature of Yang Ming disease and its absence is a reflection of accumulated damp in the interior which constrains the heat and blocks the issue of sweat. Because the damp has combined with the constrained heat, it is trapped, and urination is inhibited. This is because the heat is mingled with the damp; there is no exit for the pathogen and it surges upward harassing the heart shen, causing anguish and vexation. Further, the damp heat obstructs the qi dynamic; this impairs the dispersal of qi by the liver and gallbladder and the subsequent disordered flow of bile results in generalised yellowing and jaundice.

It must be understood by the use of the word 'will' (必) in Clause 199, that the patient is not currently jaundiced, but that the condition of yellowing is imminent. Thus the symptomatology described can be regarded as a precursor of Yang Ming jaundice. The key is to understand that the pathogenesis is damp heat locked in the interior, preventing the release of the pathogenic heat and impeding the movement of fluids. The strategy is to promote urination in order to eliminate damp, thus creating an exit for the pathogenic heat, by draining it via the urine. In this way, by simply draining damp, the cause of the potential jaundice is targeted and the yellowing will be prevented. In treating a patient who presents with the symptoms of absence of sweat, inhibited urination, anguish, and a greasy, yellow tongue coat, the appropriate formula is Xiao Chai Hu Tang omitting Ren Shen and adding Fu Ling. For optimum results it should be combined with a formula such as Zhi Zi Chi Tang or San

Ren Tang or Huo Po Xia Ling Tang in order to release the exterior, thereby facilitating the elimination of interior heat, thus providing an exit for the heat and damp.

Clause 200

阳明病，被火，额上微汗出，而小便不利者，必发黄。

Yang Ming disease, treated with fire, if there is slight sweating on the forehead, and urination is not free, there will be yellowing.

DISCUSSION: The prescribed treatment strategy for a pattern of Yang Ming interior heat is to drain heat by purging. Fire therapy is contraindicated and if used, the fire will fuel the existing heat, exacerbating the condition. If the person has a tendency to sweat heavily, and there is uninhibited urination, then the pathogen will transform into dryness and there will be no yellowing. Conversely, if there is slight sweat on the forehead and inhibited urination, it signifies that there is no exit for the damp and heat. Consequently, there is damp heat congestion in the interior which obstructs the dispersion of liver and gallbladder qi causing subsequent jaundice and yellowing.

Yang Ming disease can be differentiated as transformation into dryness or transformation into damp accumulation. The pattern of dry transformation is characterised by a stool which is dry and hard and urination which is generally uninhibited; and the pattern of damp transformation is characterised by inhibited urination. This differentiation results in diametrically opposite treatment protocols: the draining of dry heat by purging the stool on the one hand and, on the other, the draining of damp heat by promoting urination.

In *Shang Han Lun*, there are four categories of yellowing: (1) Damp heat yellowing (Clauses 134, 199, 206, 236, 260, 261 and 262); (2) Cold damp yellowing (Clauses 98, 195 and 259); (3) Fire counterflow yellowing (Clauses 111 and 200); and (4) Blood stasis yellowing (Clause 125). The patterns must be carefully differentiated and treated accordingly.

Yin Chen Hao Tang Pattern

Clause 236

阳明病，发热、汗出者，此为热越，不能发黄也。但头汗出，身无汗，剂颈而还，小便不利，渴引水浆者，此为瘀热在里，身必发黄，茵陈蒿汤主之。

Yang Ming disease, if there is fever and sweating, this means the heat is passing on, there will be no yellowing. If there is sweat only from the head, no sweat from the body, stopping at the neck, the urination is not free, there is thirst which leads to fluids, this is stasis heat in the interior, the body will turn yellow, Yin Chen Hao Tang governs.

YIN CHEN HAO TANG: Yin Chen Hao 6 liang; Zhi Zi (broken) 14 pieces; Da Huang (skin removed) 2 liang.

DIRECTIONS: First boil Yin Chen in 1 dou, 2 sheng of water, reducing to 6 sheng before adding the other two ingredients, and further reducing to 3 sheng. Strain and divide into three portions, then take one dose. Dark brownish urine the colour of the juice of Zao Jia (皂荚), also known as Zao Jiao (皂角) or honey locust fruit, will be passed. The abdominal sign will be relieved the next day.

DISCUSSION: Yang Ming and Tai Yin stand in an exterior–interior relationship. The Yang Ming channel governs dryness and the Tai Yin channel governs damp. Pathogenic heat entering the interior can either be transformed into dry heat or, if the heat combines with damp from the Tai Yin, it will give rise to damp heat.

Clause 236 points to the pathogenesis of damp heat yellowing. It first describes the mechanisms of fever and sweating which can eliminate pathogenic heat, thus forestalling the development of damp heat. In fact, the loss of fluids caused by sweating may lead to dryness, but will certainly not generate damp. However, if sweating is limited, as is shown in this clause by the fact that it issues only from the head and not from the rest of the body, and if, in addition, there is inhibited urination, then this is evidence of pathogenic damp which constrains the interior heat and prevents its elimination via sweat or urination. The constrained damp and heat in the interior block the waterways, impeding the movement of water and hindering urination. In addition, the constrained heat and damp affect the movement of qi of the liver and gallbladder, giving rise to an unregulated flow of bile, which causes yellowing and jaundice. Generally, pathogenic damp is associated with a sense of thirst where the person does not actually drink much. Here, the symptom of thirst which causes the person to drink water and other fluids is a sign of the constrained pathogenic heat having damaged fluids, giving rise to a situation where there is more heat than damp. The term stasis heat refers to the combining of pre-existing blood stasis with heat.

Yin Chen clears heat and drains damp by disinhibiting urination and is especially effective in treating yellowing or jaundice due to damp heat; Da Huang is bitter and cold, and not only purges intestinal excess heat, but is also used here to invigorate blood and resolve the stasis heat. Zhi Zi clears heat in the san jiao, diffuses the qi dynamic, and drains damp heat via the urine. The combined effect of the three herbs effectively clears heat and drains damp, thus eliminating the obstruction to the qi dynamic and alleviating the jaundice.

Promoting urination to drain damp is one of the main methods of eliminating damp heat or damp accumulation, and the formula directions affirm this when they state that after taking the decoction, dark yellow urine will be excreted of a colour resembling Zao Jia juice, which is a yellow-brown colour.

Jaundice is categorised as 'yang jaundice' caused by damp heat, or 'yin jaundice' caused by cold damp, and it is essential to make the differentiation. Yang jaundice which occurs as part of a Yang Ming pattern is characterised by a bright, orangey yellow complexion, vexation, thirst, constipation, inhibited urination, mild abdominal distension, a greasy yellow tongue coat and a rapid, soggy pulse. The governing formula is Yin Chen Hao Tang, which clears heat and drains damp. By contrast, yin jaundice is characterised by a dull, yellow complexion, no thirst, a loose stool, inhibited urination, a moist slippery tongue coat and a submerged or slow pulse. The treatment strategy is to warm the middle and drain damp using such formulas as Yin Chen Wu Ling San or Yin Chen Zhu Fu Tang.

There are two factors associated with the above pattern. (1) Damp heat congestion which is unable to be vented outward; and (2) stasis obstruction in the interior, which was mentioned by Tang Rong Chuan in *Xue Zheng Lun* when he said: "Stasis is intimately associated with yellowing at the blood level". From this, it is evident that Zhang Zhong Jing's use of Da Huang is not for its purgative properties alone, but also because of its function of invigorating blood to eliminate stasis. In modern times, Da Huang has been found to have an anti-viral effect useful in the treatment of hepatitis and is also used in the treatment of neonatal jaundice due to damp heat. In order to focus on Da Huang's function of invigorating and cooling blood, it is cooked together with the other herbs.

Clause 260

伤寒七八日，身黄如桔子色，小便不利，腹微满者，茵陈蒿汤主之。

Shang han for seven or eight days, if the body is yellow like the colour of a mandarin, the urination is not free, and the abdomen is slightly distended, Yin Chen Hao Tang governs.

DISCUSSION: Clause 236 discusses the aetiology and pathogenesis of damp heat yellowing, while here Clause 260 focuses on the symptoms. The comparison of the yellow colour to a mandarin orange is a direct reference to the bright orangey yellow of the yang jaundice associated with Yang Ming. The inhibited urination is attributed to constrained damp heat impairing the qi dynamic and obstructing the water passages of the san jiao; abdominal fullness is the result of the combined constraint of damp and heat obstructing and stagnating the qi of the intestines; on the basis of the presence of damp heat in the interior, it can be deduced that there would also be yellowing of the sclera, dark urine and a dry stool. Yin Chen Hao Tang clears heat, drains damp and eliminates stasis, thereby resolving the jaundice.

Based on Clauses 199, 200, 236 and 260, all of which relate to damp heat yellowing, inhibited urination will always be part of the pattern. Irrespective of whether this occurs before or after the appearance of jaundice, the key treatment strategy for damp heat yellowing is to promote urination. Therefore, apart from the use of herbs which clear heat and relieve toxicity, herbs such as Che Qian Zi, Jin Qian Cao and Sheng Yi Ren should be added to further promote urination and enhance the clinical outcome.

Ancient Application of Yin Chen Hao Tang

- *Pu Ji Ben Shi Fang:* For the treatment of damp heat in the stomach accompanied by food stagnation.
- *Ji Yang Gang Mu:* For the treatment of stasis heat with generalised yellowing.

Modern Application of Yin Chen Hao Tang

- *Acute infectious hepatitis:* Guo Zi Guang et al reported in *Shang Han Lun Tang Zheng Xin Pian* that Yin Chen Hao Tang was used to treat 2973 cases of hepatitis with a recovery rate ranging from 82.6% to 100%. The average treatment time was between 6.7 and 17.2 days.
- Treatment of acute cholecystitis, cholelithiasis, acute pancreatitis and damp heat hepatitis. The key points are as follows.
  - (i) Identifying the degree of damp accumulation: if it is severe, there will be a sensation of fullness and oppression in the chest, nausea, aversion to greasy food, fatigue, heaviness in the limbs, a loose stool and a thick greasy yellow tongue coat. The treatment must be focused on draining damp. Yin Chen Hao Tang can be modified by reducing the dose of Da Huang and adding Xing Ren, Hou Po, Jin Qian Cao, Che Qian Cao, Fu Ling and Sheng Yi Ren.
  - (ii) Identification of blood stasis: if stasis is pronounced, there will be a palpable mass below the ribs, pain which is aggravated by pressure and dark, distended sub-lingual veins. The treatment is to invigorate blood and transform stasis. Yin Chen Hao Tang can be modified by adding Dan Shen, Chi Shao, Chuan Xiong, Qian Cao Gen or, if warranted, Hong Hua, Tao Ren, San Leng, E Zhu, Tu Bie Chong etc.
  - (iii) Identification of heat: if the heat signs are pronounced, there will be fever which spikes in the afternoon, thirst with no desire to drink, a dry stool or difficult bowel movement, a dry yellow tongue coat and a wiry, rapid pulse. The treatment must be focused on clearing heat, relieving toxicity and drying damp. A modified version of Yin Chen Hao Tang adding Huang Qin, Huang Bai, Long Dan Cao, Sheng Shi Gao, Zhi Mu and Shi Hu can be used.
  - (iv) Identification of an exterior pathogen: if there are signs of an exterior pathogen with aversion to wind cold, Yin Chen Hao Tang can be combined with Ma Huang Lian Qiao Chi Xiao Dou Tang. If there is wind heat, add Chai Hu, Bo He, Jin Yin Hua and Lian Qiao to release the exterior.
  - (v) Identification of the strength of spleen and stomach: prolonged damp heat accumulation in the middle with constrained liver and gallbladder qi may damage the spleen and stomach and a pattern of complex heat and cold can then arise. In this case, Yin Chen Hao Tang can be combined with Xiao Chai Hu Tang in order to address both the liver and spleen.

Case Study

Acne

Extracted from Guo Yi Lun Tan 1997; (3):14

A 23-year-old male patient had suffered from dermatitis for more than six months. He had received both Western medication and Chinese medicine but his condition had not improved significantly. Other symptoms were fullness in the epigastrium, vexation, irritability and a dry stool once every three days. His urination was dark yellow. His complexion was oily and his tongue coat was yellow and greasy and he had a slippery, soggy pulse. The diagnosis was acne due to stomach and intestinal damp heat. He was prescribed seven packs of a modified version of Yin Chen Hao Tang: Yin Chen 30g, Sheng Da Huang (to be added later) 10g, Zhi Zi 10g, Huang Qin 10g, Yin Hua 15g, Ye Ju Hua 15g, Pu Gong Ying 15g, Sheng Yi Ren 15g. After this course of medication, the acne improved and his complexion was less oily. Fourteen packs of the same core formula was prescribed, omitting Da Huang, and adding Dan Shen 15g, Hong Hua 10g, Chi Shao 10g. His skin cleared.

Zhi Zi Bai Pi Tang Pattern

Clause 261

伤寒身黄，发热。栀子柏皮汤主之。

Shang han the body is yellow, and there is fever. Zhi Zi Bai Pi Tang governs.

ZHI ZI BAI PI TANG: Zhi Zi 15 pieces (broken); Zhi Gan Cao 1 liang; Huang Bai 2 liang.

DIRECTIONS: Boil all three ingredients in 4 sheng of water, reducing to 1½ sheng and then strain.

DISCUSSION: Yellowing and fever in shang han disease are an indication of damp heat constrained in the interior, with the heat surfacing as fever. This pathogenesis is representative for yang jaundice, where the damp heat is locked in the interior and unable to exit. The congealed damp heat affects the gallbladder causing a disordered flow of bile and jaundice to appear, whilst the fever is an expression of the exuberant interior heat.

Both Zhi Zi and Huang Bai are bitter and cold. Zhi Zi drains fire from the san jiao via urination and together, the two herbs clear constrained heat and dry damp, thus effectively relieving the damp heat jaundice; Gan Cao harmonises the middle and moderates the cold and bitter properties of the other two herbs. The efficacy of Zhi Zi Bai Pi Tang can be enhanced with the addition of Yin Chen, Ban Lan Gen, Yu Jin and Chai Hu.

Ancient Application of Zhi Zi Bai Pi Tang

- *Zhou Hou Fang:* For the treatment of febrile warm diseases with yellowing.
- *Xuan Ming Lun:* For the treatment of damp heat patterns characterised by mild jaundice with a slight sweat issuing from the head and uninhibited urination.

Modern Application Zhi Zi Bai Pi Tang

- Used for damp heat jaundice where there is more heat than damp and no exterior symptoms. Chen Bo Tao et al used Zhi Zi Bai Pi Tang plus Yin Chen and Yu Jin for the treatment of infectious hepatitis (*Jiang Su Zhong Yi* 1962; 2:17).
- Dysentery: Chen Shi Xing et al used Zhi Zi Bai Pi Tang in the treatment of 21 cases of dysentery (*Fu Jian Zhong Yi* 1964; 4).

Case Study

Treatment of Yellow Sweat

Extracted from Shang Han Lun Tang Zheng Lun Zhi

A 65-year-old male had suffered from spontaneous sweating on slight exertion for over six months The sweat was yellow and stained his clothes. His appetite was poor and his urination normal but with nocturnal frequency. His tongue was pale red with a thin, yellow and white tongue coat and his pulse was thready and wiry. The diagnosis was exterior deficiency with interior damp heat and the treatment principle was to augment qi and secure the exterior, clear heat and drain damp. The formula used was Yu Ping Feng San combined with Zhi Zi Bai Pi Tang modified: Sheng Huang Qi 30g, Bai Zhu 10g, Fang Feng 10g, Chao Zhi Zi 10g, Huang Bai 10g, Che Qian Zi 10g. After seven packs, the yellow sweat stopped but relapsed a week later. His pulse was thready and his tongue was pale red with a thin, white tongue coat. A modified version of Yu Ping Feng San was then prescribed: Sheng Huang Qi 30g, Bai Zhu 10g, Fang Feng 10g,

Che Qian Zi 10g, Dang Gui 10g. After five packs, the yellow sweat was gone and he was given the same formula made into pills to take for the next two months, after which there was no recurrence.

Discussion: The cause of the yellow sweat in the above case was damp heat and the diagnosis was exterior deficiency with interior damp heat. Yu Ping Feng San was used to augment qi and secure the exterior and Zhi Zi Bai Pi Tang was used to clear heat and disinhibit damp. Che Qian Zi was added to enhance the function of clearing heat and draining damp, whilst the blood invigorating property of Dang Gui was used to assist with the expulsion of damp.

Ma Huang Lian Qiao Chi Xiao Dou Tang Pattern

Clause 262

伤寒瘀热在里，身必黄， 麻黄连轺 赤小豆汤主之。

Shang han with stasis heat in the interior, the body will turn yellow, Ma Huang Lian Qiao Chi Xiao Dou Tang governs.

MA HUANG LIAN QIAO CHI XIAO DOU TANG: Ma Huang (nodes removed) 2 liang; Lian Qiao 2 liang; Xing Ren (tips removed) 40 pieces; Chi Xiao Dou 1 sheng; Da Zao 12 pieces (broken); Sheng Zi Bai Pi (sliced) 1 sheng; Sheng Jiang (sliced) 2 liang; Zhi Gan Cao 2 liang.

DIRECTIONS: First boil Ma Huang in 1 dou of rain water (liao shui) and skim off the foam before adding the other ingredients. Continue boiling and reduce to 3 sheng. Strain and take warm in three doses so as to finish the medication in half a day. Note: (1) Lian Qiao (连轺) in the original text referred to Lian Qiao Gen or root, but Lian Qiao (连翘), which is the fruit, is used in the modern application. (2) Zi Bai Pi 梓白皮 (cortex catalpae fargesii) clears heat and resolves damp and today is substituted with Yin Chen Hao. (3) In *Ben Cao Gang Mu*, Li Shi Zhen said of liao shui (rain water): "Using rain water to decoct the herbs enhances the heat clearing effect without causing more dampness."

DISCUSSION: Clause 262 describes jaundice or yellowing occurring in a shang han pattern with an unresolved exterior, and cites stasis heat as the basis of the yellowing. This is damp heat jaundice, where damp and heat have combined in the interior and, whilst not mentioned, it is understood that there would be fever due to the steaming outward of the interior heat. Interior damp heat might also be expected to manifest with vexation and inhibited urination. Here, Zhong Jing uses a formula which not only clears damp heat, but also releases the exterior and so it can be determined that the exterior pathogen is unresolved. For this reason, one would expect there to be an aversion to cold, a generalised itch and a floating pulse, but no sweating.

Together, Ma Huang, Sheng Jiang and Xing Ren resolve the exterior and diffuse and descend lung qi, thereby expelling the exterior wind cold and regulating the waterways; Lian Qiao, Chi Xiao Dou and Zi Bai Pi clear heat, promote urination and relieve toxicity; Zhi Gan Cao and Da Zao harmonise the middle. Thus this formula is indicated to treat yang jaundice with an exterior pattern.

Ancient Application of Ma Huang Lian Qiao Chi Xiao Dou Tang

- *Lei Ju Fang Guang Yi:* For the treatment of scabies (疥癣) where there is pruritus, fever, cough, wheezing, swelling and fullness.
- Xu Da Chun used this formula in the treatment of shang han where the exterior pathogen was unresolved and where there was atypical yellowing (*Shang Han Lei Fang*).

Modern Application of Ma Huang Lian Qiao Chi Xiao Dou Tang

- *Jaundice with an exterior pattern.* For an exterior pattern characterised by aversion to cold, nasal discharge and blockage, cough with white phlegm, and a moist tongue coat, use Ma Huang Lian Qiao Chi Xiao Dou Tang adding Yin Chen 30g and Fu Ling 30g. If there are signs of exterior wind heat such as fever, a blocked nose, a sore throat, cough with yellow phlegm and a dry tongue coat, then the same formula can be used omitting Ma Huang, Sheng Jiang and Da Zao and adding Jin Yin Hua, Chai Hu, Huang Qin and Yin Chen. If there are signs of summerheat damp, combine with Liu Yi San and add Huo Xiang, Xiang Ru, Bian Dou Hua and Yin Chen.

- *Acute nephritis or urinary tract infection.* For infective disease of the urinary tract accompanied by an aversion to cold, cough, watery nasal discharge, inhibited urination, facial swelling, a wet, white tongue coat and a floating pulse, use Ma Huang Lian Qiao Chi Xiao Dou Tang, substituting Sheng Jiang with Sheng Jiang Pi, omitting Da Zao and adding Bai Mao Gen, Yi Mu Cao, Qu Mai and Bian Xu. If there are traces of red blood cells in the urine, increase the dose of Lian Qiao to 15–30g. If the interior heat is severe, with a sore throat and vexation, add Shi Gao 30g or use Yue Bi Tang modified.
- *Urticaria.* For hives triggered by contact with cold air or cold water and accompanied by inhibited urination and an aversion to cold, use Ma Huang Lian Qiao Chi Xiao Dou Tang adding Chan Yi 10g, Jiang Can 10g, Bai Xian Pi 10g and Di Fu Zi 10g.

Comparison of Zhi Zi Bai Pi Tang, Yin Chen Hao Tang, Ma Huang Lian Qiao Chi Xiao Dou Tang

	Yin Chen Hao Tang	Zhi Zi Bai Pi Tang	Ma Huang Liang Qiao Chi Xiao Dou Tang
Similarities in Pathogenesis	Damp heat due to stasis heat causing constrained liver and gallbladder qi		
Differences in Pathogenesis	Equal heat and damp	More heat than damp; constraint in the muscle layer	Stagnation of damp heat with an exterior pattern
Common Symptoms	Orangey-yellow jaundice of the skin and sclera, inhibited urination, fever, no sweating		
Differentiating Symptoms	Abdominal fullness, thirst	Anguish	Aversion to cold, pruritus, floating pulse
Key Points of Diagnosis	Abdominal fullness, constipation, thirst	Anguish and restlessness	Aversion to cold, pruritus, floating pulse
Common Treatment Strategy	Clear heat and drain damp		
Differential Treatment	Clear heat and damp from the interior	Clear heat from the muscle layer	Treatment of both exterior and interior
Ingredients	Yin Chen, Zhi Zi, Da Huang	Zhi Zi, Huang Bai, Gan Cao	Ma Huang, Lian Qiao, Xing Ren, Chi Xiao Dou, Sheng Zi Bai Pi, Da Zao, Gan Cao

Summary of Yellowing due to Damp Heat in Yang Ming

The pathogenesis of jaundice is as follows. (1) Either the congestion of Yang Ming heat in the interior, or the generation of exuberant heat in the interior following the incorrect use of fire therapy. Both are characterised by "sweating from the head only which stops at the neck" or "slight sweat on the forehead", which is a result of the heat being unable to vent outward. (2) Damp heat in the interior disturbing the qi dynamic, impairing the function of the spleen and stomach and affecting the proper distribution of liver and gallbladder qi. (3) Stasis heat caused by heat entering the blood aspect combined with stasis. Thus the key pathology of jaundice is: heat, dampness and stasis, and the corresponding strategies are to clear heat, drain damp and invigorate blood to eliminate stasis.

Yin Chen Hao Tang is a leading formula in the treatment of jaundice associated with damp and heat. Zhi Zi Bai Pi Tang is principally focused on heat and Ma Huang Lian Qiao Chi Xiao Dou Tang is indicated for damp heat jaundice with an unresolved exterior. The symptom of "no sweating and inhibited urination" can be a precursor to jaundice and as such has relevance for early intervention. It is important to remember that whilst skin yellowing is characteristic of jaundice, the strategy of venting the heat and dampness is indicated even when there is no noticeable yellowing.

3.5.2 Blood Aspect Patterns

Yang Ming blood patterns are differentiated as follows.

1. An unresolved Yang Ming exterior pattern with heat sinking into the blood level causing external bleeding (Clauses 202, 227).
2. Pathogenic heat harassing the blood, where heat and blood knot in the interior causing a hard black stool (Clauses 237, 257).
3. Pathogenic heat harassing the blood in the large intestine causing blood and pus in the stool (Clause 258).
4. Yang Ming heat entering the chamber of blood and manifesting as a blood amassment pattern (Clause 216).

Unresolved Yang Ming Exterior Pattern with External Bleeding

Clause 202

阳明病，口燥，但欲漱水，不欲咽者，此必衄。

Yang Ming disease, the mouth is dry, there is a desire only to rinse the mouth, there will be external bleeding.

DISCUSSION: Thirst in Yang Ming disease is an indication of qi level heat; if, however, the mouth feels dry and there is no real thirst but just a desire to wet the mouth by rinsing with water, then this is a reflection of the pathogenic heat having fallen into the blood level. The dryness in the mouth is caused by the heat, but because fluids are being steamed upwards to the mouth and throat, there is no thirst or actual need to drink. The bleeding here is generally interpreted as nosebleed: the term 衄 (nǜ) does not refer to internal bleeding but to bleeding from external orifices and principally to bleeding from the nose.

In warm febrile disease, the symptom of a parched mouth with no desire to drink is the hallmark of heat in the nutritive or blood level. The differentiation as to whether it is nutritive level heat or blood level heat is dependent on supplementary symptoms. When there is heat in the nutritive level, apart from the dry mouth, there are supplementary symptoms of fever which worsen at night, an indistinct expression of ban or zhen (macules or papules), vexation, insomnia, delirious speech, a crimson tongue and a thready, rapid pulse. Where heat is in the blood level, the supplementary symptoms are more severe, with external haemorrhage (haemoptysis, epistaxis, haematuria, blood in the stool), a dense distribution of ban or zhen, manic behaviour, delirium and a dark crimson tongue.

In Clause 202, the reference to a dry mouth, where the person just needs to wet their mouth but not drink, signifies that there is no real thirst. This symptom narrows pattern identification to one of heat in the nutritive or blood levels. Therefore, the differentiating symptom for heat in the blood level is the presence of haemorrhage, and with the reference to bleeding, the clause positively identifies the pattern as being Yang Ming heat in the blood level. The treatment strategy is to cool blood and clear heat, drain fire and stop bleeding. Xi Jiao Di Huang Tang is the indicated formula. It can be combined with Yin Qiao San.

Clause 227

脉浮、发热、口干、鼻燥，能食者则衄。

The pulse is floating, there is fever, the mouth is parched, the nose is dry, if the person can eat, then there will be external bleeding.

DISCUSSION: The floating pulse and fever are indicative of heat in the Yang Ming channel. The dry mouth and nose are a result of the heat surging upward along the channel pathway. The ability to eat is a sign that the interior heat has not yet transformed into an excess bowel pattern and that the disorder is still at the qi level, where constrained heat in the channel has caused the flow of blood to be chaotic and leave the vessels.

The term 衄 (nǜ) does not refer to internal bleeding but refers principally to bleeding from the nose. Nosebleed in a Tai Yang shang han exterior pattern indicates a turning point in the progress of the disease and signals resolution. When constrained yang heat forces its way inward and harasses the nutritive level causing nosebleed, it is one way of resolving the constrained heat in the exterior. Because sweat and blood are of the same source, the pathogenic heat can be expelled equally well by sweating or by nosebleed, and this is what is meant by the phrase "bleeding can substitute sweating" and this is why the nosebleed heralds possible recovery.

Clause 227 is a discussion of Yang Ming channel heat where there is no interior excess and where bleeding can be interpreted as the turning point for disease resolution. There have been numerous interpretations of the significance of bleeding. If, after bleeding, the fever resolves and the dry throat and constipation are relieved, then it can be regarded as expulsion of the pathogen via bleeding. However, it must be understood that Yang Ming channel heat is not the same as a Tai Yang shang han exterior excess pattern. Channel heat in the Yang Ming generally manifests as a more severe condition, where exuberant heat damages fluids and easily transforms into dryness. And so, if after bleeding, there is an exacerbation of the heat signs accompanied by insatiable thirst and copious sweating, or by constipation with abdominal fullness, then it can be understood that resolution has not taken place, and that the channel heat has indeed transformed into an interior excess bowel pattern. In this case, Bai Hu Xi Jiao Tang (which is Bai Hu Tang with the addition of Xi Jiao) is indicated. Alternatively, in order to purge the Yang Ming excess heat, Da Cheng Qi Tang can be administered with the supplementation of herbs which clear heat and cool blood.

Heat Harassing the Blood with a Black Stool

Clause 237

阳明证，其人喜忘者，必有畜血。所以然者，本有久瘀血，故令喜忘；屎虽硬，大便反易，其色必黑者，宜抵当汤下之。

Yang Ming pattern, the person is forgetful, there must be blood amassment. The reason for this being, originally there was prolonged blood stasis, so this caused the forgetfulness. Although the stool is hard, the stool is nevertheless easily passed, since the colour will be black, Di Dang Tang is appropriate.

DISCUSSION: The reference to a Yang Ming pattern alludes to the Yang Ming symptom of a hard stool. The connection between forgetfulness and prolonged blood stasis is found in the *Su Wen: Tiao Jing Lun (Chapter 62: Discourse on Regulating the Channels)*: "If blood mingles with evil in the lower part of the body and qi mingles with evil in the upper part of the body, then qi will be disordered and there will be forgetfulness." The heart is the abode of the shen and governs blood; if blood accumulates in the lower jiao, there is insufficient to provide residence to the heart shen. If, further to that, pathogenic heat falls inward and mingles with stagnant blood which has collected in the lower jiao, when the heat then surges upward, it will harass the shen, which is already deprived of nourishment. Mental vitality will be impaired and there will be forgetfulness. If the pattern is one of Yang Ming interior heat, then there is dryness in the stomach and intestines and the stool will be hard. However, Clause 237 explains that in this case, although hard, the stool is easily excreted. The black colour of the stool is a sign of blood amassment in the lower jiao. Di Dang Tang is the appropriate formula to purge heat and dispel blood stasis.

There are two types of blood amassment, one is Tai Yang blood amassment, which is relatively mild with a short history, and the other is the more severe Yang Ming blood amassment, which has a long history of pre-existing blood stasis. Tai Yang blood amassment is characterised by acute pain in the lesser abdomen, manic behaviour, uninhibited urination and a submerged and faint pulse; the formula is Tao He Cheng Qi Tang. If the person is mentally deranged and presents with the Yang Ming symptoms of hardness and fullness in the abdomen and uninhibited urination, the appropriate formula is Di Dang Tang. Differentiation must be made between the two forms of blood amassment, mild and severe, as demonstrated by these two patterns and their corresponding formulas. The more serious Yang Ming blood amassment is characterised by forgetfulness and a black stool, which are signs of long-term pre-existing stasis.

A black stool can be attributed either to excess, as described above, or to deficiency. The deficiency pattern is generally ascribed to deficiency cold in the Yang Ming where qi fails to manage blood, resulting in bleeding. Blood is differentiated as being either 'remote', which is black in colour, or 'near', which is red. These terms may refer to the source of the bleeding or to its relative recency. Black blood in the stool is categorised as 'remote' because the bleeding is remote from the point of exit, that is, the bleeding is from the stomach or duodenum and not the large intestine or rectum. It may also refer to the fact that it has been there for a long time. Remote bleeding in the stool can also manifest as a stool which is dull, sloppy, black and greasy and is associated with a lack-lustre, pale complexion, shortness of breath, a reluctance to speak, cold limbs, abdominal pain, clear, copious urination, a pale tongue and a submerged, thready and forceless pulse. The strategy is then to warm and tonify the spleen, augment qi and stop bleeding and the indicated formula is Huang Tu Tang. However, the black stool described in Clause 237 is associated with excess blood amassment and is rarely seen.

Clause 257

病人无表里证，发热七八日，虽脉浮数者，可下之。假令已下，脉数不解，合热则消谷善饥，至六七日，不大便者，有瘀血，宜抵当汤。

The patient has neither an exterior nor an interior pattern, with fever for seven or eight days, although the pulse is floating and rapid, one may purge. If purgation was already used, the pulse is rapid and there is no resolution, there is combined heat causing rapid digestion with insatiable hunger, if for six or seven days there is no stool, there is blood stasis, Di Dang Tang is appropriate.

DISCUSSION: There are no signs of an exterior pattern, such as aversion to cold, fever, headache or nasal blockage, nor are there any interior symptoms such as abdominal fullness and delirious speech, and yet the fever has persisted for seven or eight days. Clause 257 is describing a Yang Ming pattern, where exuberant interior heat is steaming outward. The floating pulse here is a reflection of the yang heat steaming outward and does not represent an exterior pattern, and so, in spite of the floating pulse there is no exterior pattern and purgation is permitted. If the pulse is no longer floating after the purgation, then it signals that the qi aspect heat has been resolved. However, the fact that the rapid pulse persists is a sign that heat has not been cleared from the blood level. The term 'combined heat' is a reference to heat in the stomach and the intestines. Stomach heat accelerates the digestive process and results in insatiable hunger. If heat accumulates in the intestines, it will consume fluids and constipation will result. The presence of blood stasis in the intestines means that Di Dang Tang is indicated.

Following purgation, the symptoms of a rapid pulse, constipation and insatiable hunger demonstrate that most of the heat in the qi aspect has been cleared, but that the heat in the blood aspect has remained, giving rise to constraint of heat and stasis in the intestines. Di Dang Tang is therefore indicated to purge the heat from the blood aspect. It can be ascertained from the reading of earlier clauses that this pattern would be accompanied by other symptoms such as acute pain and hardness in the lesser abdomen, forgetfulness or deranged behaviour, and a black stool which is hard but easily passed. The pulse would be submerged and knotted.

Heat Harassing Blood with Blood and Pus in the Stool

Clause 258

若脉数不解，而下不止，必协热便脓血也。

If the pulse is rapid and there is no resolution, and there is incessant diarrhoea, there will be heat combined with pus and blood in the stool.

DISCUSSION: This previous clause, Clause 257, describes the case where heat has combined with blood stasis, and where blood in the stomach and intestines had produced a hard black stool. Di Dang Tang was indicated to purge the stool and eliminate the stasis. Clause 258 follows on from that, and explains that after purgation with Di Dang Tang, if the rapid pulse persists, then it is because the pathogenic heat in the blood aspect of Yang Ming has descended to the lower jiao, harassing the intestines. The result is heat diarrhoea, with blood and pus in the stool. Although purgation has cleared heat from the qi aspect, the blood aspect heat has not been resolved. The blood in the stool is the result of heat scorching the blood vessels, whilst the pus is a reflection of intestinal damp heat. This is characteristic of Yang Ming diarrhoea, which is generally attributed to damp heat in the stomach and intestines and where the indicated formula is Bai Tou Weng Tang. In this case, Bai Tou Weng Tang should be modified by adding Mu Xiang and Bai Shao in order to regulate qi, cool the blood and harmonise the ying. Ke Yun Bo proposed that Huang Lian E Jiao Tang could be used.

Heat Entering the Chamber of Blood

Clause 216

阳明病，下血、谵语者，此为热入血室。但头汗出者，刺期门，随其实而泻之，濈然汗出则愈。

In Yang Ming disease, if blood descends and there is delirious speech, it means that heat has entered the chamber of blood. If there is sweating from the head only, needle Qi Men, address the excess by purging, and a continuous sweat will bring recovery.

DISCUSSION: A Yang Ming bowel excess pattern is characterised by abdominal fullness, constipation, tidal fever and delirious speech. However, the Yang Ming pattern described in Clause 216 does not mention abdominal fullness, constipation, or tidal fever and describes instead bleeding and delirious speech. These symptoms show that the Yang Ming qi level heat is not resolved and identifies it as a blood pattern; the pathogenic heat has entered the chamber of blood where the blood level heat causes blood to be chaotic. The descent of blood refers to any bleeding from the womb which is outside the expectation of normal menstruation, and may refer to a heavy flow or to a disordered cycle. Heat in the blood ascends to the upper jiao, disturbing the heart shen and causing delirious speech; the issue of sweat from the head alone is an indication that the heat in the blood is unable to disperse and so when it flares upward, it finds its only escape in sweating from the head. The chamber of blood has an intimate relationship with the liver; in order to drain the excess and clear the pathogenic heat from the liver blood, Qi Men (Liv 14), which is the alarm point, or mu point of the liver, is needled.

The chamber of blood is generally seen to be associated with women and it is accepted by most academics that it refers to the uterus, the Chong Mai and, by implication, the liver. However, it has been the subject of much debate, with Yu Jia Yan and Ke Yun Bo maintaining that it can refer equally to the male. In *Shang Han Lun,* however, Clauses 143, 144 and 145 in the addendum to the Shao Yang chapter describe heat entering the chamber of blood in the context of a female menstrual disorder, where the menstruation either comes ahead of the normal cycle or stops due to an attack of externally contracted disease.

Summary of Blood Aspect Patterns in Yang Ming

There are four scenarios associated with Yang Ming blood aspect patterns.

1. **An unresolved channel disorder with bleeding.** There is a floating pulse accompanied by fever, a dry mouth and dry nasal passages. There is no abdominal fullness or constipation and there is external bleeding such as epistaxis or haemoptysis. The indicated formula is Xi Jiao Di Huang Tang, combined with Yin Qiao San, omitting Jing Jie and Dou Chi, in order to clear toxic heat from the blood and stop bleeding (Clauses 202, 227).
2. **Pathogenic heat harassing the blood, where heat and blood have knotted in the interior and there is a hard black stool.** There is a rapid pulse accompanied by insatiable hunger, forgetfulness and no bowel movement for six or seven days. The indicated formula is Di Dang Tang to eliminate stasis and purge heat from the blood level (Clauses 237, 257).
3. **Pathogenic heat harassing the blood in the large intestine causing blood and pus in the stool.** There is dryness in the mouth but no thirst, insatiable hunger, hardness in the lesser abdomen and forgetfulness or mental derangement. The indicated formula is Bai Tou Weng Tang modified (Clause 258).
4. **Yang Ming heat entering the chamber of blood.** This pattern is characterised by delirious speech. Qi Men (Liv 14) is needled to drain and dissipate heat from the liver channel. This treatment is followed by purging.

Differentiation of Yang Ming blood aspect patterns

Unresolved channel disorder with heat in the nutritive level	Pathogenic heat harassing the blood with a black stool	Pathogenic heat harassing blood causing blood and pus in the stool	Yang Ming heat in the chamber of blood
External bleeding (epistaxis, haematuria, haemoptysis) Dry mouth No desire to drink Dry nose Fever which is worse at night Dense rash over entire body Mental derangement Dark crimson tongue No abdominal fullness No constipation Floating pulse	Hard but easily passed black stool Forgetfulness No signs of exterior pathogen No signs of interior excess heat Floating rapid pulse Insatiable hunger	Rapid pulse Incessant diarrhoea Blood and pus in the stool	Dysfunctional uterine bleeding Delirious speech Sweating from the head
Xi Jiao Di Huang Tang combined with Yin Qiao San modified	Di Dang Tang	Bai Tou Weng Tang modified	Needle Qi Men (Liv 14)

Section Six

3.6 PROGNOSIS & RECOVERY IN YANG MING DISEASE

3.6.1 Prognosis in Yang Ming Disease

Clause 210

夫实则谵语，虚则郑声。郑声者，重语也；直视、谵语、喘满者死，下利者亦死。

Thus excess causes delirious speech, deficiency causes muttering. Muttering means repetitive speech; a fixed gaze, delirious speech, panting and fullness mean death; diarrhoea also means death.

DISCUSSION: Clause 210 describes how excess and deficiency are manifested in speech. Excess is characterised by speech which is loud and incoherent, which is what is meant by delirious speech. This is associated with the excess exuberant heat of Yang Ming, surging upwards and disturbing the shen. Deficiency is characterised by a weak or soft voice and repetitive muttering, which is attributed to deficient heart qi failing to anchor the shen. *Su Wen: Mai Yao Jing Wei Lun Pian (Chapter 17: Discourse on the Essentials of the Pulse)* states: "Where the speech is feeble and repetitive, qi is depleted". The qi here is a reference to essence qi and so muttering is a sign of serious deficiency not just of qi but also of essence.

Staring straight ahead is a sign that the liver and kidney qi is on the verge of expiry. This is understood because the eyes are the orifice of the liver and are nourished by the essence of the kidney. The inability to move the eye from left to right indicates severe exhaustion of the qi of the liver and kidney qi. Delirious speech refers to the unintelligible or nonsensical speech of a person whose mind is unclear or who is suffering from an altered state of consciousness. Panting and a sense of fullness or oppression in the chest are indicative of the desertion of lung qi, and so may herald death, as does diarrhoea, which is a manifestation of the collapse of middle qi, and which results in fluid loss, affecting yin and yang, qi and blood. Essence, qi and shen are the three treasures of life and where there is desertion of all three, the prognosis is death.

Clause 211

发汗多，若重发汗者，亡其阳，谵语，脉短者死；脉自和者不死。

Heavy sweat is promoted, if sweating is promoted again, there will be collapse of yang and delirious speech, if the pulse is short, the person will die; where the pulse is spontaneously harmonised, the person will not die.

DISCUSSION: Sweat is transformed from yin and if a person is subjected to repeated sweating, there will be desertion of yin as well as devastation of yang; because sweat is the fluid of the heart, there is depletion of heart yin and the heart qi will not be anchored, giving rise to delirious speech. A short pulse is a sign of qi and blood deficiency where there is also fluid exhaustion, and so represents a critical condition. A pulse which is not short, but recovers and is harmonious, demonstrates that zheng qi has not been devastated and so the person will not die, but will live.

Delirious speech and muttering were both mentioned in Clause 210, where delirious speech was a sign of excess, and muttering indicated deficiency. The delirious speech of Clause 211, however, is specifically associated with a pattern of yin desertion and yang devastation, and thus these two clauses show how speech can be significant in the differential diagnosis of excess and deficieny patterns.

As a general rule, Yang Ming disease is associated with patterns of heat and excess, and in Yang Ming the symptoms of delirious speech, vigorous fever, copious sweating, a rapid pulse and constipation are not signs of deficiency. Therefore, irrespective of the severity of the condition, once the heat is purged, recovery will ensue; this is reflected in the spontaneous harmonisation of the pulse. Nevertheless, it must be remembered that excess can transform into deficiency and heat into cold. If, as a result of the depletion of qi, blood, yin and yang, there is transmutation of the Yang Ming excess pattern into one of severe deficiency, with such symptoms as muttering and staring straight ahead, the pulse will be short and the prognosis will be poor.

3.6.2 Yang Ming Recovery Period

Clause 193

阳明病欲解时，从申至戌上。

The time that Yang Ming disease is ready to resolve, is from shen to xu.

DISCUSSION: Shen shi, you shi and xu shi are the three two-hour periods of the ancient Chinese system of time-keeping which cover the hours from 3pm to 5pm, 5pm to 7pm and 7pm to 9pm respectively. They preside over the period when the qi of the Yang Ming channel is at its most abundant and its capacity to resist pathogenic qi is robust. This provides the optimal time for the expulsion of pathogenic heat. It is therefore advantageous to utilise this time opportunely in order to enhance clinical outcomes.

The potential for transmission of an external pathogen to the Yang Ming is dependent on three factors.

- The nature of the pathogen: its severity and any factors which would activate the transformation of pathogenic wind cold into heat and dryness and potentiate its transmission into the Yang Ming.
- The physical constitution of the individual: a person with underlying yang excess, particularly where it is accompanied by food stagnation, are more prone to stomach and intestinal dryness.
- Incorrect or inappropriate treatment: inadequate diaphoresis may result in the pathogenic influence not being released or, on the other hand, excessive sweating or purging can cause the exterior pathogen to fall inward and transform into heat, damaging fluids and generating dryness.

Section Seven

3.7 SUMMARY OF THE YANG MING CHAPTER

The chapter on Yang Ming covers six topics, detailing sixteen different patterns, discussing the prognosis of Yang Ming disease, and concluding with an explanation of the recovery time in Yang Ming.

Yang Ming Disease Outline

Yang Ming disease is characterised by stomach excess with fever, spontaneous sweating, no aversion to cold but aversion to heat and a big pulse.

Key Points of Yang Ming Disease Aetiology and Pathogenesis

(i) *Aetiology and pathogenesis.* The aetiology of Yang Ming disease can be a direct attack on the Yang Ming by the pathogen or may be an indirect attack, due to transmission from another channel. An important factor in the contraction of or resistance to disease in any individual is their health status and constitutional balance, as for instance, whether they tend to yang exuberance or yin deficiency.

(ii) *Pathogenesis.* The focus of Yang Ming disease is primarily the stomach and large intestine. The pathogenesis is transformation to dryness, fluid damage, excess stagnation, intestinal excess heat and bowel obstruction. It must be noted that, depending on the severity of the pathogen and individual constitutional differences, Yang Ming disease can convert to patterns of cold or deficiency.

Key Points of Diagnosis in Yang Ming Disease

The initial stage of Yang Ming disease is characterised by aversion to cold, but as the disease progresses, there is fever with no aversion to cold. Therefore the key point of diagnosis is fever and, if the exterior pathogen falls inward, there will be spontaneous sweating. Heat damages the body fluids causing intestinal dryness and constipation; the interior heat pushes qi and blood to the surface giving rise to a big pulse.

Treatment of Yang Ming disease

(i) *Yang Ming channel patterns.* Where a Yang Ming channel pattern with obstruction of channel qi combines with both a Tai Yang exterior pattern and a Shao Yang half exterior and half interior pattern, it is characterised by a pulse which is wiry, floating and big, dry nasal passages, no sweating, somnolence, yellowing of the skin and sclera, difficult urination, tidal fever, belching, swelling around the ears, shortness of breath and abdominal fullness. These symptoms do not respond well to needling and Xiao Chai Hu Tang is the indicated formula to expel the pathogen. For a Yang Ming channel disorder with sweating and aversion to cold, Gui Zhi Tang should be used to promote sweating and release the pathogen from the muscle layer; if there is no sweating, but there is wheezing, Ma Huang Tang is used to promote sweating and release the exterior.

(ii) *Yang Ming heat patterns.* Yang Ming is rich in qi and blood and possesses strong anti-pathogenic qi. This causes a Yang Ming heat pattern to be characterised by vigorous fever, spontaneous sweating, aversion to heat but not to cold, vexation, thirst and a pulse which is floating, slippery and flooding. The guiding formula is Bai Hu Tang and if there is fluid damage characterised by slight coldness felt in the back, aversion to wind or insatiable thirst, Bai Hu jia Ren Shen Tang should be used. If there is vexation and anguish, insomnia, hunger with no desire for food or sweating from the head only and a slightly yellow tongue coat, Zhi Zi Chi Tang is indicated to dissipate heat in the diaphragm. If the pulse is floating and there is fever, thirst and inhibited urination, Zhu Ling Tang is indicated.

(iii) *Yang Ming excess patterns.* When an exterior pathogen enters the interior and transforms into heat, the subsequent fluid damage manifests as dryness bind or pathogenic heat knotted with stagnant food in the intestine, forming a dry stool. Symptoms include abdominal fullness and distension, no bowel movement, a dry yellow tongue coat and a submerged and excess pulse. If there is a preponderance of heat characterised by steaming fever, or vexation with delirious speech, the indicated formula is Tiao Wei Cheng Qi Tang to purge the heat, alleviate the excess and regulate the stomach qi. If there is Yang Ming bowel excess dominated by glomus and fullness, the indicated formula is Xiao Cheng Qi Tang to purge heat and move qi in order to alleviate the fullness. A third presentation is a hard stool with mild dryness bind where the indicated formula is Da Cheng Qi Tang, but only after first trialling the treatment with Xiao Cheng Qi Tang. If there is tidal fever, delirious speech, sweating from the hands and feet, abdominal hardness and fullness, no bowel movement, and a submerged and forceful pulse, Da Cheng Qi Tang is indicated. The other indication for Da Cheng Qi Tang is where urgent purgation is needed to preserve the yin fluid. This occurs in the situation where exuberant heat has consumed and exhausted body fluids and the person suffers from an inability to recognise people, constantly picks at the bedclothes, has blurred vision, or fever with copious sweat, abdominal fullness etc, urgent purgation to drain the heat is required.

(iv) *Pi Yue or Spleen Restraint.* This is a pattern attributed to stomach heat and intestinal dryness characterised by a hard stool, frequent urination, a floating and choppy Fu Yang pulse, absence of tidal fever, delirious speech, abdominal fullness and pain. Treatment is Ma Zi Ren Wan to moisten the intestines and move the bowel. If there is severe depletion of intestinal fluid characterised by either a hard stool or difficult bowel movement, a suppository such as Mi Jian Dao or pig's bile as an enema can be administered to moisten the intestines and facilitate defaecation. Bitter, cold and purging herbs are contraindicated.

(v) *Contraindications in Yang Ming disease.* (a) Bai Hu Tang is contraindicated in an unresolved exterior pattern and in interior patterns of deficiency cold. (b) Cheng Qi Tang is contraindicated if there is no interior excess and the disease location is not in the abdomen but in the epigastrium. Purgation is contraindicated in the following circumstances: if there is no passing of abdominal wind after taking Xiao Cheng Qi Tang; if there is fluid damage and scant urination; if there is qi and blood deficiency and a pulse that is faint and choppy; and if there is a Shao Yang pattern with incessant vomiting. The criterion for prescribing Cheng Qi Tang is the presence of heat excess in the bowel and intestinal dryness.

Transmuted Patterns of Yang Ming

(i) *Yang Ming disease with yellowing.* Yang jaundice is due to damp heat stagnation in the interior with symptoms of yellowing of the skin and sclera, dark, scant urination, fever, a dry throat, vexation, an oppressed sensation in the chest, fatigue, a greasy yellow tongue coat and a rapid, soggy pulse. The indicated formula is Yin Chen Hao Tang. If heat is predominant, Zhi Zi Bai Pi Tang is used, and if there is an exterior pattern with interior damp heat characterised by the absence of sweat and generalised itching, Ma Huang Lian Qiao Chi Xiao Dou Tang is used. For the treatment of yin jaundice due to damp cold, which is characterised by a yellow complexion, the absence of fever, aversion to cold, a sloppy stool, a bland taste in the mouth, a white tongue coat and a submerged, slow pulse, Yin Chen Wu Ling San or Yin Chen Zhu Fu Tang is indicated.

(ii) *Yang Ming blood aspect patterns.* There are four types of blood aspect patterns associated with Yang Ming. (a) The further development of qi aspect heat falling inward, affecting the blood aspect is a pattern characterised by a dry mouth, no thirst, and external bleeding; the treatment is to clear heat and cool blood by using Qing Ying Tang or Xi Jiao Di Huang Tang. (b) Prolonged long-term blood stasis characterised by a hard black stool which is passed without much trouble, uninhibited urination, forgetfulness and hardness in the lesser abdomen; the indicated formula is Di Dang Tang. (c) Unresolved pathogenic heat in the blood aspect of Yang Ming having descended to the lower jiao, harassing the intestines; this results in heat combining with diarrhoea, with blood and pus in the stool, tenesmus, abdominal pain and a greasy yellow tongue coat; modified Bai Tou Weng Tang can be used. (d) Heat in the chamber of blood. This is due to unresolved Yang Ming blood heat harassing the blood chamber and is characterised by bleeding and delirious speech; the treatment is the needling of Qi Men followed by purging.

Yang Ming Disease Prognosis

Shang Han Lun records the prognosis of disease in respect of various manifestations. Where there is delirious speech, a frequently encountered symptom in a heat excess pattern, it is noted that timely treatment will bring about recovery. Where Yang Ming exuberant heat with yin fluid damage is characterised by a forward staring gaze, delirious speech, panting and fullness and incessant diarrhoea, we are told that death will ensue. If incessant sweating is accompanied by delirious speech and a short pulse, indicating yin exhaustion, death will also ensue. We are told that when a Yang Ming pattern of cold and deficiency is accompanied by muttering, this is a sign of the heart shen not being anchored because of the exhaustion of essence qi. Therefore it can be understood that the condition is critical.

Yang Ming Recovery Period

Yang Ming channel qi peaks between the hours of shen to xu (3pm to 9pm) and so this is the optimal time for recovery.

少陽

Shao Yang 4

Section One

4.1 OUTLINE OF SHAO YANG

Pathway of the Shao Yang Channel

The Shao Yang channel comprises both the foot Shao Yang gallbladder and hand Shao Yang san jiao channels which stand in an exterior–interior relationship with the foot Jue Yin liver and hand Jue Yin pericardium channels respectively. The pathway of the channel covers the side of the body from head to foot and is relevant in the understanding and treatment of Shao Yang disease. The external pathway of the foot Shao Yang gallbladder channel starts at the outer corner of the eye, encircles the ear and traverses the head in zig-zag fashion, intersecting the Du meridian before continuing its zig-zag path down the side of the body to the tip of the fourth toe. An internal channel passes through the jaw and enters the chest, passing through the pericardium channel before meeting the liver and gallbladder and continuing to the hips. A luo connecting channel joins it to its yin partner the liver. The external pathway of the hand Shao Yang san jiao channel travels from the tip of the fourth finger to the shoulder, intersects the Du meridian and encircles and enters the ear. An internal channel enters the upper jiao and descends through the middle jiao to the lower jiao. The luo connecting channel leads to the chest and its yin partner, the pericardium.

Physiology of the Shao Yang Channel

The Shao Yang channel incorporates the gallbladder and the san jiao. The main function of the gallbladder is to store and secrete bile which is formed from the surplus qi of the liver. The ministerial fire residing within the gallbladder assists in the dispersion of qi and the release of bile. The gallbladder is housed within the liver and it supports the liver's function of spreading qi. The harmony of the liver, spleen and stomach and the proper function of the qi dynamic are dependent on the unimpeded dispersion of qi which, in turn, is dependent on the gallbladder. The san jiao holds the office of the sluices and governs the waterways and qi transformation. It is the avenue of qi and the pathway of fire and water.

The significance of the Shao Yang channel being located between the Tai Yang and Yang Ming channels is explained in the *Su Wen: Yin Yang Li He Lun Pian (Chapter 6: The Separation and Union of Yin and Yang)* which states: "Tai Yang governs the exterior and is in charge of opening and dispersal; Yang Ming governs the interior and is in charge of closing and storage; Shao Yang governs the space between exterior and interior and is in charge of the pivot mechanism. The activities of the three channels are not in conflict but are intimately related, and their combined name is one yang." This explains the spreading of yang qi by Tai Yang to guard the exterior, the reception and storage of yang qi by Yang Ming to sustain the interior, the co-ordinating of the movement of qi between the exterior and interior by Shao Yang, and its role of governing the pivot mechanism. This is the means by which the three yang channels act in concert to rule vital functions.

Pathology of the Shao Yang Channel

Pathogenic attacks on the Shao Yang represent the progression of disease as it goes from the exterior to the interior; as such, Shao Yang disease represents the conflict between the zheng qi and the pathogenic qi, where the ministerial fire has been constrained, adversely affecting its pivoting function. The resulting disorder is one of constrained gallbladder heat which gives rise to alternating chills and fever, a bitter taste in the mouth, a dry throat, vexation and dizziness. There is also pain in the hypochondrium, fullness in the chest, a reluctance to speak, poor appetite and nausea.

The struggle between the zheng qi and the pathogenic qi obstructs the qi dynamic, thus affecting the function of the spleen and stomach. The chills and fever are a reflection of this conflict, with fever occurring when zheng qi prevails and chills occurring when the pathogen prevails. The bitter taste, dry throat, vexation and dizziness are manifestations of the gallbladder fire rising to the mouth and head; the fullness in the chest and pain in the hypochondrium are caused by the gallbladder constraint; and the reluctance to speak, poor appetite and nausea demonstrate the adverse effects of the impaired pivoting mechanism on the middle jiao. Because the Shao Yang channel is located between the Tai Yang and Yang Ming channels, the disease pathology has significant potential to lead to concurrent patterns such as Shao Yang Tai Yang or Shao Yang Yang Ming patterns, which manifest as complexes of deficiency and excess.

Shao Yang Disease and Its Transmission Pathway

Shao Yang is located between the Tai Yang and Yang Ming channels. Shao Yang diseases, therefore, are often accompanied by Tai Yang or Yang Ming patterns, and Shao Yang disease can also represent a transitional stage as the pathogen passes from the Tai Yang exterior to the Yang Ming interior. With the exception of direct attack, the pathogen is generally transmitted to the Shao Yang from Tai Yang and Yang Ming as a result of incorrect or inappropriate treatment. Inappropriate treatment of a Shao Yang pattern can also give rise to fluid damage which subsequently transforms into dryness, as seen in Yang Ming bowel excess. Alternatively, if yang is damaged, yin will be exuberant, as seen in diseases of the three yin channels. Because Shao Yang and Jue Yin have an exterior–interior relationship, there is the tendency for Shao Yang disease to transmit to Jue Yin or, in the case of the return of yang qi in the recovery phase of Jue Yin disease, the reverse can occur and the pathogen can transfer from Jue Yin to Shao Yang. For this reason, it is said that excess patterns are associated with Shao Yang while deficient patterns are associated with Jue Yin.

Key Manifestations of Shao Yang Disease

There are three key manifestations:

- a bitter taste in the mouth;
- a parched throat; and
- dizziness.

Classification of Shao Yang Disease

Shao Yang disease has two classifications: (1) Disease originating in the Shao Yang channel as a result of a direct attack on the channel; in this case the pathogen has invaded successfully because of constitutional weakness and deficiency. This principle is described in Clause 97: "Blood is weak and qi exhausted, the interstices are open, because evil qi enters, it vies with the zheng qi, knotting below the ribs". (2) Disease transmitting to Shao Yang from another channel. This often follows incorrect or inappropriate treatment of disease in the Tai Yang or Yang Ming, causing transmission of the pathogen to the Shao Yang or, because of the interior–exterior relationship of the liver and gallbladder, it can be part of the recovery process of Jue Yin disease, where there is reversion back through the Shao Yang, producing a complex pattern such as Shao Yang Tai Yang or Shao Yang Yang Ming.

The principal pattern representing Shao

Yang disease manifests with a bitter taste in the mouth, a dry throat, dizziness, alternating chills and fever, fullness in the hypochondrium, reluctance to speak, poor appetite, vexation and nausea. The guiding formula is Xiao Chai Hu Tang and so it is often known as a Xiao Chai Hu Tang pattern. A transmuted pattern of Shao Yang characterised by fever, a slight aversion to cold, joint pain, mild nausea, knotted bind below the heart and a pulse which is floating and wiry is a Chai Hu Gui Zhi Tang pattern. If there is incessant vomiting, distress below the heart and constrained vexation, it is a Da Chai Hu Tang pattern, and if there is tidal fever with a hard stool, then it is a Chai Hu jia Mang Xiao Tang pattern. Fullness in the hypochondrium with a slight bind, inhibited urination, thirst, no vomiting, sweating from the head, and alternating chills and fever indicate a Chai Hu Gui Zhi Gan Jiang Tang pattern. Symptoms of fullness in the chest, vexation, fright, inhibited urination, delirious speech and heaviness of the body indicate a Chai Hu jia Long Gu Mu Li Tang pattern.

Treatment of Shao Yang Disease

The treatment principle in Shao Yang disease is to harmonise and Xiao Chai Hu Tang is the representative formula. This is because Shao Yang disease is neither an exterior nor an interior disorder.

Contraindications in Shao Yang Disease

The promotion of sweat, purgation and emetic therapy are contraindicated, except where justified in a concurret pattern.

Section Two

4.2 PRINCIPAL FEATURES OF SHAO YANG DISEASE

Clause 263

少阳之为病，口苦、咽干、目眩也。

Shao Yang disease, the mouth has a bitter taste, the throat is dry, the eyes are dizzy.

DISCUSSION: Shao Yang disease is caused by pathogenic cold transforming to heat. It is associated with the gallbladder, which stores and secretes the bitter gall essence or bile. A pathogenic attack on the Shao Yang will constrain the gallbladder, resulting in the non-dispersal of gallbladder qi and this constraint transforms into fire. When the fire flares upwards, there is a concurrent upsurge of bile, causing a bitter taste in the mouth and, because the fire scorches fluids, there is a parched throat. The foot Shao Yang channel arises from the inner canthus of the eye and flows into the outer canthus. Furthermore, it is connected to the liver channel, which opens into the eye. Because of these connections, the upward surge of heat enters and harasses the eye leading to dizziness and blurred vision. It should be noted that the term *mu xuan* (目眩), which is referred to here as dizziness in the eyes, refers to the purely visual form of dizziness as distinguished from the vertigo associated with an inner ear problem.

Of the three main characteristic symptoms of Shao Yang disease, bitter taste, a parched throat and dizziness, bitter taste is the most significant, as may be inferred from the fact that it is mentioned first. The *Nei Jing* states that fire is associated with a bitter taste, thus confirming that the bitter taste in Shao Yang symptomises gallbladder fire and is, indeed, the hallmark of Shao Yang disease. A dry throat and dizziness, on the other hand, may equally be associated with liver and kidney yin deficiency.

Due to the fact that the Shao Yang channel qi peaks from yin shi to chen shi (3am to 9am), the symptom of bitter taste in the mouth can be more pronounced during these hours. The Shao Yang gallbladder is housed by the liver, connects to the stomach channel and is the pivot which connects Tai Yang and Yang Ming. For this reason, both Jue Yin liver patterns and Yang Ming stomach heat patterns can manifest with an upsurge of bile causing a bitter taste in the mouth. All three symptoms of a bitter taste, a dry throat and dizziness can be seen in concurrent patterns of Shao Yang or Yang Ming and also in Jue Yin liver heat patterns. Therefore, although bitter taste is a significant symptom in Shao Yang, diagnosis can not be made on that symptom alone.

In describing a concurrent pattern of the three yang, Clause 189 reads: "Yang Ming zhong feng, a bitter taste in the mouth, a parched throat, abdominal fullness, slight panting, fever, aversion to cold, and a pulse that is floating and tight". Clinical observation has shown that an upsurge of bile with a bitter taste in the mouth is often associated with damp heat in the stomach or excess heat in the liver. The differential symptoms for damp heat in the spleen and stomach are a stifling sensation in the chest, nausea, and either constipation or diarrhoea; the identifying symptoms for excess heat in the liver are irritability, a flushed face, redness in the eyes and sometimes yellowing of the skin. Therefore, although a bitter taste is a significant feature of Shao Yang disease, diagnosis can not be made on the basis of bitter taste alone, or even two or three symptoms. In order to diagnose Shao Yang disease accurately, apart from the symptoms of bitter taste, parched throat and dizziness, one must consider all symptoms described in Clause 96 to ensure a comprehensive diagnosis and also have an understanding of the pathogenesis.

Section Three

4.3 CONTRAINDICATIONS IN SHAO YANG DISEASE

Clauses 26, 265 and 267 outline treatments contraindicated in Shao Yang disease.

Clause 264

少阳中风，两耳无所闻、目赤、胸中满而烦者，不可吐下，吐下则悸而惊。

Shao Yang zhong feng, the two ears can not hear, the eyes are scarlet, if there is fullness in the chest and vexation, one should not induce vomiting or purgation, vomiting and purgation will cause palpitations and fright.

DISCUSSION: The foot Shao Yang gallbladder channel circles the ear; wind is a yang pathogen with a tendency to rise. When pathogenic wind and fire in the Shao Yang surge upward, they harass the orifices causing deafness and red eyes. The foot Shao Yang gallbladder channel also flows through the chest and diaphragm and the pathogenic qi obstructs the Shao Yang channel as it descends through the chest, causing fullness in the chest and vexation. Shao Yang is neither exterior nor interior: this is not a pattern of interior excess but one of disharmony due to the disturbance of Shao Yang's pivoting function. It is not appropriate to purge or to induce vomiting and a harmonising formula must be chosen. Xiao Chai Hu Tang is the guiding formula.

Clause 264 alludes to the fact that the symptom of fullness in the chest and vexation may lead the practitioner to a mistaken diagnosis of stomach and bowel excess, where purgation or emesis might be the therapies chosen. However, the consequences of such wrong treatment would result in injury to qi and blood, which would lead to heart deficiency, palpitations and fright and the possibility of even more serious consequences.

Deafness is differentiated according to whether it is due to excess or deficiency. *Shang Han Gong Mu* states: "Any deafness and pain in the ears attributed to Shao Yang disease is treatable; if the deafness is accompanied by cyanosed lips and retraction of the tongue, it indicates a Jue Yin pattern and the condition is not treatable".

Excess patterns of deafness are largely due to pathogenic invasion of the Shao Yang channels by exterior wind cold or wind heat originating in another channel, and where incorrect or inappropriate treatment has resulted in the transmission of the pathogen into the Shao Yang channel. The initial stage resembles a common cold and is characterised by a cough. This can later be followed by deafness or a milder hearing impediment which is accompanied by a bitter taste in the mouth, headache, an oppressed sensation in the chest, fullness in the hypochondrium, a thin, yellow tongue coat and a wiry, rapid pulse. Some patients may experience nausea, lack of appetite and a dry stool. The guiding formula is Xiao Chai Hu Tang modified with the addition of such herbs as Sang Ye, Ju Hua, Sheng Ma, Gua Lou and Fu Ling.

Deafness due to deficiency is generally associated with deficiency of liver and kidney yin. This is based on the theory that the kidney opens in the ears; if kidney essence is depleted, the ears will not be nourished and will not hear the five sounds. The deficiency can be associated with the waning of kidney qi and essence in old age or may be the result of inappropriate and excessive use of acrid and dispersing herbs which have damaged the yin. In practice, it is often preceded by a long history of kidney deficiency, possibly manifesting as tinnitus. Because the underlying pathogenesis is kidney deficiency, it is characterised by such differentiating symptoms as an aching back, fatigue, dizziness, insomnia or disturbed sleep and a weak, thready pulse in the cubit position. Suitable guiding formulas are Qi Ju Di Huang Wan and Er Long Zuo Chi Wan (Shu Di Huang, Shan Zhu Yu, Shan Yao, Dan Pi, Fu Ling, Ze Xie, Chai Hu, Ling Ci Shi). The formulas must be appropriately modified and customised to the patient's individual presentation.

Deafness or hearing problems must not be assumed to belong to a Shao Yang pattern of gallbladder heat harassing the ear. The prescription of Xiao Chai Hu Tang must be based on such differentiating symptoms as bitter taste, red eyes, a dry throat, vexation and an oppressed sensation in the chest.

Clause 265

伤寒，脉弦细、头痛发热者，属少阳。少阳不可发汗，发汗则谵语。此属胃，胃和则愈；胃不和，烦而悸。

Shang han, if the pulse is wiry and fine and there is headache and fever, it pertains to Shao Yang. In Shao Yang, one should not promote sweat, the promotion of sweat can cause delirious speech. This pertains to the stomach, harmony of the stomach will bring recovery; if there is disharmony of the stomach, there will be vexation and palpitations.

DISCUSSION: Shang han disease of the Tai Yang channel is characterised by headache and fever, a pulse which is floating and tight; as an exterior pattern, the indicated treatment is to promote sweat and release the exterior. However, when headache and fever are accompanied by a wiry pulse, it is a sign of Shao Yang disease; as a pattern which is neither exterior nor interior, the indicated treatment is to harmonise, using Xiao Chai Hu Tang. If a sweat promoting formula such as Gui Zhi Tang is used to promote sweat, the fluid loss will give rise to stomach dryness and delirious speech. Because the delirious speech is the result of stomach dryness, drinking a little water will harmonise the stomach and resolve the disorder; however, if the physician fails to harmonise the stomach, fluids will be further depleted, the condition will deteriorate and the exacerbation of stomach heat and dryness will lead to vexation and palpitations.

Although Zhang Zhong Jing did not elaborate on the treatment for a transmuted Shao Yang pattern caused by incorrect treatment, treatment strategies have been suggested by various practitioners who followed him: Xu Shu Wei suggested that a treatment regimen of Mu Li Si Ni Tang followed by Gui Zhi Chai Hu Ge Ban Tang would bring recovery. Wei Li Tong did not propose an alternative treatment but relied on the modifications of Xiao Chai Hu Tang for treatment of heart palpitations which were included in a footnote to Xiao Chai Hu Tang. Cheng Wu Ji suggested that Tiao Wei Cheng Qi Tang was suitable to harmonise the stomach. The authors feel that in a pattern of stomach heat and dryness where delirious speech is a feature, the appropriate strategy is to harmonise the stomach and purge heat.

Both stomach heat and deficiency of the heart or gallbladder can give rise to delirious speech which is associated with fright or timidity. If, after purgation, there are signs of heart and gallbladder qi deficiency where the patient is timid or easily started, and suffers from insomnia or dream-disturbed sleep, and has a pale tongue with a thin coat and a thready, weak pulse, the indicated formula is Tian Wang Bu Xin Dan or An Shen Ding Zhi Wan with the addition of Suan Zao Ren and Bai Zi Ren. If the tongue is red with a greasy, yellow coat, and the patient has a dry throat, a bitter taste in the mouth and vexation due to phlegm heat harassing the shen, then Xiao Chai Hu Tang with the addition of Shi Chang Pu, Yu Jin and Huang Lian or Hao Qin Qing Dan Tang can be used.

A Shao Yang transmuted pattern due to incorrect treatment is rarely seen in the clinical situation, but even where not caused by incorrect treatment, the formulas cited above can be used to address a pattern characterised by palpitations, vexation and delirious speech caused by stomach dryness and heat.

Clause 267

若已吐、下、发汗、温针、谵语，柴胡汤证罢，此为坏病。知犯何逆，以法治之。

If after vomiting, purgation, sweat promotion or warm needling, there is delirious speech, the Chai Hu Tang pattern is finished, this is transmuted disease. Know the error commited, and treat according to the rule.

DISCUSSION: The correct treatment strategy in Shao Yang disease is harmonisation. Emetics, purgation, sweat promotion and warm needling all lead to fluid damage, which results in the pathogenic heat falling inward, where it harasses the heart shen and gives rise to delirious speech. This is an example of adverse treatment causing a transmuted pattern or 'huai bing' and so the pattern is no longer a Xiao Chai Hu Tang pattern. Because transmuted patterns are complex and may manifest differently, it is essential to identify precisely what error has been made in order to understand the pathogenesis of the transmuted pattern and treat it appropriately.

As it can be seen by Clause 267, transmuted patterns or huai bing are not confined to Tai Yang but are seen in diseases of the other channels as well. A similarity can be seen between this clause, in its description of Shao Yang huai bing, and Clause 16A, which, when describing Tai Yang huai bing, states: "Observe the pulse and signs, know the error committed, treat according to the pattern". The maxim to be learnt is that, when treating a transmuted pattern, it is essential to understand the pathogenesis and devise the treatment accordingly.

Summary of Contraindications in Shao Yang Disease

The outline of Shao Yang at the beginning of this chapter identifies the key symptoms of Shao Yang disease as a bitter taste, a dry throat and dizziness. Secondary symptoms include fullness in the chest, vexation, nausea and poor appetite. Shao Yang is located in the mid-stage between the Tai Yang and Yang Ming channels and the indicated treatment is harmonisation. Although there may be headache and fever, the promotion of sweat is contraindicated. Emetic and purgative therapies are also contraindicated and, if used instead of harmonisation, the subsequent fluid loss will cause the pathogenic heat to fall inwards into Yang Ming. The resulting pattern is stomach excess characterised by delirious speech, vexation and palpitations. If purgation injures qi and blood, causing the gallbladder to be deficient, there will be timidity, palpitations or jumpiness, signalling transformation into a transmuted pattern, where the practitioner must observe the pulse and signs and treat according to the pattern in the light of the pathogenesis.

Section Four

4.4 SHAO YANG DISEASE PATTERNS

Shao Yang patterns are neither interior nor exterior and are therefore not classified as being either channel patterns or fu patterns.

Xiao Chai Hu Tang Pattern

Clause 96

伤寒五六日中风，往来寒热，胸胁苦满、默默不欲饮食、心烦喜呕，或胸中烦而不呕，或渴，或腹中痛，或胁下痞硬，或心下悸、小便不利，或不渴、身有微热，或咳者，小柴胡汤主之。

Shang han zhong feng for five or six days, alternating chills and fever, if there is pain and fullness in the chest and ribs, the patient is untalkative with no desire for food or drink, vexation and nausea, or vexation in the chest with no vomiting, or thirst, or pain in the abdomen, or hard glomus beneath the ribs, or palpitations below the heart and urination which is not free, or no thirst and a slight fever, or a cough, Xiao Chai Hu Tang governs.

XIAO CHAI HU TANG: Chai Hu ½ jin; Huang Qin 3 liang; Ren Shen 3 liang; Ban Xia ½ jin; Zhi Gan Cao 3 liang; Sheng Jiang (sliced) 3 liang; Da Zao 12 pieces (broken).

DIRECTIONS: Boil the above ingredients in 1 dou 2 sheng of water, reducing to 6 sheng. Strain, bring to the boil again and reduce to 3 sheng of liquid. Take one sheng warm three times a day.

(1) If there is vexation in the chest without vomiting, omit Ban Xia and Ren Shen and add one piece of Gua Lou Shi (Quan Gua Lou). (2) If there is thirst, omit Ban Xia increase Ren Shen to 4½ liang and add 4 liang of Gua Lou Shi. (3) If there is pain in the abdomen, omit Huang Qin and add 3 liang of Shao Yao. (4) If there is hard glomus in the hypochondrium, omit Da Zao and add 4 liang of Mu Li. (5) If there are palpitations below the heart with inhibited urination, omit Huang Qin and add 4 liang of Fu Ling. (6) If there is no thirst but there is a mild fever, omit Ren Shen, add 3 liang of Gui Zhi and take the decoction warm to produce a mild sweat in order to release the exterior. (7) If there is a cough, omit Ren Shen, Da Zao and Sheng Jiang and add ½ a sheng of Wu Wei Zi and 2 liang of Gan Jiang.

DISCUSSION: Clause 96 is remarkable for its listing of the many variations in the manifestation of Shao Yang disease, all of which may share the aetiology of shang han zhong feng, or cold damage wind strike. If it is still unresolved after five or six days, and there are additional symptoms of alternating chills and fever with painful distension in the chest and side of the ribs, then the pathogen must be affecting the Shao Yang channel and its fu organ. The manifestation of alternating chills and fever is characteristic of Shao Yang and represents the struggle between the zheng qi and the pathogenic qi. The fluctuation in the advance and retreat of these two entities is seen in the manifestation of chills and aversion to cold when the pathogenic qi prevails and, when exuberant zheng qi prevails over the pathogenic qi, fever breaks out.

The Shao Yang qi has a natural tendency to disperse, thereby facilitating the movement of qi between exterior and interior and between upper and lower. It abhors constraint and so when the pathogen invasion obstructs the qi of the liver and gallbladder, its failure to flow freely results in pain and distension in the side of the chest, which represents the course of the channel. The qi constraint manifests as an unwillingness to talk or interact with others and also vexation or restlessness. The Shao Yang gallbladder stores bile essence and supports the digestive process. Pathogenic constraint of the Shao Yang results in the wood energy attacking the spleen earth. The resulting disharmony of the spleen and stomach affects the digestion and appetite, so that there is no desire to eat or drink and there is also nausea or vomiting.

The mutability of manifestations in Shao Yang disease is due to the waxing and waning of the pathogenic qi; the variation and range of symptoms is due to the location of the disease. Apart from the chills and fever, the painful distension in the chest, the reluctance to speak, distaste for food, vexation and nausea just described, there follows a list of alternative symptoms, each preceded with a definitive 'or': a) vexation without vomiting which is due to heat constraint in the chest causing counterflow of stomach qi; b) thirst which is a result of heat consuming the body fluids; c) abdominal pain which is due to gallbladder constraint stagnating liver qi, harassing the stomach and causing stagnation in the middle jiao; d) hard glomus in the hypochondrium which is due to qi constraint leading to blood stasis forming a mass; e) palpitations below the heart with inhibited urination due to water retention in the epigastrium; f) a slight fever with no thirst which is due to an unresolved exterior with pathogenic constraint in the Tai Yang; and g) a cough which could be caused by pathogenic water harassing the lung. For all of these alternative patterns and manifestations of Shao Yang, Xiao Chai Hu Tang is the indicated formula.

The pathogenesis of Shao Yang disease is qi constraint of the gallbladder and san jiao transforming into fire and disturbing the pivoting function of the Shao Yang. The herbal ingredients of Xiao Chai Hu Tang can be viewed in three functional partnerships. (1) Chai Hu and Huang Qin, where Chai Hu disperses constrained qi in the Shao Yang and Huang Qin clears heat from the gallbladder; their combined effect disperses qi in the channel and the fu, thus facilitating the clearing of heat from both the exterior and the interior. (2) Ban Xia and Sheng Jiang, which constitute the small formula known as Xiao Ban Xia Tang; Ban Xia, due to its acrid nature, helps to descend stomach qi and has the specialised function of alleviating vomiting, and when combined with Sheng Jiang its function of harmonising the stomach is enhanced. (3) Ren Shen, Gan Cao and Da Zao strengthen the spleen, augment qi and warm the middle. The rationale of incorporating these sweet and tonifying herbs is based on the need to support the zheng qi. This is because Shao Yang is the last of the three yang channels and its yang qi is much weaker than Tai Yang and Yang Ming. Moreover, the strategy of strengthening the middle qi can forestall transmutation because, if the spleen is strengthened, it will resist attack from the liver: "liver disease may affect the spleen and therefore in diseases of the liver, one should tonify the spleen" (*Jin Gui Yao Lue)*. Finally, the addition of these sweet, warm herbs can counter the bitterness and coldness of Chai Hu and Huang Qin, thus preventing damage to the spleen.

The dose of Chai Hu in the original text is ½ jin (8 liang), which is 24g and may appear excessive. However, in the treatment of Shao Yang disease, Chai Hu is not used in its capacity of releasing the exterior, but to clear constrained heat from the gallbladder, and a small dose will simply not be effective. In *Shen Nong Ben Cao Jing* it is written, "Chai Hu is bitter and neutral and is indicated in the treatment of knotted qi of the stomach and intestines associated with food stagnation". It is the view of some practitioners that the clinical effect of Xiao Chai Hu Tang is unsatisfactory. The reason for this is the modern trend to halve the dose of Chai Hu and Ban Xia, reducing it to about 12g which is inadequate. Some practitioners use a reduced dose because they fear that the dispersing nature of Chai Hu will damage the liver yin; however, if the diagnosis is correct and the appropriate dosages are used, there will be no necessity for prolonged administration and the possibility of injury to yin will not be a consideration. A dose of only 6g of Chai Hu is the dosage for Bu Zhong Yi Qi Tang, where its purpose is to raise the clear yang, and not, as in Xiao Chai Hu Tang, to vent constrained gallbladder heat.

It is not only the dosage of individual herbs, but their ratios which are important. According to Shang Han specialists, the dose of Chai Hu can be double that of Ren Shen, and the dose of Ren Shen must never exceed that of Chai Hu. The dosage of Sheng Jiang, Ren Shen and Da Zao should be equal, and should not be large. This applies in particular to Da Zao. The original formula prescribes 12 pieces, which amounts to some 30 to 40g, depending on the size of the fruit, and certainly exceeds the normal recommended dose. Such a large dose tends to generate both heat and damp and is therefore not suitable for applications of Xiao Chai Hu Tang where heat and damp are a significant factor as represented by a bitter taste and thirst, or where there is nausea, vomiting or inhibited urination. In these circumstances, the dose of Da Zao should be reduced as a large dose would defeat the purpose of the formula, and in the case of heat or damp heat in the liver and gallbladder, Da Zao is better omitted altogether. It is also important to follow the decoction method as outlined in the original text, which entails reboiling the strained liquid in order to further concentrate the decoction and enhance its functions.

Xiao Chai Hu Tang has a broad clinical application and its flexible application and high efficacy are attributed to the following.

- The formula comprises both warm and cool herbs and supplementing and draining herbs; combined, these regulate the ascent and descent of qi. Because its function is to harmonise, it can treat a range of disorders in patients presenting with either deficiency or excess patterns.
- The herbal combinations target the constrained qi of the Shao Yang and restore its function as the pivot for qi to move between the exterior and interior, and to connect the upper and lower jiao. Based on the understanding that qi obstruction is the underlying cause of many patterns, such as damp accumulation or blood stasis, the unlocking of the constrained pivot mechanism is able to address the root of many disorders.
- Because it can clear heat, tonify deficiency, harmonise the stomach and support the zheng qi, Xiao Chai Hu Tang can be used in the treatment of a wide range of disorders, and its flexible application is further increased by modification: herbs to invigorate blood and eliminate stasis, herbs to nourish yin and clear empty heat, or additional herbs to augment qi. If there is damp accumulation with inhibited urination, herbs to promote urination can be added, or if there is deficient or constrained yang qi, warming herbs can be added to tonify or unblock the yang.

Clause 97

血弱气尽，腠理开，邪气因入，与正气相搏，结于胁下。正邪分争，往来寒热，休作有时，默默不欲饮食。脏腑相连，其痛必下，邪高痛下，故使呕也，小柴胡汤主之。服柴胡汤已，渴者属阳明，以法治之。

Blood is weak and qi exhausted, the interstices are open, evil qi enters, it vies with the zheng qi, knotting below the ribs. The upright battles the evil, chills and fever come and go, off and on periodically, the patient is untalkative with no desire to eat or drink. The zang fu are interconnected, the pain will be below, the evil is high and the pain is low, hence causing vomiting, Xiao Chai Hu Tang governs. If, having taken Chai Hu Tang, there is thirst pertaining to Yang Ming, treat according to the rule.

DISCUSSION: Clause 97 elaborates on what was said in Clause 96 and explains the disease mechanism. Of particular note is the reference to constitutional deficiency being an aetiological factor, with deficiency of qi and blood having resulted in deficiency in the body's defences. The term *cou li* (腠理) or interstices refers to the openings in the layer running between the skin and muscle, which may include, but are not limited to, the pores of the skin. It is these interstices which provide a means for pathogens to pass into or out of the body. The deficiency has left the *cou li* or interstices open and the outer layer of the body unguarded. The exterior pathogen gains entrance and is subsequently locked and knotted in the area under the ribs, which is traversed by the Shao Yang channel. As the zheng qi contends with the pathogen, there is fever, and when the activity of the zheng qi abates, the evil prevails and there are chills. This periodic fluctuation is reflected in the recurrence of chills and fever. The untalkativeness is not a sign of deficiency but of qi constraint, and the lack of appetite is a sign of the impaired pivot mechanism affecting the middle qi. The interconnection between the zang and the fu means that an attack on one part of the body can affect another part and so, when the pathogen invades the Shao Yang and constrains the qi of the liver and gallbladder, the affect flows through to the spleen and stomach, which are lower down, causing abdominal pain, qi counterflow and vomiting. This is the way the clause explains the course of disease from the exterior to the interior in terms of the zang fu. Thirst following the administration of Xiao Chai Hu Tang is uncharacteristic of a Shao Yang pattern, and indicates that the pathogen has entered the Yang Ming. Xiao Chai Hu Tang is no longer appropriate and a different treatment strategy is required.

In regard to transmuted changes following the administration of Xiao Chai Hu Tang, Zhong Jing did not elaborate beyond saying that thirst is associated with Yang Ming and should be treated in accordance with that pattern. This naturally entails further differentiation. If there is formless heat in the stomach with dryness, Bai Hu Tang should be used to clear heat; if there is heat with coincident fluid damage characterised by insatiable thirst, aversion to wind and a hollow, forceless pulse, Bai Hu jia Ren Shen Tang is indicated; if there is an accumulation of formed heat in the intestines characterised by abdominal fullness, constipation, tidal fever and delirious speech, then Cheng Qi Tang should be applied to purge the intestinal heat. However, if the Shao Yang pattern is unresolved when the Yang Ming pattern manifests, Da Chai Hu Tang is the formula; if the Shao Yang pattern is resolved and the external heat pathogen has abated, but there is thirst and a dry, red tongue, then this indicates unresolved residual interior heat and Zhu Ye Shi Gao Tang is the appropriate formula to clear the residual heat, augment qi and generate fluids. In other words, the treatment strategy must be based on any change in the symptoms and signs.

Clause 266

本太阳病不解，传入少阳者，胁下硬满，干呕不能食，往来寒热，尚未吐下，脉沉紧者，与小柴胡汤。

Originally Tai Yang disease was not resolved, if it transmits to Shao Yang, there is hardness and fullness under the ribs, dry retching and an inability to eat, alternating chills and fever, and there is neither emetic nor purgation, the pulse is submerged and tight, give Xiao Chai Hu Tang.

DISCUSSION: Clause 266 describes a situation where unresolved Tai Yang disease has eventually been transmitted to Shao Yang. This is evidenced by the hard distension in the hypochondrium, which coincides with the path of Shao Yang, and the alternating chills and fever, which reflect the struggle between the zheng qi and the pathogenic qi at the mid-stage between the exterior and interior. Because the gallbladder and stomach are linked via the network vessels, the pathogenic invasion of Shao Yang disturbs the qi dynamic, causing disharmony of the spleen and stomach; hence there is dry retching and an inability to eat and keep food down. It is important to understand the significance of the fact that no emetics or purgatives have been used. If they had been used, the pathogen could have fallen inwards, injuring the zheng qi, and since they have not been used, the zheng qi is still robust.

Because the pulse is not floating, but is submerged, it is understood that the pathogen is no longer in the exterior but has passed to the Shao Yang. The term 'tight' in this context is used to refer to the wiry pulse of Shao Yang and for that reason, Xiao Chai Hu Tang can be given.

Unresolved Tai Yang disease can transmit either to Yang Ming or to Shao Yang. When it transmits to Shao Yang, it is generally due to weakness of the spleen qi. This clause demonstrates how the transmission of disease in the six channel diseases does not always follow the nominal sequence from Tai Yang through to Yang Ming before reaching Shao Yang.

Clause 99

伤寒四五日，身热、恶风、颈项强、胁下满，手足温而渴者，小柴胡汤主之。

Shang han for four or five days, if there is fever, aversion to wind, stiffness of the neck, fullness under the ribs, warm hands and feet and thirst, Xiao Chai Hu Tang governs.

DISCUSSION: Fever, aversion to wind and a stiff neck show the presence of an unresolved Tai Yang exterior disorder; fullness under the ribs is a sign of a Shao Yang pattern; the warm limbs and thirst represent a Yang Ming interior pattern. In this way, Clause 99 describes a concurrent pattern of the three yang channels. Although both Tai Yang and Yang Ming patterns are present, Xiao Chai Hu Tang is prescribed. As the guiding formula for Shao Yang disease, representing disease which is mid-stage between the exterior and the interior, it is well suited to treat a mixed pattern, because it harmonises. The rationale of this choice is as follows.

1. In Shao Yang, sweating, which is the strategy used in Tai Yang disease, and purgation, the strategy employed in Yang Ming, are both contraindicated. The promotion of sweat in either Shao Yang or Yang Ming can exacerbate heat and may result in a transmuted pattern; the use of purgation in any but a Yang Ming bowel excess pattern will similarly cause deterioration. Therefore the most appropriate treatment for a concurrent pattern of the three yang is to harmonise.
2. Owing to its location halfway between the exterior and the interior, one of the main physiological functions of Shao Yang is to act as a pivot and regulate the qi dynamic of the three yang channels; if the pivot mechanism is restored then the exterior pathogen of Tai Yang can be vented outward and the interior heat of Yang Ming can be cleared. It is interesting to note that modern research has shown that Xiao Chai Hu Tang is anti-pyretic and effective in resolving fever.
3. Xiao Chai Hu Tang is the emperor of harmonising formulas: it can release the exterior pathogen from Tai Yang, and also facilitate the distribution of body fluids in the interior, thus harmonising the stomach qi.

Contemporary practitioners regularly prescribe Xiao Chai Hu Tang when treating a concurrent pattern of the three yang. This is because, as a harmonising formula, it lends itself well to modifications. For example, where there is fever and an unresolved exterior, Ren Shen is omitted and Gui Zhi is added; where there is thirst, Ban Xia is omitted and Gua Lou Ren is added to generate fluids. Better results are obtained by such modifications because the formula then addresses both primary and secondary symptoms.

Clause 100

伤寒，阳脉涩，阴脉弦，法当腹中急痛，先与小建中汤；不差者，小柴胡汤主之。

Shang han, the yang pulse is choppy, the yin pulse is wiry, there must be acute pain in the abdomen, first give Xiao Jian Zhong Tang; if it is not despatched, Xiao Chai Hu Tang governs.

DISCUSSION: The yang pulse refers to the superficial level of the pulse which should be floating in a shang han disorder, but is choppy. This indicates blood deficiency with impeded circulation. The yin pulse refers to the deeper palpation of the pulse, which is wiry and characteristic of a Shao Yang pulse.

The acute abdominal pain is a result of pathogenic invasion of the Shao Yang, which has caused wood to invade earth on a background of pre-existing spleen deficiency. The excess qi of the Shao Yang harasses the deficient earth, giving rise to pain. Because the root of the pain is middle qi deficiency, Xiao Jian Zhong Tang is given first, the rationale being to ease the acute pain before pursuing other strategies. Once the pain is resolved by taking Xiao Jian Zhong Tang, a spleen tonifying formula can then be administered to effect full recovery. If, however, the pain remains, it means that there is still constraint of the liver and gallbladder qi, the Shao Yang has not been resolved and Xiao Chai Hu Tang should then be given.

The above use of Xiao Jian Zhong Tang demonstrates the principle of supporting earth to restrain wood, where, by strengthening deficient earth, it is able to resist the attack of excess wood. This offers an alternative method of addressing excess in the liver and gallbladder and was proposed in the *Su Wen: Zang Qi Fa Shi Lun Pian (Chapter 22: Discourse on the Law of Organ Qi and the Seasons)*: "When there is constraint in the liver, sweet food can be used to moderate the constraint". This is based on the principle of sweetness corresponding to earth in five phase theory, and being tonifying in nature. Xiao Jian Zhong Tang contains Yi Tang, Zhi Gan Cao and Da Zao, which are sweet and tonify the spleen; Gui Zhi and Sheng Jiang scatter cold and the combination of Gui Zhi, Bai Shao and Sheng Jiang together, harmonise ying and wei. Yi Tang, Da Zao, Zhi Gan Cao and Bai Shao moderate spasm; the blood tonifying herbs also serve to soften the liver. Thus Xiao Jian Zhong Tang warms and tonifies with sweet herbs and also eases pain caused by liver constraint.

There are two scenarios of Shao Yang disease accompanied by abdominal pain, each with a different treatment strategy.

1. Abdominal pain which is part of a Xiao Chai Hu Tang pattern and cited as one of the alternative symptoms in Clause 96: the abdominal pain is secondary to the main Shao Yang pattern symptoms and the main formula is modified by omitting Huang Qin and adding Shao Yao in order to relax the spleen network vessels, thereby easing the pain.
2. Abdominal pain due to deficiency and cold in the middle jiao with an associated insufficiency of qi and blood: the Shao Yang pattern is secondary to the primary pattern of cold and deficiency in the spleen, which gives rise to pain. The strategy is to warm and tonify the middle and to ease pain.

Clause 101

伤寒中风，有柴胡证，但见一证便是，不必悉具。凡柴胡汤病证而下之，若柴胡证不罢者，复与柴胡汤，必蒸蒸而振，却复发热汗出而解。

Shang han zhong feng, with Chai Hu signs, observing just one sign will do, there is no need for all to be present. Where there is purgation in a Chai Hu Tang pattern, if the Chai Hu pattern is not finished, give Chai Hu Tang again, there will be steaming and shivering, followed by fever and sweating then recovery.

DISCUSSION: The essence of the first statement in Clause 101 is not, literally, that Xiao Chai Hu Tang can be prescribed on the basis of only one sign or manifestation. The point being made is that on the appearance of one or two symptoms, and before a pattern of Shang Han zhong feng, or wind strike, is fully developed, Xiao Chai Hu Tang can be used pre-emptively. This is because it is appropriate to use the strategy of harmonisation at an early and anticipatory stage. The clause also explains that the administration of Chai Hu Tang is equally appropriate in a case where adverse purgation has been used, providing some Chai Hu Tang pattern signs are present. Where purgation has damaged the interior, Xiao Chai Hu Tang strengthens the spleen qi, thus supporting the zheng qi in its struggle against the pathogen. The reference to steaming and shivering is an allusion to the alternating chills and fever which signal this struggle, whilst the fever and sweating are signs of robust zheng qi eliminating the pathogen. The phrase "steaming and shivering followed by fever and sweating" describes a condition often referred to as 'shivering sweat' which identifies this struggle and heralds recovery. The implications of shivering sweat are described at the end of this discussion.

The interpretation of precisely what is meant by 'just one sign' has been the subject of much debate. Cheng Wu Ji interpreted it as referring to any one of the alternative symptoms listed in Clause 96; Cheng Jiao Qian believed the 'one sign' referred to the principal manifestations of a bitter taste in the mouth, dry throat, and dizziness, which are signs of fire in the Shao Yang; Yun Tie Qiao, on the other hand, believed the 'one sign' could refer to a combination of any two or three symptoms indicating constraint in the Shao Yang, namely: alternating chills and fever, pain and fullness under the ribs, an unwillingness to talk or interact with others, lack of appetite, vexation and nausea or vomiting. Modern scholars tend to concur with this last interpretation. The reference to 'just one sign' is simply a reminder that not all signs have to be present to make a diagnosis; one sign may lead us toward a particular diagnosis but further signs are needed to confirm that the pattern diagnosis is indeed true to the pathogenesis and symptomatology. The authors believe that if all eight signs have to appear before using Xiao Chai Hu Tang, this may cause unnecessary treatment delay with subsequent undesirable transmutations. This principle is not peculiar to a Xiao Chai Hu Tang pattern but is a general principle which is also seen in Ma Huang Tang, Gui Zhi Tang, Cheng Qi Tang and Bai Hu Ren Shen Tang patterns, to name but a few.

Shivering and Sweating in Shao Yang Disease

In regard to the symptoms of shivering and sweating which arise after the repeat administration of Xiao Chai Hu Tang, as cited in Clause 101, there are four points to bear in mind.

1. *The identification of shivering sweat.*
   - (i) Shivering sweat refers to severe shivering and trembling, where there are brief periods of aversion to cold which are followed by generalised copious sweating.
   - (ii) This represents an externally contracted disease which has arisen from incorrect or inappropriate treatment; the result is constrained yang qi with unresolved fever. The shivering sweat can be preceded by vexation and, occasionally, a hidden pulse or cold extremities.
   - (iii) The pulse image associated with shivering sweat will be floating, indicating that the pathogen is still in the exterior, and moderate, which indicates that the stomach qi is harmonious. This bodes well for a full recovery. If the pulse sign is hidden, submerged or scattered, one should not assume that the pulse is verging on expiry, but must observe the person's spirit. A bright spirit demonstrates that the submerged pulse is only a temporary sign; shivering sweat demonstrates that the pathogen is being vented outwards and there will be recovery and full restoration to the circulation of qi and blood. Conversely if after the episode of shivering sweat, there is a rapid pulse, accompanied by coarse breathing, numbness of the limbs, an inability to ingest fluids, sudden cramps and a fixed gaze with an inability to speak, the prognosis is poor because these are signs of depletion of essence and imminent death.
   - (iv) Apart from the manifestation of shivering and sweat, prognosis is also determined by signs of heat and cold. If the shivering sweat is followed by coldness and then by heat, the prognosis is good; however, if there is shivering but no sweating, then it indicates severe yang deficiency with exuberance of yin cold. The yang deficiency, further hampered by exuberant yin is then unable to vent the pathogen. There may be a clouded spirit and impaired consciousness and this reflects a final struggle with death.
2. *Prognosis in shivering sweat.* If, following shivering sweat, the fever persists and there is a rapid pulse, fatigue, vexation, an oppressed sensation in the chest with abdominal fullness and no desire for food, then there may be recurrence of shivering sweat; this is because the residual pathogen is not resolved. However, following the shivering sweat, if the pulse is subdued and the fever has abated, the appetite returns and the spirit is bright, then recovery is imminent. Sometimes, after shivering sweat, the person falls into a sound sleep and the pulse is harmonious and moderate. This, too, heralds recovery and no further treatment is required.
3. *Treatment of shivering sweat.* No medication is required during the actual episode of shivering sweat, but hot gruel should be given at regular intervals in order to nourish the middle and replenish qi. If the patient is not lucid and the pulse is floating in all six positions, shivering sweat is more likely to take place and hot ginger juice should be given to assist the process.
4. During an episode of shivering sweat, in addition to giving hot rice gruel and ginger soup to support the zheng qi, one should ensure the patient is in a room which is neither too hot nor too cold.

Clause 229

阳明病，发潮热、大便溏、小便自可、胸胁满不去者，与小柴胡汤。

Yang Ming disease, if there is tidal fever, the stool is sloppy, urination is as usual, and fullness in the chest and ribs does not abate, give Xiao Chai Hu Tang.

Clause 230

阳明病，胁下硬满，不大便而呕，舌上白胎者，可与小柴胡汤。上焦得通，津液得下，胃气因和，身濈然汗出而解。

Yang Ming disease, if there is hardness and fullness under the ribs, no stool but vomiting, and a white tongue coat, one may give Xiao Chai Hu Tang. The upper jiao is freed, body fluids descend, the stomach qi is therefore harmonised, there is continuous sweat and recovery.

DISCUSSION: A Yang Ming bowel excess pattern is characterised by tidal fever, a hard stool and uninhibited urination. In contrast, Clause 229 describes Yang Ming disease where the tidal fever is accompanied by a sloppy stool and uninhibited urination, indicating that the Yang Ming disease has as yet not developed into a bowel excess pattern; at the same time, there is the Shao Yang symptom of fullness and pain under the ribs. The pattern thus described is a concurrent pattern of an unresolved Shao Yang disorder occurring with a Yang Ming pattern which has not yet proceeded to bowel excess. Although there is tidal fever, there is no bowel excess and so purging is contraindicated and Cheng Qi Tang is inappropriate. The correct strategy is to adhere to the principle of releasing the exterior before treating the interior. Xiao Chai Hu Tang fulfills those requirements by releasing the pathogen from the Shao Yang, and also freeing the upper jiao to restore the proper distribution and descent of body fluids, thus harmonising the stomach qi. The tidal fever is resolved as a result of the venting of constrained heat and restoration of the qi dynamic.

Shang Han Lun outlines contraindications for purgation even in the presence of Yang Ming symptoms. The specific circumstances are the presentation of tidal fever and a sloppy stool, and the absence of a stool when the tongue coat is white. The latter indicates that the constipation is not due to dry heat bind but is a milder disorder, ascribed to the qi constraint of a Shao Yang pattern, where the stool is dry due to non-distribution of body fluids. The Shao Yang channel and network vessels are distributed over the side of the chest and hypochondrium. Obstruction to the flow of channel qi results in hardness and fullness under the ribs, and can also affect the descent of fluids, causing disharmony of the stomach and manifesting as vomiting. The white tongue coat demonstrates that there is no heat. Therefore Xiao Chai Hu Tang is used to harmonise Shao Yang and, by dissipating constrained liver qi, free the movement of vital substances in the triple jiao.

Clauses 229 and 230 both describe a concurrent pattern of Yang Ming and Shao Yang. Clause 229 describes a pattern where there is tidal fever, a sloppy stool and uninhibited urination; Clause 230 describes symptoms of constipation and vomiting. Both patterns exhibit the classic Shao Yang symptoms of fullness and oppression in the hypochondrium, and since there is no evidence of bowel excess, the treatment is focused on Shao Yang. This is an expansion of the scope of prescribing Xiao Chai Hu Tang.

Differentiation must be made between the tidal fever of Shao Yang and that of Yang Ming and their respective treatments. Tidal fever associated with a Yang Ming pattern is a manifestation of interior heat knotted in the stomach and intestines; it is characterised by abdominal distension, constipation and sweating from the extremities. The strategy is to clear interior heat and purge the knotted bind and so Cheng Qi Tang is used. In contrast, the tidal fever of Shao Yang is the result of gallbladder constraint affecting the qi dynamic; it is characterised by fullness in the hypochondrium. There is no constipation and the treatment strategy is to vent the constrained heat and restore the qi dynamic with the harmonising formula Xiao Chai Hu Tang. Constipation, a dry stool or the absence of a stool is one of the main indications for Cheng Qi Tang or Ma Zi Ren Wan, and yet Xiao Chai Hu Tang is frequently used to treat constipation. Although most practitioners are aware of Cheng Qi Tang in this application, Xiao Chai Hu Tang, which can free qi obstruction and promote the distribution of fluids, is often overlooked. The key symptoms indicating this application are a white, slippery tongue coat, nausea, and hardness and fullness under the ribs.

Clause 148

伤寒五六日，头汗出、微恶寒、手足冷、心下满、口不欲食、大便硬、脉细者，此为阳微结，必有表，复有里也。脉沉，亦在里也。汗出，为阳微；假令纯阴结，不得复有外证，悉入在里，此为半在里半在外也。脉虽沉紧，不得为少阴病。所以然者，阴不得有汗，今头汗出，故知非少阴也，可与小柴胡汤；设不了了者，得屎而解。

Shang han for five or six days, if there is sweating from the head, mild aversion to cold, cold hands and feet, fullness below the heart, no desire to eat, a hard stool and a thready pulse, this is a mild yang bind, there will be both exterior and interior signs. A submerged pulse, it is also in the interior. Sweating indicates the mild yang; if it were pure yin bind, there would be no more exterior signs, it would have entirely entered the interior; this is half in the exterior and half in the interior. Although the pulse is submerged and tight, it does not mean a Shao Yin disease. The reason being, yin has no sweat, here there is sweating from the head, and so we know it is not Shao Yin, one may give Xiao Chai Hu Tang; if it is not fully cleared, once a stool is passed, it will resolve.

DISCUSSION: Clause 148 describes a pattern where there are both exterior and interior signs: shang han disease where there is still an aversion to cold after five or six days shows that the exterior is unresolved; the fullness below the heart, lack of appetite, the hard stool and submerged pulse are manifestations of an interior disharmony, occurring as a result of disharmony between the exterior and interior. The qi dynamic has been affected by the yang constraint in the interior, referred to as 'mild yang bind', where the pathogen has obstructed the dispersal of qi. This yang constraint and non-dispersal of qi result in cold extremities. Furthermore, because the constrained interior heat obstructs the outward diffusion of yang qi, the steam which should vent the pathogenic heat is not perfused throughout the body but instead can only percolate upwards, so there is sweating from the head only. The statement in the clause "A submerged pulse, it is also in the interior" refers to the submerged pulse being a sign of the pathogen having entered the interior. This is because yang qi is constrained and fails to support the movement of qi and blood; the impeded flow then gives rise to obstruction in the interior, hence the submerged pulse. However, although it has entered the interior, it is not a purely interior pattern like yin bind of Shao Yin, where cold is knotted in the interior but there are no exterior symptoms. This is a case of mild yang bind, as shown by the sweating from the head explained above, so "this is half in the exterior and half in the interior." By reactivating the pivot mechanism, Xiao Chai Hu Tang unblocks the constrained yang and frees the yang bind, thus restoring the distribution of body fluids. By unblocking the constrained yang, it assists in the venting of the pathogenic heat yang, and so there is sweating, which will bring recovery.

The pathogenesis of mild yang bind is disharmony between the exterior and interior. Yang constraint, which represents a condition of mild pathogenic heat, manifests as constipation. This is differentiated from the constipation of a Cheng Qi Tang bowel excess pattern on the basis of the absence of the key symptoms of that pattern, namely: tidal fever, sweaty hands and feet, abdominal distension or periumbilical pain and delirium. It is also differentiated from the constipation of a Ma Zi Ren Wan pattern, where stomach heat dries the body fluids and the spleen is deficient and unable to distribute them, resulting in an insufficiency of fluids in the intestines, and giving rise to constipation due to dryness.

Clause 379

呕而发热者，小柴胡汤主之。

If there is vomiting and fever, Xiao Chai Hu Tang governs.

DISCUSSION: Shao Yang and Jue Yin stand in an exterior–interior relationship which sets the stage for further development of Shao

Yang disease to affect Jue Yin. Similarly, the restitution of yang in Jue Yin can cause Jue Yin disease to revert to Shao Yang. This restitution of yang represents a return from deficiency, and this is the basis of the saying: "Excess pertains to Shao Yang and deficiency pertains to Jue Yin". In Shang Han Lun, vomiting and fever are identifying signs of Shao Yang, as seen in Clause 149: "Shang han for five or six days, with vomiting and fever, Xiao Chai Hu Tang signs are present". The vomiting and fever described in this clause are an indication that the pathogen in Jue Yin is being vented outward to the Shao Yang and so is a reflection of the transformation of the disease from yin to yang. Vomiting in Shao Yang is attributed to the constrained qi of the gallbladder harassing the stomach.

Ancient Application of Xiao Chai Hu Tang

- *Shang Han Lun*. Clinical applications in the original text include the following.
- For Shao Yang half exterior and half interior pattern with hyperactive liver qi and spleen deficiency characterised by abdominal pain. After the administration of Xiao Jian Zhong Tang, if the disease is not resolved, Xiao Chai Hu Tang is given.
- For a concurrent pattern of the three yang where a Shao Yang pattern predominates.
- For Yang Ming disease either where there is tidal fever, a sloppy stool and distension in the hypochondrium, or where there is hardness in the hypochondrium accompanied by constipation and a white tongue coat.
- For Jue Yin disease characterised by fever and vomiting.
- For a mild Yang bind due to qi obstruction, as described in Clause 148, where there is a hard stool, cold extremities, fullness below the heart, aversion to cold and sweating from the head.
- For women presenting with blood stasis caused by heat entering the chamber of blood, Xiao Chai Hu Tang can be used with modifications.
- For the convalescent phase of shang han disease where there is fever.

In other classic texts, the applications are as follows.

- *Shang Han Huo Ren Shu:* For the treatment of a phlegm heat headache, accompanied by warm extremities, vexation, disharmony of ying and wei, leg cramps, body aches, fatigue and sleepiness and no appetite, Chai Hu Ban Xia Tang was used, modified with the addition of Bai Zhu and Mai Dong.
- *Su Wen: Bing Ji Qi Yi Bao Ming Ji* (written by Liu Wan Su, also known as Liu He Jian): For the treatment of post-partum amenorrhoea, accompanied by leg cramps and the grinding of teeth, Zeng Xun Chai Hu Tang was used, which is Xiao Chai Hu Tang with the addition of Shi Gao, Zhi Mu and Huang Qi.
- *Su Shen Liang Fang:* For alternating chills and fever, generalised fever, vexation and distension in the hypochondrium with or without thirst, and also in convalescence from shang han disease with fever.
- *Jing Yue Quan Shu:* For the treatment of damp heat malaria characterised by aching in the body, heaviness of the limbs, and where there is more cold than heat and a soggy pulse. The strategy is to parch and drain damp, harmonise the spleen and restore the qi dynamic. Chai Ping Tang was used, which is Xiao Chai Hu Tang combined with Ping Wei San.
- *Shang Han Liu Shu:* For a wind cold pattern with transformation to heat, shown by diminished aversion to cold, increased sensations of heat, the absence of sweat, headache, a dry nose, vexation, insomnia, sore eyes and a floating, slightly flooding pulse. Chai Ge Jie Ji Tang was used, which is Xiao Chai Hu Tang omitting Ren Shen and Ban Xia and adding Qiang Huo, Ge Gen, Jie Geng, Shao Yao and Bai Zhi. The original text suggests if there is an aversion to cold with no sweating, Huang Qin should be replaced by Ma Huang. In the winter months, Ma Huang should be added; in spring the dosage of Ma Huang should be reduced; in summer, Ma Huang should be replaced by Su Ye.
- *Liu Ke Zhun Sheng:* For the treatment of post-partum deficiency detriment disorder, characterised by fever which does not respond to acupuncture and moxibustion, San He Tang was used, which is Xiao Chai Hu Tang combined with Si Wu Tang and the addition of Bai Zhu, Fu Ling and Huang Qi.

Zhang Shi Yi Tong: For Shao Yang glomus and fullness accompanied by chills and fever, Chai Hu Jie Geng Tang was used, which is Xiao Chai Hu Tang with the addition of Zhi Qiao and Jie Geng.

Modern Application of Xiao Chai Hu Tang

Xiao Chai Hu Tang is a versatile formula with minimal side effects and has the potential for application in a wide range of disorders.

Fever. Zhou et al used Xiao Chai Hu Tang with modifications in the treatment of infantile rheumatic fever. Where there was more heat, Qing Dai and Qing Hao were added; where there was joint pain, Gui Zhi, Niu Xi and Qin Jiao were added; where there were palpitations, Mai Dong and Wu Wei Zi were added. The fever was resolved within 2–6 days and there was no recurrence in the following 3–6 months. (*Zhong Yi Nian Jian* 1984).

Febrile disease. Yin Hui He used a modification of Xiao Chai Hu Tang in the treatment of externally contracted febrile disease characterised by chills and fever, using Chai Hu, Huang Qin and Ban Xia as the base formula. If there was no bowel movement, Shi Gao and Da Huang were added; for a sore throat and blocked nose, Shan Dou Gen and Yu Xing Cao were added; for absence of sweat, Bo He was added (*Guang Dong Yi Xue* 1982; 9:26).

Angina pectoris. Shao et al used a modification of Xiao Chai Hu Tang to treat 46 cases of angina pectoris, where in 30 cases Western medication had brought some relief but there was a recurrence of chest pain. The core formula was Chai Hu 20g, Ban Xia 15g, Zhi Gan Cao 15g, Fu Zi 15g, Dang Gui 15g, Ren Shen 10g, Huang Qin 9g, Chuan Xiong 25g, Sheng Jiang 12g, Da Zao 12 pieces. For qi deficiency, the dose of Ren Shen was increased; for yang deficiency, the dose of Fu Zi was increased; for qi and blood stagnation, the dosage of Chai Hu, Dang Gui and Chuan Xiong were increased; for phlegm turbidity, the dosage of Sheng Jiang and Ban Xia were increased. After five packs it was found that 11 cases experienced substantial relief in chest pain and after a total of twenty packs, 35 of the 46 subjects were completely pain free (Shao Gui Zhen: *He Nan Zhong Yi* 1986; (3):18).

Cough. Wang et al used a modified version of Xiao Chai Hu Tang in the treatment of 50 cases of night coughing associated with constrained gallbladder fire and characterised by foamy sputum or watery phlegm, a pale red or red tongue with a thin, moist, white or yellow coat and a pulse which was fine and wiry or wiry and rapid. The formula used was Chai Hu 12g, Huang Qin 10g, Ban Xia 10g, Xi Xin 6g, Wu Wei Zi 10g, Sheng Jiang or Gan Jiang 10g, Xing Ren 10g, Zhi Qiao 10g, Gan Cao 6g. The result was 23 cases with total resolution of cough after three packs, two cases with substantial relief after two packs and 21 cases with full recovery after six packs of medication (*Zhong Yi Za Zhi* 1986; 4:283).

Morning sickness. Wang et al used a modification of Xiao Chai Hu Tang to treat morning sickness. The formula used was Chai Hu 4.5g, Hong Zao 5 pieces, Huang Qin 10g, Xi Dang Shen 12g, Sheng Jiang 3 pieces, Fa Ban Xia 10g, Zhi Gan Cao 3g. For spleen and stomach qi deficiency, they added Chao Bai Zhu 10g, Fu Ling 10g. For spleen qi deficiency with abdominal distension, they added Mu Xiang 6g, Sha Ren 4.5g, Chen Pi 10g. For the accumulation of phlegm fluids characterised by chest fullness, nausea and the vomiting of phlegm fluids, they increased the dose of Ban Xia to 15g and added 10g each of Fu Ling and Chen Pi. For disharmony of the liver and stomach characterised by acid reflux, abdominal fullness, belching, vexation and a bitter taste in the mouth, they added Su Geng 4.5g, Huang Lian 10g, Zhu Ru 15g. For stomach yin deficiency characterised by a red tongue and a dry mouth, they added Bei Sha Shen 15g, Mai Dong 15g, Lu Gen 24g, Shi Hu 25g. For qi and yin deficiency characterised by emaciation, fatigue and haemoptysis, they substituted Ren Shen with Dang Shen 10g, and added Wu Mei 10g, Mai Dong 15g, Dai Zhe Shi 30g (broken and decocted first), Xian He Cao 24g and E Jiao 15g (melted and mixed with decoction) (*Zhong Yi Za Zhi* 1986; 5:347).

Xiao Chai Hu Tang can be used in the treatment of jaundice which manifests as a Shao Yang pattern. The core formula should be modified by omitting Da Zao and adding Yin Chen Hao, Long Dan Cao and Bai Jiang Cao.

Modifications for additional symptoms can be made as follows. For headache: Man Jing Zi was added; for high fever and thirst: Xuan Shen and Shi Gao were added. After 3 days, the fever was reduced but a low grade fever remained, with sweating which was more pronounced at night. The core formula was then modified as follows: Da Zao was omitted and Jin Yin Hua, Xuan Shen, Di Gu Pi were added to address the empty heat. Where nausea was a pronounced symptom, Zhu Ru was also added.

The authors have found Xiao Chai Hu Tang to be effective in the treatment of gall stones and cholecystitis, where it soothes the uncomfortable digestive symptoms whilst addressing the underlying disorder. Appropriate herbs such as Jin Qian Cao, Wei Ling Xian, Yu Jin, Di Long, Mang Xiao, Qing Pi, Zhi Shi, Da Huang and Dan Shen can be used to promote the expulsion of the stones if they are small, like sand. However, larger stones must first be reduced in size with such herbs as Jin Qian Cao, Ji Nei Jin, Mang Xiao and E Zhu. For gallbladder disorders characterised by nausea and vomiting, Xiao Chai Hu Tang can be combined with Wen Dan Tang; where there is hypochondriac or epigastric pain associated with infection or inflammation of the gallbladder, Xiao Chai Hu Tang can be combined with herbs which clear toxic heat and relieve food stagnation. In addition, Xiao Chai Hu Tang can be used to treat patients with a lingering upper respiratory infection, which seems to be resolved but resurfaces. Herbs appropriate to the individual patient are added. However, the core formula can be used as part of the treatment protocol following treatment of the common cold, even where symptoms have subsided, in order to ensure full eradication of the pathogen and prevent resurgence.

Because it supports the pivot mechanism, thereby regulating the middle qi, Xiao Chai Hu Tang is also useful in digestive upsets and gastrointestinal disease as follows. Where there is externally contracted gastroenteric disease, it can be combined with Huo Xiang Zheng Qi Tang; where there is damp accumulation, it can be combined with Ping Wei San; where there is a poor appetite or epigastric distension or indigestion and bloating, Xiao Chai Hu Tang can be combined with Kai Wei Tang. Where there is constipation due to qi stagnation, Xiao Chai Hu Tang can be used with the addition of such herbs as Xuan Shen and Zhi Shi.

Professor Liu Du Zhou's Use of Xiao Chai Hu Tang in the Treatment of Hepatitis

(Extracted from *Ming Yi Jing Yan Lu* 1996.)

Professor Liu Du Zhou frequently uses Xiao Chai Hu Tang in the treatment of liver disease. In the acute phase, he uses Chai Hu Jie Du Tang (Chai Hu, Huang Qin, Yin Chen, Zhi Gan Cao, Tu Fu Ling, Cao He Che, Fung Wei Cao, Tu Yuan, Qian Cao), which disperses liver qi, clears heat, relieves toxicity drains damp, and cools and invigorates blood. In the chronic phase, he uses Chai Hu Huo Luo Tang, which is Chai Hu Jie Du Tang with the addition of Dang Gui, Bai Shao, Ze Lan, Hong Hua. For toxic damp heat or hyperactive liver and gallbladder fire, he uses San Cao Chai Hu Jie Du Tang, which is Chai Hu Jie Du Tang with the addition of Chui Pen Cao, Jin Qian Cao and Long Dan Cao.

His modifications are as follows. If there is cold in the middle jiao, add Pao Jiang and Gan Jiang to warm the middle. For dark yellow urination, add Jin Qian Cao and Hu Zhang in order to clear heat, drain damp, invigorate blood and stop pain. For abnormally high alkaline phosphatase (ALP) levels, add Chui Pen Cao. For a low ratio of albumin to globulin (where the normal ratio is 2:1) use an increased dosage of Tu Yuan and Qian Cao. If jaundice is severe, add Yin Chen Hao Tang or Zhi Zi Bai Pi Tang. For latent heat in the ying aspect, use Zhi Zi Bai Pi Tang. If there is a predominance of damp accompanied by thirst and a thick greasy yellow tongue coat, add Shi Gao, Hua Shi and Han Shui Shi, which is known as San Shi Chai Hu Jie Du Tang. For pain in the liver or hypochondrium, add Jing Ling Zi San (Chuan Lian Zi, Yuan Hu). For a loose stool due to spleen qi deficiency, add Bai Zhu and Fu Ling. If the pain in the hypochondrium is severe, use Chai Hu Zhi Tong Tang (Chai Hu, Yuan Hu, Chuan Lian Zi, Dang Gui, Bai Shao, Liu Ji Nu, Tu Yuan, Qian Cao, Zao Jiao Ci, Pian Jiang Huang, Hai Piao Xiao, Zhi Ke, Zi Wan). The focus of this formula is on nourishing and invigorating blood and regulating qi, based on the theory of qi and blood being interdependent. For yin deficiency with blood heat manifesting as vexation, five heart heat, epistaxis and seminal emission with a crimson tongue and a rapid, thready pulse, use Chai Hu Bie Jia Tang, which is Xiao Chai Hu Tang with the addition of Bie Jia, Mu Li, Yu Zhu, Sheng Di Huang, Mai Dong, Sha Shen and Bai Shao to nourish yin and soften the liver, and Tu Bie Chong, Qian Cao to invigorate blood and unblock the network vessels.

Professor Liu Du Zhou's Use of Xiao Chai Hu Tang in the Treatment of Cirrhosis of the Liver

The core formula used for liver cirrhosis is Chai Hu Huo Luo Tang modified. At this stage there is an overlap of the pathogenesis of early liver cirrhosis and that of chronic, viral hepatitis.

- For abnormal alanine aminotransferase (ALT), use Chai Hu Jie Du Tang.
- For reduction of albumin and elevated globulin, add Tu Bie Chong and Qian Cao.
- For persistent sloppy stools, use Chai Hu Gui Zhi Gan Jiang Tang to disperse liver qi, harmonise the network vessels, warm the middle and disperse cold.
- For ascites, use Dr. Liu's Bai Yu Tang 白玉汤 (Fu Ling, Yu Mi Xu, Bai Mao Gen, Dong Gua Pi, Da Fu Pi, Yi Mu Cao, Che Qian Cao, Tu Yuan, Qian Cao, Chuan Lian Zi, Yuan Hu, Zi Wan, Zhi Qiao.) This formula regulates the qi dynamic, harmonises blood and invigorates the network vessels. It has the ability to drain and expel the retained water without injuring the zheng qi.

Case Study

Emotional Distress

Source unknown

A 24-year-old woman had experienced a failed love affair and was emotionally distressed and bitter. She heard voices and imagined someone talking to her. Other symptoms were distension below the ribs, sighing, restlessness, anxiety and insomnia. Her appetite was poor, her menstrual cycle was irregular and her breasts were tender and distended prior to and during the menstrual period. Her pulse was submerged, wiry and slippery and her tongue coat was white and greasy. The diagnosis was constrained liver and gallbladder qi transforming into fire with phlegm harassing the heart shen. The formula prescribed was Xiao Chai Hu Tang combined with Wen Dan Tang: Chai Hu 12g, Huang Qin 10g, Ban Xia 16g, Sheng Jiang 12g, Zhi Gan Cao 6g, Dang Shen 6g, Da Zao 7 pieces, Zhu Ru 20g, Zhi Shi 10g, Chen Pi 12g, Fu Ling 20g. After 3 packs, she coughed up a lot of phlegm. She was given a further 3 packs and her appetite improved. In all, she was given 20 doses and her recovery was complete.

Case Study

Belching and Dyspepsia

Extracted from Greta Young's case studies

A 35-year-old female patient suffered from a liver and stomach disharmony with distension under the ribs and frequent belching. Some days previously, she experienced a stressful situation which made her very angry and since then she had had a cough with blood-streaked sputum, and suffered from dizziness, insomnia and vexation. Her pulse was wiry, fine and rapid and her tongue was red with a thin white coat. The diagnosis was liver and gallbladder fire harassing the lung. She was prescribed Chai Dai San (Chai Hu 12g, Huang Qin 10g, Ban Xia 10g, Sheng Jiang 3g, Zhi Gan Cao 6g, Dang Shen 6g, Da Zao 5 pieces, Hai Ge Qiao 20g, Qing Dai 10g (wrapped in gauze)). After seven doses the condition was resolved.

Case Study

Infertility Due to Liver Constraint

Extracted from Robin Marchment's case studies

A 36-year-old woman had been trying to conceive for four years. She had a history of an irregular menstrual cycle (26-35 days) and mid-cycle pain. The menstrual blood was dark and stagnant during the first two to three days, gradually becoming thinner in consistency and turning a bright red for the next three days, before becoming scant, sludgy and brown on the last day. The failure to conceive increased her premenstrual symptoms, and she was depressed and irritable, and also suffered mild nausea and bloating and an oppressive sensation in the chest. Her tongue was pale red with a purplish tinge and the pulse was fine and wiry on the left-hand side and slightly slippery on the right. The diagnosis was liver constraint and the treatment principle was to harmonise qi and blood and nourish the spleen and kidneys. The formula prescribed was a modified version of Xiao Chai Hu Tang: Chai Hu 8g, Huang Qin 10g, Ban Xia 8g, Dang Shen 15g, He Shou Wu 15g, Nu Zhen Zi 10g, Bai Shao 8g, Yu Jin 10g, Tu Si Zi 10g, Fu Ling 12g, Xiang Fu 8g, ZhiGan Cao 6g. This prescription, with slight variations, was administered in the weeks following the menstrual flow in each cycle. After two months, the cycle was 30 days, stabilising to 28-30 days over the next two months. The premenstrual irritability diminished significantly and there was no more pain at midcycle. The flow was a deep red colour and was no longer brown and sludgy at the end of the period. She conceived in the sixth cycle and gave birth to a healthy child later that year.

Case Study

Chronic Unresolved Exterior Syndrome Affecting the Interior

Extracted from Greta Young's case studies

A 35-year-old female patient had been suffering from fever for two months, with the temperature hovering at about 38°C before noon, rising to about 39°C in the afternoon and returning to normal in the evening. Just before the fever rose in the afternoon, she would experience an aversion to cold then there would be sweating in the late afternoon before the fever subsided. Her mouth and throat were dry and she often felt fatigued and dizzy. She also suffered from pain in the hypochondrium, a dry stool and occasional nausea. Her tongue was red with a yellow, greasy coat and the pulse was fine and wiry. She brought the reports of a blood test showing an elevated white blood cell count. The Western diagnosis was fever requiring further investigation. The Chinese medicine diagnosis was disharmony of exterior and interior with constrained damp heat in the interior. The formula prescribed was Xiao Chai Hu Tang combined with Ping Wei San to harmonise Shao Yang and aromatically transform turbidity: Chai Hu 18g, Huang Qin 10g, Ban Xia 10g, Cang Zhu 10g, Hou Po 9g, Dang Shen 8g, Huo Xiang 10g, Xuan Shen 20g, Xiang fu 10g, Gan Cao 3g. After five packs, the fever had reduced to 38°C and her bowel movement was normal but her throat was still dry and she had noticed a bitter taste in her mouth. The same formula was prescribed again, omitting Huo Ma Ren, and repeated for two more weeks. At the third consultation, there was no fever but she complained of feeling irritable. Two weeks of Xiao Yao San was prescribed with good results.

Xiao Chai Hu Tang Contraindications

Clause 98

得病六七日，脉迟浮弱、恶风寒、手足温，医二三下之，不能食而胁下满痛，面目及身黄、颈项强、小便难者，与柴胡汤，后必下重。本渴饮水而呕者，柴胡汤不中与也，食谷者哕。

Ill for six or seven days, the pulse is slow, floating and weak, there is aversion to wind and cold, the hands and feet are warm, the physician purged two or three times, if there is an inability to eat and fullness and pain under the ribs, the face, eyes and skin are yellow, the neck is stiff, and urination is difficult, give Xiao Chai Hu Tang, later there is heaviness below. If originally there was thirst and after drinking water there was vomiting, Chai Hu Tang should not be given, if the patient eats, he will vomit.

DISCUSSION: If a shang han pattern is still unresolved after six or seven days, then the possibility of transmission or transmutation must be considered. The floating pulse, aversion to wind and cold and the stiff neck are all evidence of an exterior condition which would normally be treated with an exterior-releasing formula such as Gui Zhi Tang. However a slow pulse and warm extremities are not manifestations of an exterior pattern, so it can be seen that there is both an exterior and an interior pattern. The slow, weak pulse is indicative of an interior deficiency, and in this case, it is associated with Tai Yin. The symptoms are those of an exterior pathogenic attack on a background of underlying spleen yang deficiency and the required strategy is to warm the yang. The practitioner has disregarded the interior deficiency; instead, he has mistaken the warm extremities as a sign of a Yang Ming interior excess pattern and has used purgation. This has further damaged the spleen yang and given rise to a transmuted pattern; the deficient spleen yang fails to transform and transport fluids, giving rise to an accumulation of damp cold; this obstructs the flow of qi causing constraint in the liver and gallbladder channel. The constraint manifests as pain and distension in the hypochondrium; the failure of the impaired liver and gallbladder to disperse qi results in a disordered flow of bile, giving rise to jaundice and inhibited urination. The thirst is not due to heat or dryness but to the non-dispersal and non-production of fluids by the deficient spleen yang; the spleen's failure to transform and transport fluids has also resulted in an accumulation of yin fluids in the stomach, impeding its function of receiving grain and water. Hence there is vomiting after drinking.

This must not be assumed to be a Shao Yang pattern simply on the basis of the fullness and pain in the hypochondrium. This is a pattern of interior cold and Xiao Chai Hu Tang is not warm enough; its cold, bitter herbs will further damage the spleen yang, and there will be a loose stool and a heavy sensation in the rectum. If it is given in the presence of the accumulation of yin fluids, which are demonstrated by the inability to keep water down, then there will be further deterioration of the transmuted pattern with greater damage to the middle qi, where there is vomiting of food as well as water. The pattern described in Clause 98 is an exterior pattern combined with spleen yang deficiency and Gui Zhi Ren Shen Tang is the appropriate formula to warm the middle, strengthen the spleen and release the exterior.

Summary of Shao Yang Channel Patterns

The foregoing section is a discussion of the aetiology and pathogenesis of Shao Yang disease, its key symptoms and signs, methods of pattern identification, treatment and contraindications. The cause of Shao Yang disease can be either unresolved Tai Yang disease or a direct attack from an external pathogen. The latter is described in Clause 97, which describes a direct attack associated with an underlying deficiency: "Blood is weak and qi exhausted, the interstices are open, evil qi enters, it vies with the zheng qi, knotting below the ribs". The pathogenesis is thus described as a struggle between zheng qi and pathogenic qi manifesting as alternating chills and fever, with nausea and vomiting being attributed to constraint and fire in the gallbladder which has disturbed the qi dynamic of the spleen and stomach. The principal manifestations of Shao Yang disease are alternating chills and fever, fullness under the ribs, untalkativeness, vexation, nausea and vomiting, a bitter taste in the mouth, a dry throat, dizziness and a wiry and thready pulse.

Xiao Chai Hu Tang harmonises the exterior and interior, acts as a pivot for qi moving between Tai Yang and Yang Ming, and regulates yin and yang. Because it restores the qi dynamic and facilitates the smooth flow of qi and water in the triple jiao, it is not confined to the treatment of Shao Yang patterns, but is versatile in its application and can be used for such disorders as the following:

1. Abdominal pain associated with a hyperactive liver and a weak spleen.
2. A concurrent pattern of the three yang channels where the focus is Shao Yang.
3. Yang Ming and Shao Yang disease characterised by tidal fever and constipation.
4. Disease in Jue Yin reverting to Shao Yang characterised by gallbladder heat, vomiting and fever.

5. A disharmony of the exterior and interior with yang constraint and qi stagnation.

Xiao Chai Hu Tang is contraindicated where there is a pattern of cold and deficiency in the spleen and stomach; in such circumstances its use may result in the transmuted pattern of yin jaundice. The focus of Xiao Chai Hu Tang is harmonisation; it does not warm the spleen yang or transform cold damp. Gan Cao and Da Zao, although tonifying, tend to be cloying and can generate more damp; Chai Hu and Huang Qin are bitter and cold and will cause further damage to the spleen. Further depletion of spleen yang and exacerbation of cold damp will result in diarrhoea with rectal heaviness. The appropriate formula is Yin Chen Zhu Fu Tang for the treatment of yin jaundice due to yang deficiency with damp cold.

Although Xiao Chai Hu Tang has a broad range of applications, it must not be thought of as being suitable for all disorders. There is particular potential for mistaken application if the diagnosis is based on only one symptom, as highlighted in Clause 98. Therefore, it can be concluded that the suggestion in Clause 101 to base the decision to use Xiao Chai Hu Tang on a single symptom should not be taken literally, and proper evaluation should be made using the four examinations.

Section Five

4.5 CONCURRENT PATTERNS OF SHAO YANG

The principal formula used in treating Shao Yang disease is Xiao Chai Hu Tang; however, a Xiao Chai Hu Tang pattern can be accompanied by symptoms of the other channels and therefore modifications of Xiao Chai Hu Tang are required to address the changes in the pattern. The concurrent patterns are:

- Shao Yang disease accompanied by an exterior pattern (Chai Hu Gui Zhi Tang);
- Shao Yang disease with an interior excess pattern (Da Chai Hu Tang);
- After purgation, Shao Yang disease and an interior excess pattern (Chai Hu jia Mang Xiao Tang);
- Shao Yang disease where there is impaired qi transformation (Chai Hu Gui Zhi Gan Jiang Tang);
- Shao Yang disease with disharmony of qi in the triple jiao (Chai Hu jia Long Gu Mu Li Tang).

Chai Hu Gui Zhi Tang Pattern

Chai Hu Gui Zhi Tang is a combination of Xiao Chai Hu Tang and Gui Zhi Tang and is indicated for an exterior and Shao Yang concurrent pattern.

Clause 146

伤寒六七日，发热微恶寒、支节烦痛、微呕、心下支结，外证未去者，柴胡桂枝汤主之。

Shang han for six or seven days, there is fever and a slight aversion to cold, vexing joint pain in the limbs, mild vomiting, a sustained knot below the heart, the exterior pattern has not been resolved, Chai Hu Gui Zhi Tang governs.

CHAI HU GUI ZHI TANG: Chai Hu 4 liang; Gui Zhi (bark removed) 1½ liang; Huang Qin 1½ liang; Ren Shen 1½ liang; Zhi Gan Cao 1 liang; Ban Xia (washed) 2½ ge; Shao Yao 1½ liang; Da Zao 6 pieces (broken); Sheng Jiang (sliced) 1½ liang.

DIRECTIONS: Boil the ingredients in 7 sheng of water, reducing to 3 sheng. Strain and take 1 sheng warm.

DISCUSSION: When shang han disease is still unresolved after six or seven days, there is a possibility of inward transmission. The fever, aversion to cold and joint pain are symptomatic of a Tai Yang Gui Zhi Tang pattern, while the knotted bind below the heart and mild vomiting are associated with a Shao Yang

Chai Hu Tang pattern. This is an example of a lagover pattern or bing bing: the first pattern (Tai Yang) is not yet resolved when a second pattern (Shao Yang) has arisen. The strategy is then to address both patterns simultaneously by combining half a dose each of Gui Zhi Tang and Xiao Chai Hu Tang. These two formulas respectively release the exterior and harmonise the interior. The ingredients of Da Zao, Sheng Jiang and Zhi Gan Cao are common to both formulas; Gui Zhi releases the exterior, disperses wind cold, and together with Shao Yao, regulates ying and wei. By resolving the Tai Yang exterior pathogen, it addresses the fever, the aversion to cold and the vexing joint pain. Xiao Chai Hu Tang harmonises the Shao Yang and so addresses the vomiting and the knotted bind below the heart. This is a commonly used formula as it supplements the spleen and stomach, harmonises the exterior and interior, unblocks the triple jiao and regulates yin and yang.

Ancient Application of Chai Hu Gui Zhi Tang

- *Wai Tai Mi Yao:* For the treatment of hernia with abdominal pain due to cold in the liver channel.
- *San Yin Fang:* For the treatment of Shao Yang disease characterised by fever, aversion to wind, stiffness of the neck, fullness under the ribs, warm extremities, a bitter taste in the mouth, thirst, and a pulse which is floating in the yang position and wiry in the yin.
- *Shang Han Zhun Sheng:* For the treatment of malaria presenting with fever and profuse sweating.

Modern Application of Chai Hu Gui Zhi Tang

- *Common cold or influenza due to a weak constitution.* Patients with a poor immune system tend to suffer recurrent exterior invasions of wind cold manifesting as upper respiratory tact infections, colds or influenza. These may proceed to a chronic condition where there is a raised temperature, mild aversion to cold, joint pain, nausea, poor appetite, a sense of distension in the hypochondrium and a greasy tongue coat which is either white or slightly yellow, reflecting the constrained defence yang. Other symptoms are a sore throat and rapid pulse. If the fever is more pronounced, the dosage of Chai Hu should be increased; for a sore throat, such herbs as Jie Geng, Xuan Shen and Bo He can be added.
- *Early stage cirrhosis of the liver.* Cirrhosis of the liver is a chronic disorder affecting the blood aspect and manifesting as abdominal distension and pain, a dusky or sooty complexion, a purplish tongue body with stasis spots and a submerged and wiry pulse. Liver function tests will show abnormally elevated levels of alanine transaminase (ALT) and aspartate transaminase (AST). Chai Hu Gui Zhi Tang can be modified by omitting Ren Shen, Da Zao and adding Bie Jia, Mu Li, Hong Hua, Qian Cao, Tu Bie Chong in order to invigorate blood and soften and dissipate the abdominal mass.
- *Chronic cholecystitis or cholelithiasis.* In chronic cholecystitis, prolonged administration of cold, bitter herbs to clear toxic heat can damage spleen yang and give rise to a Xiao Chai Hu Yang pattern with such symptoms as loss of appetite, fatigue, a loose stool and a white greasy tongue coat. In this situation Chai Hu Gui Zhi Tang can be used with the following modifications: for gallbladder damp heat, add such herbs as Jin Qian Cao and Yin Chen; to eliminate food stagnation, add Shan Zha and Zhi Qiao; if diarrhoea is severe or persistent, add Bai Zhu and Gan Jiang to warm and strengthen the spleen.
- *Viral influenza.* Influenza can present as a concurrent pattern of Tai Yang and Shao Yang characterised by high fever and a rapid pulse. In this case, Jin Yin Hua and Lu Gen can be added to Chai Hu Gui Zhi Tang; if there is a cough, Xing Ren, Jie Geng and Qian Hu can be added.

Chai Hu Gui Zhi Tang in the Treatment of the Common Cold and Influenza

Patent formulas which are specifically indicated for acute exterior patterns are readily available in pill form. Most, however, contain cold, bitter herbs designed for an excess pattern where there is an invasion of wind heat and a robust constitution. However, not all acute upper respiratory tract infections are a heat pattern, and many patients are of the deficiency type. The use of inappropriate cold formulas, especially for deficient patients, will fail to expel the pathogen, and it will remain in the body, manifesting with a low grade fever, and if herbs are then used which nourish yin and clear heat, it may result in further penetration of the exterior pathogen. Chai Hu Gui Zhi Tang is a useful formula to use because it releases the exterior using both cool and warm herbs and regulates ying and wei, thus expelling the pathogen.

Case Study

Diarrhoea

Extracted from the lecture notes of Prof. Fu Yan Ling, Melbourne, October 2007

A 45-year-old male had been treated for hepatitis with bitter, cold herbs which damaged the spleen yang. He suffered from abdominal distension, no appetite, diarrhoea up to three times a day, occasional dull abdominal pain, pain in the hypochondrium and lower back, slightly red eyes with aversion to light, and discharge from the eyes and gums. Following the prolonged administration of bitter cold herbs to purge liver fire, his liver function test was abnormal. His pulse was wiry and moderate and the tongue was pale with a white coat. The diagnosis was liver harassing the spleen with heat in the liver and cold in the spleen. The formula prescribed was Chai Hu Gui Zhi Gan Jiang Tang modified: Chai Hu 12g, Huang Qin 6g, Zhi Gan Cao 9g, Gan Jiang 9g, Gui Zhi 8g, Tian Hua Fen 10g, Jiang Xiang 9g, Mu Li 30g. After seven packs, the diarrhoea stopped, his appetite improved, and there was relief of the pain in the hypochondrium and lower back. The original formula, replacing Jiang Xiang with Pian Jiang Huang 12g, was repeated for a further seven packs. Follow-up treatment based on Xiao Yao San was given to regulate the liver and spleen.

Discussion: This was a pattern of liver heat and spleen cold. The liver heat manifested as pain in the back and hypochondrium, red, gritty eyes with excessive discharge and aversion to light. The spleen cold was diagnosed on the basis of the prolonged administration of bitter, cold herbs following which there was abdominal distension, dull abdominal pain, poor appetite, a wiry, moderate pulse and a pale tongue with a white coat. The treatment principle was to clear heat from the upper jiao, warm the lower jiao and scatter cold. The dose of Huang Qin was reduced to 5 to 6g in order not to further damage the spleen yang. Jiang Xiang disperses qi and blood in the liver channel and eases pain. In the second prescription, Jiang Xiang was replaced by Jiang Huang to invigorate blood and move qi so as to address the pain under the ribs and in the back.

Case Study

Low-grade Fever

Extracted from Shang Han Shi Jian Lun by Chen Rui Chun

A 46-year-old female patient had been suffering from low-grade fever which was worse at night for over a month. Her temperature ranged between 37.5 and 38.3°C. Three weeks earlier, she had succumbed to a cold with a fever. She self-medicated with Yin Qiao Pian and Ban Lan Gen granules. The fever receded but was followed shortly afterwards by a persistent low-grade fever. She had body aches and pains, aversion to cold and fever, which at night would spike up to 38.6°C before abating in the morning. There was no thirst but there was fatigue, a poor appetite, nausea, a difficult bowel movement and aversion to wind. The tongue coat was thin and moist and the pulse floating, deficient and wiry. The diagnosis was an unresolved exterior pattern with a disharmony of ying and wei. The formula used was Xiao Chai Hu Tang: Chai Hu 6g, Gui Zhi 6g, Dang Shen 15g, Bai Shao 10g, Ban Xia 10g, Huang Qin 10g, Sheng Jiang 3 pieces, Zhi Gan Cao 5g, Da Zao 3 pieces. She was given two packs, after which the peak temperature was lower

(37.6°C) and its duration shorter. Her body pain eased and there was no nausea. Her tongue coat was white and moist and the pulse was moderate, wiry and deficient.

The formula was repeated with an increase in the dose of Chai Hu to 10g and the addition of Ge Gen 15g. She was given a further four packs. After the two courses of medication, the patient's overall condition had improved, her appetite was better and the pulse moderate. Bu Zhong Yi Qi Tang modified was given for consolidation.

Da Chai Hu Tang Pattern

Clause 103

太阳病，过经十余日，反二三下之。后四五日，柴胡证仍在者，先与小柴胡汤。呕不止、心下急、郁郁微烦者，为未解也，与大柴胡汤下之则愈。

Tai Yang disease, having passed through the channel for more than ten days, nevertheless purgation was used two to three times. Four or five days later, if a Chai Hu pattern is still present, first give Xiao Chai Hu Tang. Vomiting is ceaseless, there is urgency below the heart, depression and mild vexation, this means there is no resolution, give Da Chai Hu Tang and purging will bring recovery.

DA CHAI HU TANG: Chai Hu ½ jin; Huang Qin 3 liang; Shao Yao 3 liang; Ban Xia (washed) ½ jin; Sheng Jiang (sliced) 5 liang; Zhi Shi (fried) 4 pieces; Da Zao 12 pieces (broken). Lin Yi's version advocates that 2 liang of Da Huang should be included.

DIRECTIONS: Boil the ingredients in 1 dou 2 sheng of water, reducing to 6 sheng. Strain and boil again to further concentrate the liquid. Take 1 sheng warm three times a day.

NOTE: The inclusion of Da Huang is now accepted as being part of the formula but, in the past, this was a matter of debate. In the Song edition, Lin Yi and Sun Qi recorded the inclusion of 2 liang of Da Huang and they held that without Da Huang, it was not Da Chai Hu Tang. Xu Shu Wei was of the opinion that Da Huang should not be included, and Ke Yun Bo maintained that, because the formula was intended for the treatment of formless heat and not bowel excess, Da Huang should not be in the formula. Professor Fu Yan Ling of Beijing University of Chinese Medicine suggests that the inclusion or exclusion of Da Huang in Da Chai Hu Tang should be based on the circumstances, as follows. In the case of pronounced intestinal excess Da Huang must be included to purge the excess; however, where the intestinal excess is mild or where a patient's weakened zheng qi must be considered, Da Huang can be omitted or the dosage reduced. Zhang Zhong Jing's use of Da Chai Hu Tang was for Shao Yang disease with exuberant pathogenic qi and intestinal excess, where the zheng qi was intact; where zheng qi is weak, the alternative of Xiao Chai Hu Tang jia Mang Xiao is recommended. From this it can be seen that the clinical application of Da Huang is subject to the patient's constitution and the relative severity of the intestinal excess. The authors believe that the inclusion of Da Huang is dependent on the presence of Yang Ming bowel excess.

DISCUSSION: The significance of the disease having passed through the channel is that the pathogen is no longer in the Tai Yang but has transmitted to Shao Yang; therefore the indicated treatment is harmonisation with Xiao Chai Hu Tang, and purgation is contraindicated. Where the patient's zheng qi is strong and, even where purgation has taken place two or three times, providing there is no transmutation, and providing that the Xiao Chai Hu Tang pattern persists, then Xiao Chai Hu Tang can be given. If, following the administration of Xiao Chai Hu Tang, the condition deteriorates, with symptoms such as incessant vomiting, epigastric pain, depression or irritability, then Xiao Chai Hu Tang has failed to resolve the pathogen in Shao Yang and a concurrent pattern has developed, where there is the additional complication of Yang Ming intestinal excess. Da Chai Hu Tang should then be used to resolve the pathogenic bind in Yang Ming and Shao Yang.

Da Chai Hu Tang is one of the more important Chai Hu formulas. It is Xiao Chai

Hu Tang without Ren Shen and Gan Cao, and with the addition of Da Huang, Zhi Shi and Shao Yao. Xiao Chai Hu Tang is used to harmonise Shao Yang, but where there is Yang Ming excess, Ren Shen and Gan Cao are inappropriate and the inclusion of Da Huang and Zhi Shi in Da Chai Hu Tang are needed to purge the Yang Ming heat excess. Shao Yao and Da Huang work together to sedate the counterflow of gallbladder and liver qi and the dosage of Sheng Jiang is larger than that of Xiao Chai Hu Tang so as to dissipate the knotted bind and harmonise the stomach to stop the vomiting.

The implication of Clause 103 is that Shao Yang disease is mutable and treatment principles must have the flexibility to follow pathogenic changes. This is seen in the choosing of a purgative therapy over diaphoresis, a seeming contradiction in the face of purgation being contraindicated in Shao Yang disease. However, where transmutation has carried the disease into Yang Ming, resulting in a pattern of Yang Ming excess which combines with the Shao Yang pattern, the principles of harmonisation and purgation are used together. In choosing a treatment principle therefore, it is essential to observe the signs and symptoms, understand the pathogenesis and treat accordingly.

Clause 165

伤寒发热，汗出不解，心中痞硬，呕吐而下利者，大柴胡汤主之。

Shang han with fever, sweating with no resolution, hard glomus in the heart, vomiting and diarrhoea, Da Chai Hu Tang governs.

DISCUSSION: When fever in shang han is unresolved by sweating, it is a sign that the pathogen has fallen inward to the Shao Yang. There it disturbs the pivot mechanism and the ensuing qi stagnation gives rise to hard glomus in the chest. The phrase in the original text "hard glomus in the heart" (心中痞硬) is, in fact, a reference to the chest and epigastric area, where knotted qi manifests as a palpable mass causing local discomfort. This clause thereby describes an interior pattern of exuberant heat which has obstructed the ascent and descent of qi, manifesting with vomiting and diarrhoea as well as glomus.

It is interesting to compare Clause 103, where Da Chai Hu Tang is used for a Shao Yang pattern presenting with constipation, with Clause 165, where it is used in the treatment of a Shao Yang pattern presenting with diarrhoea. This is an example of the adage: "Same disease, different treatment; different disease, same treatment" (同病异治,异病同治). This relates to the circumstances where the pathogenesis is the same, even if some symptoms differ. If the pathogenesis is the same, the same formula will apply and for this reason, Da Chai Hu Tang can treat both constipation and diarrhoea.

In *Shang Han Lun,* purgation is mentioned a number of times as a method for treating diarrhoea. The pattern differentiation and pathogenesis often differ. In addition to the application of Da Chai Hu Tang in Shao Yang diarrhoea, both Da Cheng Qi Tang and Xiao Cheng Qi Tang are cited in the treatment of foul, watery diarrhoea associated with intestinal heat bind known as Re Jie Pang Liu (热结旁流), for which a direct translation is 'knotted heat with collateral flow', and which is the emission of faecal fluid flowing down and bypassing a hard constipated stool. Further, the diarrhoea described in Clause 163, which is part of a Gui Zhi Ren Shen Tang pattern, must be differentiated from the diarrhoea of a Da Chai Hu Tang pattern. The former is a symptom of a Tai Yang Tai Yin concurrent pattern, where the diarrhoea is associated with the interior cold of the Tai Yin. Although there is fever, the fever is associated with the exterior pattern and is not representative of interior heat. The treatment strategy is to release the wind cold pathogen of the Tai Yang exterior pattern and warm the interior. The diarrhoea of a Da Chai Hu Tang pattern, as described in Clause 165, on the other hand, is associated with a concurrent Shao Yang Yang Ming pattern, and is due to heat constraint in the interior. The fever in this case is a reflection of interior heat. The corresponding treatment strategy for this concurrent pattern is to harmonise the Shao Yang and purge heat from the Yang Ming. Both these concurrent patterns present with epigastric symptoms: in the Tai Yang Tai Yin pattern, there is hard glomus below the heart; in the Shao Yang Yang Ming pattern, there is extreme discomfort described as "urgency below the heart" (Clause 103).

In a similar way, glomus associated with Xie Xin Tang patterns must be differentiated both from the glomus described in Clause 103 and from that in Clause 165. The phrase "below the heart" refers to the epigastric and hypochondriac regions and includes the liver, gallbladder and pancreas. Hard glomus below the heart refers to glomus in the chest and epigastric area. This is described here in Clause 165, and also in Clause 103, and is associated with a concurrent Shao Yang and Yang Ming disease, manifesting with acute upper abdominal pain and exhibiting the symptoms of fever, vomiting and sticky, foul smelling diarrhoea or constipation.

Ancient Application of Da Chai Hu Tang

- *Zhi Shi Fang Fu Yi:* In the treatment of dysentery with fever, abdominal distension, thirst, a dry throat, delirious speech and a yellow tongue coat.
- *Zheng Zhi Hui Bu:* For the treatment of hiccoughing.

Modern Application of Da Chai Hu Tang

- *Cholecystitis.* In Chinese medicine, cholecystitis can often fall into a concurrent pattern of Shao Yang and Yang Ming, where there are alternating chills and fever, pain in the hypochondrium, a bitter taste in the mouth, nausea and a dry stool or constipation. Da Chai Hu Tang addresses the symptoms of both patterns and offers a satisfactory clinical outcome (*Fu Jian Zhong Yi Yao* 1961; 3:1).
- *Acute abdominal pain.* For acute abdominal pain in such disorders as acute pancreatitis or intestinal obstruction due to qi stagnation, with the clinical features of a Da Chai Hu Tang pattern, Da Chai Hu Tang can be used as the core formula with the addition of Yu Jin and Mu Xiang. For damp heat with jaundice, add Yin Chen and Shan Zhi Zi; for Yang Ming bowel excess characterised by abdominal distension and constipation, increase the dose of Da Huang and add Da Fu Pi and Yuan Ming fen (Mang Xiao treated with water melon); for liver and stomach disharmony with epigastric pain, add Chuan Lian Zi and Chen Pi (*Jiang Su Zhong Yi* 1997; 3:18).

In order to determine the efficacy of Da Chai Hu Tang, the practitioner must look for the persistence of any heat signs following administration: for instance, whether there is still vomiting, pain or constipation. If a stool is passed and urination is normal, one may expect the fever to resolve and the vomiting to ease, with ultimate recovery. If, however, there is no substantial reduction in symptoms after taking two or three packs, the practitioner should review his examination and diagnosis. The poor result may also be attributed to an inadequate dose of the qi moving herbs, thus failing to eliminate severe stagnation. It must be remembered that the principal focus is on moving the bowel and if the constipation is not cleared, a good result will be unlikely.

Case Study

Crohn's Disease

Extracted from Professor Fu Yan Ling's case studies

A 63-year-old male had suffered from recurrent bouts of fever once every one or two months for the previous three years; the patient presented with fever. His temperature ranged from 37.8 to 38.3°C and he had a slight aversion to cold, abdominal pain and diarrhoea. After antibiotic treatment the superficial symptoms of fever and diarrhoea appeared resolved within ten days. However, colonoscopy revealed that he suffered from Crohn's disease, which remained unresolved over the next three years. He then looked to Chinese medicine for further treatment. His complexion was pale and he was thin. He had a bitter taste in the mouth, slight nausea, epigastric fullness and pain, intermittent chills and fever, a red tongue with a greasy, yellow coat, and a slippery, wiry pulse. These are symptoms of Shao Yang constrained heat combined with Yang Ming stagnation. The formula prescribed was Da Chai Hu Tang: Chai Hu 15g, Huang Qin 15g, Ban Xia 15g,

Sheng Jiang 12g, Bai Shao 15g, Zhi Shi 12g, Jiu Da Huang 5g, Da Zao 25g, Bai Jiang Cao 30g. After seven packs, all symptoms were relieved.

Discussion: The prescription of Da Chai Hu Tang with a dose of 6g of Da Huang targets the damp heat, represented by the red tongue with a greasy, yellow tongue coat, and also the excess accumulation in the stomach and intestines represented by the slippery, wiry pulse. Da Huang purges heat and unblocks the intestinal obstruction; Bai Jiang Cao clears heat and relieves toxicity. At the second consultation, Xiao Chai Hu Tang was prescribed with 12g of Shao Yao and Zhi Shi, and 30g of Bai Jiang Cao for seven packs. Ren Shen, Gan Cao and Da Zao tonify and augment qi and although the formula is similar to Da Chai Hu Tang, there is no Da Huang. The follow-up treatment was Xiao Chai Hu Tang with the addition of Bai Shao and combined with Huang Qin Tang, which was modified with the addition of Pu Gong Ying, Bai Jiang Cao and Ma Chi Xian to clear toxic heat. The entire course of treatment was three months and there was no recurrence.

Chai Hu jia Mang Xiao Tang Pattern

Clause 104

(一) 伤寒十三日不解，胸胁满而呕，日晡所发潮热，已而微利。(二) 此本柴胡证，下之以不得利；今反利者，知医以丸药下之，此非其治也。(三) 潮热者，实也。先宜服小柴胡汤以解外，后以柴胡加芒硝汤主之。

(1) Shang han for thirteen days with no resolution, the chest and ribs are full and there is vomiting, late afternoon tidal fever, then mild diarrhoea. (2) This is actually a Chai Hu pattern, purgation should not cause diarrhoea; but now there is diarrhoea, know it is because the physician used a pill to purge, this is not the treatment. (3) If there is tidal fever, it is excess. First it is appropriate to take Xiao Chai Hu Tang to release the exterior, afterwards Chai Hu jia Mang Xiao Tang governs.

CHAI HU JIA MANG XIAO TANG: Chai Hu 2 liang 16 zhu; Huang Qin 1 liang; Ren Shen 1 liang; Zhi Sheng Jiang (sliced) 1 liang; Ban Xia (washed) 20 zhu; Da Zao 4 pieces (broken); Mang Xiao 2 liang. Note that the earlier measure for Ban Xia was 5 pieces.

DIRECTIONS: Boil the ingredients in 4 sheng of water, reducing to 2 sheng. Strain, add Mang Xiao and boil again lightly. Divide into two and take warm twice a day. If not resolved, take again.

DISCUSSION: This describes a shang han disorder which has lasted for thirteen days. In such a protracted case it can be expected that the pathogen has fallen inward; the Shao Yang is affected, causing fullness in the chest and hypochondrium, and also the Yang Ming, causing vomiting and tidal fever. If this is so, the stool will be hard and the administration of the guiding formula Da Chai Hu Tang is appropriate and should purge without causing diarrhoea. The diarrhoea in this case, is not due to using the correct purging formula, but is an adverse consequence of inappropriate administration of purging pills. Purging pills used in the Han dynasty were made from hot acrid herbs which were not suitable either to harmonise the Shao Yang or to drain Yang Ming heat. The final statement explains that the tidal fever is indicative of an excess pattern, referring to Yang Ming excess. However, the exterior must first be released with a dose of Xiao Chai Hu Tang, which will also harmonise the Shao Yang, following which, Chai Hu jia Mang Xiao Tang is given to harmonise the interior by draining internal heat.

Chai Hu jia Mang Xiao Tang and Da Chai Hu Tang are both indicated for a Shao Yang Yang Ming concurrent pattern. Da Chai Hu Tang is not a harmonising formula, but contains many of the herbs found in Xiao Cheng Qi Tang and is thereby able to eliminate the knotted bind and ease the abdominal pain. Chai Hu jia Mang Xiao Tang, by comparison, is closer in composition to Tiao Wei Cheng Qi Tang, and so has the function of purging and dissipating the knotted heat.

Chai Hu jia Mang Xiao Tang is suitable for treating a pattern of Shao Yang combined with

Yang Ming interior excess following purgation. The hot acrid herbs of the purgative pill are inappropriate and have damaged stomach qi and consumed stomach yin, resulting in a mild bind due to dryness. Nevertheless, this interior excess is relatively mild, as can be seen by the symptoms of fullness in the chest and hypochondrium, vomiting and tidal fever, as opposed to the profuse sweating and severe constipation of a more serious bind. Because there is damage to stomach qi, Xiao Chai Hu Tang is used first, to harmonise the stomach and normalise its function, with Ren Shen and Gan Cao supplementing the deficiency. Da Chai Hu Tang can then be used to purge the dry heat.

Mang Xiao's function of purging heat and softening hardness is used also in the formulas Da Cheng Qi Tang, Tiao Wei Cheng Qi Tang and Da Xian Xiong Wan. The *Ben Cao Gang Mu* describes it thus: "Mang Xiao is salty and cold it enters the blood aspect and has a moistening effect as well as sweeping the excess heat in the triple jiao, stomach and intestines". The *Mei Shi Ji Yan Fang* says: "It has a heat clearing and toxin relieving function and can be used to treat erysipelas or *dan du* (丹毒)." There are nine formulas in *Shang Han Lun* which use Mang Xiao, with the dose ranging from 10 to 15g. Examples of modern clinical application are:

1. For viral hepatitis, Da Huang 9g and Mang Xiao 15g were steeped in warm water for 10 minutes and taken twice daily (Zheng Xian Re: *Zhong Yi Za Zhi* 1985; (4):44).
2. For acute pancreatitis with severe abdominal pain, a combination of Da Cheng Qi Tang and Da Chai Hu Tang was used, where Da Huang and Mang Xiao were the chief herbs (Jiang Jun Ming et al: *Zhong Yi Zha Zhi* 1980; (1):23).

Chai Hu Gui Zhi Gan Jiang Tang Pattern

Clause 147

伤寒五六日，已发汗而复下之，胸胁满微结、小便不利、渴而不呕、但头汗出、往来寒热、心烦者，此为未解也，柴胡桂枝干姜汤主之。

Shang han for five or six days, following the promotion of sweat, there has then been purgation, if the chest and ribs are full with a slight bind, urination is not free, there is thirst but no vomiting, sweating only from the head, alternating chills and fever, and vexation, this means there is no resolution, Chai Hu Gui Zhi Gan Jiang Tang governs.

CHAI HU GUI ZHI GAN JIANG TANG: Chai Hu ½ jin; Gui Zhi (bark removed) 3 liang; Gan Jiang 2 liang; Gua Lou Gen 4 liang; Huang Qin 3 liang; Mu Li (dry fried) 2 liang; Zhi Gan Cao 2 liang.

NOTE: Gua Lou Gen is the same part of the herb used for Tian Hua Fen.

DIRECTIONS: Boil the ingredients in 1 dou 2 sheng of water until reduced by 6 sheng. Strain and re-boil, reducing to 3 sheng. Take 1 sheng warm three times a day. Following administration, there will be mild vexation and further doses will bring sweating with subsequent recovery.

DISCUSSION: When purgation has been used in addition to the promotion of sweat, the resulting leakage of yang qi and damage to fluids allows the pathogen to fall inward to the Shao Yang. The ensuing constraint of the qi dynamic and inhibited flow of channel qi are reflected in the characteristic symptoms of alternating chills and fever and a sense of fullness in the chest and hypochondrium. The lodgement of the pathogen between the exterior and interior also affects the movement of qi and water in the san jiao; the non-distribution of fluids manifests as thirst in the upper jiao and inhibited urination in the lower jiao. Because the constrained interior heat obstructs the outward diffusion of yang qi, the steam is not perfused throughout the body but instead percolates upwards, so there is sweating from the head and not from the rest of the body.

Shang Han Lun mentions the symptom of sweating only from the head in Clauses 111, 134, 147, 148, 165, 216, 228 and 236. There are five different types of sweating. (1) Shao Yang fire constraint with non-diffusion of yang qi as described in Clauses 148, 147 and 165. (2) Heat constraint in the chest as found in Clause 228, which describes a Zhi Zi Chi Tang pattern. (3) The inability to vent the heat and damp outward, giving rise to yellowing as seen in Clauses 134 and 236. (4) Yin deficiency in the lower jiao with yang blazing upward to the upper jiao, and characterised by difficult urination as described in Clause 111. (5) Constrained heat in the blood aspect as found in Clause 216, where Yang Ming heat is entering the chamber of blood.

These symptoms reflect the pathomechanism of Shao Yang disease where the impaired qi dynamic has resulted in the non-transformation of qi and non-dispersal of fluids and is also demonstrated by the inhibited urination. Accumulated fluids, manifesting as a mild knotted bind in the hypochondrium, further affect the Shao Yang pivot mechanism, and so the essential strategy is to free the pivot mechanism and disperse the constrained qi in order to facilitate the transformation and transportation of fluids.

Chai Hu Gui Zhi Gan Jiang Tang is a modification of Xiao Chai Hu Tang best suited to this disorder. Chai Hu and Huang Qin harmonise the Shao Yang and clear gallbladder heat; Gua Lou Gen generates fluids and moistens dryness; Mu Li softens hardness in order to facilitate dispersion of the knotted bind; the warmth and sweetness of Gui Zhi combined with Gan Cao transforms yang, whilst the warm and dispersing properties of Gui Zhi and Gan Jiang transform fluids and dissipate the bind; since there is no vomiting, Ban Xia is omitted; Ren Shen and Da Zao are also omitted because they tend to be cloying and would cause further congestion. This is a formula which harmonises Shao Yang and also scatters cold damp in the spleen.

Chai Hu Gui Zhi Gan Jiang Tang can be used irrespective of the presence of an exterior pathogen. This is because the principle of Gui Zhi and Gan Jiang in this formula is based on their capacity to warm the spleen yang, and the purpose of Gan Jiang in this formula is specifically to address the damage to spleen qi caused by incorrect purgation. *Shen Nong Ben Cao Jing* recorded that the combination of Gui Zhi and Gan Jiang tonify the middle, augment qi and warm the spleen yang. The implication is that by supporting the spleen and spleen yang, they can prevent further deterioration which would lead to depletion of the kidney yang. According to *Shang Han* experts, this formula can be applied to any pattern featuring the symptoms of a bitter taste in the mouth, vexation, abdominal distension and diarrhoea, as long as the pattern is associated with constrained liver and gallbladder heat with deficiency and cold in the spleen.

Ancient Application of Chai Hu Gui Zhi Gan Jiang Tang

- *Huo Ren Shu:* Gan Jiang Chai Hu Tang, which is Chai Hu Gui Zhi Gan Jiang Tang with the omission of Huang Qin, was used to treat women suffering from shang han when it had caused cessation of menstruation during the menstrual cycle and which presented with alternating chills and fever, and a disturbed mental state.
- *Tong Shu Shang Han Lun:* Chai Hu Qing Ge Tang (Chai Hu, Da Huang, Zhi Qiao, Bo He, Zhi Zi, Jie Geng, Lian Qiao, Gan Cao, Dan Zhu Ye), which is Chai Hu Gui Zhi Gan Jiang Tang with the omission of Gui Zhi, Gan Jiang, Gua Lou Gen, Huang Qin and Mu Li and where Gan Cao replaces Zhi Gan Cao, was advocated for a Shao Yang exterior pattern characterised by a burning sensation in the diaphragm, malaria-like fever and chills, vexation, anguish and constipation.

Modern Application of Chai Hu Gui Zhi Gan Jiang Tang

- This formula is useful in the treatment of the common cold, pleurisy, cholecystitis, acid reflux and chronic hepatitis characterised by Tai Yin spleen cold.
- Professor Liu Du Zhou alternated this formula with Chai Hu Jie Du Tang (Chai Hu, Huang Qin, Yin Chen, Zhi Gan Cao, Tu Fu Ling, Cao He Che, Feng Wei Cao, Tu Bie Chong, Qian Cao) in the treatment of hepatitis with spleen cold and diarrhoea.

Case Study

Shao Yang with Retained Fluids
Extracted from Yuan Hu Zhong Yi College: Shang Han Lun Supplement: 80

A male patient had suffered alternating chills and fever for six months. Antibiotics and aspirin were prescribed but were not effective. At the consultation, he presented with chills and fever, a bitter taste in the mouth, a dry throat, vexation, fullness in the hypochondrium, stomach rumbling and inhibited urination. His tongue was pale red with a white, slippery tongue coat and the pulse was wiry and thready. The diagnosis was a Shao Yang pattern with retained fluids. The treatment principle was to harmonise Shao Yang and disinhibit water. The prescribed formula was Chai Hu Gui Zhi Gan Jiang Tang modified: Chai Hu 9g, Huang Qin 9g, Gui Zhi 6g, Gan Jiang 4.5g, Fu Ling 9g, Chen Pi 6g, Ze Xie 6g, Zhi Gan Cao 3g. After two packs, the sense of fullness in the hypochondrium and rumbling in the stomach were gone and urination was normal; however, the patient felt fatigued and his appetite was poor. Xiang Sha Liu Jun Zi Tang was prescribed to consolidate the treatment by strengthening the spleen and resolving damp.

Chai Hu jia Long Gu Mu Li Tang Pattern

Clause 107

伤寒八九日，下之，胸满、烦惊、小便不利、谵语、一身尽重，不可转侧者，柴胡加龙骨牡蛎汤主之。

Shang han for eight or nine days, with purgation, if the chest is full, there is vexation and fright, the urination is not free, there is delirious speech, the whole body feels heavy, so that the patient can not turn over, Chai Hu jia Long Gu Mu Li Tang governs.

CHAI HU JIA LONG GU MU LI TANG: Chai Hu 4 liang; Long Gu 1½ liang; Huang Qin 1½ liang; Sheng Jiang (sliced) 1½ liang; Qian Dan 1½ liang; Ren Shen 1½ liang; Gui Zhi (bark removed) 1½ liang; Fu Ling 1½ liang; Ban Xia (washed) 2½ ge; Da Huang 2 liang; Mu Li (dry fried) 1½ liang; Da Zao 6 pieces (broken).

DIRECTIONS: Boil the ingredients in 8 sheng of water, reducing to 4 sheng. Add Da Huang (cut into the size of Qi Zi) and bring to the boil once or twice. Strain and take 1 sheng warm. The original text notes: "This is Chai Hu Tang with addition of Long Gu etc."

NOTE: Qi Zi are the stones used in an ancient form of chess which enjoyed universal popularity in China. It was known as *wei qi* 围棋 or 'encircling chess' and played on a board divided into 361 squares, using black and white stones as chessmen. The object was for one player to surround the opponent's stones with his and claim the squares thus occupied as his 'territory'. The stones measured about one inch in diameter. *Qian Jin Fang* records them as being the size of a 方匕 or 'square inch spoon'. The *Shang Han Lun Da Ci Dian (The Complete Shang Han Lun Dictionary)* explains it is the equivalent of 10–12g in modern measurement. A reference to bigger stones used for chess pieces, known as *bo qi zi* (博棋子), as a form of measurement is found in Clause 393, where the footnote to Zhi Shi Zhi Zi Chi Tang reads: "If there is food stagnation, add Da Huang equalling the size of five or six bo qi zi, and recovery will follow after medication". *Qian Jin Fang* says: "The size of bo qi zi measure 2 inch by 1 inch square".

DISCUSSION: Inappropriate use of purgation in a shang han disorder has damaged the zheng qi and disturbed the Shao Yang pivot mechanism and impaired the movement of qi in the Shao Yang. The impaired Shao Yang pivot mechanism has affected communication between the exterior and interior, causing exterior–interior disharmony, and has also affected the function of the san jiao. Impeded flow of qi in the Shao Yang causes constraint of the Shao Yang ministerial fire which then surges upward, harassing the heart shen and causing vexation, fright and delirious speech. The impeded flow of qi and water in the san jiao results in a sensation of fullness in the chest and inhibited urination. The stagnation of yang qi in the interior leads to body aches and pains manifesting as an inability to change position in bed.

Chai Hu jia Long Gu Mu Li Tang not only harmonises the Shao Yang but also calms the heart shen. This is a modification of Xiao Chai Hu Tang with additional herbs to calm the shen, clear heat and free the water passages. Xiao Chai Hu Tang harmonises the Shao Yang and clears heat from the liver and gallbladder. Gan Cao is omitted because of its potential to cause further stagnation and thus protract the condition. Long Gu, Mu Li and Qian Dan settle the shen and sedate the vexation, fright and restlessness; the combination of Gui Zhi, Da Huang and Fu Ling clear heat, disinhibit urination and free the water passages of the san jiao. Chai Hu jia Long Gu Mu Li Tang can be used in the treatment of bipolar disorder, epilepsy and infantile food stagnation where the pathogenesis is liver and gallbladder constraint.

Ancient Application of Chai Hu jia Long Gu Mu Li Tang

- *Shang Han Lun Lei Fang:* For the treatment of epilepsy.
- *Jing Yan Ji Lu:* For the treatment of infantile fever with excess heat and stagnation characterised by chills and fever, fright and palpitations.

Modern Application of Chai Hu jia Long Gu Mu Li Tang

With the appropriate presentation, this formula is widely used in the treatment of externally contracted febrile disease and various neural disorders, bipolar disorder, insomnia, epilepsy, as well as hypertension and infantile nocturnal crying. With appropriate modifications, it is suitable for the treatment of shen disturbance where there is constraint of liver and gallbladder qi which has transformed into heat.

- Qian Dan is toxic and can be replaced by Hu Po; additional qi herbs such as Xiang Fu to regulate qi and Gua Lou or Shi Chang Pu to scour phlegm and open the orifices of the heart can enhance treatment outcomes.
- If there is qi stagnation with fullness and pain in the chest and hypochondrium, constipation, a purplish tongue with a greasy, white coat and a slow, choppy pulse, add such herbs as Tao Ren, Hong Hua, Chi Shao, Chuan Xiong, Xiang Fu, to move qi and blood.
- For hyperactive liver fire with damp heat pouring downward, characterised by dark, scant urination, vexation, irritability, a flushed face and constipation, omit Ren Shen, Gui Zhi, Sheng Jiang, Da Zao and add Long Dan Cao, Shan Zhi Zi, Che Qian Cao, Xia Ku Cao, Sheng Di to drain damp heat.
- For Yin deficiency with hyperactive fire, Chai Hu jia Long Gu Mu Li Tang can be used with the omission of Gui Zhi, Ren Shen, Sheng Jiang and Da Zao, and with the addition of Meng Shi, Chen Xiang and Shi Chang Pu.
- For manic behaviour associated with phlegm fire harassing the heart shen, the formula can be used omitting Ren Shen and Gui Zhi, substituting Ban Xia for Dan Nan Xing, and combining with Dian Kuang Meng Xing Tang (颠狂梦醒汤).

Case Study

Fullness in the Chest

Extracted from Liu Du Zhou Yi Xue Quan Ji

The patient was a 34-year-old male who complained of fullness in the chest and hypochondrium, restlessness, dream-disturbed sleep, spontaneous sweating and constipation. He suffered from epilepsy as a result of fright. The patient's face was expressionless, the complexion was dull and pale, his tongue was red with a yellow and white tongue coat and his pulse was submerged and wiry. The diagnosis was constrained qi of the liver and gallbladder with Yang Ming bowel heat harassing the heart shen. The treatment principle was to disperse constrained liver qi and purge stomach heat. The formula used was Chai Hu jia Long Gu Mu Li Tang: Chai Hu 12g, Huang Qin 9g, Ban Xia 9g, Sheng Jiang 9g, Long Gu 15g, Mu Li 15g, Da Huang 6g (added at the end), Fu Shen 9g, Qian Dan 4.5g (wrapped in gauze), Gui Zhi 4.5g, Da Zao 6 pieces. After one pack, the bowel movement was regular and the pain in the hypochondrium eased. The original formula was repeated with the addition of Zhu Ru and Chen Pi to resolve phlegm damp.

Summary of Formulas for Transmuted Patterns of Shao Yang

Xiao Chai Hu Tang is the representative formula for Shao Yang disorders and modifications can be made to accommodate the treatment of additional symptoms or a transmuted pattern.

- Chai Hu Gui Zhi Tang can be used for a combined pattern of Shao Yang and Tai Yang pattern characterised by vexing joint pain, fever and a slight aversion to cold.
- Da Chai Hu Tang can be used for a pattern of Shao Yang and Yang Ming interior excess characterised by acute discomfort below the heart, constipation, incessant vomiting and mild vexation, and also for vomiting and diarrhoea.
- Chai Hu jia Mang Xiao Tang can be used for Shao Yang and Yang Ming interior excess with tidal fever.
- Chai Hu Gui Zhi Gan Jiang Tang can be used for Shao Yang with impaired qi transformation resulting in an inability to move water and characterised by thirst, heart vexation and inhibited urination.
- Chai Hu jia Long Gu Mu Li can be used when, after purgation, there is chest fullness, vexation, fright, inhibited urination, delirious speech and a sensation of heaviness in the body.

Section Six

4.6 PROGNOSIS AND RECOVERY IN SHAO YANG DISEASE

Prognosis In Shao Yang Disease

Clause 269

伤寒六七日，无大热，其人躁烦者，此为阳去入阴故也。

Shang han for six or seven days, without a high fever, if the person is agitated and vexed, this is because the yang is receding and entering yin.

DISCUSSION: When the person has already had a shang han disorder for six or seven days, the lower fever is a sign that the yang, or exterior pattern, has abated; the agitation and irritability, however, are a sign of the exterior pathogen having fallen inward to the interior, which is what is meant by "the yang is receding and entering the yin."

Agitation and vexation can be classified as yin or yang. Yang pertains to the exterior, to heat, to excess and to upward and outward movement. Here, it is yang vexation, caused by the exterior heat having entered the interior and flaring upward to disturb the heart shen. Where vexation is part of a pattern of body aches, aversion to cold and an absence of sweat, it is attributed to cold constraint in the muscle layer which having transformed into heat, then enters the interior, disturbing the heart shen; Da Qing Long Tang is indicated. Where there is thirst, excessive sweating and a big, flooding pulse, the vexation is caused by Yang Ming exuberant interior heat and Bai Hu Tang is indicated. If shang han disease has been treated with emesis and purgation, and there is insubstantial vexation, insomnia, restlessness or anguish, Zhi Zi Chi Tang is indicated. If there is constipation with periumbilical pain and vexation, it is attributed to the knotting of heat and dryness in the intestine and Cheng Qi Tang is indicated.

Yin pertains to the interior, to cold and to deficiency, and to downward, inward movement. Vexation in a yin pattern is associated with deficiency caused, for instance, by the loss of sweat. In this case, there is no thirst and, although the person is restless and finds it difficult to fall asleep, once asleep, they sleep peacefully. The pulse is submerged and faint, reflecting the interior deficiency of yang. This is Shao Yin disease where exuberant cold in the interior has displaced and upcast the true yang. The indicated treatment is Gan Jiang Fu Zi Tang to warm the interior. If a Shao Yin pattern presents with deficiency cold in the interior, and there is an upsurge of turbid yin manifesting as vomiting, then Wu Zhu Yu Tang is the indicated formula, to warm the interior and direct qi downwards.

Clause 270

伤寒三日，三阳为尽，三阴当受邪。其人反能食而不呕，此为三阴不受邪也。

Shang han for three days, the three yang are ended, the three yin must contract the evil. The person can nevertheless eat and there is no vomiting, this is because the three yin do not contract the evil.

DISCUSSION: The *Shan Han Lun* theory of transmission states that on the first day, the pathogen is in the Tai Yang; on the second day, it is in the Yang Ming; on the third day it is in the Shao Yang; on the fourth, the Tai Yin; the fifth, Shao Yin and on the sixth day, it reaches the Jue Yin. According to this theory, if the person has contracted shang han or cold injury for three days, then the pathogenic influence should have gone past the three yang channels and would be about to affect the three yin channels. However, if the pathogen is in the yin channels, the middle qi will be affected. The Tai Yin channel is at the front line of the three yin channels and will be first affected, with symptoms of an inability to eat, vomiting, and also abdominal fullness and diarrhoea. The absence of these signs, the fact that there are no eating problems or vomiting, shows that the middle qi is unaffected and the interior is harmonised. This is testimony to the pathogen not having been transmitted to the yin channels and is therefore a sign of recovery.

The classic theory defines the course of the development of disease as being from yang to yin and from exterior to interior. Shao Yang is the pivot between the exterior and interior and therefore plays a significant role in the understanding of disease mechanism, transmission and treatment. Based on the theory of Shao Yang as the pivot, the administration of Xiao Chai Hu Tang can produce amazing results in a pattern of externally contracted cold with fever, aversion to wind and general malaise. This is because it has the dual effect of expelling the pathogen and supporting the zheng qi. Modifications can be made as required.

Because of its role as a pivot between the exterior and interior, Shao Yang also acts as a barrier to disease before its transmission into the yin channels. However, Shao Yang diseases are changeable. They can transform into heat as in a Da Chai Hu Tang pattern, which is a concurrent pattern of Shao Yang and Yang Ming; they can also transform into cold, as in a Chai Hu Gui Zhi Gan Jiang pattern, which is a concurrent pattern of Shao Yang and Tai Yin. Diagnosis, therefore, should not be based on the pattern symptomatology alone, but must also be based on the person's constitution and the geographical environment in order to understand the pathomechanism and select the appropriate treatment.

Clause 271

伤寒三日，少阳脉小者，欲已也。

Shang han for three days, if the Shao Yang pulse is small, it is about to end.

DISCUSSION: The characteristic Shao Yang pulse is wiry, so if after three days, the pulse becomes small, it is a sign that the pathogen is on the wane and the disease will soon resolve. Although this line refers only to the pulse sign for the prognosis, the pulse alone can not be relied upon as a sign of recovery if other Shao Yang signs have not abated. These include fullness in the hypochondrium, alternating chills and fever, a bitter taste, a dry throat, vexation or a lack of appetite. A patient with a constitutional deficiency may not have a wiry pulse but may present with other Shao Yang symptoms. For this reason, the four examinations must be used for a thorough diagnosis.

Shao Yang Recovery Period

Clause 272

少阳病欲解时，从寅至辰上。

The time that Shao Yang disease is ready to resolve, is from yin to chen.

DISCUSSION: Yin to chen refers to the period of time between 3am and 9am when there is a gradual return of yang qi. This corresponds to the time when the ascending and outward movements of the Shao Yang gallbladder qi are at their peak, and so the ability of the anti-pathogenic qi of the Shao Yang to expel the pathogen is greatest. For this reason, it is known as the optimum time for recovery from Shao Yang disease.

Section Seven

4.7 ADDENDUM: HEAT ENTERING THE CHAMBER OF BLOOD

There are three patterns associated with Shao Yang discussed in *Shang Han Lun* where heat enters the chamber of blood at the time of menstruation. At this time there is deficiency due to menstrual loss; the vessels are open and vulnerable to attack. In one case, the attack comes at the beginning of the period, in the second, the attack occurs towards the end of the menstrual flow, and in the third, when the menstrual flow is over.

Clause 143

妇人中风，发热恶寒，经水适来，得之七八日，热除而脉迟、身凉、胸胁下满，如结胸状、谵语者，此为热入血室也，当刺期门，随其实而取之。

A woman has zhong feng, there is fever and aversion to cold, coinciding with the arrival of the menstrual flow, having been sick for seven or eight days, if the fever is resolved and the pulse is slow, the body is cool, there is fullness beneath the chest and the ribs, it is like chest bind, with delirious speech, this means the heat is entering the chamber of blood, one must needle qi men, selecting it to suit the excess.

DISCUSSION: Here, the contraction of zhong feng, identified by fever with aversion to cold, has coincided with the arrival of the menstrual period. Because of the menstrual loss, not only is a woman relatively deficient in qi and blood but, at the time of menstruation, the network vessels are open and vulnerable to attack. At this time, therefore, there is a potential for an exterior pathogen to exploit this deficiency by attacking the chamber of blood. The abatement of fever is a sign that the exterior pattern is resolving; however, although the pathogen has left the exterior, it has not been eliminated but has left the exterior only to enter the interior. There it knots with the blood of the womb; this impedes the flow of blood, hence the pulse is slow. The chamber of blood has a close connection to the liver channel, and so this knotting also impedes the free flow of qi. Because of the distribution of the gallbladder and liver network vessels over the thorax, the impediment to the dispersal of qi manifests as fullness and distension in the chest and hypochondrium, similar to chest bind. The pathogen transforms into heat in the blood, which harasses the heart shen, resulting in delirious speech. The recommendation is to needle Qi Men (Liv 14), as this is the mu alarm point of the liver, and can be used to drain heat from the liver channel, thus bringing recovery.

Clause 144

妇人中风，七八日续得寒热，发作有时，经水适断者，此为热入血室，其血必结，故使如疟状，发作有时，小柴胡汤主之。

A woman has zhong feng, for seven or eight days it continues with chills and fever, occurring periodically, coinciding with the cessation of the menstrual flow, this is heat entering the chamber of blood, the blood will become knotted, thus causing malaria-like symptoms, occurring periodically, Xiao Chai Hu Tang governs.

DISCUSSION: Clause 144 describes a case of zhong feng contracted at the end of the menstrual period, and must be read as a sequel to Clause 143 preceding it, which describes zhong feng occurring at the beginning of the menstrual flow. Clause 144 describes what happens at the end of the menstrual flow. This may coincide with the natural cessation of flow or, as interpreted by He Lian Chen, may take place before this natural cessation, with the knotting of pathogenic heat with blood causing stasis which stops the flow. In either case, the pathogen has knotted with the blood of the uterus which, at the end of the period, lacks vigour and is more easily transformed into stasis. Because of the relationship between the uterus and the liver, the dispersion of qi in the liver and gallbladder channels is affected and this, in turn, affects the Shao Yang, as evidenced by the alternating chills and fever. Because the pathogen is no longer in the exterior, the chills and fever have more serious significance than the chills and fever characteristic of a Shao Yang pattern, taking on the guise of malaria. Xiao Chai Hu Tang modified with blood invigorating herbs can be used to harmonise the Shao Yang and disperse constrained liver and gallbladder qi, thus alleviating the bind caused by heat knotting with the blood.

Clause 145

妇人伤寒，发热，经水适来。昼日明了，暮则谵语，如见鬼状者，此为热入血室。无犯胃气，及上二焦，必自愈。

A woman has shang han, there is fever, coinciding with the arrival of the menstrual flow, if in the daylight hours she is lucid, and in the evening there is delirious speech, as if seeing ghosts, this is heat entering the chamber of blood. Without attacking the stomach and the upper two jiao, there will be spontaneous recovery.

DISCUSSION: Clause 145 describes a woman who has contracted an exterior shang han disease with fever at the time her menstruation starts. The exterior pathogen exploits the deficiency, transforms into heat and enters the chamber of blood. The daylight hours are dominated by yang qi whilst the hours of darkness are dominated by yin qi. Because blood is yin, the manifestations of heat in the blood aspect are more pronounced at night, and it is at this time that the blood heat surges upward disturbing the heart shen, and causing delirious speech and hallucinations. Lucidity in the daylight hours shows that the pattern does not involve Yang Ming, where delirium would be expected to occur in the daytime. Because the pathogenic heat has entered at the beginning of the period, and the pattern is one of heat exploiting the deficiency and not one of constrained qi, the heat can be expelled from the body via the menstrual flow and recovery will take place without treatment. The clause further explains that the upper two jiao (by which it refers to the upper and middle jiao), should not be 'attacked'; by this injunction, Zhong Jing cautions the physician not to mistake the shen disturbance for one due to Yang Ming excess where the physician might attempt to use purgation or sweat promotion or needling Qi Men. This is a Shao Yang pattern where erroneous purgation or sweating could lead to transmutation.

The term 'chamber of blood' was the subject of much debate by past *Shang Han* specialists. Cheng Wu Ji and Fang You Zhi suggested that it referred to the Chong Mai; Ke Yun Bo believed it referred to the liver; Zhang Jie Bing proposed that it was the uterus. Cao Bing Zhang said: "The chamber of blood is where the ying blood is stored and is the meeting place of blood; it is the Chong Mai". The collective inference of the above three clauses confirms that the correct interpretation is in fact the womb and its network vessels. Nevertheless, signs and symptoms evidencing heat in the chamber of blood are not limited to the uterus alone, but to the channels and organs pertaining to it. The liver has an intimate relationship with the uterus: it is the reservoir of blood and its channels encircle the reproductive organs; the Ren Mai and Chong Mai also pass through the uterus and have an inseparable relationship with it. These inter-relationships must be taken into consideration when interpreting what is meant by the chamber of blood.

Pattern Identification of Heat Entering the Chamber of Blood

He Lian Chen, in his annotation of *Tong Shu Shang Han Lun* proposed three differential patterns for heat entering the chamber of blood in a Shao Yang pattern.

1. The heat pathogen knots with the blood on the arrival of menstruation causing immediate cessation of the menstrual flow. This is a pattern of heat knotting with blood causing stasis and obstruction. The treatment should be focused on clearing heat and eliminating stasis. The suggested formula is Xiao Chai Hu Tang, omitting Ren Shen and Da Zao and adding Mu Dan Pi, Tao Ren, Gui Wei, Chuan Shan Jia (Clause 143).
2. The pathogenic heat enters the chamber of blood, stirring the blood and causing a shortened cycle with the menstrual flow arriving early. The strategy is to cool blood and harmonise the ying. The recommended formula is Xiao Chai Hu Tang, omitting Ren Shen and Da Zao, and adding such herbs as Sheng Di, Mu Dan Pi, Tao Ren, Chi Shao or Shui Niu Jiao to cool and invigorate blood, thus preventing it from becoming knotted with the heat.
3. The pathogenic attack comes at the end of the menstrual flow when blood is depleted. The strategy is to nourish and invigorate blood and the recommended formula is Xiao Chai Hu Tang combined with Si Wu Tang, adding Dan Shen.

Case Study

Fever During Menstruation

Extracted from Shaan Xi Zhong Yi 1976; Vol 2 (22)

The patient was a female student who normally enjoyed good health. Menarche had occurred at the age of fifteen and apart from mild lower back pain during menstruation, there were no other complaints. Six months previously, at the time of her menstrual period, she had contracted a cold with a headache, alternating chills and fever, nausea, and aches and pains in the body. She was admitted to the emergency department at hospital for observation and treatment. The chills and fever were milder in the morning but reached 40.3°C in the afternoon, dropping again in the evening following a bout of sweating. Extensive tests were conducted for tuberculosis, typhoid fever and malaria. The results were inconclusive and the treatment given in the hospital was not effective. This condition continued for the next five menstrual cycles where, at the onset of each menstrual cycle, there would be alternating chills and fever lasting for about ten days before abating only to resume at the next menstrual cycle. She was thin and her face had a red flush. The tongue was crimson with stasis spots and she had a temperature of 39°C with alternating chills and fever where the fever predominated. She was irritable, had a bitter taste in her mouth, poor appetite, slight nausea, thirst, lower abdominal fullness, a normal bowel movement and yellow urine. Her menstrual flow was scant and her pulse was wiry, thready and rapid. She noted that her period had actually stopped when she first contracted the cold six months earlier. The diagnosis was heat entering the chamber of blood. The treatment principle was to harmonise Shao Yang, clear heat from the ying, invigorate blood and transform stasis. The formula used was Tai Zi Shen 12g, Chai Hu 6g, Huang Qin 9g, Sheng Di 12g, Dan Pi 9g, Xuan Shen 12g, Lian Qiao 9g, Huang Lian 4.5g, Zhu Ru 9g, Dan Shen 9g, Tao Ren 9g, Chi Shao 9g, Gan Cao 6g. After four packs, the chills and fever diminished and her temperature dropped to 37.6°C. However, there was abdominal distension with pain, and her tongue was still red and her pulse faint, wiry and thready. Modifications were made: omit Huang Lian; add Hong Hua 9g; Yan Hu Suo 9g. After the third dose of that formula, her menstruation resumed with dark, purplish menstrual blood and clots. Her appetite improved slightly. The tongue was slightly red and the pulse thready and rapid. She also complained of fever at night. This was diagnosed as unresolved residual heat and the treatment principle was to support the yin and harmonise ying. The formula used was Tai Zi Shen 12g, Dang Gui 9g, Sheng Di 9g, Shan Yao 12g, Yu Zhu 12g,

Xuan Shen 9g, Dan Shen 9g, Tao Ren 9g, Hong Hua 9g, Di Gu Pi 9g, Gan Cao 6g. Four packs were given and a follow-up one year later showed no recurrence.

Discussion: The disorder of chills and fever in this case are attributed to the contraction of exterior cold during menstruation. In *Shang Han Lun*, this is understood as pathogenic heat entering the chamber of blood and knotting with the blood of the uterus. The treatment principle is to clear heat, cool blood and vent the pathogenic heat. The formula used was a modified version of Xiao Chai Hu Tang, omitting Ren Shen and Da Zao, and adding Mu Dan Pi, Sheng Di, Xuan Shen, Liao Qiao and Huang Lian to cool blood and clear heat from the uterus; Dan Shen, Tao Ren, Chi Shao were included to transform blood stasis. The second formula omitted Huang Lian in order to prevent damage to yin; Yuan Hu and Hong Hua were added to eliminate blood stasis more effectively.

Section Eight

4.8 SUMMARY OF THE SHAO YANG CHAPTER

The Shao Yang chapter covers six Shao Yang patterns and their associated aetiology, pathogenesis, key symptoms, treatment and contraindications.

SHAO YANG AETIOLOGY AND PATHOGENESIS: Shao Yang disease is mainly attributed to a pathogenic exploitation of a deficiency in zheng qi or, as described in Clause 97: "Blood is weak and qi exhausted, the interstices are open, evil qi enters, it vies with the zheng qi, knotting below the ribs. The upright battles the evil, chills and fever come and go". There may be transmission from Tai Yang, whether of shang han (cold injury) or zhong feng (wind strike), or there may be an attack directly on Shao Yang. Because of it being seated between the Tai Yang in the exterior and Yang Ming in the interior, there is a great potential for Shao Yang concurrent patterns to arise. These include concurrent patterns of Tai Yang and Shao Yang, Shao Yang and Yang Ming and concurrent patterns of the three yang.

KEY SYMPTOMS OF SHAO YANG DISEASE: The characteristic identifying symptoms are alternating chills and fever, pain and distension in the hypochondrium, unwillingness to talk, no desire for food, vexation, vomiting, a bitter taste in the mouth, a dry throat, dizziness and a wiry pulse.

THE SCOPE OF XIAO CHAI HU TANG: Disruption to the pivot mechanism of Shao Yang has the potential to give rise to a variety of manifestations apart from those described in Clause 96. The 'or' symptoms in Clause 96 are a list of possible developments arising from qi obstruction and include heart palpitations with inhibited urination, where qi obstruction causes water retention and a subsequent upsurge of water qi which harasses the heart causing palpitations and also results in inhibited urination. Apart from heat in the gallbladder, qi constrained in the liver and gallbladder, and the liver harassing the spleen and stomach, Xiao Chai Hu Tang can also address disharmony of the liver and spleen, and this alone significantly expands the range of gastrointestinal disorders which can be treated with Xiao Chai Hu Tang. Clause 101's suggestion that only one symptom is needed in order to use Xiao Chai Hu Tang, must not be taken literally. The actual intended meaning is that only a few symptoms are needed, not all, in order to justify prescribing that formula.

CLINICAL APPLICATION OF XIAO CHAI HU TANG: *Shang Han Lun* indicates the following applications for Xiao Chai Hu Tang: (i) Shao Yang half exterior and half interior pattern; (ii) hyperactive liver and spleen deficiency with abdominal pain; (iii) a concurrent pattern of the three yang with no signs of Yang Ming interior excess; (iv) a Yang Ming pattern with tidal fever, loose stools and unresolved distension in the hypochondrium; (v) Yang Ming disease with hardness and fullness in the hypochrondrium, constipation and a white tongue coat; (vi) Jue Yin disease with vomiting and fever; (vii) slight yang bind with a hard stool; (vii) heat entering the blood chamber; (viii) recovery of shang han where there is residual fever.

HARMONISING STRATEGY: The treatment strategy for Shao Yang disease is harmonisation. Sweat promotion, purgation and emetic therapy are contraindicated. The use of purgation for Shao Yang disease can damage the qi of the heart and gallbladder, manifesting with palpitations and fright; the promotion of sweat can damage body fluids, causing dryness of the stomach manifesting with such symptoms as vexation and delirious speech. If, in addition to the adverse treatments of purgation and sweat promotion, warm needling is employed to further promote sweating, fluid damage will be substantial and can result in the heat pathogen falling inward, and the disorder proceeding to huai bing or a transmuted pattern.

TREATMENT OF A SHAO YANG TRANSMUTED PATTERN: (i) For a concurrent pattern of Shao Yang and Tai Yang with joint pain, epigastric pain, mild vomiting, fever, and a slight aversion to cold: Chai Hu Gui Zhi Tang. (ii) For a Shao Yang and Yang Ming pattern where, following the administration of Xiao Chai Hu Tang, there is incessant vomiting and acute discomfort below the heart: Da Chai Hu Tang. (iii) If the pattern is characterised by tidal fever and slight diarrhoea: Chai Hu jia Mang Xiao Tang. (iv) For a Shao Yang Tai Yin pattern characterised by alternating chills and fever, vexation, distension of the hypochondrium and epigastrium, inhibited urination and thirst but no vomiting: Chai Hu Gui Zhi Tang. (v) Shao Yang disease affecting Tai Yang and Yang Ming with vexation, fright, chest distension, inhibited urination, delirious speech and a sense of heaviness with an inability to turn over in bed: Chai Hu jia Long Gu Mu Li Tang.

PROGNOSIS OF SHAO YANG DISEASE: (i) Further progression of Shao Yang disease is reflected in mild fever and vexation, which are indications of the exterior pathogen having fallen inward. (ii) Abatement of Shao Yang disease is reflected in the ability to eat and the absence of vomiting, which are indications that the stomach qi is in harmony. This recovery pattern is accompanied by a small pulse, indicating that the Shao Yang pattern is passing and so the prognosis is good.

SHAO YANG RECOVERY PERIOD: Shao Yang channel qi peaks between the hours of yin and chen (3am to 9am) and so this is the optimal time for recovery.

太陰

Tai Yin 5

Section One

5.1 OUTLINE OF TAI YIN

Pathway of the Tai Yin Channel

The Tai Yin channel comprises the hand Tai Yin lung and foot Tai Yin spleen channels and stands in an interior–exterior relationship with the Yang Ming channel, comprising the stomach and large intestine channels. The external pathway of the foot Tai Yin spleen channel travels from the tip of the first toe, and up the inside of the leg, the abdomen and the chest. Internally, a channel arises in the inguinal region and connects to the Ren meridian before crossing the liver channel and joining the lung channel near the shoulder. The luo connecting channel leads to its yang partner, the stomach channel. The internal pathway of the hand Tai Yin lung channel starts in the middle jiao and passes through its yang partner the large intestine before intersecting with the channel of its partner, the spleen, near the shoulder. It then exits to become the external channel and from there, travels down the arm to the tip of the thumb. The luo connecting channel connects to its yang partner, the large intestine channel.

Physiology of the Tai Yin Channel

The spleen and stomach are connected by the channel network and have a physiological relationship: the spleen's yang partner, the stomach, governs the reception and decomposition of grain, which is then transformed into a refined essence by the spleen and transported to the zang and the fu as qi and blood, thus nourishing the organs and maintaining the integrity of the four limbs. Thus it is said that the spleen rules transformation and transportation and is considered to be the source of the formation of qi and blood. The complementary relationship of the spleen and stomach is further demonstrated by the fact that the spleen ascends qi whilst the stomach descends qi. Their combined and complementary functions rule the digestion of food and the assimilation and absorption of the refined essences and nutrients. When their functions are disturbed, digestive disorders arise.

Pathology of the Tai Yin Channel

Tai Yin is the first of the three yin channels and disease in the Tai Yin therefore represents the early stage of disease in the three yin channels. The pathogenesis of Tai Yin disease is spleen yang deficiency caused either by an exterior invasion of cold or by direct injury to the interior yang by the immoderate consumption of cold foods or liquids. Tai Yin disease can also be caused by any incorrect or inappropriate treatment of disease of the three yang channels; this can damage the spleen yang and result in the transmission of an exterior pathogen to the Tai Yin. In this regard, premature or excessive purgation is often a contributing factor in Tai Yin disease; similarly, prolonged use or an inappropriately high dosage of bitter, cold herbs in the treatment of Yang Ming disease can also be a factor.

The zheng qi of Tai Yin is relatively weak and the yang qi is easily depleted. Just as the stomach depends on yin and tends to suffer from yin deficiency and dryness, so the spleen depends on yang for its function of transformation and transportation and tends to suffer when there is yang deficiency or damp. In Tai Yin disease, the spleen's function of raising the clear yang is also affected. Tai Yin pathology therefore manifests as spleen yang deficiency with an accumulation of damp cold in the interior due to the non-transformation of fluids; the impaired raising function will manifest as diarrhoea.

Tai Yin Disease and Its Transmission Pathway

One of the causes of Tai Yin disease is transmission resulting from the incorrect treatment of disease in the three yang channels, Tai Yang, Yang Ming and Shao Yang. Due to the fact that Tai Yin and Yang Ming stand in an interior–exterior relationship, there is potential for pathogenic interchange between Tai Yin and Yang Ming. However, because the stomach tends to dryness and heat and the spleen to yang deficiency and cold, they present with diametrically different manifestations, giving rise to the saying: "Excess is Yang Ming and deficiency is Tai Yin". A further progression of Tai Yin spleen yang deficiency may involve deficiency of kidney yang, producing a pattern of kidney and spleen yang deficiency, for which Zhang Zhong Jing nominated Fu Zi Li Zhong Wan as the appropriate treatment. It should be noted that a Shao Yin deficiency cold pattern can also be accompanied by symptoms of spleen yang.

Key Manifestations of Tai Yin Disease

The principal identifying features of Tai Yin disease are abdominal distension with periodic pain, vomiting and an inability to eat, diarrhoea, a pale tongue with a greasy or slippery white tongue coat, and a slow, submerged pulse.

Classification of Tai Yin Disease

Tai Yin disease is associated with spleen yang deficiency and is classified as either a Tai Yin channel pattern, where there is an exterior attack associated with the interior deficiency, a Tai Yin abdominal pattern, or a Tai Yin yellowing pattern.

Treatment of Tai Yin Disease

Tai Yin disease is characterised by spleen yang deficiency with damp constraint manifesting as periodic or occasional abdominal distension and pain, nausea, vomiting, an inability to eat, and diarrhoea or a loose stool. The general principle of treatment is to warm the spleen yang, strengthen the spleen and dry damp. Indicated formulas are Li Zhong Wan and the Si Ni Tang group of formulas. In addition, there is abdominal pain due to disharmony of qi and blood, and excess abdominal pain due to stasis, for which the indicated formulas are Gui Zhi jia Shao Yao Tang and Gui Zhi jia Da Huang Tang respectively.

Contraindications in Tai Yin Disease

Sweating is permitted only were there is a concurrent exterior pathogen, when mild sweating only must be promoted. Heavy sweating is not permitted and purging and emesis are contraindicated at all times.

Section Two

5.2 PRINCIPAL FEATURES OF TAI YIN DISEASE

Clause 273

太阴之为病，腹满而吐，食不下，自利益甚，时腹自痛，若下之，必胸下结硬。

Tai Yin is diseased, the abdomen is full and there is vomiting, there is an inability to eat, extreme spontaneous diarrhoea, periodic spontaneous pain in the abdomen, if there is purging, there will be a knotted hardness below the chest.

DISCUSSION: Tai Yin disease is attributed to deficiency and coldness of the spleen, where the impaired transformation and transportation results in an accumulation of damp cold in the interior. The damp cold accumulation obstructs the flow of qi, giving rise to glomus which manifests as pain with a sense of fullness in the abdomen. The disrupted descending function of the stomach results in qi reversal which manifests as nausea, vomiting and an inability to eat. The terms "spontaneous diarrhoea" (自利) and "spontaneous pain" (自痛) refer to diarrhoea not caused by purging, and pain without a somatic cause. The diarrhoea is a direct result of spleen yang deficiency, where the transformation process is impaired and the clear yang does not rise. Because the damp accumulation obstructs and further disrupts the spleen function, the diarrhoea, vomiting, abdominal distension and pain, and the inability to eat, will not resolve spontaneously, but will progressively worsen. The pain is described as periodic because vomiting and diarrhoea give only temporary relief as the accumulation of cold damp is reduced but, because the Tai Yin pattern is one of spleen yang deficiency, the emptiness left in the wake of vomiting or diarrhoea results in the return of pain and discomfort.

Because this is representative of a Tai Yin pattern and manifests with interior coldness due to spleen yang deficiency, the strategy is to warm the spleen yang and transform dampness. If the periodic abdominal pain is mistaken for Yang Ming bowel excess and purgation is used, it will devastate the already depleted qi of the spleen and stomach and result in an exacerbation of the cold damp accumulation and there is further stagnation of the middle qi, which together with the yin accumulation, gives rise to hard glomus in the chest.

Differentiation of Tai Yin abdominal pain from that of Yang Ming abdominal pain is made as follows. Tai Yin abdominal pain is attributed to deficiency and coldness characterised by fullness, vomiting and diarrhoea; because it is due to deficiency, the abdominal pain is not relieved by vomiting or diarrhoea but rather progressively worsens as the deficiency is exacerbated. The abdominal pain of a Yang Ming pattern is the result of heat and excess and is characterised by fullness, distension and constipation; because the pain is associated with excess, it is relieved when a stool is passed, which alleviates the fullness and distension.

SUMMARY: The key points for diagnosis of Tai Yin disease are: abdominal fullness, vomiting, an inability to eat, diarrhoea, periodic abdominal pain, a pale tongue with a white tongue coat which is greasy or slippery, and a submerged, slow pulse. If there is abdominal fullness and diarrhoea which worsens over time, one should consider the diagnosis of a Tai Yin pattern of deficiency and cold. The corresponding treatment is to warm and tonify the spleen, scatter cold, and dry damp, using Li Zhong Wan as the key indicated formula. If the pattern is one of spleen and kidney yang deficiency where there is a pronounced aversion to cold, then Fu Zi Li Zhong Wan should be used. If dampness is a significant factor, Ping Wei San can be incorporated.

Section Three

5.3 TAI YIN DISEASE PATTERNS

Tai Yin Channel Pattern

Clause 276

太阴病、脉浮者，可发汗，宜桂枝汤。

Tai Yin disease, if the pulse is floating, one may promote sweat, Gui Zhi Tang is appropriate.

DISCUSSION: Tai Yin disease is associated with a spleen disorder where one expects to find the pulse submerged and weak. To find a floating pulse is an indication of the zheng qi venting the pathogen outward; sweat promotion is therefore appropriate. *Su Wen: Ping Re Bing Lun Pian (Chapter 33: Discourse Evaluating Hot Disease)* states: "Sweating all emanates from grain, grain emanates from essence." Apart from its function of releasing the exterior, Gui Zhi Tang has a regulating effect on the spleen and stomach and harmonises qi and blood. In this way, it strengthens the spleen qi and bolsters the zheng qi, facilitating the expulsion of the pathogen, to "support the zheng qi and expel the evil" simultaneously.

Deficiency patterns of the spleen and stomach are common disorders with a range of potential diagnoses. Before Gui Zhi Tang is used, correct diagnosis must be made by considering all manifestations and not on the basis of the pulse sign alone. Specifically, Gui Zhi Tang is indicated in spleen yang deficiency with cold in the stomach and where there is a symptom complex of stomach pain, poor appetite, vomiting, nausea, an aversion to cold, cold extremities, a slippery, white tongue coat and a floating, moderate pulse. When a patient with this presentation contracts an upper respiratory tract infection and the aversion to cold persists and there are additional symptoms of headache, nasal discharge and a cough with white phlegm, or when a patient presents with a recurrent or lingering upper respiratory tract infection, Gui Zhi Tang is suitable and effective. However, when a spleen deficient patient who has a head cold or influenza presents with fatigue and heaviness in the arms and legs, a reduced appetite where eating even a small meal causes epigastric bloating and discomfort, and there are loose stools, a lack-lustre complexion, low body weight and a slow, submerged pulse, then a more appropriate formula is Bu Zhong Yi Qi Tang to strengthen the spleen, with an increased dosage of Chai Hu and Sheng Ma to enhance its function of raising qi, combined with such herbs as Fang Feng and Chan Yi. In treating a pattern where there is an externally contracted pathogen, one does not simply release the exterior, but must consider the underlying pattern, and differentiate between qi deficiency, where one must tonify qi, and yang deficiency, where the strategy is to warm the spleen and disperse cold.

Tai Yin Cold Pattern

Clause 277

自利不渴者，属太阴，以其脏有寒故也，当温之。宜服四逆辈。

If there is spontaneous diarrhoea without thirst, this pertains to Tai Yin, because there is cold in the zang organ, and one should warm. It is appropriate to administer a Si Ni type of formula.

DISCUSSION: Clause 273, cited earlier, gives a good overview of the main symptoms of Tai Yin disease, namely: fullness in the abdomen, vomiting, an inability to eat, severe diarrhoea and abdominal pain. Clause 277 mentions the additional symptoms of diarrhoea and an absence of thirst, which are ascribed to cold in the spleen, thus also providing an insight into the pathogenesis. Spleen yang has the function of transforming and transporting damp and of carrying the clear yang upwards. Diarrhoea and an absence of thirst can be attributed to spleen yang deficiency with an accumulation of cold and damp; the clear yang fails to ascend and diarrhoea is the result; fluids are not depleted by heat, and so there is no thirst. The treatment for a pattern of empty cold in the middle jiao, which is generally characterised by a loose stool with no thirst, is based on a warming strategy using warming formulas such as Li Zhong Wan; where there is both spleen and kidney yang deficiency, Fu Zi Li Zhong Wan is appropriate. Parallels can be drawn between the diarrhoea of a Tai Yin deficiency pattern with contemporary diagnoses of chronic digestive tract diseases such as colitis with impaired digestion and diarrhoea.

Spontaneous diarrhoea can be associated with Tai Yin, Yang Ming and Shao Yin diseases and must be differentiated. Tai Yin diarrhoea is due to spleen and stomach deficiency cold; impaired transportation and transformation result in a sloppy stool with undigested food. Due to the deficiency cold in the middle jiao, apart from the diarrhoea there are abdominal fullness, fatigue, stomach pain, a bland taste in the mouth, no thirst, a slow pulse, and a moist and slippery tongue coat. Shao Yin diarrhoea is the result of kidney yang deficiency failing to warm the spleen earth, therefore Shao Yin diarrhoea is diarrhoea with undigested particles of food, cold extremities, aversion to cold, a lack-lustre complexion, and a pale and swollen tongue with a white, slippery tongue coat. Unlike the diarrhoea of Tai Yin and Shao Yin, Yang Ming diarrhoea is the result of knotted heat in the intestines; there is a foul smelling, watery stool, thirst, and a red tongue with a yellow tongue coat.

Case Study

Incessant Diarrhoea

Extracted from Shang Han Wu Shi Lun by Pei Yong Qing

Dr. Pei Yun Qing treated a patient in Beijing who had suffered incessant diarrhoea for 7 years, with the condition being worse in the morning. She had had treatment from numerous Chinese medicine practitioners but to no avail. Formulae such as Si Shen Wan, Li Zhong Wan, Shen Ling Bai Zhu San had all been used without satisfactory effect. Dr Pei prescribed Wu Mei Wan on the basis that it was a chronic condition which had not responded to a range of treatments. This was also ineffective. At the next consultation, Gan Cao Xie Xin Tang was prescribed, also without effect. At the third consultation, it became apparent that the Tai Yin yang deficiency diarrhoea pattern was accompanied by an absence of thirst. Dr Pei was immediately reminded of Clause 277 and she prescribed Fu Zi Li Zhong Tang. After three days there was a noticeable improvement and at the end of seven days the diarrhoea stopped. In order to consolidate the recovery, a further 20 packs of Fu Zi Li Zhong Tang jia Huang Lian, Fu Ling was prescribed. At the end of this time, her face took on a healthier hue and her energy and appetite also improved.

Section Four

5.4 TRANSMUTED PATTERNS OF TAI YIN

5.4.1 Tai Yin Abdominal Pain
Gui Zhi jia Shao Yao Tang Pattern
Gui Zhi jia Da Huang Tang Pattern

Clause 279

本太阳病，医反下之，因尔腹满时痛者，属太阴也，桂枝加芍药汤主之。大实痛者，桂枝加大黄汤主之。

Originally there was Tai Yang disease, the physician nevertheless purges, if because of this the abdomen is full and there is periodic pain, it pertains to Tai Yin, Gui Zhi jia Shao Yao Tang governs. If there is strong excess pain, Gui Zhi jia Da Huang Tang governs.

GUI ZHI JIA SHAO YAO TANG: Gui Zhi (bark removed) 3 liang; Shao Yao 6 liang; Zhi Gan Cao 2 liang; Da Zao 12 pieces (broken); Sheng Jiang (sliced) 3 liang.

DIRECTIONS: Boil the ingredients in 7 sheng of water, reducing to 3 sheng. Strain and take warm three times a day. This is Gui Zhi Tang with an increased dose of Shao Yao.

GUI ZHI JIA DA HUANG TANG: Gui Zhi (bark removed) 3 liang; Da Huang 2 liang; Shao Yao 6 liang; Sheng Jiang (sliced) 3 liang; Zhi Gan Cao 2 liang; Da Zao 12 pieces (broken).

DIRECTIONS: Boil the ingredients in 7 sheng of water, reducing to 3 sheng. Strain and take 1 sheng warm three times a day.

DISCUSSION: Clause 279 describes the damage caused to the interior by incorrect purgation in a Tai Yang exterior pattern. The adverse use of purgation has two potential outcomes. (1) The exterior pathogen will fall inward and transform into heat, as found in a Yang Ming pattern. (2) The pathogen falls inward and, instead of affecting Yang Ming, affects the Tai Yin, further depleting an already deficient interior and injuring the yang qi. The insufficiency of yang qi results in an accumulation of cold damp which impedes its flow, and the accumulation of cold results in periodic abdominal pain. The periodic nature of the abdominal pain is attributed to the fluctuation of the yang qi, with the pain occurring when the yang qi recedes and easing on its return. Deficient yang fails to transform and transport fluids and so leads to an accumulation of damp, which is reflected in the abdominal fullness. Whilst not specified in the clause above, where cold and damp obstruct the descent of qi, there will be vomiting, and it can also be understood that the yang deficiency and non-transformation of qi would result in diarrhoea.

When Gui Zhi Tang is taken without the hot gruel described in the original directions, it is no longer a formula which promotes sweat, but is considered to be a formula which harmonises the interior. Gui Zhi Tang regulates the spleen, augments qi and blood and harmonises yin and yang. Gui Zhi jia Shao Yao Tang is Gui Zhi Tang where the dose of Shao Yao is doubled, augmenting the spleen yin, harmonising blood and, most importantly in this application, easing the abdominal pain.

The term "strong excess pain" in the last sentence indicating Gui Zhi jia Da Huang Tang contrasts with the term "periodic pain" mentioned in the first sentence, impressing upon the reader that this pain is more severe and requires more intense treatment. The excess referred to is the congealing of blood due to cold and the ensuing stagnation of qi. Da Huang is used to free the obstruction in order to normalise the flow of qi and blood and alleviate the pain. It has been suggested that the term "strong excess pain" implies that the pathogen has been transmitted to the Yang Ming: that the pain is associated with a Yang Ming bowel excess pattern and that Da Huang is used to purge the interior heat. However, the standard dose of Da Huang in a purging formula is 4 liang, whilst here, in Gui Zhi jia Da Huang Tang, it is only 2 liang. Further, its combination with Gui Zhi shows the purpose is not to clear heat but to invigorate blood and transform stasis, a function which is described in *Shen Nong Ben Cao:* "Da Huang governs the transformation of blood stasis."

Clause 280

太阴为病，脉弱，其人续自便利，设当行大黄芍药者，宜减之，以其人胃气弱，易动故也。

Tai Yin is diseased, the pulse is weak, the person continues to have spontaneous diarrhoea, if Da Huang and Shao Yao are to be given, it is appropriate to reduce, because the person's stomach qi is weak, so it is easily affected.

DISCUSSION: The weak pulse is the characteristic pulse of Tai Yin disease and is a reflection of spleen and stomach deficiency and the failure of post-natal qi to adequately produce qi and blood. The implication of the phrase "the person continues to have spontaneous diarrhoea" is that this is a pattern of chronic spleen deficiency and, whether or not the person is currently suffering from diarrhoea, he or she has already had episodes of diarrhoea and will again in the future. For this reason, caution must be taken in prescribing Da Huang because of its potential to affect the stomach qi; Shao Yao should also not be prescribed in a large dose because, although a small dose can support the zheng qi, a larger dose of this cool herb may damage the spleen and, therefore, may also damage the zheng qi. Whilst it is accepted that Gui Zhi jia Shao Yao jia Da Huang Tang is indicated for abdominal pain associated with a Tai Yin pattern, and the function of the herbs in that formula is to regulate the stomach qi, nevertheless, Da Huang is cold and Shao Yao is cool and their combined effect drains heat and can affect the yang qi. Caution must therefore be exercised as to dosage, particularly if the patient's stomach qi is weak. The Chinese word 減 can mean 'reduce' and can also mean to 'omit'. Whether the dose is reduced, or the herbs omitted entirely, is clearly subject to the discretion of the practitioner and dependent on the condition of the patient.

Differentiation of Abdominal Pain

Abdominal pain can be ascribed to heat, cold, deficiency or excess. Excess patterns discussed in *Shang Han Lun* may be associated with heat, knotted water, damp heat, qi constraint, blood stasis or food stagnation, whilst the deficiency pain of Tai Yin is mainly attributed to the deficiency of yang qi. The differentiation of abdominal pain in *Shang Han Lun* and its pathogenesis and treatment follows.

1. ABDOMINAL PAIN DUE TO EXCESS. The nature of excess abdominal pain is pain which is aggravated by pressure. The indicated formulas are Cheng Qi Tang, Da Xian Xiong Tang, Da Chai Hu Tang, Tao He Cheng Qi Tang, Si Ni San and Zhi Shi Dao Zhi Wan.

Cheng Qi Tang is indicated to purge heat where there is a hard stool bind obstructing intestinal qi. The pain is generally located in the periumbilical region and is characterised by distension, a palpable mass (the hard stool), tidal fever, irritability, constipation, a dry, yellow tongue coat and a submerged, forceful pulse.

Da Xian Xiong Tang is indicated to eliminate water and purge heat where the abdominal pain is the result of water and heat knotting together and forming a glomus in the hypochondrium and epigastrium. The location of the pain is difficult to pinpoint and is associated with fullness and hardness.

Da Chai Hu Tang is indicated to harmonise and purge where there is an unresolved Shao Yang pattern combined with a Yang Ming pattern. The pain will be located in the hypochondrium and abdomen and accompanied by a sense of fullness. Other symptoms will be alternating chills and fever, a bitter taste in the mouth, a dry throat, constipation, dark urination and a rapid, wiry pulse.

Tao He Cheng Qi Tang is indicated to purge and eliminate blood stasis where an unresolved Tai Yang channel disorder falls inward, resulting in the pathogenic heat knotting with the blood in the lower jiao. There will be fixed pain in the lesser abdomen accompanied by symptoms of mental derangement.

Si Ni San is the core formula to ease pain by dispersing constrained liver qi. This is used where constrained qi in the Jue Yin results in a disharmony of the liver and spleen. This results in the impaired movement of qi and there is a distending pain in the abdomen, accompanied by irritability, a poor appetite and a difficult bowel movement.

Zhi Shi Dao Zhi Wan is the indicated formula when food accumulation causes pain and distension in the abdomen. This is accompanied by belching, acid reflux and a greasy, white tongue coat.

2. ABDOMINAL PAIN DUE TO DAMP AND HEAT. The pathogenesis of heat in the abdomen can have two quite different outcomes. It can generate dryness and accumulation which causes abdominal pain due to constipation, as seen in the Cheng Qi Tang patterns above, and can also be associated with dampness and bleeding associated with severe diarrhoea. The indicated formulas for diarrhoea associated with damp heat are Ge Gen Qin Lian Tang and Bai Tou Weng Tang. Abdominal pain is not a characteristic feature but is often a presenting symptom.

The Ge Gen Qin Lian Tang pattern is a result of incorrect purgation in a Tai Yang Gui Zhi Tang pattern, where pathogenic heat has fallen inward causing diarrhoea. This is often accompanied by abdominal pain, fever, and a rapid pulse.

Bai Tou Weng Tang is indicated where toxic heat has lodged in the intestines causing diarrhoea with pus and blood in the stool. It is accompanied by fever, abdominal pain, thirst and a red tongue with a yellow coat. Both Bai Tou Weng Tang and Ge Gen Qin Lian Tang patterns represent acute disorders, and both are characterised by a sense of faecal urgency followed by a sensation of incomplete evacuation. The treatment strategy is to clear toxic heat and dry damp.

3. ABDOMINAL PAIN DUE TO YANG DEFICIENCY. The identifying characteristic of pain due to cold from deficiency is that it is alleviated by warmth and pressure. The indicated formulas are Xiao Jian Zhong Tang, Li Zhong Wan, Si Ni Tang, Zhen Wu Tang and Tao Hua Tang which all address yang deficiency with interior coldness.

Xiao Jian Zhong Tang is principally indicated for spleen deficiency where there is insufficiency of qi and blood. The yang deficiency is not severe and there is a dull pain in the stomach.

Li Zhong Wan is indicated for yang deficiency of the spleen with pronounced signs and symptoms of cold. There is periodic cramping abdominal pain, cold extremities and a slow, submerged pulse.

Si Ni Tang, Zhen Wu Tang and Tao Hua Tang are all indicated in the treatment of Shao Yin kidney yang deficiency. Si Ni Tang is used where the abdominal pain is relatively mild and is accompanied by cold extremities, diarrhoea with undigested food particles, an absence of thirst and a submerged, faint pulse. Zhen Wu Tang is used when the deficient kidney yang fails to govern water, and the abdominal pain is accompanied by inhibited urination, oedema, heaviness in the limbs and diarrhoea with undigested food particles. Tao Hua Tang is used when the abdominal pain is accompanied by blood and pus in the stool, constant watery diarrhoea, tenesmus and a bland taste in the mouth.

4. ABDOMINAL PAIN DUE TO A COMPLEX OF HEAT AND COLD. Complex patterns of heat and cold are those where there are mixed signs and symptoms of heat, cold, deficiency and excess, with no clear predominance of any one. Indicated formulas are Xiao Chai Hu Tang and Huang Lian Tang.

Xiao Chai Hu Tang is used for abdominal pain associated with a Shao Yang pattern where pathogenic constraint causes pain in the chest and hypochondrium which is accompanied by alternating chills and fever, nausea, irritability, a bitter taste in the mouth and a wiry pulse.

Huang Lian Tang is the formula indicated for abdominal pain associated with a complex pattern of heat in the stomach and cold in the lower jiao which manifests with vomiting and abdominal pain.

Comparison of Xiao Jian Zhong Tang with Gui Zhi jia Shao Yao Tang and Gui Zhi jia Da Huang Tang

Formula	Aetiology	Pathology	Symptoms	Treatment
Gui Zhi jia Shao Yao Tang	Incorrect purgation in Tai Yang disease with the pathogen falling inward and the exterior not resolved	Incorrect treatment has damaged the spleen; qi stagnation with impaired transportation	Abdominal fullness with periodic pain; unresolved exterior	Regulate the spleen and ease pain by using a large dose of Shao Yao
Gui Zhi jia Da Huang Tang	Incorrect purgation in Tai Yang disease with the pathogen falling inward and the exterior not resolved	Obstruction of qi and blood in Tai Yin with blood stasis	Acute abdominal pain which resists pressure	Warm the spleen and transform stasis
Xiao Jian Zhong Tang	Deficiency of yin, yang, qi and blood	Spleen deficiency with insufficiency of qi and blood	Abdominal pain and cramps, alleviated by warmth and pressure; palpitations, irritability	Warm the middle Tonify the deficiency Ease abdominal pain with a large dose of Shao Yao and Yi Tang (malt sugar)

Ancient Application of Gui Zhi Tang Variations

- *Lei Ju Fang Guang Yi:* Gui Zhi jia Shao Yao Tang is cited in the treatment of abdominal cramps and Gui zhi jia Da Huang Tang in the treatment of dysentery with fever, aversion to cold, abdominal pain and tenesmus.
- *Huo Ren Shu:* Gui Zhi jia Da Huang Tang is cited in the treatment of abdominal fullness and constipation with an excess pulse.
- *Sheng Hui Fang:* Chi Shao Yao San, which is Gui Zhi jia Da Huang Tang omitting Sheng Jiang and Da Zao and adding Bai Zhu, is cited in the treatment of persistent infantile crying at night, where the child's sleep is disturbed by colicky abdominal pain.

Modern Application of Gui Zhi Tang Variations

- Gui Zhi jia Shao Yao Tang can be combined with Ren Shen Tang to treat anaemia caused by colitis or chronic diarrhoea.
- Gui Zhi jia Da Huang Tang can be used in the treatment of dysentery and colitis characterised by tenesmus, and also constipation associated with paralytic ileus. (The practitioner must be aware of the need to refer to the emergency department of a hospital if it has persisted past 2 or 3 days.)

Case Study

Chronic Stomach Pain

Extracted from Liu Jing Bian Zheng Shi Yong Jie 2002

A 67-year-old woman had suffered for several years from stomach pain which was worse whenever she caught the common cold. The stomach pain came and went during the day and eased when she went to bed with an electric blanket. Her pulse was soggy and moderate. Xiang Sha Liu Jun Zi Tang was administered to warm the spleen and regulate qi; however, the pain was only temporarily alleviated and the condition relapsed a few days later. Based on Zhang Zhong Jing's theory that the abdominal pain of a Tai Yin pattern can be treated with Gui Zhi jia Shao Yao Tang, the following modified formula was prescribed: Gui Zhi 10g, Bai Shao 15g, Zhi Gan Cao 6g, Sheng Jiang 10g, Da Zao 4 pieces, Bai Dou Kou 6g, Sha Ren 6g. She was given three packs and one pack was decocted each day and taken warm in two doses.

Discussion: Stomach pain aggravated by cold and alleviated by heat is generally associated with yang deficiency. Xiang Sha Liu Jun Zi Tang augments the spleen and regulates qi but does not specifically tonify spleen yang and is not effective in dispersing cold. Gui Zhi jia Shao Yao Tang addresses the deficiency cold and also relieves the pain. A follow-up consultation several weeks later showed that after taking the three packs, there was no recurrence of the stomach pain.

Case Study

Dysentery

Extracted from Xin Bian Shang Han Lun Lei Fang

A 36-year-old male presented with dysentery and tenesmus. The frequent diarrhoea contained blood and pus. His pulse was wiry and his tongue was red with a yellow coat. The diagnosis was cold damp obstruction of the spleen and stomach with disharmony of qi and blood. The formula prescribed was Gui Zhi jia Da Huang Tang: Gui Zhi 6g, Bai Shao 18g, Sheng Jiang 9g, Zhi Gan Cao 6g, Da Zao 7 pieces, Da Huang 5g. After taking one pack, the patient passed a foul sticky stool with pus and mucus. After two more packs, the diarrhoea was resolved.

5.4.2 Tai Yin Yellowing Pattern

Clause 259

伤寒发汗已，身目为黄，所以然者，以寒湿在里不解故也。以为不可下也，于寒湿中求之。

Shang han where sweat was promoted, the body and eyes are yellow, the reason for this being, cold damp is unresolved in the interior. Presumably one should not purge, seek the cold and damp.

DISCUSSION: Clause 259 describes a situation where promoting sweat in shang han disease has resulted in yellowing of the skin. Zhang Zhong Jing explains that it is due to cold damp in the interior. From this, we can conclude that the promotion of sweat has eliminated the heat, but that there must have also been damp which has not been eliminated. Furthermore, the sweating has damaged the yang qi. Because the deficient spleen yang is unable to transform and transport fluids, cold and damp accumulate in the interior, obstructing the flow of qi and manifesting as yin jaundice, with yellowing of the skin and sclera.

Differentiation must be made between yin jaundice, which is yellowing due to cold damp, and yang jaundice which is associated with Yang Ming and is due to damp heat. Damp heat in the Yang Ming is treated with purgation to drain heat and eliminate damp, but this is not appropriate in a Tai Yin pattern. The pathogenesis of yin jaundice is spleen yang deficiency leading to an accumulation of cold damp. It is characterised by aversion to cold, cold extremities, a loose stool, a pale, swollen tongue and a submerged, slow and forceless pulse. In treating yin jaundice, the strategy is to warm yang, disperse cold and eliminate damp, and this is what is meant by 'seek the cold and damp'. By eliminating the accumulation of damp cold, there is no longer an obstruction to the spleen; the movement of qi is freed, and the normal flow of bile restored. In mild cases, this can be achieved with the formula Yin Chen Wu Ling Tang, where Yin Chen is added to Wu Ling San in order to promote urination and drain damp. For more serious cases, where cold is a significant factor, Yin Chen Zhu Fu Tang (Yin Chen, Bai Zhu, Gan Jiang, Fu Zi, Rou Gui, Zhi Gan Cao) or Yin Chen Si Ni Tang (Yin Chen, Pao Jiang, Fu Zi, Gan Cao) can be used to warm and strengthen the spleen, supplement yang, eliminate damp cold and thereby reduce yin jaundice.

Clause 278

伤寒，脉浮而缓，手足自温者，系在太阴；太阴当发身黄，若小便自利者，不能发黄；至七八日，虽暴烦下利，日十余行，必自止，以脾家实，腐秽去故也。

Shang han, the pulse is floating and moderate, if the hands and feet are spontaneously warm, this is in the Tai Yin; in Tai Yin the body should become yellow, if urination is spontaneously free, there can be no yellowing; on the seventh or eighth day, despite sudden vexation and diarrhoea, occurring over ten times a day, it will stop spontaneously, due to the spleen's domain being in excess, putrid filth is being eliminated.

DISCUSSION: The floating moderate pulse described in Clause 278 is identical to that of Tai Yang zhong feng, however there is no fever characteristic of that pattern; further, the hands and feet are described as warm, differentiating it from a Shao Yin disorder. Thus a floating and moderate pulse with warm extremities and vexatious pain of the four limbs can be regarded as a sign of Tai Yin disease. This is because the spleen governs the four limbs and pertains to Tai Yin, and so such symptoms as "vexatious pain of the four limbs" or "warm extremities" are an indication of disease in the Tai Yin.

The statement "in Tai Yin the body should become yellow" alludes to the potential for yellowing in Tai Yin disease. This is because the pathogenesis of Tai Yin disease is closely linked to spleen deficiency, where the failure of the transformation and transportation function results in damp accumulation. Consequently, if urination is free and uninhibited, the damp will be drained naturally and there is no need to use herbs to promote urination. The disease will therefore not proceed to yin jaundice, which is the result of severe damp accumulation inhibiting the movement of qi and further impairing the function of the spleen.

The significance of sudden vexation occurring on the seventh or eighth day is that this is a manifestation of heat generated by the zheng qi battling against the evil. The repeated episodes of diarrhoea are also a reflection of the return of spleen yang, which can now perform its function of raising the clear and descending the turbid, and it is the turbid which is expelled downward in the foul and putrid stool. For this reason, these symptoms are signs of recovery. The "excess" mentioned in the clause is the excess of turbid yin which has accumulated as a result of spleen deficiency. It must not be confused with the excess associated with Yang Ming in the form of food stagnation or constipation.

The restoration of spleen yang is generally assessed on the basis of the return of the appetite and the change in the tongue coat from white and greasy to a healthy, thin white coat. The reliance on sudden vexation and diarrhoea as a sign of the return of zheng qi as described in Clause 278 is only one of the signs of imminent recovery in *Shang Han Lun*. Others are seen in the shivering and sweating associated with a Xiao Chai Hu Tang pattern described in Clauses 101 and 230, and the nosebleeds associated with a Ma Huang Tang pattern described in Clauses 46 and 47.

Clause 187

伤寒，脉浮而缓，手足自温者，是为系在太阴。太阴者，身当发黄。若小便自利者，不能发黄；至七八日大便硬者，为阳明病也。

Shang han, the pulse is floating and moderate, if the hands and feet are spontaneously warm, it is then in the Tai Yin. If it is Tai Yin, the body should become yellow. If urination is spontaneously free, there can be no yellowing; if on the seventh or eighth day the stool is hard, this is Yang Ming disease.

DISCUSSION: Clause 187 describes the potential of disease transmission from Tai Yin to Yang Ming. In his book *Shi Re Bing Pian* Xue Sheng Bai said, "Excess is Yang Ming and deficiency is Tai Yin". Tai Yin and Yang Ming are connected by their mutual association with the earth and their location in the middle jiao. Their relationship is nevertheless both paradoxical and complementary: Tai Yin governs dampness while Yang Ming governs dryness. From this it is understood that the spleen, through its dependence on yang, is responsible for the elimination of damp and by inference, if it fails in this duty, is responsible for its generation. Ironically, it is also adversely affected by damp. Yang Ming, on the other hand, is reliant on yin, and tends to dryness and heat, which adversely affect the stomach. From this it is clear that the damp of Tai Yin disease is intimately related to the strength of the middle qi. If the spleen yang of Tai Yin is restored, and the stomach qi of Yang Ming is intact, damp may be resolved by the yang qi, and then transformed into dryness, and if yin is deficient, heat will be generated. This exemplifies the transformation of deficiency into excess; the manifestation of a hard stool signifies that the disease is now in the Yang Ming. In this clause, the spontaneously uninhibited urination has facilitated the elimination of damp to the extent that it has instigated such a transformation.

Clause 187 reminds us of possible disease transformation from the exterior to the interior, and from the interior back to the exterior; from cold to heat and from heat to cold; from excess to deficiency and from deficiency back to excess. The practitioner should be aware of potential transformation, firstly to avoid deterioration of disease, and also to take advantage of any opportunity to reverse the situation and expedite recovery.

Case Study

Hepatic Cirrhosis with Jaundice

Extracted from Liao Ning Zhong Yi Vol 30, No. 2 Feb 2003

In 1998, a 62-year-old male had been treated for ascites associated with hepatic cirrhosis. He was hospitalised for two months, after which the ascites was resolved but the jaundice persisted, with yellowing of the skin and sclera. The urine was dark and he suffered from fatigue, a poor appetite, abdominal distension, loose stools, oedema of the lower limbs, a pale tongue with stasis spots on the margin of the tongue, a white tongue coat and a submerged, thready pulse. The liver function test showed elevated levels of liver enzymes and bilirubin: gamma glutamyl transferase (GGT) 100 IU/L (N: 30-115 IU/L); aspartate aminotransferase (AST) 120 IU/L (N: 5-43 IU/L); alanine aminotransferase (ALT) 150 IU/L (N: 5-60 IU/L); serum bilirubin 5 mg/dL (N: 0.2-1.5

mg/dL). The diagnosis was qi deficiency with cold damp congealed in the spleen and blood stasis. The treatment principle was to warm the spleen, transform dampness, tonify qi and invigorate blood. The formula used was Yin Chen Si Ni Tang: Yin Chen 80g, Fu Zi 10g, Rou Gui 10g, Gan Jiang 10g, Dan Shen 30g, San Qi Fen 4g, Fang Ji 15g, Chi Xiao Dou 30g, Hua Shi 15g, Da Fu Pi 30g, Sheng Gan Cao 10g (five packs). The directions were to soak the Yin Chen in cold water for 10 minutes; bring to the boil and simmer for 10 to 15 minutes. Soak the remaining ingredients for 30 minutes then boil for 25 to 30 minutes. Combine the two decoctions and re-boil for another 15 minutes, reducing to 600 mL. The dose was 300 mL twice a day, taken warm. After taking the five packs, there was improvement in most of the symptoms. The same formula was repeated adding Huang Qi 80g and Dang Shen 100g to supplement the zheng qi. At the third consultation, there was a noticeable reduction in the jaundice and oedema. The original formula was repeated with the dose of Hua Shi increased from 15g to 30g.

Section Five

5.5 PROGNOSIS AND RECOVERY IN TAI YIN DISEASE

Prognosis in Tai Yin Disease

Clause 274

太阴中风，四肢烦疼，阳微阴涩而长者，为欲愈。

Tai Yin zhong feng, there is vexing pain in the four limbs, if yang is faint, yin is choppy but long, it is about to recover.

DISCUSSION: The pain in the limbs of Tai Yin zhong feng must be differentiated from that of Tai Yang zhong feng. In Tai Yang zhong feng, the joint pain and body aches are accompanied by fever and aversion to cold, which are the manifestation of constrained defence yang and disharmony of ying and wei. The pain in the limbs of Tai Yin zhong feng, on the other hand, is the result of spleen deficiency with devitalised yang which is then unable to warm the extremities. Because it is associated with interior cold, there is aversion to cold but no fever. Vexing pain in the limbs is a characteristic of Tai Yin disease. This is based on the theory that the spleen Tai Yin governs the four limbs, which reflect the state of yang qi. If spleen yang is deficient, and if damp cold subsequently invades, the limbs will be affected.

"Yang is faint, yin is choppy but long" is a reference to the pulse sign which Zhang Zhong Jing uses to determine recovery of Tai Yin disease. 'Yang' refers to the superficial level of the pulse, felt under light palpation, and 'yin' to the pulse felt on deeper pressure. The detection of a faint pulse at the superficial level is a positive sign that the yang qi is returning, the inference being that previously, there was none. The subsequent return of yang qi ensures the normal flow of qi and blood which will warm the extremities and resolve the pain in the limbs, and thus predicts recovery. The choppy pulse felt at the deeper level indicates spleen disharmony where cold damp is congealing and stagnating the flow. When the pulse sign is not just choppy but becomes long, it is a sign of the augmentation of spleen qi, which will result in the resolution of damp. Changes in the pulse will be matched by corresponding changes in the tongue coat from greasy and white to thin and white.

Tai Yin Recovery period

Clause 275

太阴病欲解时，从亥至丑上。

The time that Tai Yin disease is ready to resolve, recovery is from hai to chou.

DISCUSSION: The qi of the foot Tai Yin peaks during the period of hai shi to zi shi (9pm to

1am), continuing through to the beginning of chou shi. At this time, the yang qi of the Tai Yin is at its peak and is able to contend more effectively against the pathogenic qi, thus optimising recovery.

Section Six

5.6 SUMMARY OF THE TAI YIN CHAPTER

The Tai Yin chapter covers five points which need to be understood in order to diagnose Tai Yin disease.

PRINCIPAL PATTERNS AND TREATMENT STRATEGIES OF TAI YIN: Tai Yin disease is attributed to deficiency and cold in the spleen and stomach. Impaired transformation and transportation and the accumulation of damp disrupt the qi dynamic, producing the characteristic manifestations of abdominal fullness, nausea and vomiting, a poor appetite, diarrhoea, periodic abdominal pain, a wet, white tongue coat and a moderate or slow pulse. The key point of diagnosis is abdominal fullness and pain which feels worse after diarrhoea. The treatment strategy is to warm the middle and disperse cold. The recommended formula is Li Zhong Wan when the condition is mild, and Fu Zi Li Zhong Wan or Si Ni Tang when the accumulation of cold is more severe. Purging is contraindicated in Tai Yin disease because of its potential to damage the spleen and stomach further and thus exacerbate the accumulation of cold and damp, which will manifest as knotted hardness in the epigastrium.

TAI YIN CHANNEL PATTERN: A Tai Yin channel pattern is associated with weak spleen yang and the contraction of an exterior wind cold pathogen. The cold constraint in the exterior manifests as a floating pulse, headache, aversion to wind, a blocked nose, and aching joints and limbs. The treatment strategy is to warm the channels, unblock the constrained yang, regulate the middle and release the exterior pathogen from the muscle layer. Gui Zhi Tang is the indicated formula.

TAI YIN TRANSMUTED PATTERN: The two key symptoms commonly ascribed to the transmutation of disease in the Tai Yin are abdominal pain and jaundice.

- The abdominal pain of a Tai Yin transmuted pattern is the result of incorrect purgation in shang han disease which has caused the pathogen to fall inward, damaging the Tai Yin spleen. This results in a disharmony of qi and blood causing periodic abdominal fullness and pain, and the indicated formula is Gui Zhi jia Shao Yao Tang. It is differentiated from the periodic pain of the Tai Yin pattern which is due to yang deficiency. For severe pain associated with the stagnation of qi and blood, the indicated formula is Gui Zhi jia Da Huang Tang, where consideration must be given to the underlying deficiency of the patient, and the dose of Da Huang and Shao Yao correspondingly reduced.
- The second symptom, Tai Yin yellowing or yin jaundice, is attributed to the inappropriate or excessive promotion of sweat in shang han disease, which has damaged spleen yang and led to the accumulation of cold damp obstructing the interior. The text states that naturally uninhibited urination in the earlier stage of Tai Yin is a sign that it will not proceed to jaundice. The text does not cite a guiding formula, but Yin Chen Wu Ling San or Yin Chen Zhu Fu Tang can be used.

TAI YIN RECOVERY PATHWAYS: There are two pathways in the spontaneous recovery of Tai Yin disease.

- In a pattern where the yang deficiency has resulted in an accumulation of turbidity, a return of the yang qi manifests as sudden vexation, which is a reflection of the zheng qi contending against the pathogen, and also results in the elimination of the turbidity in the form of a putrid stool.
- In a pattern where the mechanism of recovery is the transmission of the pathogen from the

Tai Yin to the Yang Ming, Yang Ming signs of a hard stool and a floating, moderate pulse will appear.

SIGNS OF TAI YIN RECOVERY: Tai Yin recovery is heralded by signs such as: (i) a pulse which is faint at the superficial level, demonstrating the return of yang qi, and a pulse image which is no longer just choppy, but has changed to being long, indicating the augmentation of spleen qi; (ii) vexing pain in the limbs with a faint yang pulse and a choppy yin pulse which indicate the return of the flow of yang qi; (iii) a change of tongue coat from thick and greasy to thin and white; and (iv) increased appetite and reduced diarrhoea.

TAI YIN RECOVERY PERIOD: Tai Yin channel qi peaks between the hours of hai and chou (9pm to 1am) and so this is the optimal time for recovery.

少陰

Shao Yin 6

Section One

6.1 OUTLINE OF SHAO YIN

Pathway of the Shao Yin Channel

The Shao Yin channel incorporates the hand Shao Yin heart and foot Shao Yin kidney channels; these stand in an interior–exterior relationship with the hand Tai Yang small intestine and foot Tai Yang urinary bladder channels. The internal pathway of the hand Shao Yin heart channel emerges from the heart, surrounds the vessels and leads to its yang partner, the small intestine. A second channel travels from the heart to the root of the tongue and upwards to the brain. The external channel runs from the axilla down the arm to the tip of the fifth finger. The internal pathway of the foot Shao Yin kidney channel travels from the tip of the coccyx to the kidneys and urinary bladder, ascending via the liver and lungs to the throat and the root of the tongue. The external channel emerges at the tip of the little toe and ascends the inside of the leg to the abdomen, continuing up the chest to the throat.

Physiology of the Shao Yin Channel

The Shao Yin channel incorporates the heart and kidney and by thus governing the organs of fire and water, constitutes the source of yin and yang for the whole body. The heart pertains to fire, governs blood and provides residence for the shen; the kidney pertains to water, stores essence which is the foundation of true yin and true yang, and is the root of preheaven qi from which life emanates. The physiological interaction of heart fire and kidney water is the basis of the mutual supplementation of fire and water and ensures the equilibrium of these two opposing forces upon which good health depends.

Pathology of the Shao Yin Channel

Because of its relationship to the heart and kidney, Shao Yin disease is regarded as a serious and even life-threatening stage of disease. It is the result of insufficiency of the heart and kidney and substantial weakening of the zheng qi. It is characterised by a faint and thready pulse, a desire to sleep, vomiting, and diarrhoea. Two significant features of Shao Yin pathology which must be borne in mind are firstly, the kidneys tend to deficiency but not to excess and secondly, kidney yin and kidney yang are mutually engendering and depletion of one will eventually lead to deficiency of the other.

Pathology in the Shao Yin channel is attributed either to a direct attack from an exterior pathogen made possible by weak zheng qi associated with aging or poor health, or to transmission from other channels where incorrect treatment has depleted the qi of the heart and kidneys. Deficiency of the heart and kidneys most commonly manifests as a yang deficiency with exuberant cold in the interior. This is known as a Shao Yin cold conversion pattern and the strategy is to scatter cold and warm the interior yang. When deficient yang fails to transform damp, water is not controlled and the required strategy is to tonify yang, drain damp and promote urination. Where yang is further depleted and becomes devastated, yin is not controlled and the resulting exuberant yin cold repels the deficient yang, which will manifest as false heat. If the yang qi is not rescued, this pattern can proceed to a pattern of desertion of yang and exhaustion of yin. Where kidney yin is deficient, ministerial fire will flare in the heart and the strategy is to nourish yin and clear empty fire. Insufficiency of kidney yin with hyperactive heart fire is known as a heat conversion pattern. Where there is a pre-existing heart and kidney yin deficiency, the ensuing deficiency heat in the interior will knot with water in the urinary bladder and manifest as inhibited urination, thirst, vexation and insomnia.

In brief, Shao Yin patterns are primarily cold patterns associated with yang deficiency, but also include heat patterns associated with yin deficiency. Where there is an underlying yang deficiency in the Shao Yin, an exterior attack will present as Shao Yin disease with an exterior pattern. Exuberant deficiency heat in the Shao Yin channel, or excessive yang return consuming yin, can both lead to dryness and manifest as a Shao Yin interior excess pattern.

Shao Yin Disease and Its Transmission Pathway

Shao Yin disease is the penultimate stage of standard transmission in six channel theory. The transmission pathways are as follows. (1) Exterior to interior channel transmission, when yang deficiency in the Shao Yin channel is accompanied by insufficiency of zheng qi and the external pathogen attacking the Tai Yang can bypass the Tai Yang channel and attack the Shao Yin channel directly. This exemplifies 'yue jing chuan' or 'transmission by skipping channels'. (2) Tai Yin spleen yang deficiency has the potential to affect the kidney yang, resulting in transmission to Shao Yin. This exemplifies 'xun jing chuan' or 'transmission in sequence of the channels'. (3) Correct treatment can cause the pathogen to return to the yang channels and can eventually expel the pathogen.

Key Manifestations of Shao Yin Disease

The key identifying symptoms for Shao Yin disease are: diarrhoea with undigested food particles, aversion to cold, cold extremities, a desire to sleep, a pulse which is submerged, faint and thready.

Classification of Shao Yin Disease

Shao Yin disease falls into two categories: cold conversion and heat conversion. Conversion patterns refer to patterns of deficiency which are characterised by manifestations of either extreme cold (cold conversion) or extreme heat (heat conversion). The pattern descriptions are as follows.

1. *Shao Yin cold conversion.* No fever, aversion to cold, a desire to sleep curled up, somnolence, vomiting, a watery stool with undigested food particles, and a faint and thready pulse. Where exuberant yin cold repels the true yang, resulting in a pattern of true cold with false heat, there will be a flushed face and no aversion to cold.
2. *Shao Yin heat conversion.* Vexation, insomnia, a dry or sore throat, a red tongue with a scant coat and a thready, rapid pulse.

Treatment of Shao Yin Disease

Treatment is differentiated according to whether the pattern is one of a yang deficiency with exuberant cold, when the strategy is to supplement yang and disperse yin, or a pattern of deficiency heat, when the strategy is to nourish the yin and clear heat. The warming and tonifying formulas are Si Ni Tang, Tong Mai Si Ni Tang, Bai Tong Tang; the heat clearing and nourishing formulas are Huang Lian E Jiao Tang and Zhu Ling Tang. If Shao Yin disease is combined with an exterior pattern, the treatment will be directed towards warming yang and promoting sweat, using a formula such as Ma Huang Fu Zi Xi Xin Tang. For a concurrent pattern of Shao Yin and Yang Ming, the strategy is to preserve the yin by purging with Da Cheng Qi Tang.

Contraindications in Shao Yin Disease

In Shao Yin disease which is characterised by cold and deficiency, sweat promotion, purgation and fire therapy are all contraindicated.

Section Two

6.2 PRINCIPAL FEATURES OF SHAO YIN DISEASE

The principal features of Shao Yin disease have their root in yang deficiency of the heart and kidneys with an accumulation of yin cold. Clause 281 describes a typical Shao Yin cold pattern, Clause 282 describes a cold conversion pattern, and Clause 283 identifies a Shao Yin sore throat pattern.

Clause 281

少阴之为病，脉微细，但欲寐也。

Shao Yin is diseased, the pulse is faint and thready, the person desires only to sleep.

DISCUSSION: Shao Yin disease involves the heart and kidney which are the organs of fire and water and the root of yin and yang. The heart houses shen; the kidneys store essence and are the abode of true yin and true yang. Shao Yin disease is associated with prolonged illness which has affected the heart and kidneys and drained yin, yang, qi and blood, resulting in a substantial weakening of zheng qi. It often parallels the Western medical diagnosis of late stage chronic heart and kidney disease.

The faint and thready pulse and the desire to sleep reflect a severe depletion of vital substances. The faint pulse is a sign of yang deficiency and the thready pulse indicates deficiency of blood. Constant somnolence represents an altered state of consciousness brought about by an insufficiency of yang qi. The *Nei Jing* attributes somnolence to a deficiency of yang qi thus: "Wakefulness is associated with the emergence of defence yang while sleep is associated with the retreat of defence yang". The signs described in Clause 281 are an allusion to the pathology of Shao Yin disease being founded in heart and kidney yang deficiency with insufficiency of qi and blood; the associated inadequacy of zheng qi leaves the body without the resources to fight the pathogen. This is the key point to be grasped by the practitioner so as to ensure adoption of the appropriate strategy; this is aimed at fortifying the yang of the heart and kidneys in the early stage of Shao Yin, thereby warming the yang and dispersing the accumulated cold.

The sequence of describing the pulse images corresponds to their diagnostic priority. In other words, the faintness of the pulse being mentioned first implies that the deficiency of yang qi should be read as being the primary factor in considering the cause of Shao Yin disease. The deficiency of yin and blood represented by the thready pulse, is the secondary factor. Finally, the insufficiency of kidney essence, which is a result of the debilitating effects of chronic illness, is seen as a third aspect of the illness; insufficient essence fails to transform blood to nourish the spirit, and the three treasures, essence, qi and spirit, are all in deficit, and so the person wants only to sleep.

The symptom of extreme somnolence (但欲寐 dan yu mei) in this clause must be differentiated from the mild somnolence (嗜卧 shi wo) described in Tai Yang and Yang Ming, which might better be translated as 'feeling sleepy' or 'wanting to have a lie down'. This is more clearly illustrated by contrasting the severe somnolence described here in Clause 281, with the milder sleepiness mentioned in Clause 37, which reads: "Tai Yang disease, ten days have passed, where the pulse is floating and fine and the patient is sleepy, the exterior pattern has resolved." This sleepiness is a sign that the pathogen is already resolved; the patient is recovering and simply wants to rest. A third type of somnolence is described in Clause 231: "Yang Ming zhong feng, the pulse is wiry, floating and big, and there is shortness of breath, distension throughout the abdomen, pain under the ribs and in the heart, a sense of qi blockage under prolonged pressure, a dry nose, an absence of sweat, a desire to lie down…". This type of somnolence, found in Yang Ming disease and expressed as a desire to lie down, results from exuberant heat clouding the spirit and the prognosis is good. In contrast with the milder somnolence of Tai Yang and Yang Ming, Clause 281 describes a situation in Shao Yin disease where consciousness is impaired and the condition is critical; the pattern is not one of heat, but one of yang deficiency.

Cold Conversion in Shao Yin

Cold conversion refers to a pattern of kidney and heart yang deficiency with exuberant cold in the interior characterised by aversion to cold, cold extremities, a desire to sleep, a loose stool with undigested food particles, vomiting and a submerged, faint and thready pulse.

Clause 282

少阴病，欲吐不吐，心烦但欲寐，五六日自利而渴者，属少阴也。虚故引水自救；若小便色白者，少阴病形悉具，小便白者，以下焦虚有寒，不能制水，故令色白也。

Shao Yin disease, there is an urge to vomit but no vomiting, the heart is vexed and the person wants only to sleep, if on the fifth or sixth day there is diarrhoea and thirst, this pertains to Shao Yin. There is deficiency so taking water will give spontaneous relief; if the colour of the urine is clear, the signs of Shao Yin are all there, if urine is clear, it is because there is deficiency and cold in the lower jiao, an inability to control water, and so it causes the colour to be clear.

DISCUSSION: The urge to vomit, vexation and thirst are reminiscent of a heat pattern, but we are told that this is a pattern of deficiency and cold. This is confirmed by the symptom of wanting to do nothing but sleep, and at the end of the clause with the symptom of clear, copious urination, which is a key indicator of a cold pattern. In Shao Yin disease, an urge to vomit is ascribed to yang deficiency and yin cold accumulation in the lower jiao causing qi reversal. The qi surges upwards causing an urge to vomit; however, there is no actual vomiting, because the stomach is empty. Exuberant yin in the lower jiao displaces and repels the deficient yang, which harasses the heart when it surges upwards, causing vexation. As explained earlier, the desire to do nothing but sleep indicates severe yang deficiency, which leaves the patient sleepy and listless with neither the physical nor mental energy to do anything. This pattern is thus associated with heart and kidney yang deficiency with exuberant yin cold in the interior.

After five or six days, the disease progresses, with continuing deterioration of the heart and kidney yang. The kidney yang does not warm the spleen, and its transformation and transportation functions are not supported; impaired transformation results in diarrhoea, and impaired transportation results in the non-distribution of fluids; this results in thirst, which, because it is not due to heat, is easily relieved by drinking water. The clear urination is a sign of cold, and the inability to control urination is a reflection of the kidney yang deficiency. Clear copious urination is a characteristic symptom of deficiency cold and is a key feature of a Shao Yin cold conversion pattern.

Key Points of Diagnosis of Cold Conversion

1. *Differentiation of thirst.* Thirst is often attributed to heat, whether due to excess or deficiency. However, as in the pattern described above, thirst can also be due to yang deficiency. The reference to diarrhoea and thirst in the one phrase draws attention to the fact that they both have a single cause, namely insufficient yang: the failure to transform leads to diarrheoa, and the failure to distribute fluids causes thirst. A second cause of the thirst is the loss of fluids in the watery stool. Thirst due to heat is characterised by urination which is yellow and scant as opposed to the clear and copious urination described in Clause 282. Furthermore, a heat pattern is generally characterised by a strong thirst, whereas the thirst of a Shao Yin pattern is easily quenched with a little water.
2. *Differentiation of vexation.* Vexation can be differentiated according to whether it is caused by heat or by cold. The vexation of a Shao Yin pattern is associated with cold and is accompanied by an urge to vomit and a desire to sleep; it is the result of

deficient yang. The desire to sleep is a sign of yang deficiency and the urge to vomit is a manifestation of the counterflow of turbidity caused by the accumulation of yin cold in the interior. There are accompanying symptoms of diarrhoea and cold hands and feet, the pulse is weak and submerged, and the tongue is pale with a white coat; the indicated formula is Si Ni Tang. By contrast, in vexation due to excess heat, as seen in a Yang Ming pattern, there is no vomiting and no desire to sleep. Instead there are such symptoms as pain and distension in the abdomen, constipation, a yellow tongue coat, a dry mouth and a flooding, big or slippery and rapid pulse; the indicated formula is Zhi Zi Chi Tang.

3. *Differentiation of diarrhoea.* Diarrhoea due to heat is generally characterised by a foul sloppy stool and a burning sensation in the anus. The tongue coat is turbid and yellow. In contrast, Shao Yin diarrhoea is due to yang deficiency and cold. The stool is watery with undigested food particles and the tongue coat is moist and white.

Sore Throat in Shao Yin

Clause 283

病人脉阴阳俱紧，反汗出者，亡阳也，此属少阴，法当咽痛而复吐利。

The patient's yin and yang pulse are both tight, nevertheless there is sweating, this is devastation of yang, it pertains to Shao Yin, there will be a sore throat and then vomiting and diarrhoea.

DISCUSSION: The tightness of the yin and yang pulse is a reference to the pulse across all three positions including the guan pulse, not just the chi and cun positions. A tight or tense pulse is an indication of excess cold and in this case it reflects the exuberant internal yin cold of a Shao Yin pattern. By contrast, Tai Yang shang han is characterised by yin and yang pulses which are floating and tight, accompanied by headache, fever, aversion to cold and an absence of sweat. The yin and yang pulses of Shao Yin are not only tight but would also be submerged, since they are a reflection of an interior pattern. The sweating in such a pattern is not the sweating of an exterior disorder, but is the result of excess yin and deficient yang; it demonstrates that the deficient yang is unable to secure the exterior: the sweating is a sign of yang desertion. The vomiting and diarrhoea are features of Shao Yin disease which have been discussed with Clause 282. A sore throat is not always due to toxic heat; it is also associated with Shao Yin disease because the kidney channel passes through the throat, terminating at the root of the tongue. No specific formula is suggested in Clause 283, but based on the pattern of yang deficiency with exuberance of yin, the appropriate treatment is to warm and resuscitate the devastated yang using such herbs as Gan Jiang and Fu Zi. To address the sore throat, *Huo Ren Shu* proposes that suitable formulas are: Gan Cao Tang, Jie Geng Tang, Ban Xia San and Tong Mai Si Ni Tang combined with Jie Geng Tang, or Ma Huang Sheng Ma Tang.

Summary of the Principal Features of Shao Yin

Shao Yin disease is characterised by a pulse which is faint and thready and a strong desire to sleep. These manifestations reflect the pathology of heart and kidney deficiency, where the deficiency is one of both yin and yang, but predominantly of kidney yang. Symptoms which demonstrate deficiency cold of the kidneys are: an urge to vomit with no vomitus, vexation, a strong desire to sleep, spontaneous diarrhoea, mild thirst, a sore throat, and a tight or tense pulse spanning all three positions. The sweating of Shao Yin is a manifestation of yang desertion and persistent diarrhoea further demonstrates the exhaustion of true yang failing to support transformation.

Section Three

6.3 SHAO YIN DISEASE PATTERNS

6.3.1 Shao Yin Cold Conversion Patterns

Cold conversion is a pattern of yang deficiency with exuberant cold in the interior. The term cold conversion, or *han hua* (寒化) refers to the development of extreme cold as a result of yang deficiency. There are nine patterns of Shao Yin cold conversion, all attributed to heart and kidney yang deficiency with accumulation of yin cold in the interior. Their indicated formulas are: Si Ni Tang, Tong Mai Si Ni Tang, Bai Tong Tang, Bai Tong jia Zhu Dan Zhi Tang, Zhen Wu Tang, Fu Zi Tang, Wu Zhu Yu Tang and Tao Hua Tang, and finally, the Shao Yin moxibustion pattern.

Si Ni Tang Pattern

Clause 323

少阴病，脉沉者，急温之，宜四逆汤。

Shao Yin disease, if the pulse is submerged, one must urgently warm, Si Ni Tang is appropriate.

SI NI TANG: Zhi Gan Cao 2 liang; Gan Jiang 1½ liang; Fu Zi (raw, skin removed, broken into 8) 1 piece.

DIRECTIONS: Boil all three the ingredients in 1 sheng 2 ge of water. Strain and take warm twice a day. Patients of robust constitution can be given a large piece of Fu Zi and 3 liang of Gan Jiang.

DISCUSSION: Clause 323 is better read in conjunction with Clause 281 which outlines Shao Yin disease, describing the Shao Yin pulse as being not only submerged, but also faint and thready, and also citing the symptom of extreme somnolence. Thus we are reminded that Shao Yin disease represents a condition of kidney yang deficiency with exuberant interior yin cold. The Shao Yin channel relates to the heart and kidneys and is therefore the root of source qi and governs the body's yang qi. An attack on Shao Yin damages the source yang; Shao Yin disease is therefore characterised by a depletion of yang, aversion to cold, cold extremities and a potential for the disease to proceed to yang desertion. The treatment is Si Ni Tang to warm and support the kidney yang and disperse the cold.

Si Ni Tang can be translated as 'Four Reversals Soup' and is so named in reference to the symptom of cold conversion, where the four limbs are cold as a result of the severe depletion of yang and its inability to reach and warm the extremities. Zhi Gan Cao is sweet and warm; it warms the middle and assists yang qi, which is pivotal in the function of raising qi and dispersing cold. Fu Zi is acrid and hot and is the most effective herb to disperse cold and restore devastated yang. It unblocks the vessels in the upper jiao, tonifies heart yang, and supplements the fire of ming men in the lower jiao, thus fortifying the kidney yang. Gan Jiang is acrid and hot and is especially effective in dispersing cold and warming the interior; thus it assists Fu Zi in its action of warming the channels and dissipating cold in the middle jiao. Fu Zi targets the lower jiao by warming the kidney yang, and Gan Jiang targets the middle jiao by warming the spleen yang. Together they disperse cold, augment the yang of the spleen, stomach and kidneys, and rescue devastated yang.

The key principle in the treatment of Shao Yin disease is to warm the interior and restore devastated yang as a matter of urgency. This is based on the following. (1) The Shao Yin channel pertains to the heart and kidney. When the yang qi of these two vital organs is depleted, the condition is serious and treatment aimed at fortifying yang is required to preserve life. (2) The underlying cause of Shao Yin disease is yang deficiency with exuberant yin cold, and therefore potent warming strategies are urgently needed. (3) The faint and thready pulse of Shao Yin combined with a strong desire to sleep reflects the critical nature of the condition.

Clause 324

（一）少阴病，饮食入口则吐；心中温温欲吐，复不能吐。始得之，手足寒，脉弦迟者，此胸中实，不可下也，当吐之。（二）若膈上有寒饮，干呕者，不可吐也，当温之，宜四逆汤。

(1) Shao Yin disease, as soon as food and drink are eaten, there is vomiting; there is discomfort in the heart and an urge to vomit, then an inability to vomit. In the beginning if the hands and feet are cold, the pulse is wiry and slow, this is excess in the chest, one should not purge, one must induce vomiting. (2) If there is cold fluid above the diaphragm, and dry retching, one should not induce vomiting, one must warm, Si Ni Tang is appropriate.

DISCUSSION: Clause 324 compares the condition of cold phlegm excess in the chest with that of the accumulation of cold fluids above the diaphragm. The first sentence explains how to identify the presence of pathogenic excess in the chest. The phenomenon of discomfort in the heart where the patient has an urge to vomit but can not, is the result of obstruction caused by pathogenic excess in the chest. The initial manifestations were cold extremities and a slow and wiry pulse. The wiry pulse is a reflection of the phlegm obstruction in the chest, and the slow pulse indicates pathogenic cold. Because there is excess cold phlegm obstructing the yang qi of the chest, the pulse is likely to be not only wiry and slow, but also forceful. The constrained chest yang can not reach the extremities and so the hands and feet are cold. The obstruction of phlegm in the chest prevents the zheng qi from flowing downwards, and results in an upward impulse of qi, or qi reversal, where food and drink are ejected as soon as they enter the digestive tract. There is an uncomfortable sensation in the chest with an urge to vomit but an inability to do so, due to the stubborn phlegm bind in the chest. This uncomfortable sensation in the chest represents the accumulation of phlegm which is congealed by cold and therefore not easily expectorated. The treatment therefore, is not to purge, but to induce vomiting with a formula such as Gua Di San.

In contrast, an accumulation of cold fluids above the diaphragm is the result of devitalised yang which is unable to transform water. In this case, there is dry retching but no vomiting of food. Because this pattern represents a pattern of Shao Yin yang deficiency with interior yin cold, there would also be a watery stool with undigested food particles. It is a matter of urgency to disperse cold, warm the interior and restore the yang. Emetic treatment is inappropriate and the treatment must address the devitalised yang. Si Ni Tang is the formula chosen to fortify and resuscitate yang, and to warm the interior and scatter cold.

Clause 324 differentiates between two patterns which affect the chest. The first is associated with excess phlegm in the chest, where Gua Di San can be used to expel the phlegm by inducing vomiting. The second pattern is one of cold fluids retained in the chest, where the appropriate formula is Si Ni Tang to warm the interior, fortify yang and transform water. The urge to vomit where the patient is not able to vomit, mentioned in Clause 324, must be differentiated from the similar situation mentioned in Clause 282. In Clause 324, the inability to vomit is attributed to pathogenic obstruction: there is vomitus which must be ejected, but it is obstructed by the accumulation of phlegm; this is reflected in the wiry slow pulse and the discomfort in the chest. The failure to vomit in Clause 282, on the other hand, is due to Shao Yin yang deficiency where insufficent yang has not dispersed cold and the yin accumulation causes a reverse flow of qi, resulting in nausea and an urge to vomit. However, there are no stomach contents to eject and so there is no vomiting. Deficiency is the predominant factor in this pattern, and is reflected in the faint and thready pulse, the desire to sleep and the spontaneous diarrhoea.

Si Ni Tang comprises three herbs and is a guiding formula used in the restoration of yang. The interpretation of its constituent herbs has been a subject of some debate. Ke Yun Bo suggested that since there is yang desertion, Ren Shen should be included, however the contemporary view is that Ren Shen is not included. Cheng Wu Ji proposed that the chief herb is Gan Cao, that Gan Jiang is the deputy and Fu Zi the envoy. *Yi Zong Jin Jian* shares the same view. In his book *Jin Jing Nei Tai Fang Yi*, the Ming dynasty practitioner Xu Hong suggests that the chief herb is Fu Zi, Gan Jiang is deputy and Gan Cao is the assistant, explaining that Fu Zi warms the interior and disperses cold while Gan Jiang warms the middle; thus their combined effect can resuscitate yang.

Contemporary Research on Si Ni Tang

1. Si Ni Tang has been shown to improve cardiovascular function and promote circulation. Fu Zi extract has been used in the treatment of cardiac failure.
2. Si Ni Tang has been shown to elevate blood pressure and has been used in the integrated Western and Chinese medical treatment of hypotension associated with acute myocardial infarction (*Tianjin Yi Yao* 1973; 1:10).
3. The application of Fu Zi, both alone and in combinaton with other herbs, is as follows.
   - Fu Zi is used to warm and dissipate the cold and warm the interior in such formulas as Wu Mei Wan.
   - Fu Zi and Ren Shen are combined to resuscitate devastated yang, augment qi and generate fluids in formulas such as Si Ni jia Ren Shen Tang and Fu Zi Tang.
   - Fu Zi and Gan Jiang are used to restore yang and treat cold extremities due to the devastation of yang in such formulas as Si Ni Tang, Tong Mai Si Ni Tang and Bai Tong Tang.
   - Fu Zi and Bai Zhu are used to warm the channels, disperse cold, strengthen the spleen and eliminate damp in such formulas as Gan Cao Fu Zi Tang, Zhen Wu Tang and Fu Zi Tang.
   - Fu Zi and Gui Zhi are used to warm the channels, unblock the yang, dispel cold and ease pain in such formulas as Gan Cao Fu Zi Tang and Gui Zhi Fu Zi Tang.
   - Fu Zi can be used with Ma Huang to warm the channels, support yang and release the exterior in such formulas as Gui Zhi Qu Shao Yao jia Fu Zi Tang.
   - Fu Zi is used with Shao Yao to warm the channels, astringe yin and moderate pain in such formulas as Gui Zhi Fu Zi Gan Cao Tang, Zhen Wu Tang and Fu Zi Tang.
   - Fu Zi and Da Huang are used to simultaneously purge heat and alleviate glomus in the formula Fu Zi Xie Xin Tang.
   - Fu Zi and Sheng Jiang are used to warm the channels, disperse cold and release the exterior in Gui Zhi Fu Zi Tang and Gui Zhi Fu Zi qu Gui jia Zhu Tang.
4. The difference between raw and baked Fu Zi: in *Shang Han Lun* there are 23 formulas containing Fu Zi with some using Fu Zi as the chief herb and others as a secondary herb. Processed Fu Zi is generally used to disperse cold and processing reduces its toxicity. However, the raw form is seen as being more effective in emergency use for the restoration of yang, which is its primary function in the formulas Si Ni Tang, Tong Mai Si Ni Tang, Tong Mai Si Ni jia Zhu Dan Zhi Tang, Bai Tong Tang, Bai Tong jia Zhu Dan Zhi Tang, Si Ni jia Ren Shen Tang, Fu Ling Si Ni Tang and Gan Jiang Fu Zi Tang. In addition to this precept, there are strict rules regarding the combination of Fu Zi with other herbs. When combined with Gan Jiang, the raw form is used, but when combined with other herbs, baked Fu Zi is always used to warm the channels, dissipate cold or eliminate water qi.
5. The dosage and toxicity of Fu Zi: due to its toxicity, it is recommended to start with a small initial dose before gradually increasing it to a dose of between 6 and 10g. The side effects can include numbness of the lips as well as of the hands and feet, nausea, vomiting, diarrhoea, dizziness, and in extreme cases, palpitations, dyspnoea, tremor and hypotension. However, the toxicity is substantially reduced by processing, especially when prepared with Gan Cao, Gan Jiang or Lu Dou (mung beans). Traditionally, Xi Jiao was also used to reduce toxicity. In *Xin Zhong Yi* (1981; 1:49) Li et al reported that when Fu Zi was combined with Gan Jiang, it effectively raised blood pressure and improved cardiac function with a reduction in toxic effects.

Ancient Application of Si Ni Tang

- *San Yin Fang* cited Si Ni Tang in the treatment of Shao Yin disease characterised by spontaneous diarrhoea, an absence of thirst, nausea and incessant vomiting, scant urination, diarrhoea, excessive sweating, abdominal pain and distension, cold extremities. And a faint pulse verging on expiry.
- *Yi Jing Hui Yuan* cited Si Ni Tang with the addition of Chao Wu Zhu Yu, Ban Xia, Sheng Jiang for the treatment of yin toxins characterised by nausea, incessant salivation or lower abdominal pain. For incessant vomiting Ban Xia, Sheng Jiang Zhi should be added; for incessant diarrhoea, Bai Zhu, Ren Shen, Huang Qi, Fu Ling and Sheng Ma should be added.
- *Wan Bing Hui Chun* recommended Si Ni Tang for the treatment of Tai Yin disease characterised by spontaneous diarrhoea, an absence of thirst, and disease of the three yin channels characterised by cold extremities and a faint pulse verging on expiry. Si Ni Tang was to be taken warm to produce a mild sweat in order to bring about recovery.

Modern Application of Si Ni Tang

- Myocardial infarction with cardiac failure.
- Acute and chronic gastroenteritis, oedema or prolapse of the stomach attributed to spleen and kidney yang deficiency.
- Wang et al used Si Ni Tang with the addition of Huang Lian in the treatment of 70 cases of infantile diarrhoea. Results: 58 cases recovered; 9 cases substantial improvement; 4 cases not effective. The scope of this formula includes the treatment of diarrhoea due to heat and stagnation in the stomach and intestines in the presence of spleen and kidney yang deficiency, characterised by a sloppy stool, cold extremities, fatigue, mild fever, a faint and weak pulse and a thin, white tongue coat. Si Ni Tang is not indicated where the bowel movement is foul and there is tenesmus (*Zhejiang Zhong Yi Za Zhi* 1964; 8:14).
- Si Ni Tang can substantially improve blood supply to the heart. Tang Shan Hospital in Guang Dong province used an extract of Fu Zi in an intramuscular injection to treat 13 cases of cardiac failure attributed to cardiogenic shock and pulmonary cardiac disease with satisfactory results (*He Bei Xin Yi Yao* 1973; 3).

Modifications

1. For deficiency of the spleen and stomach due to kidney yang deficiency, characterised by an upsurge of cold qi, hiccoughs, a pale complexion, fatigue, poor appetite, cold extremities, a soft voice, cold in the abdomen, clear copious urination, a loose stool and a weak, thready pulse, add Dang Shen, Bai Zhu, Gao Liang Jiang, Sha Ren, Jiang Ban Xia, Chen Pi, Su Geng.
2. For seminal emission or spermatorrhoea due to excessive sexual acitivity, and accompanied by a pale lack-lustre complexion, fatigue, tinnitus, back pain, weakness in the knees, a slippery white tongue coat and a submerged thready pulse, add Tu Si Zi, Wu Wei Zi, Jin Ying Zi, Xian Ling Pi, Duan Long Gu, Duan Mu Li or combine with Gui Zhi jia Long Gu Mu Li Tang.
3. For bi syndrome attributed to an insufficiency of kidney yang characterised by muscle and joint aches, stiffness, a thready pulse and a pale tongue with a white, greasy coat, add Du Huo, Sang Ji Sheng, Gui Zhi, Fang Feng, Dang Gui, Chuan Xiong and Ji Xue Teng.

Case Study

Diarrhoea

Extracted from Xin Zhong Yi 1995; (2):14

A 52-year-old male had suffered from chronic diarrhoea for six years. The condition was exacerbated in cold weather or following the ingestion of cold food. One month ago, a further episode of diarrhoea had been caused by eating cold food and also catching a cold. He suffered from abdominal pain and diarrhoea with undigested food particles in the early hours of the morning and he also suffered borborygmus. He had a preference for warmth, a pale, lack-lustre complexion, cold extremities, a poor appetite and fatigue. His tongue was pale with a thin, white coat and his pulse was thready, faint and forceless.

The treatment principle was to tonify the spleen and warm the kidney yang. The formula used was Si Ni Tang modified: Zhi Fu Pian, Jiao San Xian (Shan Zha, Shen Qu, Mai Ya) 15g each; Gan Jiang, Zhi Gan Cao, Chao Dang Shen, Chao Bai Zhu, Bu Gu Zhi, Rou Dou Kou, Mu Xiang, Ge Gen 10g each. After five packs, the patient's condition improved and a further 30 packs were prescribed to consolidate the treatment.

Tong Mai Si Ni Tang Pattern

Clause 317

少阴病，下利清谷，里寒外热，手足厥逆，脉微欲绝，身反不恶寒，其人面色赤，或腹满，或干呕，或咽痛，或利止脉不出者，通脉四逆汤主之。

Shao Yin disease, there is diarrhoea with undigested food, the interior is cold and the exterior is hot, there is desertion reversal of the hands and feet, the pulse is faint and about to expire, the body is nevertheless not averse to cold, if the person's face is crimson, or there is abdominal distension, or there is dry retching, or the throat is sore, or the diarrhoea ceases and the pulse is not palpable, Tong Mai Si Ni Tang governs.

TONG MAI SI NI TANG: Zhi Gan Cao 2 liang; Fu Zi (raw, skin removed) 1 large piece (broken into eight); Gan Jiang 3 liang (for a person with a strong constitution, 4 liang can be given).

DIRECTIONS: Boil all three ingredients in 3 sheng of water, reducing to 1 sheng 2 ge. Strain and take twice a day. A return of the pulse is a sign of recovery. If the face is flushed, add nine stems of spring onion; if there is abdominal pain, omit the spring onion and add Shao Yao 2 liang; for vomiting add Sheng Jiang 2 liang; for a sore throat omit Shao Yao and add Jie Geng 1 liang; if the diarrhoea stops but the pulse is hidden, omit Jie Geng and add Ren Shen 2 liang. The formula must be appropriate for the disease manifestations.

DISCUSSION: Diarrhoea with undigested food particles, as found in Shao Yin disease, reflects a severe depletion of kidney yang to the point where it is unable to support the transformation of water and grain. 'Desertion reversal' refers to a desertion pattern where the devastation of yang has resulted in cold extremities. A faint and thready pulse represents deficiency and is characteristic of Shao Yin disease. When the pulse is so faint that it verges on expiry, this indicates a further deterioration with exuberant yin cold and exhaustion of yang. If the expiring pulse is accompanied by a flushed face with no aversion to cold, then this is a manifestation of severe yin cold repelling the yang to the exterior. In this case, interior cold is the true condition, and the exterior heat is a false sign, because it is not excess heat, but is deficient yang which is floating because it is not anchored to its source.

Clause 317 depicts a serious condition of deficient yang being repelled by exuberant yin, and as such, is an example of the non-interaction of yin and yang. The possible manifestations of deficient yang with exuberant yin are: abdominal pain due to pathogenic cold congealing the flow of qi and blood; an upsurge of cold qi harassing the stomach causing dry retching; a sore throat due to deficient yang floating upward and harassing the throat; sudden cessation of diarrhoea with no palpable pulse due to the exhaustion of body fluids and depletion of qi. Tong Mai Si Ni Tang is an effective formula to resuscitate the devasted yang in these urgent situations.

Tong Mai Si Ni Tang is Si Ni Tang with an increased dosage of Fu Zi (using a large piece) and 3 liang of Gan Jiang (instead of 1½ liang) to enhance the action of resuscitating yang and resolving yin. The term 'tong mai' can be translated as 'to open, unblock or penetrate the channels'. The significance of the name of the formula relates to its objective of breaking up the yin cold by restoring and fortifying yang, warming the channels and promoting the flow of qi and blood, and scattering cold and warming the interior in order to facilitate the return of the pulse.

The original text nominates some modifications as follows. (1) For a flushed face, add Cong Bai (the bulb of a spring onion) in order to disperse the yang which has been pushed to the exterior by the yin. (2) For abdominal pain, omit Cong Bai and add Shao Yao to moderate pain and ease spasm. (3) For vomiting, add Sheng Jiang to warm and harmonise the stomach in order to dissipate the cold and stop the vomiting. (4) For a sore throat, omit Shao Yao, which is sour and astringent, and add Jie Geng to disseminate qi and disinhibit the throat. (5) If the pulse is hidden, omit Jie Geng and add Ren Shen to supplement qi and blood and generate the pulse.

The indication for Tong Mai Si Ni Tang is a pattern complex of interior cold and exterior heat, which represents true cold and false heat. The key to understanding a pattern of true cold and false heat is that the true pattern can be reconciled with the fundamental nature or the 'root' of the disease. The false signs relate to the fact that the progress of extreme cold can lead to the appearance of heat signs (flushed face, irritability etc) and, conversely, cold signs can appear in a pattern of extreme heat. This is sometimes referred to as extreme yin mimicking yang, or extreme yang mimicking yin, where some of the signs are in diametric opposition to the basic pattern.

The difference between Si Ni Tang and Tong Mai Si Ni Tang patterns is found in the respective pathogenesis of each. A Si Ni Tang pattern is the result of a yang deficiency with subsequent exuberant yin, whilst a Tong Mai Si Ni Tang pattern is a pattern of exuberant interior cold subsequently repelling the true yang, pushing it to the exterior via the upper jiao, from where it might finally depart, and thus giving rise to signs of false heat.

Clause 370

下利清谷，里寒外热，汗出而厥者，通脉四逆汤主之。

Diarrhoea with undigested food, the interior is cold and the exterior is hot, if there is sweating and reversal, Tong Mai Si Ni Tang governs.

DISCUSSION: Clause 370 is better read in conjunction with Clause 317 because of the similarity in the pathogenesis. This is a pattern of Shao Yin yang deficiency affecting the yang of both the spleen and the kidneys and manifesting as a loose stool where, because food is not properly digested, particles are visible in the stool. The exterior is hot as a result of exuberant yin pushing deficient yang outwards to the exterior. The sweating is a reflection of yang deficiency, potentially proceeding to yang desertion.

Diarrhoea with undigested food particles is characteristic of Shao Yin yang deficiency with interior yin cold. In *Shang Han Lun*, diarrhoea is differentiated according to whether it pertains to the yang channels or the yin channels. Diarrhoea associated with the three yin channels is generally due to yin cold and is referred to as being 'spontaneous' because it is not the result of purgatives. It is generally a symptom of deficiency cold of the spleen and stomach. Middle jiao diarrhoea which is part of a spleen yang deficiency pattern can be treated with Li Zhong Wan; lower jiao diarrhoea attributed to kidney yang deficiency can be treated with Si Ni Tang or Fu Zi Li Zhong Wan.

Ancient Application of Tong Mai Si Ni Tang

- *Shang Han Lun Bian Zheng Guang Zhu:* For a flushed face due to counterflow of deficient yang, add Cong Bai to redirect the yang qi.
- *Yi Zong Bi Du:* For the treatment of Tai Yin spontaneous sweating, with no thirst, a submerged pulse and body pain: Fu Zi 3 qian; Gan Cao 1.5 qian; Gan Jiang 1.5 qian; Sheng Jiang 8 fen.

Modern Application of Tong Mai Si Ni Tang

Xu et al treated 16 cases of late stage infectious disease which presented with signs of Shao Yin false heat, and characterised by aversion to cold, fever and a white greasy coat at the root of the tongue. Cardiac and lung functions were normal. Antibiotics were administered but the response was insignificant. Key points of diagnosis of a Shao Yin pattern with yin repelling yang were: fever, aversion to cold, abdominal pain, cold extremities, a big pulse which scattered on pressure, verging on expiry. Tong Mai Si Ni Tang can be used with addition of Shao Yao or Mai Dong and Zhi Mu (*Zhong*

Yi Za Zhi 1962; 2:14). The results were not published.

Case Study

Diarrhoea Due to Spleen Yang Deficiency

Extracted from Shang Han Lun Lin Chuang Shi Yan Lu

A 53-year-old male patient had suffered from diarrhoea following the consumption of too much watermelon in the summer. His condition improved after hospital treatment but since then, he had suffered periodically from diarrhoea. He was thin with a pale complexion, he was fatigued, had a poor appetite and spontaneous sweating, a loose stool, and vexation with difficulty falling asleep. At times, his complexion was flushed and his extremities were cold. His pulse was submerged and faint, verging on expiry at the cubit position. The treatment principle was to warm the middle and supplement the kidney yang. The formula was Jia Wei Tong Mai Si Ni Tang: Zhi Gan Cao 15g, Zhi Fu Pian 10g, Gan Jiang 18g, Chi Shi Zhi 10g, Ren Shen 6g, Fu Ling 10g. After three packs, the diarrhoea eased and the extremities were warmer. After three further packs, the diarrhoea stopped. He was given a further 20 packs to consolidate treatment.

Bai Tong Tang Pattern

Clause 314

少阴病，下利，白通汤主之。

Shao Yin disease, there is diarrhoea, Bai Tong Tang governs.

BAI TONG TANG: Cong Bai 4 pieces (bulb and stem); Gan Jiang 1 liang; Fu Zi (raw, skin removed and broken into 8) 1 piece.

DIRECTIONS: Boil the ingredients in 3 sheng of water, reducing to 1 sheng. Strain and take warm twice a day.

DISCUSSION: The Shao Yin outline describes Shao Yin disease as being characterised by a faint and thready pulse and a desire to sleep, and a Si Ni Tang pattern as being characterised by cold extremities. Clause 314 describes Shao Yin disease presenting with diarrhoea. Based on the ingredients of Bai Tong Tang and the fact that it is a formula associated with Si Ni Tang, it is clear that the diarrhoea in this clause is that of a Shao Yin yang deficiency pattern with yin accumulation in the interior. By referring to the directions attached to Clause 317, where it is recommended to add 9 stems of Cong Bai to Tong Mai Si Ni Tang when the face is flushed, it can be seen that Bai Tong Tang, which contains 4 stems of Cong Bai, is based on that modification of Tong Mai Si Ni Tang. From this, it may further be inferred that Clause 314 also describes a pattern where true yang is being pushed upward and outwards, and for this reason, the face could be flushed in this pattern also.

Bai Tong Tang is a modification of Si Ni Tang where Cong Bai is added, Gan Cao is omitted, and the dose of Gan Jiang is reduced. The addition of Cong Bai supports the main action of the formula in warming the interior and restoring yang; additionally, its warm, acrid and dispersing nature not only disperses cold, but also frees and promotes the ascent of yang qi, thus facilitating the interaction of the upper and lower jiao, thereby breaking up the yin. Zhi Gan Cao is omitted because its moderating property would inhibit the potent warming action of Gan Jiang and Fu Zi.

The application of Bai Tong Tang for Shao Yin deficiency cold diarrhoea is based on two factors. (1) Diarrhoea is generally a feature of the early stage of Shao Yin disease, at which time Si Ni Tang can be used. However, Si Ni Tang is sometimes not potent enough for a more serious condition of stubborn or persistent diarrhoea. (2) The diarrhoea associated with Bai Tong Tang is more serious, and is characterised by undigested food particles in a watery stool. Other manifestations are cold extremities, a flushed face, a faint and thready pulse verging on expiry and a pale tongue with a slippery white tongue coat. The flushed face is a result of yang being cast upward by exuberant yin; it stands out, amidst the many cold signs, as the key indicator that this is a pattern of true cold and false heat.

Modern Application of Bai Tong Tang

- Zhao et al (Zhao Lin Tang: *Harbin Zhong Yi* 1960; 2:22) reported that a large dose of Bai Tong Tang was used to treat a case of Raynaud's syndrome, which is a chronic disease of the circulatory system characterised by fingers and toes which turn white with cold.
- Bai Tong Tang was used to treat critical hypertension associated with devastated heart and kidney yang and the repulsion of yang by exuberant yin. Additional herbs were: Dan Qiu Shi, Zhi Wu Wei Zi, Duan Long Gu, Duan Mu Li (*Shang Han Lun Tang Zheng Lun Zhi* 2000).

Case Study

Critical Hypertension Due to Upcast Yang

Extracted from Zhong Yi Za Zhi 1987; (8):16

A 48-year-old male with a history of hypertension for over ten years presented with severe dizziness aggravated by standing up. He was photophobic, his face was flushed, and he suffered from palpitations and vexation. There was strong aversion to cold with cold extremities; his pulse was submerged, thready and faint and his tongue was pale and swollen. His blood pressure was 200/120mmHg. The diagnosis was hypertension due to heart and kidney yang deficiency. He was given Bai Tong Tang modified: Pao Fu Pian 9g (decocted first), Gan Jiang 4.5g, Cong Bai 4 stems, Dan Qiu Shi 9g, Zhi Wu Wei Zi 3g, Duan Long Gu 30g, Duan Mu Li 30g. After one pack, the dizziness and palpitations subsided. His pulse was moderate and forceful. He was given another pack and his condition was stabilised.

Bai Tong jia Zhu Dan Zhi Tang Pattern

Clause 315

(1) 少阴病，下利，脉微者，与白通汤。(2) 利不止，厥逆无脉，干呕，烦者，白通加猪胆汁汤主之。(3) 服汤，脉暴出者死，微续者生。

(1) Shao Yin disease, if there is diarrhoea and the pulse is faint, give Bai Tong Tang. (2) If the diarrhoea does not stop, there is desertion reversal and no pulse, dry retching and vexation, Bai Tong jia Zhu Dan Zhi Tang governs. (3) Having taken the decoction, if the pulse suddenly rises the person will die, if a faint pulse continues, they will live.

BAI TONG JIA ZHU DAN ZHI TANG: Cong Bai 4 stems; Gan Jiang 1 liang; Fu Zi (raw, skin removed, broken into 8) 1 piece; human urine 5 ge; Zhu Dan Zhi (pig's bile) 1 ge.

DIRECTIONS: Boil the ingredients in 3 sheng of water, reducing to 1 sheng. Strain, add the pig's bile and human urine, blend thoroughly and take warm twice a day. The formula can still be used if the pig's bile is unavailable.

DISCUSSION: The first statement of this clause is very similar to that of Clause 314 which precedes it, reinforcing that Bai Tong Tang is the indicated formula for Shao Yin diarrhoea. In Clause 315, however, there is emphasis on the pulse sign, with the faint pulse being a reflection of weak yang which in this pattern is accompanied by exuberant yin cold. If Bai Tong Tang has not been effective and the diarrhoea does not stop, then the condition is serious: 'desertion reversal' refers to cold extremities resulting from the devastation of true yang, which is further demonstrated by a pulse which is not palpable. Exuberant yin obstructs the descent of stomach qi causing dry retching, and the counterflow of yin cold surges upwards, harassing the heart so there is vexation. Bai Tong Tang has failed to resuscitate the yang, the disease has deteriorated, and the absence of a palpable pulse not only indicates desertion of yang, but also demonstrates serious debilitation of the heart and kidney, which fail to fill the vessels with qi and blood.

The reason for the deterioration is not that Bai Tong Tang was inappropriate, but because the yin cold accumulation is so extreme that it has repelled the hot herbs. For this reason, the same formula is used with the addition of Zhu Dan Zhi (pig's bile) and human urine, which augment the yin and harmonise the yang, thus leading the yang herbs to the interior. This type of treatment, where yin is treated with yin, is known as paradoxical treatment and here it enables the extreme yin condition to accept the hot herbs in order to restore the yang.

The third statement describes the prognosis following medication. If the pulse suddenly surfaces as a big, floating and stirring pulse, this is a false sign of vitality; it is the last flicker of the flame, indicating the imminent extinguishment of true yang. The prognosis is poor. However, if the hidden pulse seeks a gradual return, and is weak, but palpable, this is the normal pattern of gradual recovery from a serious condition and the prognosis is relatively good.

Bai Tong Tang breaks up the knotted yin and resuscitates the devastated yang by facilitating interaction between the upper and lower jiao. Human urine is salty and cold and is added to nourish yin and drain fire. Its immediate action of draining fire whilst conserving the yin prevents the exhausted yin from being further consumed by the yang herbs. Zhu Dan Zhi is bitter and cold, it generates fluids and clears empty heat. The objective of adding the urine and pig's bile is to guide the yang herbs to the yin interior so that they can exert their function of warming the interior and dissipating the yin cold.

The principle of paradoxical treatment (反治) by treating like with like, as opposed to the conventional approach (zheng zhi 正治) of treatment based on the opposite properties of the presenting pattern or pathogen, is found in *Su Wen: Zhi Zhen Yao Da Lun Pian (Chapter 74: Essential Great Discourse to Reach the Truth):* "逆者正治, 从者反治" and "逆而从之, 从而逆之", which may be translated as, "Opposite is correct treatment, concordant is reverse treatment" and "If it is reverse, it is concordant, when concordant, it is reverse". This refers to conventional allopathic treatment, where heat is used to treat cold, and cold to treat heat. To treat heat with heat, or cold with cold, is known as paradoxical treatment and is often employed when treating disease of a serious nature. However, when applied to the use of cold herbs in Bai Tong jia Zhu Dan Zhi Tang, this explanation is somewhat simplistic and misses the point. The function of the cold, salty, bitter herbs in the treatment of a severe yang deficiency in fact has a more intelligent explanation.

The heart and kidney yang deficiency which is the root of Shao Yin disease results in an accumulation of yin cold, which manifests as incessant diarrhoea. Consequently, there is a heavy loss of body fluids and the pattern becomes one of dual yin and yang deficiency. Bai Tong Tang is a yang resuscitating formula containing hot and acrid herbs; however, it has no yin nourishing herbs. Yin and yang are interdependent and mutually engendering. Therefore, the addition of salty, bitter cold herbs is needed to nourish the yin and moderate the hot acrid properties of Gan Jiang and Fu Zi. The objective of adding human urine (which is relatively sterile when it leaves the body) and Zhu Dan Zhi are twofold. (1) By moderating the acrid, hot properties of Gan Jiang and Fu Zi, the yin substances make the hot herbs acceptable to the interior, ensuring they reach their target destination without being repelled by the extreme yin cold. (2) The two yin substances also augment the yin, supplementing body fluids and enhancing the harmonisation of yin and yang. On a similar note, in wen bing or warm disease, mid-stream urine of young boys was used extensively in the treatment of febrile diseases characterised by high fever and delirium.

Modern Application of Bai Tong Tang jia Zhu Dan Zhi Tang

Liao et al (*Xin Zhong Yi* 1975; 3: 24) reported that this formula was used in the treatment of infantile diarrhoea associated with a pattern of exuberant yin repelling yang. Apart from diarrhoea, the child suffered from fever, restlessness, thirst, retching of stomach fluids, a pale complexion, sunken eyes, a greasy, white tongue coat and a thready, rapid and forceless pulse. He was given Bai Tong Tang jia Zhu Dan Zhi Tang: Fu Pian 15g, Gan Jiang 4.5g, Cong Bai 2 inches, human urine 30mL, Zhu Dan Zhi 6mL. After one decoction, the fever receded. The treatment was consolidated with a formula which warmed the spleen, augmented qi and generated fluids.

Case Study

Diarrhoea Due to Deficiency Cold

Extracted from Shang Han Lun Lin Chuan Shi Yan Lu,

Tianjin Ke Ji Publications 1984

A 48-year-old male patient suffered from diarrhoea due to deficiency cold. It was initially triggered by an improper diet. Earlier treatment with cold bitter herbs was not effective. He presented with vexation, abdominal fullness and pain, red eyes, parched lips, a clouded spirit, and he was untalkative. This condition had lasted for more than 20 days. His cun pulse was big and forceless and the cubit pulse was submerged and faint. He was given Bai Tong Tang jia Zhu Dan Zhi: Gan Jiang 15g, Hei Fu Zi 10g, Zhi Gan Cao 12g, Cong Bai 15g, human urine ½ cup; Zhu Dan Zhi 3g. He was given 4 packs and after taking the first, there was a noticeable reduction in the frequency and severity of the diarrhoea. After finishing the 4 packs, for the next three weeks he was given a formula to strengthen the spleen and tonify qi in order to consolidate the treatment.

Zhen Wu Tang Pattern

Clause 316

少阴病，二三日不已，至四五日，腹痛，小便不利，四肢沉重疼痛，自下利者，此为有水气。其人或咳，或小便利，或下利，或呕者，真武汤主之。

Shao Yin disease, not finished on the second or third day, if by the fourth or fifth day, there is abdominal pain, the urination is not free, the four limbs are heavy and aching, and there is spontaneous diarrhoea, this is because of water qi. If the person either has a cough, or the urination is free, or there is diarrhoea, or vomiting, Zhen Wu Tang governs.

ZHEN WU TANG: Fu Ling 3 liang; Shao Yao 3 liang; Bai Zhu 2 liang; Sheng Jiang (sliced) 3 liang; Fu Zi (skin removed, broken into 8 and dry-fried) 1 piece.

DIRECTIONS: Boil all five ingredients in 8 sheng of water, reducing to 3 sheng. Strain and take 7 ge warm three times a day. If there is a cough, add Wu Wei Zi ½ sheng, Xi Xin 1 liang, Gan Jiang 1 liang; if the urination is uninhibited, omit Fu Ling; if there is diarrhoea, omit Shao Yao and add Gan Jiang 2 liang; if there is vomiting, omit Fu Zi and add Sheng Jiang to give a total of ½ jin.

DISCUSSION: When Shao Yin disease has persisted for two or three days and is still not resolved by the fourth or fifth day, the progession of disease will bring additional symptoms of abdominal pain and heaviness, aching in the arms and legs, inhibited urination and diarrhoea. These symptoms represent a further depletion of kidney yang, failing to support the transformation function. Damp accumulation in the intestines causes diarrhoea, the congelation of damp cold retards the flow of qi and blood causing cramping pain in the sinews and abdomen; the damp also causes a heavy sensation in the limbs, and the inability to transform qi will cause inhibited urination. These are all manifestations of water qi, which is the pathological accumulation of water and retention of damp.

Water is a yin pathogen which can be carried by qi to harass various zang fu. If the water qi harasses the lungs, there will be cough; if it harasses the stomach, there will be vomiting; if the water qi descends to the lower jiao and harasses the intestines, there will be diarrhoea; where deficient yang is unable to control water, there will be copious or frequent urination. The formula to use is Zhen Wu Tang to warm the yang, transform qi and to drain damp by promoting urination. The urination associated with kidney yang deficiency is an ambiguous issue. There are two possibilities: the first is where deficient yang fails to warm and transform fluids, resulting in inhibited or scant urination; the second possibility is where inadequate yang is unable to control water, resulting in frequent or copious urination as described here in Clause 316.

Fu Zi is acrid and hot and its function is to fortify kidney yang, tonify the fire of ming men and support the kidney function of transforming water. *Ben Cao Zheng Yi*: "Fu Zi is a pure yang herb which penetrates the twelve channels, reaching the exterior to expel exterior cold and reaching the interior to warm the true yang." Bai Zhu is bitter and warm. It strengthens the spleen's function of transforming and transporting, dries damp and promotes urination. Fu Ling is sweet and bland and so drains damp by promoting urination. The combination of these two herbs enhances the formula's function of draining damp. Sheng Jiang is acrid and warm, it disperses the water qi, warms and harmonises the stomach and assists Fu Zi to warm the yang and transform qi. Shao Yao is sour and cold. It eases pain and nourishes yin, thus counteracting the harsh properties of Fu Zi and protecting the yin. When Shao Yao is combined with Fu Zi, the Fu Zi exerts a warming effect to counter the coldness of Shao Yao, and when combined with Shao Yao, it resuscitates the devasted yang without being too hot. Clause 316 lists additional symptoms for which modifications must be made, as follows. For cough, add Gan Jiang to warm the lungs and transform phlegm, Xi Xin to disperse cold, warm the lung and dry phlegm, and Wu Wei Zi to astringe the lung qi. Where there is copious or frequent urination, omit Fu Ling. Where there is diarrhoea, omit Shao Yao and add Gan Jiang. Where there is vomiting, omit Fu Zi and add Sheng Jiang to harmonise the stomach and redirect qi downward.

Comparison of Zhen Wu Tang, Wu Ling San and Ling Gui Zhu Gan Tang

Zhen Wu Tang differs from Wu Ling San and Ling Gui Zhu Gan Tang in that it is indicated in severe yang deficiency. Both Zhen Wu Tang and Wu Ling San are indicated for water accumulation due to the non-transformation of qi in the lower jiao; however, the inhibited urination of a Wu Ling San pattern is the result of water bind in the urinary bladder obstructing the transformation of qi. This is in contrast to the inhibited urination of a Zhen Wu Tang pattern, which is due to severe yang deficiency of the spleen and kidneys leading to damp accumulation which manifests as diarrhoea, abdominal pain, heaviness in the limbs and inhibited urination, and where the treatment is to warm the yang, transform qi and move water. If deficient yang of the kidneys affects their ability to control water resulting in frequent or copious urination, suitable modifications must be made to moderate the formula's action of promoting urination.

The difference between Zhen Wu Tang and Ling Gui Zhu Gan Tang is the disease location. Ling Gui Zhu Gan Tang is indicated where there is spleen yang deficiency manifesting as water accumulation in the middle jiao, characterised by epigastric distension, an upsurge of qi which harasses the chest, a mild headache and dizziness or vertigo. In contrast, Zhen Wu Tang is indicated for kidney yang deficiency with water accumulation in the lower jiao which surges upward and gives rise to palpitations, abdominal pain, diarrhoea, inhibited urination, heaviness of the four limbs, oedema, vomiting and cough or wheezing. From the perspective of modern medicine, this parallels congestive heart disease with tachycardia, wheezing, dyspnoea, and impaired renal function resulting in such symptoms as scant urination, oedema and nausea.

Ancient Application of Zhen Wu Tang

- *Shang Han Xu Lun:* For the treatment of insomnia following the loss of sweat, where there is insubstantial vexation and the pulse is floating and weak.
- *Wang Shi Yi Jian Fang:* Zhen Wu Tang was used under the name 'Gu Yang Tang' （固阳汤） in the treatment of deficiency detriment disorder characterised by aversion to cold, vigorous fever, cough and diarrhoea.
- *Lei Ju Fang Guang Yi:* For the treatment of *wei bi* (痿痹) or flaccid obstruction characterised by abdominal cramps, cold extremities, inhibited urination or incontinence, back pain, abdominal pain, aversion to cold and diarrhoea. Also advocated in the treatment of chronic diarrhoea, oedema, post-partum diarrhoea with borborygmus, inhibited urination, and weak or aching limbs.

Modern Application of Zhen Wu Tang

- Zhen Wu Tang can be used for any disorder where there is a pathogenesis of yang deficiency of the heart and kidney resulting in water qi, and where there is a swollen tongue with a moist, white tongue coat and a submerged, wiry pulse.

- Rheumatic heart disease, hypertension, congestive heart disease or scant urination (add Zhu Ling, Ze Xie, Gui Zhi and Ze Lan Ye).
- Acute and chronic nephritis.
- Chronic bronchitis, asthma, emphysema or other respiratory tract disease characterised by a chronic cough or wheeze, copious, white, watery phlegm, and a submerged and wiry pulse (add Wu Wei Zi, Xi Xin, Kuan Dong Hua).
- Gastrointestinal disorders such as chronic gastritis, stomach prolapse, peptic ulcers, constipation.
- Chronic colitis characterised by abdominal pain, diarrhoea and a slow, submerged pulse (add Dang Shen, Zhi Gan Cao, Chao Yi Ren and substitute Sheng Jiang for Gan Jiang).

Case Study

Oedema

Extracted from Shang Han Qie Yao

A 52-year-old female complained of generalised oedema. Her complexion was pale and her face and eyelids were puffy. Her legs were also swollen, and she suffered from abdominal distension, a loose stool, dizziness, fatigue, an oppressed sensation in the chest, shortness of breath, a poor appetite and scant urination. Her pulse was thready and moderate, and the tongue coat was wet and slippery. No back pain was reported. There was no protein in her urine and the ECG was normal. The formula used was Wu Pi San and Fang Ji Huang Qi Tang modified: Sheng Huang Qi 20g, Fang Ji 10g, Fu Ling Pi 20g, Bai Zhu 15g, Da Fu Pi 10g, Sheng Jiang 3 pieces, Chi Xiao Dou 30g, Hai Tong Pi 15g. One pack a day for five days was prescribed. After three packs her urinary output increased and the swelling subsided. After the fourth and fifth packs, however, the urination became scant again, the oedema returned as did the other symptoms: she had breathing difficulties, felt lethargic and had lost her appetite. This was because the first formula had targeted the lung and spleen, when the underlying cause was the kidneys. Two packs of Zhen Wu Tang were then prescribed: Zhi Fu Pian 10g, Fu Ling 15g, Bai Zhu 15g, Bai Shao 12g, Sheng Jiang 3 pieces. When she returned for the third visit, the oedema had subsided, she felt more energetic and her pulse was moderate and forceful. A further five packs of the Zhen Wu Tang formula were prescribed.

Case Study

Vertigo

Extracted from Shang Han Shi Jian Lun by Chen Rui Chun

A 52-year-old male patient complained of vertigo, each episode being accompanied by dizziness, aversion to cold and cold extremities. Drinking water gave him relief. The attacks were frequent and prevented him from working. He was slightly overweight, his complexion was pale, the stool was loose, the pulse was thready and weak and the tongue was pale and wet. His blood pressure was 110/70mmHg and his ECG was normal. He was given Ling Gui Zhu Gan Tang: Fu Ling 20g, Gui Zhi 10g, Bai Zhu 15g, Zhi Gan Cao 5g, Sheng Huang Qi 20g, Ling Ci Shi 15g. After five packs, the attacks were of shorter duration but his pulse was still thready and weak and the tongue pale and wet. Zhen Wu Tang was then prescribed: Zhi Fu Pian 10g, Fu Ling 20g, Bai Zhu 15g, Bai Shao 10g, Sheng Huang Qi 20g, Yuan Zhi 10g, Ling Ci Shi 15g, Sheng Jiang 3 pieces. After ten packs of that formula, the attacks of vertigo were almost gone. He was given Liu Jun Zi Tang for two weeks to consolidate the treatment.

Fu Zi Tang Pattern

Clause 304

少阴病，得之一二日，口中和，其背恶寒者，当灸之，附子汤主之。

Shao Yin disease, contracted for one or two days, there is harmony in the mouth, the back is averse to cold, moxibustion should be used, Fu Zi Tang governs.

FU ZI TANG: Fu Zi (skin removed, and dry-fried) 2 pieces broken into 8; Fu Ling 3 liang; Ren Shen 2 liang; Bai Zhu 4 liang; Shao Yao 3 liang.

DIRECTIONS: Boil the ingredients in 8 sheng of water, reducing to 3 sheng. Strain and take 1 sheng warm three times a day.

DISCUSSION: The statement that Shao Yin disease was contracted one or two days previously indicates that it is still in its early stage. The expression "harmony in the mouth" conveys the idea that there is no abnormal taste or sensation in the mouth. The significance of this is that there is no bitter taste or thirst indicative of interior heat, and so the reader may deduce that this is a Shao Yin pattern of deficiency cold. Harmony in the mouth is, in fact, a key symptom of a Shao Yin pattern of yang deficiency and damp accumulation. The Shao Yin channel is related to the kidney, which rules the back, and so, if the kidney yang is deficient and fails to warm the back, it will be prone to feeling the cold. The symptom of the back being sensitive to cold is also explained by the fact that it carries the pathways of both the Du channel, which is the sea of all yang, and the urinary bladder channel, which serves as the passage for yang qi. These traverse the back, and so when yang is deficient, cold will be felt in the back. Moxibustion is recommended as it introduces yang qi directly into the body, warming both the channels and the zang fu. The herbal decoction Fu Zi Tang primarily addresses the interior, warming it rapidly and effectively, augmenting the source of fire, and dissipating the yin cold.

Fu Zi Tang is composed of 2 pieces of Fu Zi, which is very hot, acrid, drying and dispersing. It penetrates the twelve channels and so resuscitates the devastated source yang; it serves as a guide, leading the exterior releasing herbs upward and outward to expel the pathogenic wind cold; it enters the kidney channel and leads the other warming herbs to the lower jiao to resolve the interior cold damp. Ren Shen augments qi, warms and tonifies the spleen and, when combined with Fu Zi, its function of supplementing the source yang is substantially increased. Bai Zhu warms the spleen and dries damp and, together with Fu Ling, strengthens the spleen and promotes urination. Shao Yao astringes yin and harmonises ying blood to consolidate true yin.

The instruction to use moxibustion before administering Fu Zi Tang is based on the understanding that although the decoction will have a longer lasting and deeper internal effect, in such an urgent situation, the use of moxibustion has the advantage of obtaining an immediate effect. Zhang Zhong Jing did not specify any particular acupuncture points, but in his book *Wan Bing Hui Chun*, Wang Ling You suggested Guan Yuan (Ren 4) and Qi Hai (Ren 6). Such points as Shen Que (Ren 8), Tian Shu (St 25), Zu San Li (St 36), Da Zhui (Du 14), Ming Men (Du 4), Pi Shu (UB20), Shen Shu (UB23), Da Chang Shu (UB25) can also be used.

Fu Zi Tang and Zhen Wu Tang are both indicated in patterns of Shao Yin kidney yang deficiency with cold damp accumulation. Fu Zi Tang is indicated for a more severe pattern of yang deficiency, where cold damp has accumulated in the joints and muscles, obstructing the flow of qi and blood and giving rise to painful obstruction or bi syndrome. Zhen Wu Tang is used in a pattern of yang deficiency giving rise to water accumulation, where the pathogenic water qi harasses the organs and the channels, causing palpitations and muscle twitching. The ingredients are similar and both formulas are warming and drying, but the focus is different. Fu Zi Tang eliminates damp by tonifying and dispersing: its focus is on warming and tonifying the source yang and the dosage of Fu Zi, Bai Zhu and Ren Shen is larger. Zhen Wu Tang, on the other hand, tends to be draining: its primary focus is not on tonification, but on moving water. Hence there is a smaller dosage of Fu Zi and Bai Zhu and there is no Ren Shen; the inclusion of Sheng Jiang in Zhen Wu Tang assists Fu Zi's function of warming yang and supports Bai Zhu and Fu Ling in their action of strengthening the spleen and controlling water.

Clause 305

少阴病，身体痛，手足寒，骨节痛，脉沉者，附子汤主之。

Shao Yin disease, if the body is aching, the hands and feet are cold, there is joint pain, and the pulse is deep, Fu Zi Tang governs.

DISCUSSION: Clause 305 should be read together with Clause 304, as both describe a Shao Yin disease with yang deficiency and congelation of cold damp. In this clause, however, the yang deficiency has resulted in cold and damp accumulating in the muscles and joints, giving rise to aches and pains. The cold extremities are a result of the inadequate yang qi failing to reach the hands and feet. The submerged pulse, which we may assume also to be faint and thready, is a reflection of the sinking of yang qi and the stagnation of cold damp. The indicated formula is Fu Zi Tang to warm the yang, disperse the cold, and dry the damp.

Clause 304 and Clause 305 both describe a Fu Zi Tang pattern. Clause 304 focuses on yang deficiency featuring aversion to cold in the back; Clause 305 is more focused on exuberant yin cold and features body aches and joint pain. The symptom of aversion to cold in the back has clinical significance. It differs from the aversion to cold associated with a Tai Yang exterior pattern and also the aversion to cold in the back encountered in the Bai Hu jia Ren Shen Tang pattern of Yang Ming interior heat. Tai Yang exterior aversion to cold is generalised and is accompanied by exterior symptoms such as headache, body aches and pains, and a floating pulse. In contrast to this, the aversion to cold in the back of a Shao Yin yang deficiency pattern is accompanied by interior yang deficiency symptoms such as a pale complexion, a desire to sleep, a watery stool, and a submerged, faint and thready pulse. The aversion to cold in the back associated with the Yang Ming Bai Hu jia Ren Shen Tang pattern is the result of exuberant interior heat which has damaged qi and body fluids and depleted exterior yang, causing mild insecurity of the exterior, which manifests only in the back, as the residence of yang. It is accompanied by fever, profuse sweating, thirst and a dry throat, and the aversion to cold in the back is relatively mild. Both Clause 304 and Clause 305 describe the symtoms of yang deficiency. In Clause 304, the yang deficiency manifests as the milder symptom of the back being averse to cold; Clause 305 highlights aches and pains in the body which emphasise the severity of yin cold which has arisen as a result of the yang deficiency.

In *Shang Han Lun*, reference to body pain appears in various contexts: a Ma Huang Tang pattern, Da Qing Long Tang pattern, Gui Zhi Xin Jia Tang pattern and Fu Zi Tang pattern, to name a few. The pathogenesis and clinical features of each pattern differ, as does the treatment. For example, the body pain of a Ma Huang Tang pattern is attributed to pathogenic wind cold in the exterior, obstructing wei yang and constraining ying yin; it is acccompanied by fever, aversion to cold, absence of sweat, and a floating, tight pulse; the treatment strategy is to release the exterior by promoting sweat using Ma Huang Tang. The body pain in a Da Qing Long Tang pattern is associated with exterior constraint of wind cold where there is gradual transformation of heat in the interior; accompanying symptoms are aversion to cold, fever, an absence of sweat, and vexation; Da Qing Long Tang fulfills the treatment requirements of releasing the exterior and mildly clearing interior heat. A Gui Zhi Xin Jia Tang pattern also features body pain; the pathogenesis is damage to qi and ying by the loss of sweat; the body pain is due to the subsequent disharmony of ying and wei, and the pulse is submerged and slow; Gui Zhi Xin Jia Tang is used to augment qi and blood and regulate ying and wei. The pain of a Fu Zi Tang pattern is due to yang deficiency with an accumulation of yin cold; it is characterised by aversion to cold in the back and also features cold extremities; Fu Zi Tang is used to fortify yang and disperse cold, thus resolving the cold damp. In treating any symptom, it is essential to differentiate the pattern according to the key symptoms and treat appropriately.

Ancient Application of Fu Zi Tang

- *Qian Jin Yao Fang:* For the treatment of damp bi painful obstruction syndrome add Gui Xin and Gan Cao.

- *Zhi Sheng Pian:* For the treatment of yang deficiency with cold in the qi aspect.

Modern Application of Fu Zi Tang

- Rheumatoid arthritis with severe joint pain. If there is more pain in the upper limbs, add Gui Zhi; if there is pronounced damp, add Bai Zhu 30–60g; if cold predominates, use Pao Fu Zi 30–45g (*Shang Han Lun Tang Zheng Lun Zhi*).
- Varicose veins and Raynaud's syndrome where there are cold extremities and a submerged pulse, with the addition of Tao Ren, Hong Hua; for elderly patients with a deficient constitution, add Dang Gui, Huang Qi; for severely cold extremities, add Xi Xin and Gui Zhi (*Shang Han Lun Tang Zheng Lun Zhi*).
- Modified Fu Zi Tang was used to treat 53 cases of habitual miscarriage: Fu Zi 10g, Dang Gui 10g, Zhi Gan Cao 10g, Dang Shen 30g, Huang Qi 30g, Duan Long Gu 30g, Duan Mu Li 30g, Tu Si Zi 15g, Bai Zhu 15g, Chuan Duan 12g. One pack to be taken three times a week. The patients were told to start the medication from the first month of conception and continue it for the first four months of pregnancy. The outcome was success in 52 cases, with no sign of miscarriage, and one case where the pregnancy did not proceed (*Sichuan Zhong Yi* 1993; 12:45).

Case Study

Bi Syndrome

Extracted from Zhong Yi Yan Jiu Tong Xin 1962; 3:42

A 40-year-old female presented with bi syndrome characterised by weakness and stiffness in the limbs. She had frequent, clear urination, no thirst, and a submerged, thready and forceless pulse. The diagnosis was kidney yang deficiency and the formula prescribed was Fu Zi Tang with the addition of Gui Zhi, Chuan Xiong, Dang Gui. After three packs of medication, the joint pain had eased substantially, and she was given a further five packs to consolidate the treatment. After the five packs of medication, she complained of lumbar pain and heaviness in the lower limbs. Fu Zi Tang was again prescribed, with the addition of Huai Niu Xi and Bu Gu Zhi, for a further three packs and she completely recovered.

Wu Zhu Yu Tang Pattern

Clause 309

少阴病，吐利，手足逆冷，烦躁欲死者，吴茱萸汤主之。

Shao Yin disease, if there is vomiting and diarrhoea, reversal cold of the hands and feet, vexation and agitation with a feeling one is about to die, Wu Zhu Yu Tang governs.

DISCUSSION: Clause 309 describes a Shao Yin yang deficiency pattern with exuberant yin cold harassing the spleen and stomach and an accumulation of turbid damp. The proper middle jiao dynamic of ascent and descent is disrupted, causing vomiting and vexation, and where the yin cold harasses the intestines, diarrhoea will ensue. The cold extremities are a result of deficient yang failing to warm the four limbs; the struggle between the physiological yang qi and the pathogenic yin causes vexation and a feeling that one is about to die. This is not intended to suggest that death is imminent, but is merely an expression of how badly the patient feels. The cause of the turbid accumulation which harasses the stomach is yang deficiency. Wu Zhu Yu Tang warms the middle, disperses cold and redirects qi downwards, causing the turbidity to descend.

The main feature of a Wu Zhu Yu Tang pattern is vomiting, with its secondary features being diarrhoea and cold extremities. Cold extremities and vomiting are features of both Wu Zhu Yu Tang and Si Ni Tang; however, in Wu Zhu Yu Tang patterns, vomiting is the primary feature, and in Si Ni Tang patterns, cold extremities are the predominant symptom. The cold extremities of these two patterns are differentiated by their degree of severity, which is also a measure of the degree of internal cold.

Differentiation of Cold Extremities

Coldness of the extremities in a Si Ni Tang pattern is described as extending from the fingers to the elbows and from the toes to the knees; this represents a significant depletion of yang, with the possibility of yang desertion. The cold extremities associated with a Wu Zhu Yu Tang pattern, however, follow an episode of vomiting which has damaged the yang temporarily, and the cold is relatively mild. They are therefore easily distinguished from the severely cold extremities of Si Ni Tang.

Differentiation of Vexation

In *Shang Han Lun*, symptoms of vexation, agitation and restlessness can be ascribed to external or internal factors. For example, the vexation of a Da Qing Long Tang pattern is due to exterior cold and interior constrained heat; vexation of a Zhi Zi Chi Tang pattern is the result of heat harassing the chest and diaphragm; vexation of a Cheng Qi Tang pattern is ascribed to heat bind in the intestines; vexation of a Huang Lian E Jiao Tang pattern is due to kidney yin deficiency with hyperactive heart fire; vexation of Wu Mei Wan is caused by the agitation of round worms; the vexation of a Si Ni Tang pattern is a symptom of false heat in a pattern of severe yang deficiency where exuberant yin repels true yang to the surface. Vexation and agitation with a feeling one is about to die should not be interpreted as a sign of imminent death. In *Shang Han Lun*, vexation and restlessness associated with a terminal illness are marked by impaired consciousness and the patient's sub-conscious action of tugging and twisting at the bedclothes.

It is useful to compare Clause 309 with Clause 296, which reads: "Shao Yin disease, there is vomiting, diarrhoea, agitation and vexation, if there are four reversals, the person will die." Both clauses describe vomiting and diarrhoea with vexation and cold extremities; both clauses describe patterns of yang deficiency, but the pathogenesis and prognosis are different.

In the Wu Zhu Yu pattern the yang qi is deficient but not exhausted and so can contend with the pathogen. The agitation is the result of the yang qi vying with the pathogen, the coldness in the extremities is mild, and the sensation of being near death is a subjective one, merely expressing extreme discomfort. It can be treated by warming the interior and regulating the qi using Wu Zhu Yu Tang. The yang deficiency described in Clause 296, however, is a pattern of yang desertion. The condition is critical, the coldness in the extremities is severe, and the prognosis of death is real. There is no suggested treatment.

A discussion of Wu Zhu Yu Tang and its ingredients is found in Clause 243 in Chapter 3 Yang Ming Disease. Nevertheless, it must be remembered that a Wu Zhu Yu Tang pattern is ascribed to deficiency cold of the liver and stomach causing turbidity and qi reversal; it is not associated with Yang Ming disease alone. In *Shang Han Lun* there are three situations associated with Wu Zhu Yu Tang: (1) a Yang Ming pattern of cold in the stomach where there is vomiting following the ingestion of food; (2) a Shao Yin pattern with vomiting and diarrhoea, cold extremities, vexation and a feeling of being near death; and (3) a Jue Yin pattern where there is headache, dry retching and excessive salivation and drooling. The Jue Yin headache is located at the vertex and is accompanied by symptoms of stomach cold, acid reflux, excessive salivation, dizziness, a bland taste in the mouth, a pale complexion, a white slippery tongue coat and a pulse which is submerged and wiry.

Tao Hua Tang Pattern

Clause 306

少阴病，下利便脓血者，桃花汤主之。

Shao Yin disease, if there is diarrhoea with pus and blood in the stool, Tao Hua Tang governs.

TAO HUA TANG: Chi Shi Zhi 1 jin (one half used whole in the decoction and the other half crushed and sieved for use as a powder); Gan Jiang 1 liang; Jing Mi 1 sheng. (Jing Mi (粳米), sometimes mistakenly pronounced Geng Mi, is a variety of round grain non-glutinous rice.)

DIRECTIONS: Boil the ingredients in 3 sheng of water until the rice is cooked. Strain and take

7 ge warm after adding a square inch spoonful (approx 6-9g) of Chi Shi Zhi powder. Take three times a day and if recovery occurs after one dose, do not take again.

DISCUSSION: Shao Yin diarrhoea is the result of spleen and kidney yang deficiency, and when the diarrhoea persists for a prolonged period, the subsequent damage to qi impairs the spleen's ability to maintain the integrity of the network vessels and their ability to contain blood; this results in bleeding. The depletion of yang qi will also result in the non-transformation of fluids and the non-separation of turbidity, leading to the appearance of turbid yin or pus in the stool.

The chief herb in Tao Hua Tang is Chi Shi Zhi, which warms and astringes the intestines to stop the diarrhoea, controls blood and stops bleeding due to yang deficiency; Gan Jiang is acrid and warm. It warms the interior, and together with Chi Shi Zhi is effective in treating the uncontrollable diarrhoea which is due to deficiency cold in the lower jiao. Jing Mi is sweet and warm; it warms the stomach and harmonises the middle. The purpose of reserving half of the Chi Shi Zhi to add to the decoction later as a powder, is to enable it to have a direct and local effect on the intestines, thus staunching bleeding and astringing diarrhoea. Modern research on Chi Shi Zhi has shown that it is anti-bacterial, has an anti-inflammatory effect on intestinal mucosa, and it can stop intestinal bleeding.

Clause 307

少阴病，二三日至四五日，腹痛，小便不利，下利不止，便脓血者，桃花汤主之。

Shao Yin disease, for two, three or even four or five days, if there is abdominal pain, the urination is not free, there is incessant diarrhoea, with pus and blood in the stool, Tao Hua Tang governs.

DISCUSSION: Shao Yin disease which has lasted several days is considered chronic; damage to yang is severe and has resulted in an accumulation of yin cold. The cold retards the flow of qi and blood, giving rise to abdominal pain; the resulting disruption to the qi dynamic, combined with the kidney yang deficiency, results in severe, persistent diarrhoea. The kidney yang fails to support the spleen's transformation function, giving rise to diarrhoea, and also affects the spleen's function of controlling blood, so there is bleeding due to deficiency. The inhibited urination is a result of fluid depletion caused by the diarrhoea. The indicated formula is Tao Hua Tang, which warms and astringes the intestines and stops bleeding.

There are four principal features of a Shao Yin yang deficiency pattern with exuberant yin cold.

1. Dull, persistent abdominal pain which is relieved by warmth and pressure.
2. Diminished or difficult urination due to a) waning fire in the lower jiao and the non-transformation of qi and b) fluid loss due to the severity of the diarrhoea.
3. Uncontrollable diarrhoea with extreme frequency and urgency.
4. Diarrhoea with blood and pus in the stool.

Two things should be noted. Firstly, because the inhibited urination is caused by depleted fluids, the use of herbs which promote urination and cause further loss of fluids is contraindicated. Secondly, although blood and pus in the stool are often associated with heat, the presence of blood and pus in Shao Yin diarrhoea is due to a prolonged chronic disorder where yang has transformed into yin and qi into blood. By this it is meant that the depletion of yang has given rise to the accumulation of yin, and the exhaustion of qi has resulted in loss of blood. As a pattern of cold and deficiency, there is a bland taste in the mouth, and cold signs with no signs of dry heat; the tongue is pale with a white coat and the pulse is submerged, faint and thready.

There are three patterns of diarrhoea attributed to deficiency cold. (1) Yang deficiency of the spleen and kidney where the focus is on the middle jiao; there is an absence of thirst, a reduced appetite, periodic abdominal pain, and a submerged, weak and forceless pulse. The indicated formula is Li Zhong Wan or Fu Zi Li Zhong Wan. (2) Deficiency cold in the lower jiao characterised by a watery stool with undigested food particles, cold extremities, abdominal cramps, an aversion to cold and a pulse which is submerged, faint and thready. The indicated formula is Si Ni Tang. (3) Deficiency cold in the lower jiao where there is blood and pus in a watery stool and the pulse is submerged, faint and thready. The formula to use is Tao Hua Tang.

Tao Hua Tang and Chi Shi Zhi Yu Yu Liang Tang both astringe the intestines to stop diarrhoea and promote healing. Tao Hua Tang, however, has a stronger warming effect and so is more useful in cold patterns.

The appearance of blood and pus in diarrhoea can be ascribed either to heat and excess or to cold and deficiency, and they are differentiated as follows. A pattern of excess heat harassing the intestines is characterised by a foul-smelling sloppy stool, tenesmus, abdominal pain, fever, thirst, a yellow tongue coat and a rapid pulse; the indicated formula for diarrhoea with pus and blood attributed to heat is Bai Tou Weng Tang. A pattern of yang deficiency of the spleen and kidney with an accumulation of cold damp is characterised by watery diarrhoea, mild tenesmus, dull abdominal pain, a preference for warmth and pressure, the absence of fever or thirst, a white tongue coat and a weak pulse; the formula for diarrhoea with blood and pus attributed to cold and deficiency is Tao Hua Tang. Diarrhoea associated with an excess heat pattern is generally an acute, short-lived disorder, whilst diarrhoea associated with a pattern of deficiency and cold is generally a chronic disorder occurring as a sequel to other patterns. Therefore, the initial stage of diarrhoea can generally be presumed to be a heat pattern and warm astringent herbs are contraindicated. In chronic diarrhoea due to depleted yang of the spleen and kidney however, astringent warm herbs are essential for effective treatment.

Ancient Application of Tao Hua Tang

- *Wai Tai Mi Yao:* For the treatment of diarrhoea with blood and pus, increasing the dose of Gan Jiang from 1 liang to 4 liang.
- *He Ji Ju Fang:* For the treatment of cold dysentery with abdominal pain, grinding equal parts of Duan Chi Shi Zhi and Pao Gan Jiang into powder and making pills to be taken three times a day.

Modern Application of Tao Hua Tang

Tao Hua Tang is effective in the treatment of chronic colitis, ulcerative colitis and dysentery associated with yang deficiency and cold.

- Li et al used Tao Hua Tang, substituting Jing Mi with Shan Yao and adding Long Gu, Mu Li, Sheng Di Yu and Qin Pi in the treatment of chronic amoebic dysentery (*Guang Dong Zhong Yi* 1959; 4:163).
- For chronic diarrhoea with blood and pus, a modified version of Tao Hua Tang can be used: for acute abdominal pain add Bai Shao and Wu Yao; for chronic diarrhoea with a watery stool add Fu Ling, Zhu Ling and Bai Zhu; for persistent diarrhoea add Wu Mei, Dang Shen and Rou Dou Kou.

Case Study

Irritable Bowel Syndrome

Extracted from Jilin Zhong Yi Yao 1997; (2):20

A 51-year-old male had suffered from recurrent diarrhoea for over two years. The number of episodes ranged from 2 to 6 times a day, each time accompanied by borborygmus and there was mucus in the stool. The Western diagnosis was irritable bowel syndrome. Antibiotics had had no effect and he sought Chinese medicine treatment. He presented with fatigue, a poor appetite, cold extremities, a pale and swollen tongue with teeth marks, and a submerged, thready and forceless pulse. The formula prescribed was Tao Hua Tang modified: Chi Shi Zhi 30g, Gan Jiang 10g, Shu Jiao (Chuan Jiao) 6g, Ban Xia 10g, Rou Gui 10g (ground into powder), He Zi (Ke Zi) 10g, Shi Liu Pi 10g. He took one pack a day for three days, after which there was significant improvement in the diarrhoea and borborygmus. After a further 20 packs there was full recovery. He was then given Jin Gui Shen Qi Wan for the ensuing three months to consolidate the treatment.

Shao Yin Moxibustion Pattern

Clause 325

少阴病，下利，脉微涩，呕而汗出，必数更衣，反少者，当温其上，灸之。

Shao Yin disease, there is diarrhoea, a faint and choppy pulse, vomiting and sweating, and there should be a frequent change of clothes, if instead the stool is infrequent, one should warm the upper jiao, using moxibustion.

DISCUSSION: Persistent diarrhoea damages fluids, and in Shao Yin disease, where there is already a deficiency, this can rapidly proceed to a deficiency of qi and blood, yin and yang. Such a situation is indicated by the faint and choppy pulse, where the faint pulse is a reflection of deficient yang qi, and the choppy pulse is indicative of depleted yin blood. Yang is insufficient and yin accumulates causing qi reversal which manifests as vomiting, and the insecure defence yang results in sweating. The expression "change of clothes" is a euphemism for going to the toilet and refers to passing a stool. Where there is such severe yang deficiency, a loose and frequent stool, or frequent "changing of clothes" would be expected. However, the stool is infrequent. The apparent paradox is explained by the devastation of fluids caused by the earlier diarrhoea, vomiting and loss of sweat. Remaining fluids are insufficient to result in a frequent loose stool.

This pattern is difficult to treat because although yang is deficient, warming herbs may damage the yin; the use of herbs which direct qi downwards in order to check the vomiting could cause the diarrhoea to worsen; conversely, herbs which raise qi could exacerbate the vomiting. With this dilemma in mind, moxibustion is the chosen treatment. The upper jiao is a broad concept which does not refer only to the chest, but incorporates the head. Here, the implication is that by using moxibustion on a point located on the head, the diarrhoea can be resolved without damaging yin or exacerbating the vomiting. The selection of an acupuncture point for the application of moxa has been the subject of some discussion. Some have suggested that Shao Yin Tai Xi (Kid 3) should be used, but the majority of commentators advocate Bai Hui (Du 20). Bai Hui is located at the vertex of the head and is the intersection point of the Du meridian and all the yang channels; moxa on Bai Hui causes clear yang to ascend and rescues sinking qi. Using moxa on the point invigorates the yang, and so this method is effective in tonifying and raising the sunken and deficient yang qi and can be used to resolve yang deficiency diarrhoea. Salt moxa on Shen Que (Ren 8) can also be used in the treatment of diarrhoea.

Clause 292

少阴病，吐、利，手足不逆冷，反发热者，不死。脉不至者，灸少阴七壮。

Shao Yin disease, there is vomiting and diarrhoea, if the hands and feet have no reversal cold, but there is fever, the person will not die. If the pulse does not arrive, use seven cones of moxa on Shao Yin.

DISCUSSION: The presentation of vomiting and diarrhoea in Shao Yin disease represents a sign of deficient yang. One might expect the extremities to be cold, and if they are not, then the yang deficiency is not severe as there is sufficient yang to reach and warm the extremities. In addition, if there is fever signalling the return of yang qi, then the prognosis is good and the person will not die. In order to support the yang qi, it is suggested that moxa be used on the Shao Yin channel or on Shao Yin channel points.

In Shao Yin disease, where there is vomiting and diarrhoea, the pulse should be faint and weak. Cold extremities combined with a pulse which is not palpable indicate a severe deficiency of yang, and herald the separation of yin and yang. If the pulse is hidden but the hands and feet are warm and there is fever, then the hidden pulse is not attributed to the imminent separation of yin and yang but to the non-communication of yin and yang associated with a less serious pattern of relatively mild qi and yang deficiency. The prognosis is therefore good, and the use of moxa on the foot Shao Yin kidney channel points will fortify the yang and restore the pulse.

The fever associated with a Shao Yin pattern of yang deficiency and yin exuberance can be explained in one of two ways: (1) exuberant interior yin cold repelling the yang in a pattern of true cold with false heat or (2) a sign of yang qi returning. The symptom of cold extremities is a key point of differential diagnosis. If the fever occurs in the presence of cold extremities, it is a manifestation of yang being repelled by yin in a pattern of false heat; this represents a serious condition. However, if the fever occurs in the presence of warm hands and feet, it is a sign of the return of yang qi, which bodes well for recovery and can be supported with treatment. Clause 292 mentions only the Shao Yin channel and does not specify any acupuncture points. Many suggest the use of Tai Xi (Kid 3) which is a source point of the Shao Yin channel. Ke Yun Bo suggested Tai Xi (Kid 3), Fu Liu (Kid 7) and Yong Quan (Kid 1). Others have advocated Guan Yuan (Ren 4) and Qi Hai (Ren 6), both of which support kidney qi, and points on the Shao Yin channel such as Qi Xue (Kid 13) or Huang Shu (Kid 16) can also be considered.

6.3.2 Shao Yin Heat Conversion Patterns

Heat conversion in Shao Yin disease occurs as a result of deficient kidney yin failing to control heart yang. Heart fire then flares, manifesting as vexation and insomnia; the tongue is red with a scant coat, reflecting the yin deficiency, and the pulse is rapid and thready. The indicated formula is Huang Lian E Jiao Tang which both nourishes yin and clears heat from the heart. If the pathogenic heat binds with water in the urinary bladder, the heart fire will be accompanied by scant or difficult urination as well as vexation, insomnia and thirst. The appropriate formula is then Zhu Ling Tang, which nourishes yin and promotes urination.

Huang Lian E Jiao Tang Pattern

Clause 303

少阴病，得之二三日以上，心中烦、不得卧，黄连阿胶汤主之。

Shao Yin disease, contracted for more than two or three days, there is vexation in the heart and an inability to sleep, Huang Lian E Jiao Tang governs.

HUANG LIAN E JIAO TANG: Huang Lian 4 liang; Huang Qin 2 liang; Shao Yao 2 liang; Ji Zi Huang (egg yolks) 2; E Jiao 3 liang (*Qian Jin Yi Fang* records the dose as 3 blocks).

DIRECTIONS: Boil the first three ingredients in 6 sheng of water, reducing to 2 sheng, then strain. Melt the E Jiao separately before adding. Allow the mixture to cool a little before adding the egg yolks. Blend thoroughly and take 7 ge warm three times a day.

DISCUSSION: The Shao Yin pertains to the heart, the organ of fire, and the kidney, the organ of water. The interaction of fire and water refers to the equilibrium maintained by the heart fire descending to warm kidney yang and control kidney water, and the ascent of kidney water to nourish the yin and control the heart fire. When this physiological function is properly co-ordinated, it is said that the heart and kidney are in communication (心肾交通). Their co-operative activity is also expressed in the phrase "the assistance of fire and water" (水火既济). This mutual dependence of fire and water mirrors the interdependence of yin and yang, the balance of which is the basis of both physical and psychological health, as described in *Su Wen: Sheng Qi Tong Tian Lun Pian (Chapter 3: Discourse on Qi and Heaven)*: "Only when yin is level and yang is restrained can the spirit be ordered"

Pathogenic qi attacking the Shao Yin has two possible outcomes. The first is a pattern of Shao Yin yang deficiency with an accumulation of yin cold, which is the basis of a cold conversion pattern; the second is a pattern of Shao Yin yin deficiency with hyperactive heart fire, which is a heat conversion pattern. Which of these two patterns ultimately develops is intimately related to the person's constitution.

Huang Lian E Jiao Tang is indicated for a pattern of yin deficiency: either a pre-existing yin deficiency with hyperactive yang, which lays the foundation for the pathogen in Shao Yin to transform into heat, or an exterior invasion of pathogenic heat affecting the lower jiao and damaging the kidney yin. In Clause 303, the Shao Yin pattern was contracted at least two or three days earlier. This implies that a pre-existing yin deficiency, unable to control yang, has resulted in the generation of heat or, in other words, deficient kidney water can not cool and control the heart fire. The treatment is to nourish yin and drain fire in order to re-establish the balanced interaction of fire and water. The purpose of E Jiao in Huang Lian E Jiao Tang is to nourish both the kidney yin and the yin blood; Ji Zi Huang or egg yolk nourishes heart blood and harmonises ying qi; Bai Shao nourishes blood, clears heat and harmonises and astringes yin; when combined with Bai Shao, Huang Lian clears fire from the heart without damaging the yin. Huang Lian and Huang Qin together drain fire to preserve the yin and facilitate its return.

The key indication for Huang Lian E Jiao Tang is yin deficiency characterised by vexation and insomnia where the symptoms are more pronounced at night. Other symptoms are a dry throat, thirst, urination which is dark in colour, a red or crimson tongue with a scant tongue coat and a thready, rapid pulse.

A comparison should be drawn between Huang Lian E Jiao Tang and Zhi Zi Chi Tang both of which are indicated for insomnia. The difference is found in the pathogenesis as well as the pattern. Zhi Zi Chi Tang is indicated for a pattern of residual excess heat harassing the chest and diaphragm, which manifests with symptoms of anguish, restlessness, and insomnia. There is no deficiency of yin. Huang Lian E Jiao Tang is indicated for a pattern of kidney yin deficiency where the yin of the kidneys fails to interact with the fire of the heart and results in vexation, a dry throat and insomnia.

There are two points to be borne in mind when decocting Huang Lian E Jiao Tang. (1) E Jiao must not be decocted with the other herbs but must be melted (usually over a double boiler) and, after straining, blended into the decoction when it is removed from the flame. (2) Ji Zi Huang or egg yolk should be added only after straining and after allowing the decoction to cool a little.

Ancient Application of Huang Lian E Jiao Tang

- *Zhang Shi Yi Tong:* For the treatment of blood in the stool due to heat.
- *Yi Zong Bi Du:* For the treatment of dysentery with blood and pus in the stool associated with toxic heat and accompanied by vexation and insomnia due to yin deficiency in Shao Yin.
- *Wen Bing Tiao Bian:* For a pattern of Shao Yin wen bing where true yin is exhausted and fire flares, manifesting as vexation and insomnia.
- *Shang Han Lun Bao Ming Ji:* For vexation and insomnia, omit Huang Qin, Bai Shao, Ji Zi Huang, add Huang Bai, Zhi Zi.

Modern Application of Huang Lian E Jiao Tang

Huang Lian E Jiao Tang is indicated for the treatment of mouth ulcers or dysentery attributed to yin deficiency with hyperactive fire. It can also be used for chronic cough, chronic diarrhoea.

Modifications

For thirst and a dry throat, add Mai Dong, Sha Shen; for a sore throat, combine with Jie Geng Tang; for severe insomnia, add Chao Suan Zao Ren, Long Gu and Mu Li; for insomnia with vexation, add Bai He, Sheng Di and Chao Suan Zao Ren.

Case Study

Palpitations and Insomnia

Extracted from Shang Han Lun Fang Yun Yong Fa

Zhejiang Ke Ji Publications 1985

Following exercise, a 21-year-old male athlete used a cold towel to wipe off sweat. He suffered from frequent colds which usually resolved without treatment, and he had also suffered from rheumatoid arthritis for two years. Two weeks previously, he contracted the flu and after Western medication, the fever receded. However, he did not recover fully and complained of palpitations, shortness of breath, an oppressed sensation in the chest, fatigue, a reduced appetite and excessive sweating. The symptoms were all worse at night. His face was red and he suffered from headache, a dry parched throat, vexation and insomnia. The edge and tip of his tongue were red, the tongue coat was scant, and the pulse was thready and rapid. The diagnosis was insufficiency of heart yin with empty fire blazing. The treatment principle was to nourish yin and clear heat. The formula used was Huang Lian E Jiao Tang: Huang Lian 9g, Huang Qin 9g, Bai Shao 10g, Dang Gui 10g, Sheng Di 15g, E Jiao 10g (melted and strirred in at the end), 2 egg yolks (added when mixture is slightly cooled). After three packs there was a slight improvement in his overall condition, with significant improvement in the palpitations and insomnia. The same formula was prescribed for another three packs, and followed by a month of Zhu Sha An Shen Wan to consolidate the treatment.

Zhu Ling Tang Pattern in Shao Yin

Clause 319

少阴病，下利六七日，咳而呕、渴、心烦、不得眠者，猪苓汤主之。

Shao Yin disease, there has been diarrhoea for six or seven days, if there is coughing and vomiting, thirst, heart vexation and an inability to sleep, Zhu Ling Tang governs.

DISCUSSION: Where Shao Yin disease has persisted with diarrhoea for six or seven days, the symptoms of cough, vomiting, thirst, vexation and insomnia are due to yin deficiency with interior heat. Water and heat knot together, stagnating the qi. If the water and heat bind descends to the large intestine, diarrhoea will ensue; if the water qi surges upward harassing the lungs, cough will ensue; if the pathogen harasses the stomach, vomiting will ensue; when the water and heat bind obstructs the distribution of fluids, there is thirst; when empty fire generated by yin deficiency harasses the heart shen, it causes vexation and insomnia. The indicated formula is Zhu Ling Tang, which nourishes yin, clears heat, transforms qi and promotes urination.

The pattern described in Clause 319 shares a similar aetiology and similar features with the Zhu Ling Tang pattern described in Clause 223 in the Yang Ming chapter. Both exhibit yin deficiency characterised by thirst and inhibited urination, which is the result of water and heat knotting in the lower jiao. Clause 223 describes a pattern caused by incorrect purgation in a Yang Ming pattern, which has damaged fluids and resulted in heat knotting with water. There is a floating pulse, fever, thirst and inhibited urination. Clause 319 describes Shao Yin disease accompanied by diarrhoea, cough, vomiting, thirst, vexation and inhibited urination. Because the aetiology of the inhibited urination in both patterns is the knotting of heat and water in the lower jiao, the formula for both is Zhu Ling Tang.

However, the Shao Yin pattern is differentiated by a pulse which is not floating but deep, and by continuing diarrhoea which is not due to purgation; there is also vomiting, a cough and an inability to sleep.

Comparison Between Huang Lian E Jiao Tang, Zhi Zi Chi Tang and Zhu Ling Tang Patterns

A comparison should be drawn between a Huang Lian E Jiao Tang pattern, a Zhi Zi Chi Tang pattern, and the Zhu Ling Tang pattern described in Clause 319. All three are characterised by vexation and insomnia, but differ in their pathogenesis. Huang Lian E Jiao Tang is indicated for yin deficiency with hyperactive heart yang; there is no knotting of water and heat in the lower jiao and there should be a red tongue with no coat, a parched throat and a thready and rapid pulse. A Zhi Zi Chi Tang pattern is attributed to heat constraint in the chest and diaphragm where the focus is on severe anguish and restlessness. The Zhu Ling Tang pattern described in Clause 319 is a pattern of yin deficiency where water and heat knot in the lower jiao affecting qi transformation, presenting with vomiting, thirst and inhibited urination.

Comparison Between Zhu Ling Tang and Zhen Wu Tang Patterns

A comparison of Zhu Ling Tang with Zhen Wu Tang shows that both patterns are characterised by water accumulation in the interior accompanied by a cough, vomiting, diarrhoea and inhibited urination. The pathogenesis of a Zhen Wu Tang pattern, however, is deficient yang unable to control water, whilst a Zhu Ling Tang pattern is one of yin deficiency with heat and water knotting in the lower jiao.

Differentiation of Cold and Heat Diarrhoea Patterns in Shao Yin

Shao Yin diarrhoea can be attributed either to cold or to heat. The cold pattern is characterised by cold extremities, aversion to cold and diarrhoea with undigested food particles, representing a Si Ni Tang pattern. Shao Yin diarrhoea associated with heat is due to yin deficiency; it is characterised by vexation, cough, vomiting and thirst, representing a Zhu Ling Tang pattern.

Ancient Application of Zhu Ling Tang

- *Yi Fang Ji Jie:* For the treatment of jaundice due to damp heat where there is thirst and inhibited urination.
- *Lei Ju Fang Guang Yi:* For the treatment of dribbling urination or lin zheng characterised by scant, painful urination and abdominal distension.
- *Huang Han Yi Xue:* For the treatment of urinary infection.

Modern Application of Zhu Ling Tang

This formula is commonly used in the treatment of acute pyelonephritis, urinary tract infection, chyluria, chronic nephritis and prostatic hypertrophy.

Modifications

For dysuria due to heat, add Bian Xu, Qu Mai; for haematuria, add Bai Mao Gen, Da Ji and Xiao Ji; for acute urinary tract infection, add Lian Qiao, Bai Jiang Cao and Tu Fu Ling; for acute pyelonephritis, add Han Lian Cao, Nu Zhen Zi and San Qi Fen.

Case Study

Haematuria

Extracted from Guan Ming Zhong Yi 1988; 3:17

A 53-year-old male had passed blood in his urine for ten days and also experienced lower back pain and weakness in the knees. He was treated for kidney stones but the medication was not effective. For the past few days, he had had frequent diarrhoea, and also suffered from fatigue, thirst, a heavy sensation in his body, vexation, a red tongue with a thin, yellow coat and a pulse which was wiry and tight. The diagnosis was bloody dysuria or *xue lin*. The treatment principle was to nourish yin, drain fire, cool blood and stop bleeding. The formula prescribed was Zhu Ling Tang with the addition of Qian Cao, Bai Shao, Zhi Zi Tan 10g each. He recovered after three packs.

Shao Yin Heat in the Urinary Bladder

Clause 293

少阴病，八九日，一身手足尽热者，以热在膀胱，必便血也。

Shao Yin disease, for eight or nine days, if the whole body and hands and feet are extremely hot, it is because of heat in the urinary bladder, there will be blood in the urine.

DISCUSSION: Fever is not typical of Shao Yin disease. If, after eight or nine days of Shao Yin disease, severe fever appears, it signifies heat in the urinary bladder, which will be marked by blood in the urine. This is explained by the interior–exterior relationship of Shao Yin and Tai Yang, and is a sign that the course of the disease is reverting from yin to yang, and has transmitted from the Shao Yin to the Tai Yang. The Tai Yang channel governs yang qi, so if the pathogen moves into the Tai Yang channel, it will be converted into heat under the influence of the yang qi of Tai Yang, causing fever. Because the urinary bladder is the fu of the Tai Yang, the urinary bladder will be affected by the heat, which will scorch the network vessels and cause bleeding. From the perspective of heat in the bladder, this can be categorised as a heat conversion pattern and the corresponding treatment is Huang Lian E Jiao Tang.

There are two situations where Shao Yin disease is characterised by fever. (1) Where devastated yang is proceeding to yang desertion and the fever is a manifestation of false heat. (2) Where the fever is a sign of the return of yang qi and the subsequent struggle of the zheng qi against the pathogenic qi, as found in Clause 293 which describes the attendant transformation of the nature of the disease from yin to yang and from cold to heat. It is essential to have a clear understanding of all aspects of disease transformation in order to identify the pathogenesis and determine the treatment strategy.

The Shao Yin is connected to the Tai Yang through their interior–exterior relationship, and therefore, strong zheng qi can cause the pathogen to revert from the interior Shao Yin to the exterior Tai Yang. Conversely, if there has been inappropriate treatment of Tai yang disease which damages the zheng qi, or if there is a pre-existing weakness of yang qi, the pathogen can transmit inward to the Shao Yin interior, causing the disease to be transformed from a Tai Yang exterior pattern to a concurrent pattern of Tai Yang and Shao Yin.

It should be noted that in referring to the urine, Clause 293 uses the general term 'bian' (便) which can refer both to the stool, *da bian* (大便) and the urine, *xiao bian* (小便); in this clause, because it is used in reference to the urinary bladder, it is generally accepted as referring to urine. Zhang Zhong Jing did not elaborate on this issue and different interpretations have been proposed. Ke Yun Bo maintained that if there is heat in the bladder, the blood must be in the urine; Qian Tian Lai suggested that even if the heat was in the bladder, the blood was not necessarily excreted via the urine; Fang You Zhi suggested that heat harassing the bladder can be characterised by blood in either the urine or the stool.

Shao Yin Heat Diarrhoea

Clause 308

少阴病, 下利, 便脓血之者, 可刺。

Shao Yin disease, if there is diarrhoea, with pus and blood in the stool, one may needle.

DISCUSSION: Shao Yin disease where there is blood and pus in a loose stool can be treated by both herbal medicine and acupuncture. When needling, the draining method is used to clear pathogenic heat, and the tonifying method can be used to address deficiency, with moxibustion and warm needling used to support the yang and dispel cold. The manifestations of blood and pus described in Clause 308 show that the appropriate therapy is to expel heat, and that such a formula as Tao Hua Tang would not be appropriate. For this reason, it is suggested that acupuncture be used to to drain the heat from the ying aspect.

In determining whether diarrhoea in Shao Yin disease is associated with heat or cold, the relevant signs and symptoms must be observed because the treatment strategies differ. In regard to the pattern described in Clause 308, if the pathogenesis is yin deficiency with hyperactive yang, the diarrhoea will be characterised by tenesmus, a foul odour, a burning sensation in the anus and a red tongue with a scant tongue coat. Conversely, if the diarrhoea is due to cold, there will be cold signs such as watery diarrhoea with undigested food particles, aversion to cold, cold extremities and a pale or pale red tongue. For diarrhoea due to cold in the Shao Yin, Tao Hua Tang can be prescribed, and moxa may be applied to such acupoints as You Men (Kid 21), Tai Xi (Kid 3), Fu Liu (Kid 7), Shen Shu (UB 23) or Ming Men (Du 4).

6.3.3 Summary of Shao Yin Disease Patterns

Shao Yin disease can be categorised as either a cold conversion pattern or a heat conversion pattern, with cold conversion being more characteristic of Shao Yin. The principal features are cold extremities, a strong aversion to cold, a desire to sleep, diarrhoea with undigested food particles, and a pulse which is submerged, faint and thready. The treatment strategy is to warm the interior and disperse cold, and Si Ni Tang is the key formula. Tong Mai Si Ni Tang is indicated for a pattern of exuberant yin cold repelling the true yang, where there are cold extremities, a flushed face and a faint pulse verging on expiry. Bai Tong Tang is indicated for diarrhoea with a faint pulse associated with constrained yang and knotted yin; if there is incessant diarrhoea, cold limbs, vomiting and vexation and no palpable pulse, Zhu Dan Zhi (pig's bile) or human urine should be added. Zhen Wu Tang is indicated for abdominal pain, diarrhoea, inhibited urination, heaviness of the four limbs and pain; it warms the yang and controls water. Fu Zi Tang is indicated for a neutral taste in the mouth, aversion to cold in the back, aches and pains in the body and joints, cold extremities, and a submerged pulse; the strategy is to support yang. Wu Zhu Yu Tang is indicated where there is vomiting, cold extremities, vexation and a feeling as if one is about to die; this is a formula that warms the interior and descends counterflow. Tao Hua Tang is indicated for diarrhoea due to cold and deficiency where there is blood and pus in the stool; it warms and astringes the intestines and stops bleeding.

Shao Yin heat conversion patterns are ascribed to insufficiency of kidney yin with hyperactive heart fire and are characterised by vexation and insomnia. The indicated formula is Huang Lian E Jiao Tang. If there is knotted heat in the lower jiao with inhibited urination, Zhu Ling Tang is used to nourish yin, clear heat and promote urination. Finally, a Shao Yin pattern of heat in the bladder, where there is fever and blood in the urine, is a sign of a yin pattern reverting to a yang pattern, and can be treated with either herbal medicine or acupuncture.

Section Four

6.4 CONCURRENT PATTERNS OF SHAO YIN

Concurrent patterns can appear in the course of Shao Yin disease, where Shao Yin symptoms are accompanied by symptoms associated with another channel. Such concurrent patterns are Shao Yin and Tai Yang, Shao Yin and Yang Ming, and Shao Yin and Shao Yang.

6.4.1 Concurrent Pattern of Shao Yin and Tai Yang

Ma Huang Xi Xin Fu Zi Tang

Clause 301

少阴病，始得之，反发热、脉沉者，麻黄细辛附子汤主之。

Shao Yin disease, has just started, nevertheless if there is fever and the pulse is submerged, Ma Huang Xi Xin Fu Zi Tang governs.

MA HUANG XI XIN FU ZI TANG: Ma Huang (nodes removed) 2 liang; Xi Xin 2 liang; Fu Zi (skin removed, dry roasted and sliced into 8 pieces) 1 piece.

DIRECTIONS: First boil Ma Huang in 1 dou of water, reducing by 2 sheng, then skim off the foam. Add the other ingredients and boil, reducing to 3 sheng. Strain and take 1 sheng warm three times a day.

DISCUSSION: Shao Yin disease is characterised by yang deficiency and exuberant yin, there should be cold signs but no fever. Clause 301 describes the initial onset of Shao Yin disease where there is fever. The fever is a manifestation of an exterior Tai Yang pattern; however, the pulse is not floating but is instead submerged, which is a reflection of the interior Shao Yin pattern. In this way, the clause describes a concurrent pattern of the exterior and interior, representing a concurrent pattern of Tai Yang and Shao Yin. The treatment strategy is to promote sweat in order to release the exterior, whilst simultaneously warming the interior to disperse interior cold.

Ma Huang releases the exterior and expels exterior cold, which are the actions used for its application in a Tai Yang exterior excess pattern. Fu Zi warms the interior and supports the kidney yang and enhances Ma Huang's action of expelling exterior cold. Xi Xin is acrid and warm; it dispels cold from the exterior and also warms and disperses the interior Shao Yin cold. The combination of these three herbs has the overall effect of releasing the exterior and warming the interior yang. It should be noted that Ma Huang and Xi Xin have a potent dispersing effect and prolonged use can damage the zheng qi. In this application, it is suitable because it is treating the early stage of Shao Yin disease where deficiency of zheng qi is not pronounced, and prolonged administration is unlikely.

It is essential to establish whether the general pulse image is floating or submerged, forceful or forceless, before palpating the cubit pulse alone to determine its strength. The cubit pulse relates to the kidneys and to source qi, and therefore indicates the condition of the zheng qi. At the onset of an exterior pattern, if the zheng qi is strong, the pulse will be floating and forceful. As the disease progresses, the zheng qi sustains damage and the pulse tends to become submerged, thready and forceless, or submerged and faint. The cubit pulse is a reflection of the source yang, and weakness or forcelessness in that position indicates that source yang is insufficient. As explained in Clause 49: "the cubit pulse is faint, this is interior deficiency". The pulse also establishes the location of the disease: in an exterior pattern of Tai Yang, the pulse should be either floating and tight or floating and moderate; if the pulse is submerged and thready or submerged and faint, then it must be an interior pattern, and in this case, it is disease in the Shao Yin.

Clause 301 describes a concurrent pattern of Tai Yang and Shao Yin. As such, it is characterised by the presence of both exterior and interior symptoms. The treatment principle mirrors this by treating both the exterior and the interior simultaneously. However, should the interior yang deficiency predominate, then despite the concurrent exterior symptoms, the priority must be placed on first treating the interior and then the exterior. Clause 92 says: "The disease has fever and headache, the pulse is submerged, if there is no recovery and there are body aches and pains, one must treat the interior. The formula is Si Ni Tang." Both Clauses 92 and 301 describe a concurrent pattern of Tai Yang and Shao Yin, but Clause 92 describes a more severe condition, where Shao Yin cold predominates; even though there are unresolved exterior symptoms, because of the severity of the interior cold, the priority of treatment is to warm the interior, and so Si Ni Tang is used to warm the interior first. Clause 301 describes a concurrent pattern of the exterior and interior where interior cold does not predominate and so it is appropriate to proceed with treatment to release the exterior and warm the interior simultaneously.

Ancient Application of Ma Huang Xi Xin Fu Zi Tang

- *Zheng Zhi Zhun Sheng:* For the treatment of cough known as 'kidney cough' because coughing causes pain in lower back.

Comparison of Ma Huang Xi Xin Fu Zi Tang and Gui Zhi jia Fu Zi Tang

Formula	Pathogenesis	Manifestations	Treatment
Ma Huang Xi Xin Fu Zi Tang	Tai Yang pathogenic wind constraint with Shao Yin yang deficiency	Aversion to cold, fever, no sweating, pulse is submerged	Support zheng qi and expel the pathogen; warm the yang and release the exterior
Gui Zhi jia Fu Zi Tang	Tai Yang with incorrect sweat promotion causing yang desertion with yin damage; deficiency of the exterior and interior	Incessant sweating; aversion to wind, inhibited urination, mild acute cramps of the four limbs with stiffness	Support the yang and secure the exterior, harmonise ying and wei

- *Zhang Shi Yi Tong:* For acute loss of voice characterised by a sore throat or a desire to cough or an unproductive cough and a wiry and tight pulse. Ma Huang Fu Zi Xi Xin Tang can be used to warm, but Fu Zi must be treated with honey and the decoction held in the mouth to maximise its topical effect.
- *Shi Bian Liang Fang:* Zhi Mi Fu Zi Xi Xin Tang, which is Ma Huang Fu Zi Xi Xin Tang with the addition of Chuan Xiong and Sheng Jiang, was cited for the treatment of headache due to pathogenic wind cold.
- *Yi Guan.* For the treatment of tension headache.

Modern Application of Ma Huang Xi Xin Fu Zi Tang

- A modification of Ma Huang Xi Xin Fu Zi Tang was used in the treatment of 50 cases of arrhythmia due to sinus node dysfunction. Zhi Huang Qi 24g; Gui Zhi 10g; Zhi Fu Zi (decoct first) 10g; Chuan Xiong 12g; Dang Gui 12g; Rou Gui 6g; Xi Xin 9g; Zhi Ma Huang 9g; Xi Xin 9g; Sheng Di 20g; Mai Dong 15g; Wu Wei Zi 10g. One course was 30 days and no Western medication was given. Result: very effective (alleviation of all symptoms) 14 cases; effective (reduction of symptoms with an average increase in heart rate of 2–9 beats per minute) 27 cases; not effective 9 cases. Total effective rate = 82%. (*Shi Yong Zhong Xi Yi Jie He Za Zhi* 1991; (4): 280–281).
- In the treatment of the common cold, headache due to yang deficiency, somnolence and myocarditis. Jiang et al reported treating one case of somnolence due to insufficiency of heart yang by using Ma Huang Xi Xin Fu Zi Tang plus Zhi Gan Cao and Xian He Cao (*Shang Hai Zhong Yi Za Zhi* 1979; 6:37).

Case Study

Shao Yin Headache

Extracted from Wu Pei Heng Yi An 1979

A male patient had contracted a head cold, for which he was prescribed a cool acrid formula. His condition did not improve and more than ten days later, he had a severe headache. His symptoms included aversion to cold in the afternoon, a heavy aching sensation in the body and a lack of thirst. His tongue coat was white and slippery and the pulse was faint and forceless. The diagnosis was cold in the Shao Yin channel obstructing clear yang. The formula given was Ma Huang Xi Xin Fu Zi Tang modified: Fu Pian 10g, Gan Jiang 6g, Zhi Gan Cao 6g, Ma Huang 10g, Xi Xin 5g, Qiang Huo 10g. Two packs.

Case Study

Concurrent Pattern of Tai Yang and Shao Yin

Extracted from Wu Pei Heng Yi An 1979

A 42-year-old patient caught a cold walking home in the rain on a cold day. Initially there was fever, aversion to cold, a headache, aches and pains, sleepiness and a preference for warm drinks. The tongue was slightly purple and the coat was white and slippery; the pulse was submerged, thready and tight. The treatment principle was to warm the channels, release the exterior and support the zheng qi. The formula used was Ma Huang Xi Xin Fu Zi Tang: Fu Pian 10g, Ma Huang 10g (both decocted first), Xi Xin 6g, Gui Zhi 13g. After one dose, he came out in a sweat and the fever was resolved, but he still suffered from dizziness and cough. He was then given a combination of Si Ni Tang and Er Chen Tang with the addition of Xi Xin and Wu Wei Zi, following which he recovered.

Ma Huang Fu Zi Gan Cao Tang Pattern

Clause 302

少阴病，得之二三日，麻黄附子甘草汤微发汗。以二三日无证，故微发汗也。

Shao Yin disease, contracted for two or three days, Ma Huang Fu Zi Gan Cao Tang promotes a mild sweat. Because there were no symptoms for two or three days, a mild sweat must be promoted.

MA HUANG FU ZI GAN CAO TANG: Ma Huang (nodes removed) 2 liang; Zhi Gan Cao 2 liang; Fu Zi (skin removed and dry roasted) 1 piece sliced into 8 pieces.

DIRECTIONS: Simmer Ma Huang in 7 sheng of water, bringing to the boil once or twice, then skim and add the other ingredients. Boil again, reducing to 3 sheng. Strain and take 1 sheng warm three times a day.

DISCUSSION: Clause 302 is better read in conjunction with Clause 301, because both describe concurrent patterns of exterior Tai Yang and interior Shao Yin. However, although the pulse is submerged in both, indicative of the interior pattern, there are no interior symptoms, and so the promotion of sweat is permitted. Clause 301 advocates the use of Ma Huang Xi Xin Fu Zi Tang, which is hot and dispersing and promotes a rigorous sweat, and so it is understood that the Shao Yin pattern is less advanced and heavy sweating will be tolerated. Clause 302, however, recommends the milder formula of Ma Huang Fu Zi Gan Cao Tang, which is moderated by the omission of Xi Xin and the addition of Gan Cao, and only promotes a mild sweat. This indicates that it is to be used where the Shao Yin pattern has progressed, but not to the point of manifesting with interior symptoms such as diarrhoea or cold extremities.

Ma Huang Fu Zi Gan Cao Tang is Ma Huang Fu Zi Xi Xin Tang omitting Xi Xin and adding Zhi Gan Cao. Xi Xin is hot and acrid and, combined with Ma Huang, produces a strong sweat. Zhi Gan Cao is warm and is able to moderate the harsher action of Ma Huang and Fu Zi. The reason for replacing Xi Xin with Zhi Gan Cao is to avoid damage to fluids by promoting sweat two or three days into the disease, which is no longer in the acute phase. The acrid dispersing properties of Xi Xin are too harsh and have a propensity to damage qi and fluids. Zhi Gan Cao, on the other hand, is not an exterior releasing, sweat promoting herb, but is sweet and moderate, nourishing yin and tonifying qi. This modified formula is therefore appropriate for the condition described in Clause 302, where a more moderate warming action is required, and the objective is to promote a mild sweat in order to release the exterior.

The absence of interior cold symptoms has two implications: (1) the disease has not yet progressed to the point where the interior has been affected; and (2) because the Shao Yin pattern is not severe, sweating can be promoted. However, the clause tells us that in this concurrent pattern of Tai Yang Shao Yin, only mild sweating should be promoted to release the exterior. Heavy sweating is contraindicated because it will damage both the yin and the yang and cause deterioration of the Shao Yin pattern, which at this stage is not severe. The conclusion that can be drawn is that sweat promotion in a Shao Yin exterior pattern can only be used in the absence of interior deficiency symptoms; otherwise the interior cold must be addressed first before treating the exterior pattern with a formula which promotes sweat.

There are three formulas associated with the treatment of Tai Yang Shao Yin concurrent patterns, each one suitable according to the nature and severity of the pattern. (1) Ma Huang Fu Zi Xi Xin Tang is the indicated formula for the initial stage of wind cold invading the Shao Yin, characterised by fever and a submerged pulse, where the strategy is to warm the channels and promote sweat. (2) Ma Huang Fu Zi Gan Cao Tang is used to promote a mild sweat where the disease is no longer in the acute phase, but there are no manifestations of interior cold. (3) Si Ni Tang is indicated to warm the interior when there has been no resolution following the administration of either of the preceding two formulas, and where there are manifestations of interior cold, such as aches and pains in the body, diarrhoea and cold extremities, and a pulse which is submerged and faint.

Ancient Application of Ma Huang Fu Zi Gan Cao Tang

- *Jin Gui Yao Lue:* For the treatment of water qi where the pulse is submerged and small.
- *Wei Sheng Bao Jian Bu Yi:* For a patient suffering from fever characterised by cold extremities, a lack-lustre complexion and a pulse which is not palpable or which is verging on expiry.

Modern Application of Ma Huang Fu Zi Gan Cao Tang

Ma Huang Fu Zi Gan Cao Tang is indicated for an exterior pattern with an underlying deficiency of yang and is suitable for such disorders as coronary heart disease and acute or chronic nephritis. Cheng et al (*Jiangxi Zhong Yi Yao* 1980; 4:29) used Ma Huang Fu Zi Gan Cao Tang in the treatment of coronary heart disease with arrhythmia which was characterised by palpitations, shortness of breath, sweating and an oppressed sensation in the chest, all ascribed to insufficiency of heart yang. Ren Shen and Huang Qi were added to enhance the treatment effect.

Case Study

Oedema in the Lower Jiao

Extracted from Zhejiang Zhong Yi Za Zhi 1979; (5):12

A 35-year-old female had suffered for over four months from generalised oedema which was more pronounced in the lower jiao. Other symptoms were heaviness and pain in the lower back, scant urination, constipation, cold extremities, and a dusky complexion. Her tongue was pale and swollen and the tongue coat was white. The submerged thready pulse was weak and faint in the cubit position. The diagnosis was water flooding due to yang deficiency. The formula given was Ma Huang Fu Zi Gan Cao Tang: Ma Huang 4.5g, Fu Zi 9g, Zhi Gan Cao 6g, Hei Dou (black bean) 30g, Che Qian Zi 12g. After five packs, the oedema subsided, her facial complexion improved, and her energy increased. A milder formula was then prescribed for three days, with a reduction in the dose of Ma Huang to 3g and that of Fu Zi to 6g. Following that, there was full recovery.

6.4.2 Concurrent Pattern of Shao Yin and Yang Ming

Da Cheng Qi Tang

Clause 320

少阴病，得之二三日，口燥咽干者，急下之，宜大承气汤。

Shao Yin disease, contracted for two or three days, if the mouth is parched and the throat is dry, one should urgently purge, Da Cheng Qi Tang is appropriate.

DISCUSSION: A parched mouth and throat occurring after two or three days of Shao Yin disease is attributed to the knotting of dryness and heat in the interior, which consumes fluids and scorches the kidney yin. This represents severe damage to the kidney yin and Da Cheng Qi Tang is indicated to purge heat as a matter of urgency, in order to preserve the yin. This emergency measure is employed in order to prevent further damage to yin, and is comparable to removing firewood from beneath a cauldron so as not to burn the contents.

Past annotators of *Shang Han Lun* considered this to be a transmuted pattern because the symptoms of a dry mouth and parched throat, although indicating interior heat, do not of themselves justify urgent purgation. Evidence of stomach excess and the appropriate pulse sign are necessary before implementing this strategy, and this can be seen in Clause 321, as follows.

Clause 321

少阴病，自利清水，色纯青，心下必痛，口干燥者，可下之，宜大承气汤。

Shao Yin disease, spontaneous watery diarrhoea of a greenish colour, there will be pain below the heart, if the mouth is parched, one may purge, Da Cheng Qi Tang is appropriate.

DISCUSSION: The reference to Shao Yin disease indicates that there is exhaustion of true yin by pathogenic heat. It is this which is the cause of the diarrhoea, which takes the form of a greenish watery discharge. The heat has descended to the lower jiao, producing knotted heat and dryness in the intestines. The extruded fluids run off from the dry stool, and are excreted as a foul watery discharge. The knotted dry heat obstructs the middle jiao and the stagnation of stomach qi manifests as pain below the heart, which is aggravated by pressure; the damage to yin fluids and their non-distribution results in a parched throat and mouth, and if immediate steps are not taken to stop further devastation of yin fluids, the exhaustion of yin will reach a critical point. Da Cheng Qi Tang is recommended to preserve the yin fluids as a matter of urgency.

The key point in Clause 321 is the greenish coloured watery stool. Because it is associated with constipation due to heat bind, it would be malodorous. The watery discharge does not represent a runny stool, but is separated from the dry, hard stool which can not be passed. The unusual manifestation of a dry stool with leakage of foul fluid is generally associated with excess heat in the Yang Ming, but here it is a feature of Shao Yin disease where the dry stool is a result of heat having exhausted yin. The phenomenon of a dry stool with leakage of foul fluid encountered in a Shao Yin pattern of extreme yin depletion is more serious than the simple fluid depletion and difficult defaecation of a Yang Ming pattern.

Clause 322

少阴病，六七日，腹胀、不大便者，急下之，宜大承气汤。

Shao Yin disease, for six or seven days, if the abdomen is distended and there is no stool, one should urgently purge, Da Cheng Qi Tang is appropriate.

DISCUSSION: Shao Yin disease which has lasted for six or seven days, and where there is abdominal distension and constipation, is attributed to interior dryness binding the stool. The constipation and abdominal fullness belong to a Yang Ming bowel excess pattern. The knotted heat and dryness has scorched the yin fluids, causing dryness of the mouth and throat. However, the practitioner must not rely on these symptoms alone; the pattern of urgent purging must be confirmed by the tongue and pulse.

The essential points in diagnosing a Shao Yin pattern of urgent purgation are found in three clauses, each having a different emphasis. Clause 320 is focused on the damage to yin fluids by heat and dryness which is demonstrated in the parched mouth and throat. Clause 321 demonstrates the degree of fluid loss due to the knotting of heat and dryness by mentioning the dryness in the mouth and throat and also describing the phenomenon of constipation with the leakage of faecal fluid. Clause 322 simply focuses on the abdominal distension and constipation of Yang Ming bowel excess; the potential for fluid damage is implied by the recommendation for urgent purgation. Because all three clauses have a similar pathogenesis, they share Da Cheng Qi Tang as the indicated treatment.

In the Yang Ming chapter, there are three references to patterns requiring urgent purgation, all of which are associated with the knotting of severe heat and dryness in the intestines. The three Shao Yin patterns of urgent purgation are also due to the knotting of heat and dryness in the Yang Ming, with attendant damage to the true yin of Shao Yin. The Shao Yin pattern of urgent purgation can be understood as a transmuted pattern of Shao Yin attributed to exuberant deficiency heat having caused severe damage to yin fluids. The strategy of urgent purgation can not be justified on the sole basis of interior heat with injury to yin, and must only be used in the presence of Yang Ming fu excess. Nevertheless, modern disease diagnoses such as encephalitis or epidemic meningitis bear similar clinical features, and the strategy of purgation can be justified wherever it is necessary to eliminate interior heat in order to prevent damage to yin as a matter of urgency.

There are two situations associated with urgent purgation in Shao Yin. (1) The incorrect treatment of a Yang Ming heat bind pattern resulting in the consumption of true yin. (2) A pre-existing yin deficiency where heat in the

Yang Ming has further exhausted yin fluids. It can be said that the nature of a Shao Yin urgent purgation pattern is excess and deficiency. By this it is meant that exuberant excess heat in the bowel scorches the true yin, resulting in obstruction in the large intestine.

Zhang Zhong Jing uses the phrase "excess earth and water exhaustion" to refer to excess in the Yang Ming stomach and deficiency in the Shao Yin kidney, and it is this which leads to a parched mouth and the greenish watery effluent from the large intestine. Because there is constipation and abdominal fullness, Da Cheng Qi Tang is indicated. However, although the rationale of urgent purgation in Shao Yin has a similar rationale, the objective is not the same. The aim of urgent purgation in Yang Ming disease is to preserve the yin of the stomach, whilst in Shao Yin, the aim is to preserve the yin of the kidneys. By comparing the Shao Yin urgent purgation patterns with those of Yang Ming, the reader will better comprehend the overall picture. By appreciating the urgent nature of the disease, prompt and appropriate measures can be taken.

6.4.3 Concurrent Pattern of Shao Yin and Shao Yang

Si Ni San

Clause 318

少阴病，四逆，其人或咳，或悸，或小便不利，或腹中痛，或泄利下重者，四逆散主之。

Shao Yin disease, the four are reversed, if the person has either a cough, or palpitations, or the urination is not free, or there is pain in the abdomen, or diarrhoea with heaviness below, Si Ni San governs.

SI NI SAN: Zhi Gan Cao; Zhi Shi (broken, soaked in water then dried); Chai Hu; Shao Yao (10 fen of each).

DIRECTIONS: Grind into a powder, sieve and mix well. Stir 1 square-inch-spoonful of the powder into cooled rice water and take three times a day.

MODIFICATIONS: (1) For cough or diarrhoea, add 5 fen each of Wu Wei Zi and Gan Jiang. (2) For palpitations, add 5 fen of Gui Zhi. (3) For inhibited urination, add 5 fen of Fu Ling. (4) For pain in the abdomen, add 1 piece of Fu Zi which has been dry-fried until cracked. (5) For diarrhoea with rectal heaviness, boil 3 sheng of Cong Bai in 5 sheng of water, reducing to 3 sheng. Strain and add 3 square-inch-spoonfuls of the powder. Boil and reduce to 1½ sheng. Divide into two portions and take warm twice a day.

DISCUSSION: Clause 318 describes a pattern of interior yang constraint with coldness in the extremities, referred to as 'the four are reversed'. This coldness in the hands and feet is not a direct consequence of a yang deficiency, but is the result of the Shao Yin failing to provide passage for the movement of yang qi. The Shao Yin constraint affects not only the ascent and descent of qi, but also its general dispersal. This then may give rise to coughing, to palpitations, inhibited urination, abdominal pain or diarrhoea with a heavy sensation in the rectum. Coughing is a result of lung qi not descending; palpitations are a result of the yang qi not reaching the heart, and devitalised heart yang can no longer rule the vessels; inhibited urination and rectal heaviness represent the failure of the descent of qi in the lower jiao; abdominal pain reflects the non-flow of qi in the channels; diarrhoea is the result of constrained yang not supporting transformation. These are all manifestations of the impaired Shao Yin pivot mechanism which has resulted in qi constraint.

The concept of the pivot mechanism of Shao Yin is explained on the basis of Shao Yin being located between Tai Yin and Jue Yin. If the Shao Yin pivot mechanism is impaired, liver qi can be constrained and disharmony of the liver and spleen can arise. The symptoms described in Clause 318 are all manifestations of qi constraint arising as a result of impairment to the Shao Yin pivot mechanism, and so the indicated formula is Si Ni San, which disperses constrained liver qi and promotes the flow of yang qi. Chai Hu effectively restores the pivot mechanism, thus facilitating the movement of qi and dispersing the constrained yang. The proper distribution of yang qi warms the limbs and disperses cold in the extremities; Zhi Shi regulates qi and, when combined with the ascending properties of Chai Hu, is able to disperse constraint and dissipate stagnation in all directions, thus normalising the movement of qi; Shao Yao and Zhi Gan Cao harmonise the liver and spleen and relax tension. The combined effect of the four herbs disperses constrained qi, eliminates stagnation and restores the normal distribution of yang qi.

The actions of the herbs used by Zhong Jing in the modifications are as follows. In the treatment of cough, Gan Jiang warms the lungs, promotes the flow of yang qi and resolves phlegm, while Wu Wei Zi astringes the lung qi to stop the cough. In the treatment of diarrhoea, Gan Jiang warms the middle and fortifies kidney yang, whilst Wu Wei Zi secures the kidneys and stops diarrhoea. In the treatment of palpitations, Gui Zhi supports the flow of yang qi in the vessels of the heart. In inhibited urination, Fu Ling is added because it promotes urination. Abdominal pain is treated with Fu Zi because it warms the interior and expels cold. For diarrhoea with rectal heaviness, Cong Bai is added to unblock the yang and disperse cold.

Differentiation of Cold Extremities in Si Ni Tang and Si Ni San

Shang Han Lun describes the role of the Shao Yang channel as being a pivot for the movement of qi between the exterior and interior; the role played by Shao Yin, on the other hand, serves to facilitate the movement of qi between all the yin channels. The symptom of coldness in the four limbs or 'si ni' in the Si Ni **San** pattern is not the same as that of the Si Ni **Tang** pattern. Cold extremities are a key feature of both patterns. However, the cold limbs of a Shao Yin Si Ni Tang pattern are a reflection of interior exuberant yin which is a consequence of the kidney yang deficiency. It is therefore accompanied by other yang deficiency symptoms such as aversion to cold, sleeping or lying in a curled up posture, diarrhoea with undigested food particles and a faint and thready pulse. The indicated formula is Si Ni Tang which warms the interior and dispels cold. The cold extremities of a Si Ni San pattern, however, are not accompanied by other manifestations of cold, because the pathogenesis is not cold, but impairment of the Shao Yin pivot resulting in the non-dispersal of yang qi. The cold extremities of the Si Ni San pattern are milder than those of the Si Ni Tang pattern. The cold limbs of both these patterns must also be differentiated from the cold limbs which appear in a pattern of exuberant heat constraint, referred to as 'severe heat and severe reversal', so called because the more severe the heat, the more severe the coldness of the extremities; the indicated formula is Bai Hu Tang. Thus it can be seen why it is important to have a clear understanding of the implications and differentiation of the symptom 'cold extremities'.

Past interpretations of Shao Yin disease with cold extremities have been varied. The first was Cheng Wu Ji who said it represented shang han disease with the pathogen in Shao Yang and transmission to Shao Yin. Shen Ming Zong said it was due to pathogenic qi in the Shao Yin combined with a patten of liver wood harassing the earth stomach. Zhang Lu said: "Although there is Shao Yin disease, it is actually a disharmony of the spleen and stomach with obstruction of the clear yang failing to warm the four limbs". Xu Da Chun said that it was a result of the pathogen transmitting to the Shao Yin and transforming into heat. Lu Yuan Lei said: "This is a Shao Yang type of pattern and should not be treated as Shao Yin disease".

Regardless of the various interpretations of past *Shang Han* specialists, the important thing is to differentiate the cold limbs of the Si Ni San pattern from those of the Shao Yin yang deficiency pattern which is accompanied by cold symptoms. The pivot mechanism of qi is not governed only by the Shao Yang channel, which serves to connect the exterior and interior, but also by the Shao Yin which serves as a pivot for yin and yang and has particular significance in the interaction of fire and water. The Shao Yin provides communication with the Tai Yin and Jue Yin. As with the Shao Yang, the failure of the pivot mechanism to disseminate qi will give rise to constraint and stagnation which, in turn, will lead to spleen and liver disharmony, with ensuing pain and distension in the hypchondrium, or diarrhoea, or vomiting. In the clinical situation, this may relate to emotional stress causing liver qi constraint.

Ancient Application of Si Ni San

- *Jing Yue Quan Shu:* For the treatment of hypochondriac pain, glomus below the heart, alternating chills and fever and dysmenorrhoea, substitute Zhi Shi with Zhi Qiao and add Xiang Fu, Chuan Xiong.
- *Lei Ju Fang Guang Yi:* Si Ni San was advocated for incessant dysentery characterised by hypochondriac pain, glomus and tenesmus.

Modern Application of Si Ni San

Si Ni San can be used in the treatment of chronic hepatitis, pancreatitis, enteritis, acute appendicitis, gastritis and ulceration attributed to disharmony of the liver and stomach. It can also be used to treat irregular menstruation, leucorrhoea, pelvic inflammatory disease, heart palpitations and cough. Yan et al reported using Si Ni San to treat infantile fever with cold extremities (*Hu Bei Zhong Yi Za Zhi* 1981; 6:30).

Case Study

Chronic Abdominal Pain and Diarrhoea

Extracted from Greta Young's case studies

A 40-year-old female patient had been suffering from chronic abdominal pain and diarrhoea for nearly ten years. Endoscopy and colonoscopy confirmed that she was suffering from chronic atrophic gastritis and chronic colitis. She presented with fullness in the epigastrium, persistent abdominal distension and pain, and up to five episodes of diarrhoea a day, accompanied by a sticky discharge. She had a poor appetite, and dream-disturbed sleep. Her tongue was pale with a thin, white tongue coat. Her pulse was wiry, fine and slightly slippery. The diagnosis was constrained liver qi leading to impairment of spleen yang and stomach disharmony. The treatment principle was to regulate the liver and spleen and to free the yang of the middle jiao. The patient was prescribed ten packs of Si Ni San modified: Chai Hu 10g, Zhi Qiao 10g, Bai Shao 10g, Dang Shen 10g, Pao Jiang 10g, Huang Qin 10g, Ban Xia 10g, Da Fu Pi 10g, Huang Lian 6g, Zhi Gan Cao 6g, Di Yu Tan 30g. After this course of medication, Shen Ling Bai Zhi San was prescribed to consolidate the treatment. After two months, the colonoscopy report was near normal.

Discussion: Si Ni San modified is indicated for chronic gastritis, duodenal ulcer and chronic colitis due to constrained liver qi. The gallbladder stores bile and depends upon the free coursing of liver qi to maintain its normal function. If the liver qi is constrained, this may in turn affect the normal discharge of bile, and may manifest as hypochondriac pain, a bitter taste in the mouth, a parched throat, vertigo, constipation, nausea, and a thick and greasy tongue coat.

Case Study

Infertility

Extracted from Gui Yang Zhong Yi Xue Bao 1991; (1):15

A 25-year-old woman had been married for three years and had not conceived. Her menstrual cycle was irregular and painful, and she suffered from tender painful breasts premenstrually and also from heavy leucorrhoea. Her appetite and urination were normal, her tongue was a dark purplish colour and had a thin, white coat and her pulse was submerged, fine and slightly wiry. On examination, it was found that she had a retroverted uterus and blocked fallopian tubes. The diagnosis was constrained liver qi with blood stagnation and the formula given was a modification of Si Ni San: Chai Hu, Zhi Shi, Dang Gui, Chuan Xiong, Chi Bai Shao, Sheng Di, Tao Ren, Dan Pi, Yu Jin, Chuan Shan Jia 10g each, Ze Lan Ye, Yi Mu Cao, Fu Ling 15g each, Gui Zhi, Da Huang Tan, Zhi Gan Cao 6g each. She was asked to take five doses prior to each menstrual cycle for the next three months. After three months of medication, her pulse became normal and she gave birth to a little boy the following year.

Note: Si Ni San has the potential for broad application, dispersing constrained liver qi, regulating menstruation and stemming leucorrhoea. Liver qi stagnation is extremely common in gynaecological complaints, because blood and qi form the basis of women's menstruation and the liver has an intimate connection to the uterus, and is responsible for spreading qi and storing and regulating blood. The gallbladder qi assists the liver in its function of coursing qi. The free flow of liver qi is therefore important for gynaecological and reproductive health. Where liver qi is stagnant, the strategy is to disperse liver qi, nourish blood, and regulate menstrual flow. The analysis of Tiao Jing Wan Dai Tang (Chai Hu, Zhi Shi, Shao Yao, Zhi Gan Cao, Dang Gui, Chuan Xiong, Bai Zhu, Ze Lan Ye, Yi Mu Cao) is as follows. It contains Si Ni San to spread liver qi and unblock constrained yang; it also contains Si Wu Tang to nourish yin and blood; and finally contains Bai Zhu to strengthen the spleen, resolve damp and check the leucorrhoea, and Ze Lan and Yi Mu Cao to invigorate blood and regulate the menstruation.

Case Study

Testicular Swelling

Extracted from Shang Han Shi Jian Lun

A 32-year-old male patient presented with swelling of the right testicle, which was hard and had enlarged to the size of a hen's egg. He also suffered heaviness and discomfort in the lower abdomen. His stool and urination were normal and the blood tests showed no abnormality. His pulse was wiry and moderate and his tongue coat was thin, white and moist. He was given Si Ni San modified: Chai Hu 10g, Chi Shao 15g, Zhi Qiao 10g, Zhi Gan Cao 5g, Qing Pi 10g, Ju He 15g (broken), Li Zi He 15g (broken), Xiang Fu 10g, Wu Yao 10g, Sheng Mu Li 15g, Yu Jin 10g, Hua Shi 15g. After four packs, the swelling was reduced. There was tenderness but the heaviness in the lower abdomen was gone. The same formula was repeated with the addition of Tian Hua Fen 15g, Ren Dong Teng 20g. After taking seven packs, he recovered.

Discussion: The rationale of using Si Ni San was based on the location of the disorder being in the liver channel, a branch of which encircles the genitalia. The patient's blood test was normal and there was no constrained heat toxin, so a formula focused on clearing heat and toxicity was not called for. Si Ni San with the addition of Qing Pi, Ju He, Li Zi He, Yu Jin and Xiang Fu was prescribed to move and regulate the flow of qi in the liver channel; Wu Yao was used to eliminate pain and stagnation in the lower jiao; Mu Li was added to soften hardness and reduce the swelling; Hua Shi and Gan Cao were used to drain damp heat. Ren Dong Teng was added to the second formula to resolve toxic heat from the lower jiao to ensure complete recovery.

6.4.4 Summary of Shao Yin Concurrent Patterns

1. A concurrent pattern of Shao Yin and Tai Yang is characterised by a submerged pulse and fever. There are no interior symptoms and the indicated formula is either Ma Huang Xi Xin Fu Zi Tang or Ma Huang Fu Zi Gan Cao Tang.
2. A concurrent pattern of Shao Yin and Yang Ming is characterised by abdominal fullness, a hard stool with foul watery discharge, pain below the heart, and a parched mouth and throat, and the strategy is one of urgent purgation to preserve the yin using Da Cheng Qi Tang.
3. A concurrent pattern of Shao Yin and Shao Yang is characterised by mildly cold extremities and the formula is Si Ni San to disperse constrained yang.

Section Five

6.5 SHAO YIN SORE THROAT PATTERNS

Sore throat patterns associated with the Shao Yin channel are patterns of yin deficiency with empty fire, which may or may not be accompanied by phlegm or other pathogenic processes and their manifestations. In Chinese, the term *yan* (咽) refers to the back of the throat or oral pharynx situated behind the root of the tongue and extending from the nasal pharynx to the larynx; it is linked to the stomach. The term *hou* (喉) refers to the laryngopharynx, which is directly below that, and is immediately posterior to and includes the larynx; it has a connection with the lungs. In practice, the two are closely linked and commonly both are affected.

Zhu Fu Tang Pattern

Clause 310

少阴病，下利、咽痛、胸满、心烦，猪肤汤主之。

Shao Yin disease, there is diarrhoea, the throat is sore, the chest feels full, the heart is vexed, Zhu Fu Tang governs.

ZHU FU TANG: Zhu Fu (pig's skin) 1 jin.

DIRECTIONS: Boil the above ingredients in 1 dou of water, reducing to 5 sheng. Strain and add 1 sheng of honey and 5 ge of rice flour, which has been dry-fried until the aroma is released, then blend thoroughly. Divide into six doses and take warm.

DISCUSSION: Shao Yin diarrhoea can be associated with cold conversion or heat conversion. Clause 310 describes the latter, where the diarrhoea is a result of deficiency heat harassing the intestines. Here, both the diarrhoea and sore throat are manifestations of yin deficiency in the Shao Yin channel. The fluid loss caused by the continuous diarrhoea has depleted fluids and the consumption of kidney yin results in empty heat, which flares upward to the throat along the course of the kidney channel, causing a sore throat. On its way to the throat, the kidney channel crosses the diaphragm and connects with the liver and lungs as it passes through the chest; the obstruction of these channels by the deficiency heat gives rise to fullness in the chest and a feeling of vexation in the heart. Because the heat is not due to an excess pathogen but is due to yin deficiency, the treatment strategy is to nourish the yin of the kidneys and lungs in order to clear heat.

Zhu Fu Tang or pig skin soup is made from the skin of a piece of pork with the inner layer of fatty meat removed. It is sweet and moistening and so nourishes fluids. By enriching kidney water and supplementing yin, it moistens dryness and clears heat from deficiency. Honey is sweet and cold, it moistens the lung, augments qi and soothes irritability. Rice flour harmonises the stomach and tonifies the spleen, thus addressing qi deficiency diarrhoea. Together, these ingredients enrich the kidneys, moisten the lungs, and tonify the spleen.

Because the sore throat in this pattern is due to the upsurge of empty fire, it is associated with yin deficiency and dryness. The pain is relatively mild and must be differentiated from a sore throat caused by wind heat or toxic heat where there is inflammation, swelling and a burning sensation. To focus on treating diarrhoea, the indicated formula is Tong Mai Si Ni Tang to warm the interior. Zhong Jing laid the foundation for the herbal treatment of wen bing or warm disease where the heat had damaged yin. Tian Men Dong, Mai Men Dong, Tai Zi Shen, Shi Hu, Shan Yao and E Jiao are all indicated for the treatment of a sore throat with yin deficiency, and can be used in such cases as chronic laryngitis.

Modern Application of Zhu Fu Tang

This formula is seldom used in modern times, but has been used in the treatment of chronic laryngitis due to yin deficiency and dryness, and also in primary thrombocytopenia characterised by fluid damage (*Shang Han Lun Tang Zheng Lun Zhi* 2000).

> **Case Study**
>
> **Sore Throat and Hoarseness**
> ***Extracted from Shang Han Qie Yao***
>
> A 22-year-old female patient, who was a singer by profession and due to perform, was suffering from hoarseness and taking Pang Da Hai had not helped. She was then asked to take Zhu Fu Tang mixed with egg white, which is sweet and cool and soothes the throat. Her voice returned to normal after four doses.

Gan Cao Tang and Jie Geng Tang Pattern

> **Clause 311**
>
> 少阴病二三日，咽痛者，可与甘草汤；不差，与桔梗汤。
>
> Shao Yin disease for two or three days, if the throat is sore, one may give Gan Cao Tang; if there is no relief, give Jie Geng Tang.

GAN CAO TANG: Gao Cao 2 liang.

DIRECTIONS: Boil in 3 sheng of water, reducing to 1½ sheng. Strain and take 7 ge warm twice a day.

JIE GENG TANG: Jie Geng 1 liang; Gan Cao 2 liang.

DIRECTIONS: Boil in 3 sheng of water, reducing to 1 sheng. Strain, divide into 2 portions and take warm twice a day.

DISCUSSION: Clause 311 describes a situation where heat associated with the yin deficiency of Shao Yin disease rises up the channel and harasses the throat. There are no other symptoms and so Gan Cao can be given, decocted as a single herb. If there is no relief, Jie Geng Tang is given, which is specific for its beneficial effect on the throat. When raw, Gan Cao is neutral, clears heat and relieves toxicity; it can reduce swelling and inflammation, treat abscess and benefit the throat. Xu Bing said: "Gan Cao as a single herb can harmonise yin and clear heat associated with the Chong and Ren. For the treatment of abscess, use four liang of Sheng Gan Cao to effect a speedy recovery, it clears Shao Yin deficiency heat and is a special herb to treat a sore throat" (*Shang Han Lun Annotations*).

Jie Geng is bitter and acrid; it enters the lung channel, disseminates lung qi and benefits the throat. When used together, Jie Geng and Gan Cao are effective in disinhibiting the throat and easing pain. Jie Geng Tang is also known as Gan Cao Jie Geng Tang; it is renowned for treating a sore throat and when given in frequent doses, it disinhibits the throat and loosens the chest and diaphragm.

Gan Cao appears in seventy *Shang Han Lun* formulas, with almost all specifying Zhi Gan Cao. Sheng Gan Cao is used in this formula because it is the raw form which clears heat and toxicity and it has a greater moistening effect. *Ben Cao Zheng* says: "Gan Cao is sweet and neutral, it reduces the toxicity of toxic herbs; when mixed with exterior releasing herbs, it enhances the exterior releasing function; if mixed with purging herbs, it moderates the purging action". Zhong Jing used Gan Cao in both its raw and prepared form with the objective of draining fire, relieving toxicity, stopping cough, transforming phlegm, tonifying spleen and heart qi, benefiting the throat and moistening the lungs. Its effect is mild and moderating and it is also used to alleviate glomus and ease pain.

Ancient Application of Jie Geng Tang

- *Qian Jin Yao Fang:* For the treatment of *hou bi* or throat impediment, 1 liang each of Jie Geng and Zhi Gan Cao were boiled in 1 sheng of water and taken warm to discharge pus.
- *Lan Shi Mi Cang:* For the treatment of macules with a sore throat. When given in frequent doses, it disinhibits the throat and loosens the chest and diaphragm.

Modern Application of Jie Geng Tang

- For chronic laryngitis with an inflamed, sore throat, Jie Geng Tang with Ban Lan Gen, Jin Yin Hua and Niu Bang Zi are often combined to clear toxic heat and disinhibit the throat. If the throat is red and the pulse is thready and

rapid, this indicates yin deficiency and Mai Dong and Xuan Shen can be added.
- For plumstone throat, Jie Geng Tang with Bai Mei Hua, Chai Hu, Su Zi and Ban Xia.
- For cough, Jie Geng Tang with Chuan Bei Mu, Bai Bu, Huang Qin and Qian Hu, where there is a sore throat, phlegm and a thready and rapid pulse.

Case Study

Sore Throat and Hoarseness

Extracted from Zhang Zhong JIng Yao Fa Yan Jiu 1984: 656

A 16-year-old girl competed in a track event and after the race she suddenly became hoarse. Investigations showed that she had dysfunctional vocal cord disorder. Her face was red, her throat red and swollen, her breathing was rapid, she coughed frequently and had a red tongue with a white coat. The patient had a history of recurrent sore throats and head colds. The diagnosis was toxic wind heat in the Shao Yin channel. The formula given was Jie Geng Tang combined with Qian Jin Wei Jing Tang and Zhu Ye Shi Gao Tang modified: Jie Geng 12g, Gan Cao 10g, Lu Gen 15g, Dong Gua Ren 12g, Tao Ren 9g, Zhu Ye 9g, Sheng Shi Gao 24g, Mai Dong 10g, Ban Xia 3g, Tai Zi Shen 15g, Niu Bang Zi 9g. After three packs, there was full recovery.

Ku Jiu Tang pattern

Clause 312

少阴病，咽中伤、生疮、不能语言、声不出者，苦酒汤主之。

Shao Yin disease, if there is injury to the throat, an abscess has formed, the person can not speak, or there is no voice, Ku Jiu Tang governs.

KU JIU TANG: Ban Xia (washed and broken to the size of a date seed) 14 pieces; a hen's egg (remove the yolk and add rice vinegar to the shell). Note that *ku jiu* 苦酒 refers to vinegar.

DIRECTIONS: Place the Ban Xia in the eggshell filled with vinegar, and set the eggshell in the ring of a knife handle and hold over a flame. Let it come to the boil three times then strain. Hold a little in the mouth and swallow. If there is no relief, make up three more lots. Note that the unusual cooking method of using the eggshell as a cooking utensil is done by retaining the eggwhite, adding the vinegar and then the Ban Xia which has been broken into many small pieces. The instruction to use a knife handle is merely a convenience because most knives had a big ring at the end of the handle, which was the right size for an egg, and served well to hold the eggshell over the flame while the mixture cooked. In the absence of a knife handle, a loop of wire could be used to hold the eggshell over the flame.

DISCUSSION: In Shao Yin disease, if the throat is ulcerated and the person can not speak, it means that toxic heat has attacked the throat, damaging the vessels and causing swelling and pain. The knotting of fire and turbidity obstructs the passage of qi and impedes the ability of the throat to produce sound: the person is either hoarse or has completely lost their voice. Ku Jiu Tang can reduce swelling, heal open sores, and ease pain. Ban Xia transforms phlegm and turbidity; the egg white is sweet and cool, moistens dryness and clears heat, thus countering the drying properties of Ban Xia; the rice vinegar is sweet, sour and astringent, thus reducing the toxic swelling and promoting healing. The mixture is held in the back of mouth before swallowing in order to gain benefit from the topical application.

Ban Xia San or Tang Pattern

Clause 313

少阴病，咽中痛，半夏散及汤主之。

Shao Yin disease, there is pain in the throat, Ban Xia San and Tang govern.

BAN XIA SAN: Ban Xia (washed); Gui Zhi (bark removed); Zhi Gan Cao.

DIRECTIONS: Using equal amounts of the above ingredients, pound, grind and sieve each one separately before combining. Blend with a little cooled rice water (*bai yin* 白饮) and take one square-inch-spoonful of the blended powder three times a day. If the powder can not be taken, boil 1 sheng of water seven times, add 2 square-inch-spoonfuls of powder, bring to the boil three more times, then remove from the flame, cool slightly, and drink in small amounts. Ban Xia is toxic and should not be taken in powder form; it is for this reason that the powder is blended with rice water.

DISCUSSION: By examining the ingredients of Ban Xia San, one can see that it is designed to treat an attack of wind cold in the Shao Yin channel, with constrained yang qi and the congelation of phlegm damp. The pathogenesis is constrained pathogenic cold and the swelling and pain of the throat is a result of phlegm damp obstructing the channel qi. The indicated formula is Ban Xia San or Tang to disperse the cold, open the channels and sweep congealed phlegm damp to relieve the obstruction and pain.

Ban Xia is acrid and warm and it dries damp and resolves phlegm; Gui Zhi is acrid and warm and it disperses wind cold; Gan Cao is sweet, harmonises the middle and benefits the throat. Together, these three herbs disperse cold, eliminate the phlegm obstruction and so relieve the sore throat. The rice water is sweet and warm, it tonifies the spleen and stomach, nourishes fluids and augments qi, and at the same time counters the toxicity of Ban Xia and the dryness of Gui Zhi. If preferred, Ban Xia San can be prepared as a decoction rather than taken as a powder.

Clause 313 does not elaborate on the pattern and the only symptom cited is the sore throat. However, based on the warm nature of the formula, the conclusion can be drawn that it is a pattern of cold or wind cold or wind cold damp, and because it is a Shao Yin pattern, there must be an underlying yin deficiency. The fact that it is associated with cold distinguishes it from other Shao Yin sore throat patterns; the throat would not be as red and swollen as in a heat pattern. Other symptoms would be an aversion to cold, a thin white tongue coat, watery sputum, and other manifestations of cold.

There are three points made regarding the method of administration of Ban Xia San.

1. *Taking it with rice water.* The objective of blending the powder with rice water is to protect the stomach and its fluids from the acrid dryness of the herbs in this formula. Rice water or rice gruel is also taken with Wu Ling San and San Wu Bai San with the same objective. In *Shang Han Lun,* Bai Hu Tang, Bai Hu jia Ren Shen Tang, Tao Hua Tang and Zhu Ye Shi Gao Tang are all decocted with non-glutinous rice or *jing mi* 粳米. The reason for taking rice gruel after administration of other formulas such as Gui Zhi Tang, Li Zhong Wan and San Wu Bai San is to supplement the middle qi in order to strengthen the zheng qi.
2. *Taking it in small amounts.* This is similar to the method of medication with Ku Jiu Tang to facilitate more effective application of the herbs on the affected area. In practice, this can be done by rinsing the throat or slowly swallowing the medication.
3. *The option of powder or decoction.* Either can be used.

Ancient Application of Ban Xia San

- *Qian Jin Yao Fang:* For the treatment of throat bi with an inability to speak.
- *Lei Fang Zhun Sheng:* For an acute attack of cold characterised by sore throat, Ban Xia Gui Zhi Gan Cao Tang was used with 2.5 qian of Ban Xia San, adding 5 pieces of Sheng Jiang.

Modern Application of Ban Xia San

Ban Xia San is used in the treatment of upper respiratory infection with a sore throat or laryngitis.

Summary of Sore Throat Patterns

Sore throat patterns in Shao Yin arise as a result of the pathway of the channel passing through the throat. However, it must be remembered that the sore throat of Shao Yin is just one feature of the pattern and the formulas used to treat the throat do just that, and do not address the underlying Shao Yin pattern. The four patterns are as follows.

- *Zhu Fu Tang pattern.* This is a pattern where the heat arising from yin deficiency in the Shao Yin harasses the throat and is accompanied by diarrhoea, fullness in the chest and vexation;

the strategy is to nourish lung and kidney yin and drain empty fire.

- *Gan Cao Tang or Jie Geng Tang pattern*. This is a pattern of pathogenic heat attacking the Shao Yin channel, giving rise to an inflamed and swollen sore throat. The treatment is to clear heat, relieve toxicity and disseminate lung qi.
- *Ku Jiu Tang pattern*. This is a pattern of toxic fire searing the throat and injuring the vessels; this leads to ulceration, inflammation and pain in the throat, accompanied by an inability to utter sound. The treatment is to clear heat, reduce toxic swelling, and resolve turbidity.
- *Ban Xia San or Tang pattern*. This pattern is one where pathogenic cold has attacked the Shao Yin causing a sore throat, aversion to cold, a cough due to qi reversal and profuse watery sputum. The treatment is to warm the channels, disperse cold, and sweep away the congealed phlegm damp.

These four formulas treat Shao Yin sore throat patterns attributed to the flaring of deficient heat, pathogenic heat, toxic fire with turbidity, and cold damp congelation. These formulas do not contain bitter, cold herbs conventionally used to treat a sore throat, but use warm or moistening herbs which nourish yin, clear heat, resolve phlegm and disseminate the lung qi.

Comparison of Sore Throat Patterns in Shao Yin

	Zhu Fu Tang	Gan Cao Tang Jie Geng Tang	Ku Jiu Tang	Ban Xia San and Tang
Pathogenesis	Shao Yin yin deficiency with an upsurge of deficiency fire	Pathogenic heat in the Shao Yin channel	Pathogenic heat harassing the Shao Yin channel with constrained fire due to yin deficiency	Pathogenic heat harassing the Shao Yin channel with yang constraint
Key Symptoms	Sore throat, diarrhoea, fullness in the chest and vexation	Inflamed throat (redness, swelling and heat)	Severe inflamed and ulcerated throat with loss of voice	Swelling and pain in the throat with phlegm and aversion to cold
Treatment	Clear heat, moisten dryness, nourish the lungs and kidneys	Clear heat, relieve toxicity, disinhibit the throat, ease pain	Clear heat, relieve toxicity, astringe ulceration and restore voice	Warm and dissipate the cold pathogen; disinhibit the throat and ease pain

Section Six

6.6 CONTRAINDICATED TREATMENTS IN SHAO YIN DISEASE

Clause 284

少阴病，咳而下利、谵语者，被火气劫故也。小便必难，以强责少阴汗也。

Shao Yin disease, if there is cough and diarrhoea with delirious speech, it is due to being raided by fire. Urination will be difficult, because sweating was wrongly forced in Shao Yin.

DISCUSSION: Shao Yin disease presenting with cough and diarrhoea can be attributed either to a yang deficiency associated with cold conversion, or a yin deficiency associated with heat conversion. The delirious speech, however, is not part of a Shao Yin pattern, but is a direct result of incorrect fire therapy. If the pattern is one of yang deficiency with water flooding, then Zhen Wu Tang is indicated to fortify the yang and scatter the yin cold. In heat conversion, where heat has knotted with water, Zhu Ling Tang is used to nourish yin and clear heat. Irrespective of whether the pattern is one of heat conversion or cold conversion, the underlying Shao Yin pattern is one of interior deficiency, and so the promotion of sweat is contraindicated. The phrase "raided by fire" in Clause 284 refers to the incorrect use of fire therapy to promote sweat which is compared here to a wrongful act of violence. Namely, the forcing of sweat is likened to the pillaging of yin fluids, resulting in the flaring of empty fire, with the heart yang cast upwards, causing delirious speech. Difficult urination is a reflection of the depletion of body fluids.

This clause describes a transmuted pattern caused by the incorrect use of fire therapy. The reason for this erroneous treatment can be explained by the Shao Yin's interior–exterior relationship with the Tai Yang channel, where the physician has mistaken a Shao Yin interior cold pattern for a Tai Yang exterior cold pattern. This is because the diagnosis was based only on the pulse, which can be tight or tense in both patterns, and the physician has failed to take the diarrhoea into account. Although this is a cold pattern requiring warming therapy, the fire therapy has been excessive and the extreme sweating produced is adverse; loss of fluids in a deficiency pattern can give rise to a transmuted pattern. In this clause, the cough and diarrhoea represent the original Shao Yin pattern, but the delirious speech and difficult urination are the result of fire therapy and exhaustion of yin fluid, representing disease transmutation.

Delirious speech can be ascribed to deficiency or to excess and Clause 284 clearly describes a case of yin deficiency, not of stomach excess. Clause 211 says: "Heavy sweat is promoted, if sweating is promoted again, there will be collapse of yang and delirious speech, if the pulse is short, the person will die", demonstrating that it is essential to identify the pattern correctly in order to optimise the treatment outcome. Regardless of whether the cough and diarrhoea were symptoms of a Zhen Wu Tang or a Zhu Ling Tang pattern, they are a manfestation of water qi harassing the lung and intestines. This parallels contemporary disorders such as chronic nephritis, heart or kidney failure, pleurisy or cirrhosis of the liver with ascites.

Clause 285

少阴病，脉细沉数，病为在里，不可发汗。

Shao Yin disease, the pulse is thready, submerged and rapid, the disease is in the interior, one should not promote sweating.

DISCUSSION: A thready, submerged pulse is characteristic of Shao Yin interior disease. A rapid pulse which is also thready usually indicates heat from yin deficiency, and in some situations, it can indicate severe yang deficiency. In either case, it is contraindicated to promote sweat. Such a pattern must not be confused with an exterior wind cold pattern, and the use of a formula which promotes sweat, such as Ma Huang Tang or Ma Huang Xi Xin Fu Zi Tang, is strongly contraindicated.

A submerged pulse pertains to an interior pattern, a thready or fine pulse indicates deficiency, and a rapid pulse is usually a reflection of heat but can also be attributed to deficiency. Thus, a rapid pulse can be due to heat excess or severe deficiency. The pulse described in Clause 285 could therefore be presumed to be associated with an interior pattern of deficiency heat, in other words, heat due to yin deficiency.

In the less common circumstance where the submerged and thready pulse represents a cold pattern, a slightly rapid pulse may manifest as a result of co-existing deficiency of yin and yang, qi and blood. In Shao Yin particularly, because of the mutual generation of kidney yin and kidney yang, a deficiency of yang can lead to a deficiency of yin, qi and blood, and even in a pattern of true cold, if the depletion of vital substances is severe and generalised, the pulse may be slightly rapid. In these circumstances, the pulse is close to expiry and 'scatters' on palpation. The rapid pulse represents the stirring of severely depleted yang when exuberant yin repells deficient yang, and could manifest with fever. In a pattern of severe deficiency cold, characterised by somnolence, cold extremities, diarrhoea with undigested food particles and a pale tongue, the strategy is to warm and fortify the yang and dispel interior cold.

Clause 285 cites the significance of the

pulse sign in differenting between heat and cold. If the pulse is submerged, thready, rapid and forceful, is accompanied by vexation and insomnia, and if the tongue is red with little coat, then it is a heat conversion pattern and the treatment is to nourish yin and clear heat. If the pulse is submerged, thready, rapid and forceless, disappearing under pressure and accompanied by a desire only to sleep, cold extremities, aversion to cold, and diarrhoea with undigested food particles, then it is a Shao Yin cold conversion pattern and the treatment is to warm the yang and disperse cold. Irrespective of whether it is a heat conversion or a cold conversion pattern, sweat promotion is contraindicated.

Clause 286

少阴病，脉微，不可发汗，亡阳故也。阳已虚，尺脉弱涩者，复不可下之。

Shao Yin disease, the pulse is faint, one should not promote sweat, because yang will be devastated. If yang is already deficient and the cubit pulse is weak and choppy, one should also not purge.

DISCUSSION: Shao Yin disease represents a deficiency pattern which is reflected in the Shao Yin pulse. Clause 286 mentions a pulse which is faint, thus describing the weak and thready pulse of Shao Yin disease. In this way, it underlines the fact that it is a deficiency pattern and, as such, must not be treated by sweating or purging. A faint pulse is one which is barely palpable and represents serious deficiency. In Shao Yin disease, a faint pulse is the reflection of extreme weakness of the heart and kidney, where loss of body fluids by sweating will devastate yang. The cubit pulse relates to the kidney, and if it is not only weak but also choppy, then there is severe insufficiency of yin blood, which would be further depleted by the loss of fluids caused by purgation. Thus this clause discusses the adverse outcomes in deficiencies of both yin and yang caused by sweating and purgation. No formula was nominated by Zhong Jing; however, in *Shang Han Suo Yuan Ji,* Qian Tian Lai proposed the formula Fu Zi Tang to warm the channels and fortify yang. Si Ni jia Ren Shen Tang can also be used.

Summary of Contraindicated Treatments in Shao Yin Disease

Purgation and sweat promotion are both contraindicated in Shao Yin disease. This section emphasises the pulse as an indicator of the deficiency characteristic of Shao Yin disease. A faint pulse represents deficiency of yang and qi, and a pulse which is weak and choppy reflects deficiency of yin and blood. The prohibition of sweating and purging stands regardless of whether the deficiency is one of yin or one of yang.

Section Seven

6.7 PROGNOSIS AND RECOVERY IN SHAO YIN DISEASE

6.7.1 Prognosis in Shao Yin Disease

Shao Yin cold conversion patterns are characterised by aversion to cold and cold extremities; they represent one stage in the progression of disease. If there is incessant diarrhoea with a pulse verging on expiry, the prognosis is poor; however, if the extremities become warm and the diarrhoea eases, this indicates the return of yang qi and so the prognosis is good. Emphasis is given to pulse image in determining the changes that are taking place.

Spontaneous Recovery in Shao Yin

Clause 287

少阴病，脉紧，至七八日自下利，脉暴微，手足反温，脉紧反去者，为欲解也。虽烦、下利，必自愈。

Shao Yin disease, the pulse is tight, on the seventh or eighth day there is spontaneous diarrhoea, the pulse is suddenly faint, *nevertheless the hands and feet are warm, this means it is about to resolve. Even though there is vexation and diarrhoea, there will be spontaneous recovery.*

DISCUSSION: A tight pulse in a Tai Yang pattern is a sign of cold constrained in the exterior; this generally manifests as fever, aversion to cold and an absence of sweat. A tight pulse in Shao Yin disease is a reflection of interior cold; there is no cold, but there is an aversion to cold and cold extremities. After the disease has persisted for seven or eight days, there is the additional symptom of diarrhoea, after which there are two possible developments. The first is where zheng qi is insufficient and pathogenic qi prevails, giving rise to a deterioration in the condition marked by incessant diarrhoea, aversion to cold, a preference for sleeping in a curled up position, cold extremities, spontaneous sweating and vexation. These symptoms reflect a serious condition which can lead to the desertion of yang and the exhaustion of yin. The second possible outcome is where zheng qi is strong and prevails over the pathogen, and it is this scenario which is described in Clause 287. The sudden faintness of the pulse is not a bad sign, but is a reference to the fact that it is no longer tight because the yin pathogen is on the wane; warmth in the extremities in a Shao Yin pattern is a clear sign of the return of yang qi which is able to disperse the cold, and confirms for the practitioner that the faint pulse is not a sign of deterioration. Vexation is a temporary manifestation resulting from the activity of the defence yang in combating the pathogen; and the diarrhoea is a residual symptom which will resolve once restoration of yang qi is complete and the Shao Yin pattern resolved. This clause emphasises that recovery in Shao Yin disease is conditional on the strength of zheng qi to combat the pathogen and foster the return of yang.

Clause 290

少阴中风，脉阳微阴浮者，为欲愈。

Shao Yin zhong feng, if the pulse is faint in yang and floating in yin, this means there is about to be recovery.

DISCUSSION: Clause 290 relies on the pulse sign to demonstrate the change of disease from yin to yang with subsequent gradual recovery. A pulse which is faint in the yang or distal position is contrary to the expectation of a floating yang pulse characteristic of pathogenic wind, which is a yang pathogen affecting the exterior. The change in the yang pulse from floating to faint is a sign that the wind pathogen is receding. Conversely, the yin or proximal pulse is associated with the interior and should be submerged; when it rises to the surface, becoming a floating pulse, it signals a change from yin to yang, representing the return of the yang qi.

This is a good example of how recovery can be determined by observing the pulse. In general, a big pulse in disease of any of the three yang channels signals the progression of the disease, whilst a faint pulse, which may mean a change from big to faint, or from forceful to moderate, is a sign that the disease is receding and recovery is about to take place. In disease of the three yin channels which are characterised by waning yang qi, if the pulse changes from small to big, from submerged to floating, or from forceless to forceful, it heralds the return of yang qi.

Treatable Patterns in Shao Yin

Although there are no recommended formulas for the patterns which follow here, the term 'treatable pattern' should not be interpreted as meaning a pattern which requires no treatment. Although the zheng qi is sufficient for a favourable prognosis, recovery would not be spontaneous, and a formula such as Si Ni Tang is required to resuscitate the devastated yang so the patient can recover.

Clause 288

少阴病，下利。若利自止，恶寒而蜷卧，手足温者，可治。

Shao Yin disease, there is diarrhoea. If the diarrhoea stops spontaneously, there is aversion to cold and a curled up sleeping posture, and the hands and feet are warm, it is treatable.

DISCUSSION: Shao Yin diarrhoea is attributed to deficient kidney yang unable to warm the spleen earth, and is marked by aversion to cold. Aversion to cold and sleeping in a curled up position are indications of severe interior cold with possible yang desertion. If the diarrhoea stops of its own accord, and the extremities gradually become warm, then the interior qi is harmonised, yang qi is returning, and the interior cold can be treated successfully.

The clinical features of Clause 287 and Clause 288 differ, with Clause 287 describing the presence of diarrhoea and Clause 288 describing its cessation. Nevertheless, warm hands and feet are a feature of both, showing that in each case the yang qi is returning and the yin cold retreating. In this clause, the cessation of diarrhoea in a Shao Yin pattern can signal one of two things. It can be a sign that fluids have been exhausted by the diarrhoea, so there is no watery stool; in other words, devastation of yang has led to exhaustion of yin. Or it can be a sign that the Shao Yin disease is resolving. The differential factor is the warmth of the extremities, where warm hands and feet are a sign of a favourable prognosis.

In *Su Wen: Tong Ping Xu Shi Lun Pian (Su Wen Chapter 28: Discourse on Deficiency and Excess)* Huang Di says: "What is meant by the phrase: if things are unhindered the patient will live and if perverse the patient will die? Qi Bo says: Unhindered is when the hands and feet are warm; perverse is when the hands and feet are cold". Thus, it is explained that warm hands and feet show that the qi is flowing properly and the prognosis is favourable, but cold hands and feet show that the flow of qi is perverse and the patient will die.

Clause 287 also discussed a change in the condition where the pulse suddenly became faint, but despite the continuing diarrhoea, the hands and feet were warm. This signals the return of yang and the prospect of recovery if treated. In contrast, Clause 288 relies on the cessation of the diarrhoea as confirmation of the return of yang qi and a favourable prognosis. Despite superficial differences, both Clause 287 and 288 describe a situation where the zheng qi has prevailed, and in both, warm extremities are the basis for a good prognosis.

Clause 289

少阴病，恶寒而蜷，时自烦，欲去衣被者，可治。

Shao Yin disease, there is aversion to cold and a curled up posture, if there is occasional vexation, and a desire to remove the bedclothes, the condition is treatable.

DISCUSSION: Aversion to cold is a common feature of Shao Yin disease. However, the desire to curl up is a sign of severe yang deficiency with exuberant cold, which is the root of a Shao Yin cold conversion pattern. Generally, a patient suffering from a Shao Yin pattern prefers quietness and there is no vexation; the description in Clause 289 of vexation and a desire to remove the bedclothes heralds the return of yang qi and the subsequent retreat of pathogenic yin cold, even before the limbs are warm again. The prognosis is good and therefore the condition is treatable.

In this clause, occasional spontaneous vexation and a desire to remove the bedclothes are cited as key symptoms for determining the prognosis; however, there appears to be an anomaly in the concurrence of those yang manifestations and the yin symptoms of aversion to cold and a preference for lying curled up. It is explained thus: if the pulse sign is faint and thready, even if accompanied by vexation and a desire to remove the bedclothes, it is a reflection of deficient yang; the manifestations of yang are false signs, which are a reflection of deficient yang being repelled by the exuberant yin cold. Once again, it is the pulse sign which can serve as the determining factor in establishing the prognosis.

Critical Conditions in Shao Yin Disease

Clause 294

少阴病，但厥、无汗，而强发之，必动其血。未知从何道出，或从口鼻，或从目出者，是名下厥上竭，为难治。

Shao Yin disease, there is only reversal and no sweating, but there has been forced promotion, the blood will stir. It is not known from which passage it will issue, whether from the mouth and nose, or from the eyes, it is known as lower reversal and upper exhaustion, it is difficult to treat.

DISCUSSION: Reversal refers to cold limbs due to the inadequacy of yang qi and its failure to warm the limbs; the absence of sweat is also due to the insufficiency of yang and its inability to transform fluids to provide the material foundation of sweat. This is not an exterior disease. The strategy is to support yang and expel cold, and the promotion of sweat is contraindicated. Clause 294 describes a situation where there has been forced promotion of sweat due to the interior pattern being mistaken for an exterior one. The inappropriate forcing of sweat causes further damage to both yin and yang with disastrous consequences. Damage to yang will impair the function of keeping blood in the vessels, and depletion of yin will generate empty heat, giving rise to the frenetic flow of blood. The bleeding may be from any passage, including the nose, mouth or the eyes. This phenomenon is described as reversal in the upper jiao and exhaustion in the lower jiao. This is because the cold extremities, referred to here as reversal, stem from the lower jiao and the bleeding is from the upper jiao. This is a critical condition in Shao Yin disease because of the dilemma posed by the paradox of cold in the lower jiao and heat in the upper jiao. Although warm herbs are needed for the lower jiao, they would exacerbate the bleeding in the upper jiao; and cool astringent herbs needed to treat the bleeding in the upper jiao would exacerbate the underlying Shao Yin pattern of yang deficiency. It is not only a critical condition, but one which is difficult to treat.

A comparison needs to be made between Clause 294 here, and Clause 293 earlier in this chapter, which describes heat in the urinary bladder. Bleeding is featured in both clauses, but the pathogenesis for each is different. Clause 293 describes fever with blood in the urine, which is the result of a pattern of yin and cold transforming to one of yang and heat, causing bleeding in the lower jiao. In contrast, Clause 294 describes a pattern of cold due to deficiency in the lower jiao manifesting as cold limbs, and heat due to the exhaustion of yin in the upper jiao, causing bleeding from the orifices of the upper jiao. This represents the desertion of both yin and yang and the prognosis is poor. However, the pronouncement that this condition is difficult to treat by no means implies it is untreatable. Tao Jie An suggested the combination of herbs and acupuncture with Dang Gui Si Ni Tang and the needling of Tai Xi (Kid 3), San Yin Jiao (Sp 6) and Yong Quan (Kid 1). Zhang Jing Yue proposed that Liu Wei Hui Yang Yin (Fu Zi, Gan Jiang, Ren Shen, Gan Cao, Shu Di, Dang Gui) should be used to nourish yin and resuscitate yang.

Bleeding is commonly associated with heat and excess, but is less commonly associated with a yin pattern. Li Dong Yuan cited a condition of haemoptysis being treated with Sheng Jiang and Rou Gui and here Clause 294 actually describes just such a situation: although there is exhaustion of fluids generating heat in the upper jiao, the underlying cause of the bleeding is a yin pattern of deficiency cold. The following case study is a good example of the strategy of stopping bleeding by warming the channels and supporting yang.

Case Study

Nosebleed

Extracted from Yue Mei Zhong Yi An

The patient was a driver and had a history of nosebleeds. One day, after a long and tiring journey, his vehicle broke down and took three days to repair and he was unable to return home. On the evening of the third day, he suffered from a nosebleed. His complexion was pale, his limbs were cold and his pulse was weak and faint. He consulted Dr Yue Mei Zhong who prescribed Gan Cao Gan Jiang Tang: Zhi Gan Cao 9g, Gan Pao Jiang 9g, with instructions to take it in a single dose. Two hours later, the warmth returned to his arms and legs and the bleeding stopped. The next morning, he saw Dr Yue again, who found that the pulse was stronger and prescribed 12g of E Jiao to be taken in two doses to consolidate the treatment.

Clause 295

少阴病，恶寒、身蜷而利、手足逆冷者，不治。

Shao Yin disease, if there is aversion to cold, a curled up posture and diarrhoea, and the hands and feet suffer reversal cold, it is not treatable.

DISCUSSION: Aversion to cold and sleeping curled up are characteristic features of a Shao Yin pattern of yang deficiency with interior cold; the diarrhoea is a further manifestation of the yang deficiency unable to warm the spleen earth and unable to control the exuberant yin cold. The additional symptom of cold extremities indicates a serious devastation of true yang and the condition is not treatable.

As discussed earlier in this chapter, the presence or absence of extreme cold in the extremities is significant in determining prognosis. This is because the warmth or coldness of the extremities is a measure of the vitality of yang qi and so is relied upon in prognosis. Zhang Jie Bing said: "The most precious thing in the universe is the red sun, and the most precious thing in the human body is the breath of yang qi". Both Clause 295 and 288 describe a critical pattern of Shao Yin deficiency cold marked by aversion to cold, sleeping in a curled up position and diarrhoea. In Clause 288, because the limbs are warm, the condition is deemed treatable; Clause 295 describes a condition where the limbs are cold and the condition is therefore pronounced as untreatable.

Clause 296

少阴病，吐利躁烦，四逆者，死。

Shao Yin disease, there is vomiting, diarrhoea, agitation and vexation, if the four are reversed, the person will die.

DISCUSSION: The symptoms of vomiting, diarrhoea, agitation and cold extremities (here described as 'si ni', referring to reversal cold of the four limbs) are characteristic of a Shao Yin pattern of yang deficiency with exuberant yin cold. If the zheng qi is adequate and can prevail over the pathogenic qi, then yang qi will return and the vomiting and diarrhoea will be resolved. Similarly, warming of the limbs is a sign of the return of yang. But if, as in this clause, the vomiting and diarrhoea are not resolved, and further, if there is agitation and vexation with no easing of the cold in the limbs, this shows that the situation has deteriorated to a point where recovery is unlikely. It is relevant here to note the distinction between agitation and vexation. The term vexation or *fan* (烦) generally describes a feeling, an internal sense of irritability, and is often associated with heat patterns such as Bai Hu Tang or Zhi Zi Chi Tang. Agitation or *zao* (躁), however, tends to describe restless activity which can be a demonstration of vexation. In itself, it generally reflects a more serious condition, and is not always a reflection of heat.

Clause 309 says: "Shao Yin disease, if there is vomiting and diarrhoea, reversal cold of the hands and feet, vexation and agitation with a feeling one is about to die, Wu Zhu Yu Tang governs". This pattern is relatively mild and is treatable. And yet, the symptoms described are similar to those in Clause 296, where the condition is critical and not deemed treatable. This is explained as follows. The symptom of vexation in Clause 309, where the patient feels as though they are near death, is a result of turbid yin cold causing qi reversal manifesting as frequent vomiting. In that case, although the patient feels extremely unwell, they are lucid and the indicated formula is Wu Zhu Yu Tang. By contrast, the agitation described in Clause 296 is a reflection of the devastation of true yang, as seen in the altered level of consciousness, which may even lapse into unconsciousness. This pattern can be seen in coma associated with liver failure, and other terminal diseases where patients can exhibit restlessness and agitation.

Clause 297

少阴病，下利止而头眩，时时自冒者，死。

Shao Yin disease, if the diarrhoea ceases and there is dizziness, with periodic loss of lucidity and blurred vision, the person will die.

DISCUSSION: There are two explanations for the cessation of diarrhoea in Shao Yin, one being fluid exhaustion and the other the return of yang qi. Where yang qi returns, the limbs will be warm, the appetite will return and the person will be lucid because the clear yang rises to the head. This bodes well for recovery. When the reason for the cessation of diarrhoea is fluid exhaustion, and not the return of yang, then the extremities remain cold. Not only is there desertion of fluids, but also depletion of yang, and both these factors contribute to the dizziness and loss of lucidity. Firstly, depleted yang can not rise to the head, and more seriously, because there is dual devastation of yin and yang, and because qi, blood and essence are also depleted, the spirit has neither nourishment nor vitality, and the person may slip in and out of consciousness. Thus Clause 297 describes a condition with critical depletion of the five vital substances, and so the prognosis is poor.

The situation where a patient feels dizzy or faint is also described in Clause 93: "Tai Yang disease, first there is purging but there is no recovery, and so sweating is then promoted, because of this both exterior and interior are deficient, the person will then feel dizzy. Patients who feel dizzy will sweat and recover spontaneously". This describes dizziness in Tai Yang disease caused by the incorrect sequence of treatment, where purgation and sweating have given rise to a dual exterior and interior deficiency with pathogenic constraint in the exterior. In this case, the yang qi has been mobilised in support of the zheng qi's battle against the pathogen, and so the clear yang does not rise, and there may be dizziness. This will precede the shivering sweat which ultimately brings resolution. By contrast, the dizziness described in Clause 297 is caused by exhaustion of yin and depletion of yang. This means that yin, blood and essence are insufficient to nourish the shen spirit, so there is not merely dizziness, but a loss of mental acuity and vitality. Clear differentiation must be made between the two situations.

Clause 298

少阴病，四逆、恶寒而身蜷、脉不至、不烦而躁者，死。

Shao Yin disease, the four are reversed, there is aversion to cold and a curled up posture, if the pulse does not arrive, and there is no vexation but there is agitation, the person will die.

DISCUSSION: Clause 298 describes a patient suffering from a Shao Yin pattern which is characterised by cold extremities, referred to as a reversal of qi in the four limbs, aversion to cold and a curled up posture. These are all manifestations of severe yang deficiency with exuberant yin cold. The pulse which can not be found, and the presence of agitation with no feelings of vexation, indicate the terminal nature of the condition. The yang qi is too weak to carry the blood to the pulse position, and the blood is affected by the depletion of yin, so no pulse can be felt. This is where a pulse verging on expiry is actually expiring. There is no vexation because the heart shen is devitalised and the patient has little or no awareness. The agitation refers to a semi-conscious state with involuntary restlessness and fidgeting. This indicates that devastated ying blood has failed to nourish and anchor the shen, and the meaningless and undirected activity is a sign of the scattering of depleted yang. Vexation and agitation are commonly seen together, but in the terminal stage of illness, where a patient with an altered state of consciousness exhibits restlessness and agitation, the prognosis is poor.

In Clause 298, the agitation in the absence of vexation is the main warning that the patient is in the terminal phase. Although the failure of the pulse to arrive and be palpable indicates serious deficiency, it is not a sign of imminent death. Elsewere in *Shang Han Lun* a pulse which does not arrive is described as indicating a prospect of recovery. A pulse which does not arrive is also a feature of the pattern described in Clause 292, advocating the use of moxibustion to tonify the yang. Clauses 292 and 298 both pertain to Shao Yin disease and both are characterised by a pulse which does not arrive (脉不至), but the patterns are not the same. In the condition described by Clause 292, the limbs are warm and there is fever; prospects are good. But Clause 298 describes the late stage of a terminal illness, characterised by aversion to cold and cold limbs, a curled up posture and agitation without vexation. The pattern in Clause 292 signals the return of yang; that of Clause 298 signals the expiry of yang and imminent death.

Other clauses which describe a pulse which is so faint it is not palpable are Clauses 315 and 317, which respectively refer to such a pulse as "no pulse" (无脉), and "the pulse is not palpable" (脉不出). Clause 315 describes a situation where there is "reversal cold and no pulse", for which the treatment is Bai Tong jia Zhu Dan Zhi Tang; Clause 317 describes a situation where "the diarrhoea ceases and the pulse is not palpable" for which the indicated formula is Tong Mai Si Ni Tang jia Ren Shen. From these clauses, it can be seen that the absence of a pulse means simply that it is faint and can not be felt under the fingers, and that the condition may be treatable.

Clause 299

少阴病六七日，息高者，死。

Shao Yin disease for six or seven days, if the breathing is shallow, the person will die.

DISCUSSION: The objective of Clause 299 is to describe the effects of prolonged ill health ending in a Shao Yin pattern where there is long-term depletion of zheng qi and kidney yang. The shallow breathing is a sign that the kidneys' function of grasping qi is severely impaired; the lung qi is also weak and can not descend qi. The condition is serious, and represents the imminent expiry of kidney qi and dissipation of lung qi. The person is close to death.

As a Shao Yin pattern, the pulse would be faint and thready and the person would have a strong desire to sleep. The specified period of six or seven days should not be taken literally and is merely intended to suggest that the disease is entrenched. The ineffective shallow breathing is evidence of the seriousness of the patient's condition. The lungs rule qi and govern respiration and are the tip of qi; the kidneys grasp qi and generate qi, and are known as the root of qi. Superficial breathing using only the upper portion of the lungs is referred to as breathing without root, as the qi is not able to descend to the Dan Tian in the lower jiao. This condition can find parallels in the modern disease conditions of uraemia or diabetic coma.

Clause 300

少阴病，脉微细沉、但欲卧、汗出不烦、自欲吐，至五六日自利，复烦躁不得卧寐者，死。

Shao Yin disease, the pulse is faint, thready and submerged, the person wants to do nothing but sleep, there is sweating without vexation, and an urge to vomit spontaneously, if on the fifth or sixth day there is spontaneous diarrhoea, then vexation and agitation and an inability to sleep, the person will die.

DISCUSSION: A faint, thready and submerged pulse and a desire to sleep are characteristics of Shao Yin disease. Sweating is the result of deficient yang with insecurity of the defence yang; the absence of vexation is evidence of the depth of the yang deficiency and its inability to disperse the yin cold. The term 'spontaneous vomiting' refers to vomiting which is not induced by emetic herbs; thus emphasis is given to the vomiting being a manifestation of qi reversal caused by the accumulation of yin cold. These signs and symptoms all call for warming treatment to resuscitate the yang. If the condition persists, by the fifth or sixth day there will be additional symptoms of diarrhoea, vexation, agitation and insomnia. These show a progression from yang deficiency to yang desertion and recovery is out of reach.

Summary of Prognosis in Shao Yin Disease

There are ten clauses associated with the prognosis of Shao Yin disease, which tends to represent serious and life-threatening conditions, principally associated with the cold conversion pattern. The chief criterion for a favourable prognosis in Shao Yin disease is the restoration of yang qi. Signs of the return of yang are gradual warming of the extremities, a change from aversion to cold and a curled up posture to the absence of aversion to cold and a desire to remove clothing; and the cessation of diarrhoea accompanied by warm extremities.

In confirming an unfavourable prognosis, evidence of the devastation of yin and yang must be found. Symptoms of desertion of yang with yin cold accumulation are aversion to cold, a curled up posture, uncontrollable diarrhoea, cold extremities and no pulse. Symptoms of dual exhaustion of yin and yang are cessation of diarrhoea with dizziness and loss of lucidity. Exhaustion of lung and kidney qi is evidenced by shallow and ineffectual breathing.

It must be said that many conditions deemed to be terminal in the Eastern Han era, when available treatment was limited, would now be well managed with modern medicine.

6.7.2 Shao Yin Recovery Period

Clause 291

少阴病欲解时，从子至寅上。

The time that Shao Yin disease is ready to resolve, is from zi to yin.

DISCUSSION: The optimal time for recovery in Shao Yin disease is in the period from zi to yin (11pm to 5am). Shao Yin disease is characterised by yang deficiency with exuberant yin. Recovery depends on the promotion of yang and is assisted by the ambient yang qi of that time period, which relates to the emergence of yang after its transformation from yin. The rationale is that this emerging and waxing yang qi will warm and invigorate the yang qi of the body, thus supporting recovery from the yang deficient disease of Shao Yin. Prognosis as discussed in the Shao Yin chapter is based on clinical experience and observation. Parallels can sometimes be drawn between Shao Yin cold conversion patterns and modern diagnoses such as coronary disease, emphysema, pneumonia and cardiac failure.

Section Eight

6.8 SUMMARY OF THE SHAO YIN CHAPTER

Shao Yin patterns are associated with yang deficiency where exuberant interior yin cold has accumulated and prevailed; these are known as cold conversion patterns. Heat conversion patterns are patterns where deficient kidney yin gives rise to hyperactive fire harassing the heart shen.

Principal Features of Shao Yin Disease

Features of a cold conversion pattern are a faint and thready pulse, cold extremities, and a desire to sleep; these symptoms are attributed to heart and kidney yang deficiency with interior yin cold. Formulas indicated in Shao Yin cold conversion patterns are the Si Ni Tang group (Tong Mai Si Ni Tang, Bai Tong Tang, Bai Tong jia Zhu Dan Zhi Tang); Zhen Wu Tang, Fu Zi Tang, Wu Zhu Yu Tang and Tao Hua Tang. Each governs a specific pattern of symptoms as appears below. Formulas indicated for heat conversion are Huang Lian E Jiao Tang and Zhu Ling Tang.

Shao Yin Cold Conversion Patterns

SI NI TANG PATTERN: The Si Ni Tang group comprises the principal formulas indicated for the treatment of Shao Yin cold conversion patterns. Where there are cold extremities, aversion to cold, a curled up posture, diarrhoea with undigested food particles, pale copious urination, a faint and thready pulse, and a desire to sleep, the indicated formula is Si Ni Tang to resuscitate yang. Where exuberant yin repels true yang and there is diarrhoea and cold extremities with no aversion to cold, a flushed face, and a faint pulse verging on expiry, the indicated formula is Tong Mai Si Ni Tang to resuscitate the yang and alleviate the yin cold. If the true yang is more vigorously repelled by the interior yin, it is known as upcast yang and there will be a flushed face, diarrhoea, a faint pulse, aversion to cold, and cold limbs and the most appropriate formula is Bai Tong Tang. If the yin cold rejects the warming herbs, giving rise to incessant diarrhoea, cold limbs, no pulse, dry retching and vexation, this is an extreme form of an upcast yang pattern and Bai Tong jia Zhu Dan Zhi Tang is indicated so its cold salty herbs can lead the warm herbs inwards to the interior.

ZHEN WU TANG PATTERN: This is a pattern of kidney yang deficiency with an inability to govern water, giving rise to fluid retention and oedema; it is characterised by abdominal pain, diarrhoea, inhibited urination and aching limbs. Zhen Wu Tang is the indicated formula to fortify yang and transform water.

FU ZI TANG PATTERN: This is a pattern of severe yang deficiency where damp cold has congealed in the joints and muscle layer resulting in body and joint pain, cold extremities, a submerged pulse, aversion to cold in the back and harmony in the mouth. Fu Zi Tang is indicated to warm and supplement the source yang and resolve the damp cold.

WU ZHU YU TANG PATTERN: This is caused by Shao Yin pathogenic cold harassing the stomach and causing the reverse flow of turbid qi. It is characterised by vomiting, diarrhoea, cold extremities, vexation with agitation; the patient feels so bad they think they are going to die. Wu Zhu Yu Tang is indicated to warm the middle, expel cold, and redirect qi downwards to stop vomiting.

TAO HUA TANG PATTERN: This is a pattern of spleen and kidney yang deficiency with damp cold obstructing the middle jiao. It is characterised by incessant watery diarrhoea, blood in the stool, abdominal pain and inhibited urination. Tao Hua Tang is indicated to warm the interior and astringe the intestines to stop the diarrhoea.

Shao Yin Heat Conversion Patterns

HUANG LIAN E JIAO TANG PATTERN: This is a Shao Yin heat conversion pattern associated with kidney yin deficiency and hyperactive heart fire. It is characterised by vexation, insomnia, a red tongue with a scant tongue coat and a thready and rapid pulse. Huang Lian E Jiao Tang is indicated to nourish yin and promote urination.

ZHU LING TANG PATTERN: This is a heat conversion pattern where heat arising from yin deficiency knots with water in the lower jiao, causing inhibited urination, cough, vomiting, thirst, vexation and insomnia. Zhu Ling Tang is indicated to clear heat, nourish yin and promote urination.

HEAT TRANSFERRING TO THE URINARY BLADDER: This is where a disease of the Shao Yin kidney zang has transferred to its fu partner, giving rise to a pattern of heat in the urinary bladder which is characterised by fever and blood in the urine. The strategy is to clear heat and nourish yin, cool blood and stop the bleeding.

SHAO YIN HEAT DIARRHOEA: For Shao Yin diarrhoea with blood and pus in the stool, acupuncture can be used.

Concurrent Patterns of Shao Yin

These comprise Shao Yin and Tai Yang patterns, Shao Yin and Yang Ming patterns and Shao Yin and Shao Yang concurrent patterns.

SHAO YIN AND TAI YANG CONCURRENT PATTERN: Tai Yang and Shao Yin stand in an exterior–interior relationship and so there is a relatively high incidence of a Shao Yin and Tai Yang concurrent pattern. It is characterised by fever, headache, aversion to cold and a submerged and faint pulse. Ma Huang Xi Xin Fu Zi Tang is indicated to warm the channels and release the exterior. If the disease persists, or if the constitution is weak, Ma Huang Fu Zi Gan Cao Tang is indicated to warm the channels and promote a mild sweat.

SHAO YIN AND YANG MING CONCURRENT PATTERN: This comprises three different but associated patterns of urgent purgation resulting from Shao Yin heat conversion, which has consumed yin. The clinical features are abdominal distension, constipation where the hard stool is not passed, but there is a foul watery discharge, pain below the heart and a parched throat and mouth. Da Cheng Qi Tang is indicated to purge heat so as to preserve yin fluids as a matter of urgency.

SHAO YIN AND SHAO YANG CONCURRENT PATTERN: Although this is known as Shao Yin disease, it is due to qi stagnation impairing the dispersal of yang qi and manifesting as cold extremities. The treatment is to disperse constrained liver qi and vent yang qi by using Si Ni San.

Shao Yin Sore Throat Patterns

A sore throat in a Shao Yin pattern arises because the Shao Yin channel passes through the throat. There are four main patterns.

ZHU FU TANG PATTERN: This is a pattern of yin deficiency where the pathogenesis of the sore throat is the flaring deficiency fire; heat harasses the upper jiao causing a dry, sore throat and vexation. As a Shao Yin pattern, it is characterised by diarrhoea and fullness in chest. Zhu Fu Tang is indicated to nourish the lung and kidney yin and clear deficient heat.

GAN CAO TANG AND JIE GENG TANG PATTERN: Gan Cao Tang consists of Sheng Gan Cao, which is cool and can drain fire and relieve toxicity. It is indicated to treat a sore throat with slight redness and swelling or soreness and where there are no other symptoms, making the use of either hot or cold herbs inappropriate. Xu Zong said: "Gan Cao by itself can harmonise the yin and clear heat". Jie Geng is bitter, acrid and neutral; it diffuses lung qi and disinhibits the throat. When combined with Gan Cao, it relieves the sore throat by dispersing the knotted bind.

KU JIU TANG PATTERN: This is a pattern where empty fire has scorched the throat. Phlegm heat results in ulceration and a lost voice. Ku Jiu Tang is indicated to clear heat, sweep phlegm, and reduce swelling.

BAN XIA SAN AND TANG PATTERN: This is a sore throat pattern caused by pathogenic cold harassing the throat and is characterised by aversion to cold and copious phlegm. Ban Xia San and Tang are indicated to warm the channels and disperse cold, sweep phlegm and eliminate stagnation.

There are five formulas for the treatment of sore throat in Shao Yin: Zhu Fu Tang, Gan Cao Tang, Jie Geng Tang, Ku Jiu Tang and Ban Xia San or Tang. They are all indicated for sore throat but their application is differentiated on the basis of severity. Jie Geng Tang is indicated for a throat which is swollen and inflamed. If the swelling is severe and there is an exterior pathogen or if the condition is protracted, Ban Xia San or Tang and Ku Jiu Tang are indicated; if the throat is dry and sore, Zhu Fu Tang is indicated.

Contraindicated Treatments in Shao Yin Disease

Shao Yin patterns of deficiency cold are treated by urgent warming. Sweat promotion, emesis and purgation are contraindicated. Clause 285 describes a pattern where there are palpitations and the pulse is thready, submerged and rapid. Clause 286 is a pattern of yang deficiency which is reflected in the faint pulse, and where a weak and choppy pulse in the cubit position is attributed to depleted yin blood. Clause 284 focuses on the contraindication of fire therapy. In brief, Shao Yin disease represents deficiency and requires treatment stategies which warm the yang or nourish the yin.

Prognosis and Recovery in Shao Yin Disease

PROGNOSIS: A favourable prognosis is made on the basis of the return of yang. This is characterised by aversion to cold and a curled up posture in the presence of a gradual warming of the extremities, cessation of diarrhoea, the development of vexation and a desire to remove clothing, which are a reflection of zheng qi overcoming the pathogen. An unfavourable prognosis is made on the basis of yang desertion and yin exhaustion. This is where exuberant yin prevails and there is devastation of yang, manifesting with cessation of diarrhoea, dizziness, loss of mental clarity, and severely depleted lung and kidney qi giving rise to shallow breathing. The prognosis is poor and death may be imminent.

SHAO YIN RECOVERY PERIOD: Shao Yin channel qi peaks between the hours of zi to yin (11pm to 5am) and so this is the optimal time for recovery.

厥陰

Jue Yin 7

Section One

7.1 OUTLINE OF JUE YIN

Pathway of the Jue Yin Channel

The Jue Yin channel incorporates the foot Jue Yin liver and hand Jue Yin pericardium channels and has an interior–exterior relationship with the foot Shao Yang gallbladder and hand Shao Yang san jiao channels. The external pathway of the foot Jue Yin liver channel runs from the tip of the first toe, crossing the spleen and kidney channels as it ascends the inner leg, then continues upward to the lower ribs at the side of the body. An internal channel departs from the inguinal region and connects to the Ren meridian in the lower abdomen before passing around the stomach, homing to the liver and gallbladder, and rising through the lungs and throat to the eye, then to the vertex. The luo connecting channel encircles the genital organs and a second branch leads to its yang partner, the gallbladder channel. The external pathway of the hand Jue Yin pericardium channel emerges from the chest and descends the arm, ending at the tip of the third finger. An internal channel passes from the pericardium through all three of the san jiao, and the luo connecting channel leads from the external channel to the heart.

Physiology of the Jue Yin Channel

The liver pertains to wood and wind; it houses the ministerial fire of the kidneys, whilst the pericardium houses the sovereign fire of the heart. The liver stores blood and governs the free flow of qi. Its opening is the eyes, which are therefore intimately related to the liver. The liver rules the sinews, which relate to agility and flexibility of movement, and it has an interior–exterior relationship with the gallbladder. The pericardium enshrouds the heart and is connected to the san jiao in an interior–exterior relationship. If the passages of the triple jiao are unhindered, they provide an avenue for harmonious communication between the upper and lower jiao; the san jiao facilitaties the proper interaction of heart fire and kidney water, and the nourishing of liver wood.

Pathology of the Jue Yin Channel

Jue Yin is the final stage of six channel disease; it also represents the terminal phase of illness, where zheng qi is struggling to contend with the pathogenic qi, and where there is the waxing and waning of yin and yang. Jue Yin can be translated as 'utmost yin' or 'terminal yin'. The *Su Wen: Zhi Zhen Yao Da Lun Pian (Su Wen Chapter 74: Essential Great Discourse on Reaching the Truth)* writes: "What is Jue Yin? Qi Bo said: The end stage of the interaction of the two yin". Based on the theory that extreme cold can engender pathogenic heat and can also herald the return of yang qi, these extreme states of yin and yang mean that both heat and cold can manifest in Jue Yin disease. On the one hand, there is the phenomenon of yin and yang repelling each other, with their ultimate separation spelling death; on the other, extreme yin cold can be resolved with the gradual return of yang qi. In brief, Jue Yin disease is primarily associated with unpredictable fluctuations of yin and yang due to their non-communication.

Jue Yin Disease and Its Transmission Pathway

The aetiology of Jue Yin disease can be either direct attack, which is rare, or transmission of a pathogen from another channel, for example, from Tai Yin or Shao Yin. This can occur as part of the natural progression of disease attributed to insufficient zheng qi, or it can be caused by the incorrect treatment of Shao Yang disease, or by the inappropriate administration of purgatives in Yang Ming disease, all of which can ultimately lead to a Jue Yin pattern.

Key Manifestations of Jue Yin Disease

The Jue Yin channel incorporates the liver channel and Jue Yin disease is often characterised by the relationship between wood and earth, with liver fire harassing the spleen and stomach, giving rise to heat in the upper jiao and cold in the lower jiao. This manifests with vomiting, a scorching sensation in the chest, diarrhoea and cold extremities.

Classification of Jue Yin Disease

1. **Heat and cold complex.** The non-communication of yin and yang in Jue Yin disease readily manifests as a complex of heat in the upper jiao with cold in the lower jiao. This is because in Jue Yin disease yin and yang are no longer rooted; they are therefore no longer in harmony and so are in disarray.
2. **Waxing and waning of yang qi.** This manifests respectively as fever or cold extremities. The relative balance of yang qi and yin cold can be determined by the degree and duration of each manifestation at a given time.
3. **Jue ni or desertion pattern.** A desertion pattern or *jue ni* (厥逆) is a result of the non-communication of yin and yang. There are seven desertion patterns: (a) Cold jue or *jue leng* (厥冷) which manifests as cold extremities with exuberant cold in the interior; (b) heat jue or *re jue* (热厥), where deep-seated pathogenic heat obstructs the dispersion of yang qi; (c) roundworm reversal or *hui jue* (蛔厥), where heat and cold are intermingled due to disruption to the flow of qi and blood caused by roundworm infestation; (d) blood jue or *xue jue* (血厥), where cold congeals blood, resulting in cold extremities and a pulse that is verging on expiry; (e) water jue or *shui jue* (水厥), where water accumulation obstructs the dispersion of yang qi; (f) organ jue or *zang jue* (脏厥) where the cold extremities are the result of the desertion of true yang; (g) phlegm jue or *tan jue* (痰厥), where phlegm excess in the chest obstructs the dispersion of yang qi resulting in cold extremities. This is described in Chapter 2 Tai Yang Disease in reference to a Gua Di San pattern.
4. **Diarrhoea and vomiting.** Diarrhoea and vomiting are differentiated according to whether they are caused by heat or cold. Diarrhoea and vomiting due to cold are accompanied by cold extremities, whereas diarrhoea and vomiting due to heat conversion or excessive yang return are accompanied by thirst, fever and tenesmus.

Treatment of Jue Yin Disease

Treatment in Jue Yin disease must be based on the principle of treating the cold with warmth and the heat with cold. Due to the complexity of Jue Yin disease, consideration must be given not only to the pathology, but also to the patient's constitution.

Contraindications in Jue Yin Disease

As a deficiency pattern, purgation, sweating and emetic therapy are contraindicated.

Section Two

7.2 PRINCIPAL FEATURES OF JUE YIN DISEASE

Jue Yin is associated with utmost yin, preceding its transformation into yang, as with the diurnal cycle of night and day, where the deepest part of night heralds the transformation of yin into yang as a new day is born. For this reason, yin and yang are in fluid equilibrium, with one easily transforming into the other.

Terminology in Desertion Patterns with Cold Extremities

There are two items in the terminology of Chinese medicine which are sometimes interchanged, but are not exactly the same. The first is *ni* (逆), which can be variously translated as 'opposite', 'reverse', 'counter', 'contrary', 'inverse', 'converse' and even 'rebellious' or 'perverse'; this is the term used to describe the reverse or rebellious flow of qi that manifests as coughing or vomiting. The second is *jue* (厥), which may be translated as 'final', 'ultimate', 'utmost', 'extreme', 'terminal' or 'desertion'. In Chinese medicine jue can refer to collapse or loss of consciousness, and is also used to refer to cold extremities, both of which are a result of the non-communication of yin and yang, and are characteristic symptoms of Jue Yin disease.

Developed from these two words, are the terms *jue leng* (厥冷) and *jue ni* (厥逆), which are both often translated as 'reversal cold'. A closer translation of jue leng (厥冷) would be 'desertion cold' and a direct translation of jue ni would be 'desertion reversal' or 'extreme reversal'. The problem presented by the translation of both jue leng (厥冷) and jue ni (厥逆) as 'reversal cold' is that it means that jue (厥) is translated as 'reversal', which is the primary meaning of ni (逆), and not the primary meaning of jue (厥). Nevertheless, both terms are used to refer to cold limbs, generally caused by depleted yang qi, an obstruction to the flow of yang qi, or the non-interaction of yin and yang. The simplified term 'desertion pattern' is also often used to refer to both jue leng and jue ni.

JUE LENG: In *Shang Han Lun*, jue leng is the conventional term for the symptom of coldness in the four limbs, which is also referred to by the terms 'si ni' and 'jue ni'. Clauses 340, 343, 354, 355, 362 and 388 all use the term jue leng, which is the manifestation of the non-interaction of yin and yang caused by impaired flow due either to deficiency or obstruction. There are three situations associated with jue leng.

1. Yang deficiency with exuberant yin cold as described in Clause 354: "There is profuse sweating, if there is severe diarrhoea and desertion cold, Si Ni Tang governs."
2. Phlegm accumulation obstructing the flow of yang qi as described in Clause 355: "The patient suffers from cold in the hands and feet, if the pulse is all of a sudden tight, evil is knotted in the chest, there is fullness below the heart and vexation, hunger with no ability to eat, then the disease is in the chest, one should induce vomiting, Gua Di San is appropriate."
3. Yang desertion resulting in jue as described in Clause 368: "Following diarrhoea, the pulse has expired, there is desertion cold of the hands and feet, if within one day the pulse returns, and the hands and feet are warm the person will live; if the pulse does not return the person will die". In *Wai Gan Wen Bing Pian,* Chen Bo Ping said: "Yang qi stems from the four limbs, yin qi stems from the five zang, the continuous flow of yin and yang qi is a circuit with no end. Cold jue is attributed to the yang qi not connecting with the yin, and heat jue is attributed to the yin not connecting with the yang".

JUE NI: A second term referring to coldness of the extremities is jue ni, the direct translation of which is 'desertion reversal' as explained above. This concept falls into the same category as jue, si ni and jue leng. The basic pathology of jue ni is the non-interaction of yin and yang qi. Three factors lead to jue ni.

1. Incorrect sweat promotion in Tai Yang disease resulting in yang desertion, as seen in Clause 38: "… If the pulse is faint and weak, where there is sweating and aversion to wind, one should not take medication. Medication will cause desertion reversal".

2. Dual deficiency of yin and yang as seen in Clause 29: "Shang han the pulse is floating, there is spontaneous sweating, frequent urination, there will be heart vexation, a slight aversion to cold, and cramps in the feet, but Gui Zhi Tang is given to attack the exterior, this is a mistake. Having given it, there is jue".
3. The term jue ni or desertion reversal is used in Clause 315 in reference to Shao Yin disease with yang deficiency and exuberant yin cold: "… if the diarrhoea does not stop, there is desertion reversal and no pulse, dry retching and vexation, Bai Tong jia Zhu Dan Zhi Tang governs"; and also in Clause 353: "Profuse sweating, the fever does not abate, there is spasm in the interior, pain in the four limbs. If there is also diarrhoea, and desertion reversal and aversion to cold, Si Ni Tang governs".

Some of the terms used in desertion patterns are: *han jue* (寒厥) or 'cold desertion', referring to desertion due to cold; *re jue* (热厥) or 'heat desertion', referring to desertion due to heat; *hui jue* (蛔厥) or 'roundworm desertion', referring to desertion due to roundworms; *jue ni* (厥逆) or 'desertion reversal', which describes 'reversal' or cold extremities caused by jue or desertion; and *ni leng* (逆冷) or 'reversal cold', referring to cold caused by reversal. Each of these terms indicates the cause of the desertion pattern. Nevertheless, with the exception of heat jue and jue patterns associated with a material substance such as roundworms or water, the terms jue leng or desertion cold, ni leng or reversal cold, han jue or cold desertion, and jue ni or desertion reversal, are by and large interchangeable. It should also be noted that 'hands and feet' (手足) in Chinese can refer just to the hands and feet but may also include the lower arm and leg. For this reason, the term 'extremities' is often used.

The translation of Chinese medicine terminology is fraught with problems for authors, teachers and students alike. For instance, Jue Yin is variously translated as 'Terminal Yin' and 'Reverting Yin'. Given the above discussion of the semantics of the word jue (厥), the former is closer to the original meaning, and the latter seems to allude to the imminent reversion of yin on reaching its limit. Neither interpretation is wrong, but it is useful to understand their derivation. Because of the confusion caused by problematic translation, where fitting, the authors prefer to use the original Chinese terms which encompass all these nuances.

Jue Ni or Desertion Patterns

Clause 326

厥阴之为病，消渴，气上撞心，心中疼热，饥而不欲食，食则吐蛔、下之利不止。

Jue Yin is diseased, there is quenchless thirst, qi rushes upward to the heart, there is burning pain in the chest, hunger with no desire to eat, eating causes the vomiting of roundworms and purgation causes incessant diarrhoea.

DISCUSSION: Clause 326 describes a pattern of heat and cold complex with heat in the upper jiao and cold in the lower jiao. This is highly characteristic of Jue Yin disease, where the mutual transformation of yin and yang finds expression in extreme yin heralding the return of yang.

The Jue Yin channel relates to the liver and if the flow of liver qi is impaired, the ensuing stagnation will generate heat, which will accumulate in the upper jiao; the excess liver qi will attack the stomach and intestines, resulting in cold accumulating in the lower jiao and heat in the upper jiao. This pattern generally manifests as a gastrointestinal disorder. Due to the intense liver fire, the yin of the liver and stomach is consumed, giving rise to extreme thirst. The liver fire attacking the stomach causes a burning sensation in the chest, and the transportation function of the spleen is impaired, resulting in a reduced appetite. The use of purgatives will cause further damage to the spleen qi, and then there will be continuous diarrhoea. Thus it can be seen that a Jue Yin pattern of heat and cold complex is associated with fire in the liver and gallbladder, and the cold is associated with spleen deficiency giving rise to an accumulation of yin cold.

The vomiting of roundworms after eating is a direct result of heat in the upper jiao and spleen deficiency with cold in the intestines. The heat of the upper jiao is repelled by the cold in the lower jiao. Because of this, qi can not descend, and any food eaten will be vomited up again; if there is an infestation of worms, they will be expelled with the vomiting. Purgatives are inappropriate and will further damage the yang qi.

Although Clause 326 gives an indication of some of the features of Jue Yin disease, it by no means covers the full spectrum of its various presentations, as is done with the first five channels, and it fails to describe the various categories of Jue Yin desertion patterns. The complex of heat in the upper jiao and cold in the lower jiao demonstrates a pattern of heat and cold complex, but does not demonstrate the waxing and waning of yang qi and thus does not fully reflect the full spectrum of Jue Yin disease.

No formula is specified, but based on the symptoms of heat in the upper jiao and cold in the lower jiao, the treatment principle is to clear heat from the upper jiao, warm the middle and lower jiao, and regulate qi. This strategy addresses the heat cold complex itself, and also the impaired flow of liver qi which is a major contributing factor. Jue Yin disease is the final phase of disease in the three yin channels and represents a condition of significant deficiency. In view of this, herbs to supplement the middle and augment zheng qi, as well as herbs to nourish yin, should be included. A formula such as Wu Mei Wan can be considered.

Clause 337

凡厥者， 阴阳气不顺接， 便为厥. 厥者，手足逆冷者是也.

Whenever the utmost is reached, yin and yang qi do not connect smoothly, so it is called the utmost. At the utmost, it is the hands and feet which suffer reversal cold.

DISCUSSION: Clause 337 describes the pathogenesis of a jue or desertion pattern and its associated symptoms. The reference to 'the utmost' being reached is a reference to the utmost yin channel or Jue Yin. The characteristic feature of a jue or desertion pattern is cold extremities. It is important to understand that in a jue pattern, cold extremities are not simply a reflection of yang deficiency, as in a Si Ni Tang pattern, but are a reflection of the non-interaction of yin and yang and can therefore be differentiated as associated with either heat or cold. This phenomenon is peculiar to a jue pattern.

The physiological function of yin and yang is defined by the expression "yin and yang have their root in each other" (阴阳互根). In that one phrase is incorporated the concept of mutual dependence and mutual engenderment, and thence, equilibrium. If these two entities are not in balance, and there is a preponderance of either one or the other, then health is disturbed and disease will occur. If yang is deficient, and gives rise to exuberant cold, it is not only a case of insufficient yang qi not reaching the extremities to provide warmth, but the obstruction caused by the interior yin cold is the basis for the development of a cold jue pattern. If, on the other hand, the yang qi is constrained by heat and it is this constraint which prevents yang qi from reaching and warming the extremities, then it is known as heat jue. In both cases, the underlying cause is the non-communication of yin and yang.

Clause 337 is only one of several clauses in *Shang Han Lun* which emphasise the relevance of yin and yang in pattern identification, prognosis, and pathogenesis. Clause 7 cites yin and yang as differentiating factors in the aetiology of cold and heat patterns; Clause 58 explains that if there is damage to blood or body fluids in the wake of harsh treatment, once yin and yang harmonise, recovery will occur; and Clause 337 here uses the pathological behaviour of yin and yang to explain the pathogenesis and symptoms of jue or a reversal pattern. These three clauses therefore exemplify the significance of yin and yang in understanding disease, and in disease diagnosis and prognosis.

In addition to heat and cold jue or desertion patterns, Jue Yin disease is associated with other patterns as follows: (1) the devastation of fluids and desertion of yang due to incorrect use of sweat promotion, purgatives or emetics; (2) heat in the liver and cold in the stomach causing the stirring of roundworms; (3) blood deficiency with congealed cold; (4) phlegm obstruction causing phlegm jue; (5) qi constraint causing jue; (6) water retention causing jue; (7) turbid yin cold harassing the stomach; (8) devastation of true yang; and (9) phlegm in the chest, as found in a Gua Di San pattern. Although they differ in pathogenesis, any of these can result in cold extremities, and so the treatment of cold extremities must be based on the pattern and not the symptom. Therefore, pattern differentiation is of critical importance in determining the appropriate treatment.

According to the *Huang Di Nei Jing* there are two definitions of jue or desertion: (1) sudden loss of consciousness characterised by cold extremities and dizziness; (2) cold extremities without loss of consciousness. It is this second definition to which the term jue refers in *Shang Han Lun*. Apart from the non-interaction of yin and yang, jue patterns can be caused by qi, blood, phlegm, water and food stagnation, and are named accordingly.

Section Three

7.3 JUE YIN PATTERNS

7.3.1 Patterns of Heat and Cold Complex

Wu Mei Wan Pattern

Clause 338

（一）伤寒脉微而厥，至七八日肤冷，其人躁无暂安时者，此为脏厥，非蛔厥也．（二）蛔厥者，其人当吐蛔，今病者静，而复时烦者，此为脏寒．蛔上入其膈，故烦，须臾复止，得食而呕，又烦者，蛔闻食臭出，其人常自吐蛔．（三）蛔厥者，乌梅丸主之．又主久利．

(1) Shang han with a faint pulse and jue, on the seventh or eighth day, the skin is cold, if the person is agitated without a moment's peace, this is zang jue, it is not roundworm jue. (2) In roundworm jue, the person should vomit roundworms, now the patient is quiet, but if there is repeated vexation, this is cold in the zang. The roundworms go upward and enter the diaphragm, hence the vexation, which all of a sudden stops again. If taking food causes vomiting, and also vexation, the roundworms smell the odour of the food, the person will often spontaneously vomit the roundworms. (3) In roundworm jue, Wu Mei Wan governs, it also governs chronic diarrhoea.

WU MEI WAN: Wu Mei 300 pieces, Xi Xin 6 liang; Gan Jiang 10 liang; Huang Lian 16 liang; Dang Gui 4 liang; Fu Zi (skin removed, dry-fried) 6 liang; Shu Jiao (Chuan Jiao) (sweated) 4 liang; Gui Zhi (bark removed) 6 liang; Ren Shen 6 liang; Huang Bai 6 liang. (Note: To prepare Shu Jiao, set over a low flame until water and oil begin to appear.)

DIRECTIONS: First soak the Wu Mei in vinegar overnight, remove the skin, steam with five dou of rice and when cooked, pound into a paste and mix together. Grind and sieve the other herbs and mix with the Wu Mei paste. Add honey and form into pills the size of the fruit of wu tong or the Chinese parasol tree. Take ten pills three times a day, gradually increasing to twenty pills. Refrain from eating cold or greasy food. Note: wu tong fruit are consistent in size, being approximately 2cm in diameter, and are commonly used in measurement.

DISCUSSION: The first sentence in Clause 338 describes a faint pulse occurring in the course of shang han disease, which is accompanied by jue ni or desertion, indicating cold limbs due to deficient yang and exuberant yin cold. The faint pulse indicates weakness of yang qi, which can not carry the blood to the pulse position, and the cold extremities are attributed to a yang deficiency with severe yin cold which is unable to warm the four limbs. After seven or eight days, the yang qi is further depleted so the manifestation of cold is not confined to the limbs but has spread to the surface of the body, and so the skin also is cold. Vexation is generally the result of yang qi rising and disturbing the heart. Here, there is agitation rather than vexation, which does not relate to emotional discomfort as much as it does to physical manifestations of restlessness. The first sentence therefore explains that the agitation is a result of zang jue or zang desertion, not worms. Zang jue refers to cold in the organs which obstructs the proper flow of yin and yang.

The second sentence goes on to describe the manifestations of roundworm jue, the treatment of which differs from that for zang jue described in the first sentence. The pathology of roundworm jue is a complex of heat in the upper jiao and intestinal cold in the lower jiao. If the worms are in the stomach and are expelled by vomiting, the person will feel better. However, if the worms are disturbed by the extreme internal cold and migrate through the diaphragm to the warmth of the upper jiao, their activity will cause vexation. Once the roundworm activity stops, the vexation also abates. Thus the temporary vexation relates to the migration of the roundworms as they seek the warmth of the upper jiao, after which they are quiet and the person is no longer vexed. Food entering the stomach will disturb the worms, and so there will be a recurrence of the vexation and repeated vomiting, with worms appearing in the vomitus. In roundworm jue, the roundworms obstruct the flow of qi and blood. It is this which leads to the failure of yin and yang to communicate properly, and results in the cold extremities which are the mark of a jue pattern. The indicated formula is Wu Mei Wan which contains cold herbs to cool the upper jiao and hot herbs to warm the lower jiao and also open the channels, thus promoting the flow of qi and blood. In this way, the complex of heat and cold is addressed.

Finally, the clause states that Wu Mei Wan is also indicated for chronic diarrhoea. This is because Wu Mei is sour and astringent, and by following Zhong Jing's directions and soaking it in vinegar, the astringent properties are reinforced. Wu Mei is a relatively mild herb and so the dosage is extraordinarily large. It enters the liver, and more readily gravitates to the liver when treated with vinegar. Wu Mei generates fluids and nourishes the liver yin, and astringes the intestines to stop the diarrhoea. Because it is both warm and sour, it calms the worms, having an almost paralytic effect on them. Shu Jiao and Xi Xin are hot and acrid; they unblock the yang, disperse the cold, break the congealed yin and also kill the worms. Wu Mei and Shu Jiao kill and calm parasites and ease pain. Fu Zi, Gui Zhi and Gan Jiang support the yang and dispel cold. Huang Lian and Huang Bai are bitter and cold; they drain heat and their descending action helps to expel the worms and ease the vomiting; Ren Shen augments qi and tonifies the spleen, and by supporting the earth, it restrains the liver; Dang Gui nourishes blood and softens the liver; the combination of Dang Gui and Wu Mei nourishes the yin and blood of the liver, and the addition of rice and honey, which are sweet, tonifies the stomach. This is a formula where the combined properties of the sour, acrid and hot herbs paralyse and kill the worms, while the cold and bitter herbs drain heat, leading it downwards and helping in the expulsion of the worms.

The clinical features of zang jue (organ jue) and hui jue (roundworm jue) must be assessed in order to differentiate between the two patterns and determine the correct treatment. Zang jue is a pattern of kidney yang devastation with exuberant yin cold heralding the imminent desertion of true yang; it is characterised by a faint pulse, cold extremities, cold skin and constant, unremitting agitation, which is the direct result of the exuberant yin cold. It is a pattern which is approaching a state of pure yin and complete devastation of yang, and spells death. The strategy in the treatment of zang jue is to support the yang and resolve the yin cold. Formulas such as Si Ni Tang and Tong Mai Si Ni Tang can be used to resuscitate the yang and restore the pulse, and moxibustion can be used to warm the channels and disperse cold.

Hui jue is attributed to roundworms harassing the interior, with a surging sensation in the stomach and abdomen, vexation, the vomiting of roundworms, abdominal pain and cold extremities; agitation is not a feature, there is just periodic vexation with remission. Because it does not represent a pattern of extreme devastastion of yang, the prognosis of hui jue is better than that of a zang jue pattern.

Ancient Application of Wu Mei Wan

- *Qian Jin Fang:* For the treatment of chronic diarrhoea.
- *Sheng Ji Zong Lu:* For the treatment of incessant post-partum diarrhoea.
- *Shang Han Lei Fang Hui Can:* For the treatment of abdominal pain due to cold, swelling of the testes and headache located at the vertex.

Modern Application of Wu Mei Wan

- Wu Mei Wan was used to treat 225 cases of biliary obstruction due to roundworm infestation; 97.6% had full recovery. The pattern was one of heat and cold complex. The formula used was Wu Mei 15–30g, Bing Lang 15g, Chuan Lian Zi 15g, Hua Jiao 6g, Gui Zhi 6g, Shu Fu Zi 6g, Xi Xin 3g, Gan Jiang 3g (with a reduced dose for children). Where there was more heat than cold, Huang Bai 9g and Huang Lian 6g were added and the dose of Gui Zhi was increased to 9g (*Hu Nan Yi Yao Wei Sheng Ke Ji Cheng Guo* 1971; 11).

- Wu Mei Wan can be used in the treatment of chronic enteritis, colitis and dysentery. Gao et al (*Henan Zhong Yi*, 河南中医 Henan Journal of Traditional Chinese Medicine 1978; 4:1) used Wu Mei Wan to treat acute dysentery; of 60 cases, 53 cases recovered. The formula used was Wu Mei 15g, Huang Lian 5g, Huang Bai 10g, Hua Shi 30g, Dang Gui 10g, Pao Jiang 3g, Fu Zi 1g, Gui Zhi 1g, Xi Xin 1g, Chuan Jiao 1g, Dang Shen 5g. Once the bowel movement was normal, Shen Mei Tang was used (Dang Shen 10g, Wu Mei 10g, Mu Gua 10g, Yi Ren 15g, Bian Dou 15g, Jiao Shan Zha 3g, Gu Ya 3g, Gan Cao 3g).

Case Study

Ulcerative Colitis

Extracted from Professor Fu Yanling's case studies

Pearls of Wisdom Seminar, Melbourne, October 2007

A 56-year-old male patient had suffered for about one year from persistent diarrhoea with blood and pus in the stool, tenesmus, lower abdominal pain, cold hands and feet, aversion to cold, a red tongue with a yellow coat and a submerged and rapid pulse. The Western diagnosis was ulcerative colitis. The Chinese medicine diagnosis was heat and cold complex. He was prescribed Wu Mei Wan modified (Wu Mei 9g, Huang Lian 6g, Huang Bai 6g, Pao Fu Pian 6g, Gui Zhi 6g, Mu Xiang 6g, Chuan Jiao 6g, Xi Xin 6g, Gan Jiang 6g, Dang Gui 10g, Bai Shao 10g, Jiu Da Huang 9g). After two packs, the abdominal pain eased, his hands turned warm and the diarrhoea was reduced. After a further five packs, the abdominal pain and bloody stool were resolved. Wu Mei Wan was then made into pills for a further two months. A subsequent colonoscopy showed that there was no abnormality in the epithelium of the colon.

Case Study

Non-specific Colitis

Extracted from Professor Fu Yanling's case studies

Pearls of Wisdom Seminar, Melbourne, October 2007

A 39-year-old female patient had suffered for two years from blood and pus in the stool, tenesmus and abdominal pain which was alleviated by warmth and pressure. Her condition was aggravated by cold or greasy food. Investigations showed the presence of pus and white blood cells in the stool and the Western diagnosis was non-specific colitis. She was emaciated and her complexion was sallow. She had no energy, often felt dizzy and her hands and feet were cold. The tip and margin of her tongue were red and the tongue coat was yellow. The pulse was submerged and thready. She was prescribed Wu Mei Wan modified (Wu Mei 10g, Fu Zi 6g, Gui Zhi 6g, Gan Jiang 6g, Hua Jiao 6g, Huang Bai 6g, Huang Lian 6g, Mu Xiang 6g, Dang Gui 10g, Dang Shen 10g). She took seven packs, one each day, and after a week there was no more blood or pus in the stool. The formula was administered in pill form for a further two months to consolidate the treatment.

Gan Jiang Huang Qin Huang Lian Ren Shen Tang Pattern

Clause 359

伤寒本自寒下，医复吐下之，寒格，更逆吐下；若食入口即吐，干姜黄芩黄连人参汤主之。

Shang han disease, originally with spontaneous cold diarrhoea, then the physician induced vomiting and purging, cold repels and there was further adverse vomiting and purgation; if there is vomiting as soon as food enters the mouth, Gan Jiang Huang Qin Huang Lian Ren Shen Tang governs.

GAN JIANG HUANG QIN HUANG LIAN REN SHEN TANG: Gan Jiang 3 liang; Huang Qin 3 liang; Huang Lian 3 liang; Ren Shen 3 liang.

DIRECTIONS: Boil the ingredients in 6 sheng of water, reducing to 2 sheng. Strain and take warm twice a day.

DISCUSSION: Cold diarrhoea indicates that there was an underlying pattern of severe spleen yang deficiency which preceded the contraction of shang han or cold injury. Under such circumstances, the subsequent emetic and purgative therapies were incorrect; they had a deleterious effect on the yang qi, and yin was no longer controlled. The severity of the condition is conveyed in the phrase 'cold repels', which is a reference to the accumulated yin cold repelling yang qi. This gives rise to heat in the upper jiao and cold in the lower jiao. Adverse treatment has damaged both yang qi and yin fluids, and the stomach's function of receiving food is so impaired that vomiting occurs as soon as food is swallowed. It goes without saying that the cold diarrhoea will worsen.

This is a case of damage to yang qi resulting in cold accumulation, and damage to fluids resulting in depletion of stomach yin. The diarrhoea is associated with spleen yang deficiency; the immediate vomiting after eating is ascribed to stomach heat generated as a result of the fluid damage. Gan Jiang Huang Qin Huang Lian Ren Shen Tang is the most appropriate treatment because it restores the qi dynamic of the middle jiao by clearing heat from the stomach, whilst simultaneously warming the interior. This is a strategy of using hot acrid herbs to open and cold bitter herbs to drain, thus addressing the complex of heat in the upper jiao and cold in the lower jiao. Huang Qin and Huang Lian are bitter and cold; they clear heat from the upper jiao and ease vomiting; Gan Jiang is acrid and hot; it disperses the yin accumulation and unblocks the yang qi; Ren Shen is bitter, sweet and warm; it tonifies the spleen and replenishes fluids, thus restoring the pivot mechanism of the middle jiao.

Vomiting can be attributed to heat or cold. Generally, vomiting immediately after eating is associated with stomach heat, and where food eaten in the morning is vomited later in the day, it is ascribed to stomach cold. Stomach heat often coincides with the modern diagnosis of gastritis, and the vomiting of food eaten many hours earlier can coincide with pyloric stenosis.

The formulation of both Gan Jiang Huang Qin Huang Lian Tang and Ban Xia Xie Xin Tang is based on the principle of "acrid opening and bitter draining"; the former is directed at resolving a pattern of exuberant yin repelling yang, resulting in heat in the upper jiao with cold in the lower jiao; the latter is indicated for glomus associated with a pattern of heat and cold complex. Gan Cao and Da Zao are not included in the formula because of their cloying nature, which tends to cause stagnation and aggravate rebellious stomach qi. Ren Shen, therefore, is used on its own to augment qi and benefit the middle.

Ancient Application of Gan Jiang Huang Qin Huang Lian Ren Shen Tang

- *Shang Han Fu Yi:* For patients suffering from vomiting, where such herbs as Mu Xiang, Sha Ren, Jie Geng and Ban Xia are not effective, Gan Jiang Huang Qin Huang Lian Ren Shen Tang is appropriate.
- *Shang Han Lun Yi Shi:* Effective in treating the regurgitation of sour fluids as it descends qi; also applicable for Jin Kou Li 噤口痢, which is dysentery due to deficiency and cold in the spleen, characterised by a poor appetite and vomiting anything that is swallowed.

Modern Application of Gan Jiang Huang Qin Huang Lian Ren Shen Tang

This formula is modified with the addition of Zhu Ru and Chen Pi for the treatment of diarrhoea and vomiting.

If the diarrhoea is protracted and severe, Fu Ling and Bai Zhu are added to strengthen the spleen and resolve damp.

Case Study

Chronic Gastritis

Extracted from Zhang Zhong Jing Yao Fa Yan Jiu Beijing: Ke Xue Ji Zhu Wen Xian Publications, 1984

A 45-year-old female patient had a history of acid reflux and vomiting together with other chronic stomach problems. Her appetite was poor and she suffered from epigastric and abdominal distension which was aggravated by eating cold food and also by stress. Her condition had deteriorated over the previous seven days, following family arguments. She also had mouth ulcers, a loose stool, a preference for warmth on the abdomen, a greasy, white tongue coat and a wiry and taut pulse. She was prescribed Gan Jiang Huang Qin Huang Lian Ren Shen Tang modified (Gan Jiang 9g, Huang Qin 9g, Huang Lian 6g, Dang Shen 15g, Chai Hu 10g, Chi Shao 10g, Chao Zhi Qiao 10g, Gan Cao 10g, Huo Xiang 9g). Two packs. After the two packs of medication, there was borborygmus and a subjective feeling of cold qi descending in the lower abdomen. The vomiting and distension eased. The original formula was repeated with the addition of Hou Po. After three packs, she recovered fully.

Comparison of Gan Jiang Huang Qin Huang Lian Ren Shen Tang with Ban Xia Xie Xin Tang and Ge Gen Qin Lian Tang

	Gan Jiang Huang Qin Huang Lian Ren Shen Tang	Ban Xia Xie Xin Tang	Ge Gen Qin Lian Tang
Pathogenesis	Cold repelling heat in the upper jiao, with cold in the lower jiao	Complex heat with cold glomus due to incorrect purgation	Heat in both the exterior and interior with diarrhoea
Key signs and symptoms	Vomiting immediately following the intake of food	Glomus below the heart, vomiting and diarrhoea	Diarrhoea, dyspnoea, sweating, exterior signs and symptoms
Treatment	Clear heat in the upper jiao and warm the lower jiao	Harmonise the middle and eliminate glomus	Release the exterior and clear interior heat
Formula	Huang Qin 3 liang Gan Jiang 3 liang Ren Shen 3 liang Huang Lian 3 liang	Ban Xia ½ jin Huang Qin 3 liang Gan Jiang 3 liang Huang Lian 1 liang Ren Shen 3 liang Gan Cao 3 liang Da Zao 12 pieces	Ge Gen ½ jin Huang Qin 3 liang Huang Lian 3 liang Gan Cao 2 liang

Ma Huang Sheng Ma Tang Pattern

Clause 357

伤寒六七日，大下后，寸脉沉而迟，手足厥逆，下部脉不至，喉咽不利，唾脓血，泄利不止者，为难治，麻黄升麻汤主之。

Shang han disease for six or seven days, after heavy purgation, the cun pulse is submerged and slow, there is desertion reversal of the hands and feet, the lower pulse does not arrive, the throat is not free, there is spitting of pus and blood, diarrhoea is incessant, this is difficult to treat, Ma Huang Sheng Ma Tang governs.

MA HUANG SHENG MA TANG: Ma Huang (nodes removed) 2½ liang; Sheng Ma 1 liang 1 fen; Zhi Mu 18 zhu; Huang Qin 18 zhu; Wei Rui (Yu Zhu) 18 zhu; Shao Yao 6 zhu; Tian Men Dong (hearts removed) 6 zhu; Gui Zhi (bark removed) 6 zhu; Zhi Gan Cao 6 zhu; Shi Gao 6 zhu (crushed and wrapped in cloth); Bai Zhu 6 zhu; Gan Jiang 6 zhu. Note: In one edition of *Shang Han Lun*, Wei Rui was replaced by Shi Chang Pu.

DIRECTIONS: Boil Ma Huang first in 1 dou of water, bringing to the boil once or twice. Skim the liquid then add the rest of the herbs, boiling until reduced to 3 sheng. Strain and take warm three times a day. The time between doses should be the time it takes to cook three dou of rice. The decoction should be finished in one dose, and when sweat issues, the patient will recover.

DISCUSSION: When shang han disease has already lasted for six or seven days, the pathogen will have transmitted to the interior. If the pathogen lingers in the exterior, then the exterior must be released before treating the interior. If the pathogen which has entered the interior transforms into heat but has not yet developed into an excess fu pattern, then purgation cannot be used, because if it is, it will injure the zheng qi. The resulting deficiency, combined with yang constraint, will manifest as heat in the upper jiao and cold in the lower jiao. This is mainly due to pathogenic obstruction and constrained yang. Incorrect purgation will cause heat to be constrained in the upper jiao, obstructing the flow of qi to the throat. This constrained heat subsequently scorches and injures the network vessels, and hence there is bleeding and a purulent exudate which appears in the sputum. Incorrect purgation also damages the spleen and stomach giving rise to incessant diarrhoea.

The slow and submerged cun pulse is a sign of interior cold and, combined with 'desertion reversal', which describes the condition of cold hands and feet attributed to devastated yang, clearly indicates the presence of interior cold due to deficiency. The unpalpable 'lower pulse' could refer to the chi position, representing the kidneys in the lower jiao, or it might refer to the lower pulses of the "Three Sections Nine Regions" (三部九候) schema, which would be Fu Yang (St 42) on the dorsalis pedis artery or Tai Xi (Kid 3) on the posterior tibial artery. Both these pulses are easily palpated and significant in understanding the severity of a patient's condition. If absent, they indicate a poor prognosis. Whether 'lower' refers to the kidney position on the wrist or to the feet, the non-arrival of the 'lower pulse' is further evidence of a Jue Yin desertion pattern.

This condition presents a treatment dilemma: if cold herbs are used in isolation in order to clear the heat in the upper jiao, the cold in the lower jiao will be exacerbated; if tonifying herbs are used to address the deficiency, the pathogenic excess will become stronger; and purging the excess will aggravate the deficiency. The dilemma is overcome by using Ma Huang Sheng Ma Tang to clear heat in the upper jiao, scatter cold in the lower jiao, disperse the constrained yang and nourish the yin. Ma Huang and Sheng Ma vent the constrained yang; at the same time Sheng Ma clears heat from the upper jiao and raises the sinking yang qi; Zhi Mu, Shi Gao and Huang Qin clear the lung and stomach heat; Tian Dong and Wei Rui nourish yin and generate fluids; Dang Gui and Shao Yao nourish blood and harmonise yin; Gui Zhi and Gan Jiang warm the interior and unblock the yang; Bai Zhu, Fu Ling and Gan Cao strengthen the spleen and tonify the middle qi, and thus support the interaction of yin and yang. The effect of the whole formula is to tonify deficiency and clear heat with a combination of warm and cold herbs. Many *Shang Han Lun* formulas incorporate both hot and cold herbs in order to address a complex pattern of heat and cold. Among these are: Huang Lian Tang, Ban Xia Xie Xin Tang, Wu Mei Wan and Gan Jiang Huang Qin Huang Lian Ren Shen Tang.

A peculiarity of this formula is the relatively large number of herbs, each in a relatively small dose appropriate for the dispersion of constrained yang. Ma Huang, at 2.5 liang (approx 7.5g), has the largest dose, Sheng Ma has the second largest, followed by Dang Gui and then Wei Rui, Zhi Mu and Huang Qin. Because the chief herb is Ma Huang, which is hot and acrid, the overall function of this formula is to release the exterior and so, after taking the decoction, there is sweating. The sweating releases the exterior by unblocking constrained yang and expelling the interior pathogen. This is explained in the directions, which say that when sweat issues, the patient will recover.

Ancient Application of Ma Huang Sheng Ma Tang

The principle of combining the hot and acrid Ma Huang with herbs which are sweet and cold, as seen in Ma Huang Sheng Ma Tang, is applied in the associated formula Qian Jin Wei Rui Tang, which is used to treat wind warmth with severe spontaneous sweating. That formula is composed of Ma Huang as the chief herb, with Wei Rui, Shi Gao and Zhi Gan Cao from the original formula. Other herbs in the formula are Bai Wei, Mu Xiang, Ge Gen, Xing Ren, Chuan Xiong and Du Huo.

Modern Application of Ma Huang Sheng Ma Tang

With the appropriate presentation, this formula is useful in the treatment of scarlet fever, menopausal syndrome, chronic colitis and upper respiratory tract infection.

Comparison of Wu Mei Wan, Gan Jiang Huang Qin Huang Lian Ren Shen Tang and Ma Huang Sheng Ma Tang

	Wu Mei Wan	**Gan Jiang Huang Qin Huang Lian Ren Shen Tang**	**Ma Huang Sheng Ma Tang**
Pathogenesis	Heat in the upper jiao and cold in the lower jiao with harassment of roundworms	Incorrect treatment giving rise to a pattern of heat repelling cold, impaired function of ascent and descent of the spleen and stomach	Constraint of exterior pathogen with complex heat in the upper jiao and cold in the lower jiao
Symptoms	Periodic vexation with quietness, vexation and restlessness, vomiting after ingestion of food, vomiting of roundworms and cold extremities	Vomiting immediately on the ingestion of food	Submerged and slow cun pulse, cold extremities, non-arrival of the lower pulse, inhibited throat, spitting of pus and blood and incessant diarrhoea
Treatment	Clear heat from the upper jiao, scatter cold and warm the lower jiao, calm the roundworms and ease pain	Clear heat in the upper jiao and warm the lower jiao, regulate the spleen and stomach	Release the exterior and expel the pathogen; clear heat from the upper jiao, warm the lower jiao, support the zheng qi, augment yin, dissipate the constrained yang

> **Case Study**
>
> **Chronic Diarrhoea**
>
> ***Extracted from Hu Bei Zhong Yi Za Zhi 1986; (3):36***
>
> A 44-year-old female patient had suffered from chronic diarrhoea for over ten years. This was in spite of numerous treatments, all of which were ineffective. Prior to the consultation, there had been deterioration, resulting in six or more episodes a day. There was no abdominal pain and no blood or pus in the stool. Her appetite was normal, she had a slight thirst but her intake of water was minimal. She complained of hot flushes and had cold hands and feet. Her face was flushed and her tongue was red with a white coat. Her pulse was slippery in the cun and guan positions and the chi pulse was submerged. The Western diagnosis was chronic colitis. She was prescribed Ma Huang Sheng Ma Tang with Pao Jiang Tan 20g replacing Gan Jiang 20g, and Mai Dong 10g replacing Tian Dong. After three packs, the frequency of bowel movement was reduced. The original formula was repeated with an increase in the dose of Pao Jiang from 20g to 30g. She continued her medication for another forty days and there was full recovery.

Summary of Jue Yin Patterns of Heat and Cold Complex

This section summarises the pattern identification and treatment of heat and cold complex with heat in the upper jiao and cold in the lower jiao.

1. *Wu Mei Wan pattern*. The principal clinical features of hui jue (roundworm jue) are the vomiting of roundworms, vexation which is relieved after the vomiting of the roundworms, and paroxysmal upper abdominal pain caused by roundworm harassment. Zang jue (organ jue) is differentiated from hui jue (roundworm jue) on the basis of a faint pulse, cold extremities, cold skin and unremitting as opposed to periodic agitation. Si Ni Tang can be used.
2. *Gan Jiang Huang Qin Huang Lian Ren Shen Tang pattern*. This is a condition of spleen cold deficiency with cold diarrhoea; the interior cold has been exacerbated by purgatives and emetics, and is combined with an exterior pathogenic attack which has transformed into heat. The manifestations of vomiting immediately after eating, and the diarrhoea, are both ascribed to exuberant yin repelling yang, referred to in Clause 359 as 'cold repels'. The treatment is to clear the heat in the upper jiao and dispel cold in the lower jiao by using Gan Jiang Huang Qin Huang Lian Ren Shen Tang.
3. *Ma Huang Sheng Ma Tang pattern*. This is a complex pattern of heat in the upper jiao and cold in the lower jiao associated with deficient zheng qi and the constraint of heat in the upper jiao. The cun pulse is floating and slow, and the 'lower pulse' (in general accepted as referring to the kidney pulse) is not palpable. There are cold extremities due to devastated yang, a severely inflamed throat with blood and pus in the sputum, and incessant diarrhoea. This condition is difficult to treat and the suggested formula is Ma Huang Sheng Ma Tang to vent the constrained yang whilst simultaneously clearing heat from the upper jiao and warming the lower jiao.

7.3.2 Cold Patterns in Jue Yin

Deficient Yang with Exuberant Yin

Si Ni Tang Pattern

> **Clause 353**
>
> 大汗出，热不去，内拘急，四肢疼。又下利，厥逆而恶寒者，四逆汤主之。
>
> *Profuse sweating, the fever does not abate, there is spasm in the interior, pain in the four limbs. If there is also diarrhoea, and desertion reversal and aversion to cold, Si Ni Tang governs.*

DISCUSSION: In an exterior pattern, fever should be resolved by sweating. If, even after profuse sweating, it is not resolved, then the pattern is not an exterior pattern. Simultaneous sweating and fever is reminiscent of a pattern of Yang Ming interior heat. However, this would be characterised by a strong thirst, and an absence of diarrhoea; the extremities would not be cold, and there would be no aversion to cold. It is evident that this is not a Yang Ming interior heat pattern. On the contrary, the copious sweat is a manifestation of true cold with false heat, which is characterised by severe yang deficiency with exuberant yin cold. Here the fever is a sign of deficient yang being repelled by the excess of interior yin. The yang deficiency gives rise to cold; cold congeals and contracts, preventing the fluids already depleted by copious sweating from reaching and nourishing the sinews; the two factors of yang deficiency and congealing cold give rise to cramps and spasm in the interior, and pain in the limbs. The diarrhoea, the cold extremities (referred to in the clause as 'desertion reversal' because they result from the devastation of yang) and the aversion to cold are all evidence of yang exhaustion failing to warm either the extremities or the interior zang. Therefore, the indicated formula is Si Ni Tang to warm the interior and resuscitate the devastated yang.

Clause 353 describes a jue ni pattern due to cold desertion, also known as cold jue (寒厥). It must be differentiated from that of heat desertion or heat jue (热厥), which also presents with cold extremities, where the jue which results in cold extremities is attributed to constrained heat causing impaired flow of yang qi. The cold jue pattern is characterised by cold extremities due to obstruction by cold, and presents with a range of signs of a cold pattern such as the absence of heat, aversion to cold, a preference to curl up, nausea and vomiting, diarrhoea with undigested food particles, clear urine, a pale tongue with a slippery white tongue coat, and a submerged, faint and thready pulse verging on expiry or, alternatively, a submerged, slow pulse. The strategy is to resuscitate the yang with Si Ni Tang. The heat jue pattern is attributed to exuberant interior heat constraining the yang; the yang is then unable to warm the four limbs. The cold extremities are accompanied by heat signs: fever, an aversion to heat, a burning sensation in the chest and abdomen, severe thirst, irritability, insomnia, and sometimes delirious speech. Other symptoms include constipation, abdominal distension, a parched tongue with a dry yellow or black tongue coat and a pulse which is forceful and slippery, or excess and big. The strategy is to clear excess heat by using either Bai Hu Tang or Cheng Qi Tang.

Clause 354

大汗，若大下利而厥冷者，四逆汤主之。

There is profuse sweating, if there is severe diarrhoea and desertion cold, Si Ni Tang governs.

DISCUSSION: Clause 354 describes the situation where a loss of fluids due to heavy sweating has led to yang desertion with cold extremities, referred to here as 'desertion cold'. This pattern can be the result of incorrect treatment or an exterior attack of pathogenic cold, both of which have the potential to damage the yang. In both cases, a degree of pre-existing yang deficiency can be assumed. In the first scenario, the diarrhoea and cold extremities are the result of severe damage to yang caused by the incorrect promotion of sweat, with a subsequent accumulation of yin cold in the interior. The second interpretation is that there is an exterior attack of pathogenic cold, where the damage to yang gives rise to an insecure exterior and spontaneous sweating. The sweating then further damages yang; yang can not control yin, and this leads to the additional symptoms of diarrhoea and cold extremities. In other words, the profuse sweating and diarrhoea can be either the cause or the result of yang deficiency, and may, therefore, create constant mutual deterioration. Although this pattern represents two different aetiologies, both result in the same pattern of devastated yang, and so the indicated formula for both is Si Ni Tang in order to resuscitate yang as a matter of urgency.

Although the above pattern represents depletion of both yin and yang, the treatment strategy must be focused on restoring yang because the yang deficiency is the source of the depletion of fluids. Si Ni Tang is prescribed because of the urgent need to restore the yang; once yang qi is revitalised, qi transformation will be supported and fluids will be regenerated. *Su Wen: Tian Yuan Ji Da Lun Pian* (*Chapter 66: Great Discourse on the Origin of Heaven*) expresses this principle when it says: "yang is transformation, yin is growth" (阳生阴长).

In the contemporary clinical setting, a cold reversal pattern can parallel a critical condition where there is life-threatening hypotension or hypovolaemic shock. In such a situation, a large dose of Ren Shen and Fu Zi can be given to resuscitate the yang. These herbs have been shown to raise blood pressure in hypotensive patients, and can thus reverse such a critical condition.

Blood Deficiency with Congealed Cold

Dang Gui Si Ni Tang Pattern

Clause 351

手足厥寒，脉细欲绝者，当归四逆汤主之。

If there is desertion cold of the hands and feet, and the pulse is thready verging on expiry, Dang Gui Si Ni Tang governs.

DANG GUI SI NI TANG: Dang Gui 3 liang; Gui Zhi (bark removed) 3 liang; Shao Yao 3 liang; Xi Xin 3 liang; Zhi Gan Cao 2 liang; Tong Cao 2 liang; Da Zao 25 pieces (broken).

DIRECTIONS: Boil all the herbs in 8 sheng of water, reducing to 3 sheng. Strain and take 1 sheng warm three times a day.

DISCUSSION: This pattern is characterised by cold extremities and a thready pulse verging on expiry. It differs from cold jue (寒厥) or desertion cold (厥冷), both of which refer to cold limbs due to yang deficiency with exuberant yin, and is also different from heat jue, which also results in cold limbs. A thready pulse indicates blood deficiency; a pulse which is verging on expiry is a pulse which is so faint it is barely palpable. This pulse is a sign not just of yang deficiency but also of deficient blood, where the flow is impeded by the congelation of cold. The impeded flow of qi and blood, combined with the blood deficiency, results in the non-interaction of yin and yang. Dang Gui Si Ni Tang is indicated to nourish blood, disperse interior cold and unblock the vessels.

Dang Gui Si Ni Tang is a modified version of Gui Zhi Tang where Sheng Jiang is omitted and Dang Gui, Xi Xin and Tong Cao are added. Dang Gui is sweet and acrid and Gan Cao is acrid and warm. According to *Ben Cao Zheng Yi* "sweet tonifies blood and acrid moves blood", and so Dang Gui tonifies and moves blood. Shao Yao nourishes blood and astringes yin, and these two herbs nourish the liver and regulate the ying. Xi Xin is acrid, warm and aromatic; it unknots qi and eliminates constraint, thus dispersing cold and unblocking the network vessels. Gui Zhi and Xi Xin unblock the yang, promote the flow of qi and blood, and disperse the cold; Gui Zhi and Shao Yao regulate ying, wei, qi and blood. The large dose of Da Zao nourishes blood and, combined with Gan Cao, tonifies the middle and benefits qi, thus supplementing the source of qi and blood and supporting the return of the pulse. Da Zao and Gan Cao also moderate the dispersing action of Xi Xin. Tong Cao assists the movement of the other herbs through the channels and thereby assists in the resumed interaction of yin and yang. This is a modified version of Gui Zhi Tang which not only warms the channels and dissipates cold, but also augments qi and blood to restore the pulse.

Based on the pathogenesis of blood deficiency with cold congelation, there will be a pale complexion, dizziness and other symptoms according to the location of the disorder: if there is cold stagnation affecting the channels and joints, there will be cold hands and feet and joint pain; if the congealed cold affects the lower jiao, there will be frequent, clear urination and no constipation. In spite of the variation in symptoms, the pathogenesis and treatment are the same. The thready pulse verging on expiry in this pattern must be distinguished from a faint pulse verging on expiry. A thready pulse is a pulse which feels like a thread of cotton under the fingers and which is a reflection of blood deficiency; a faint pulse is felt as a pulse without force, unable to rise beneath the fingers, and is associated with yang deficiency. This distinction is important because the treatment differs.

A Dang Gui Si Ni Tang pattern must be differentiated from a Si Ni Tang pattern. The former is a pattern of liver blood deficiency with cold accumulation and is characterised by cold extremities with a thready pulse verging on expiry; the treatment is to warm the channels and disperse cold. The latter is a pattern of kidney yang deficiency with exuberant interior yin and is characterised by cold extremities, diarrhoea with food particles and a faint pulse verging on expiry; the treatment is to resuscitate yang and eliminate yin cold.

Ancient Application of Dang Gui Si Ni Tang

- *Yi Zong Bi Du:* A patient had had an inguinal hernia for ten years. His complexion was pale and dull. Li Zhong Zhi observed a bulge in the left side of the chest as wide as the thickness of an arm. This was diagnosed as hernia jue and Dang Gui Si Ni Tang was used. After six months of medication the hernia disappeared.
- *Han Yao Shen Xiao Fang:* For the treatment of chilblains.

Modern Application of Dang Gui Si Ni Tang

Dang Gui Si Ni Tang has a broad range of applications and is useful in the treatment of inguinal hernia, cold bi pattern, Jue Yin headache, dysmenorrhoea and Raynaud's syndrome.

- Migraine headache: You et al treated 52 cases of migraine headache characterised by aversion to cold, a pale complexion and a slow pulse. The treatment course ranged from 20–30 packs. The results were: effective = 9; headache under control = 17; satisfactory = 18 and not effective = 8 (You Guo Xiong: *Zhong Hua Yi Xue Za Zhi* 1980; 1:57).
- Thrombotic angiitis: Liu et al used Dang Gui Si Ni Tang modified to treat 10 cases of thrombotic angiitis with satisfactory results (*Shang Hai Zhong Yi Yao Za Zhi* 1965; 8:19).
- Raynaud's syndrome: Zhu et al used Dang Gui Si Ni Tang with the addition of Ai Ye, Wu Zhu Yu, Tao Ren paste and Hong Hua to treat 4 cases of Raynaud's syndrome attributed to yang deficiency (*Jiang Su Zhong Yi* 1963; 6:15).
- For sciatica associated with blood deficiency and congealed cold, add Niu Xi, Di Long; for chronic pain with blood stasis, add Tao Ren and Hong Hua; for severe cold, add Fu Zi (*Shang Han Lun Yu Lin Chuang*).

Comparison of Dang Gui Si Ni Tang, Si Ni Tang and Si Ni San

	Dang Gui Si Ni Tang	Si Ni Tang	Si Ni San
Pathogenesis	Blood deficiency with cold congealing	Yang deficiency with exuberant yin cold	Constrained yang qi in the interior
Key signs and symptoms	Cold extremities, a thready pulse verging on expiry	Aversion to cold, diarrhoea, cold extremities, a faint pulse verging on expiry, a desire to sleep	Cough OR palpitations OR inhibited urination OR abdominal pain OR diarrhoea with tenesmus, cold extremities and a wiry pulse
Ingredients	Dang Gui Gui Zhi Shao Yao Tong Cao Da Zao Xi Xin Gan Cao	Fu Zi Gan Jiang Zhi Gan Cao	Chai Hu Shao Yao Zhi Shi Zhi Gan Cao.

Case Study

Chilblains

Extracted from Greta Young's case studies

A 15-year-old girl had suffered from frostbite each winter for many years. The symptoms included coldness, numbness and pain in the hands and feet and itching and swelling at the site of the chilblains. She was menstruating at the time of her consultation and also presented with lower back pain and abdominal discomfort. Her pulse was faint and thready and her tongue was pale red with a thin, white and moist tongue coat. This is an attack of exterior cold damaging interior yang and causing the blood to congeal. She was prescribed Dang Gui Si Ni Tang modified (Dang Gui 10g, Gui Zhi 10g, Xi Xin 3g, Tong Cao 5g, Zhi Gan Cao 5g, Bai Shao 10g, Chai Hu 10g, Wu Yao 10g, Sheng Jiang 3 pieces, Da Zao 5 pieces). After two packs, her hands and feet felt warm and her pulse was moderate and forceful. The original formula was repeated for five more days and the following year there was no re-occurrence of the chilblains.

Discussion: Frostbite and chilblains are attributed to blood deficiency with cold congealing blood in the channels; in this case it was also the cause of the patient's menstrual pain. The treatment strategy was to warm the channels, disperse cold and regulate the flow of liver qi. The author used this formula to treat many cases of frostbite and the best result was obtained if the herbs were prescribed when the acute symptoms of swelling and itching were present. Dang Gui Si Ni Tang is also effective in the treatment of varicose veins when combined with Si Miao Yong An Tang.

Case Study

Dysmenorrhoea

Extracted from Greta Young's case studies

A 23-year-old woman had had irregular and painful menstruation since the menarche at the age of 14. The menstrual flow was scant and pale and the pain forced her to stay in bed. She had been given Si Wu Tang and Xiao Yao San to nourish blood and regulate qi but this was not effective. On the day of the consultation, her face was pale, her hands and feet were cold, the fingers were white, and she had cramping lower abdominal pain. Her appetite was poor and she felt fatigued and tired; her stool and urination were normal, the pulse was moderate and thready, and her tongue coat was white and moist. She was prescribed Dang Gui Si Ni Tang modified (Dang Gui 15g, Bai Shao 10g, Gui Zhi 12g, Lui Ji Hu 8g, Xi Xin 3g, Wu Zhu Yu 6g, Zhi Gan Cao 5g, Sheng Jiang 3 pieces, Da Zao 5 pieces, Xiang Fu 10g, Yan Hu Suo 10g). After one month, her abdominal pain eased considerably, her hands and feet felt warm and she was more energetic. She was given two more packs and was instructed in future to take 2–3 packs each menstrual period. She continued that treatment for six months and her menstruation became more regular.

Discussion: Dysmenorrhoea can be attributed to cold in the channels, characterised by pain and cold extremities. The pattern of dysmenorrhoea due to blood heat is rarely seen. Thus the strategy is to warm and unblock the channels with Dang Gui Si Ni Tang as the guiding formula. During previous treatment, this patient had been given Si Wu Tang or Tao Hong Si Wu Tang and Xiao Yao San all of which were ineffective. Si Wu Tang can nourish blood while Xiao Yao San can disperse constrained liver qi but none of the above formulas are targeting the root cause which is blood deficiency with channel coldness.

Dang Gui Si Ni jia Wu Zhu Yu Sheng Jiang Tang Pattern

Clause 352

若其人内有久寒者，宜当归四逆加吴茱萸生姜汤。

If the person has long-term interior cold, Dang Gui Si Ni jia Wu Zhu Yu Sheng Jiang Tang is appropriate.

DANG GUI SI NI JIA WU ZHU YU SHENG JIANG TANG: Dang Gui 3 liang; Shao Yao 3 liang; Zhi Gan Cao 2 liang; Tong Cao 2 liang; Gui Zhi (bark removed) 3 liang; Xi Xin 3 liang; Sheng Jiang (sliced) ½ jin; Wu Zhu Yu 2 sheng; Da Zao 25 pieces.

DIRECTIONS: Boil in 6 sheng of water mixed with 6 sheng of clear wine, reducing to 5 sheng. Strain, divide into five doses and take warm.

DISCUSSION: This clause continues on from Clause 351 which describes cold extremities with a thready pulse verging on expiry where Dang Gui Si Ni Tang is indicated. Clause 352 goes on to describe a person who has suffered from interior cold for a prolonged period. From the recommended formula, which is Dang Gui Si Ni Tang, with the addition of Wu Zhu Yu and Sheng Jiang, it can be inferred that the condition has progressed to the point where it is affecting the liver and stomach. Accumulated phlegm fluids cause vomiting and excessive salivation, and accumulated yin cold binding the interior causes pain in the middle and lower jiao. This pattern is the result of prolonged exposure to exterior cold, and is a more serious condition than the Dang Gui Si Ni Tang pattern of Clause 351. The indicated formula is Dang Gui Si Ni jia Wu Zhu Yu Sheng Jiang Tang, which is Dang Gui Si Ni Tang with the addition of Wu Zhu Yu Sheng Jiang Tang.

Dang Gui Si Ni Tang nourishes blood and warms the channels, thus unblocking the vessels and dissipating cold. The addition of Wu Zhu Yu and Sheng Jiang dispels both interior and exterior cold. Wu Zhu Yu warms the middle, regulates the liver qi, eases pain, and directs qi downwards to alleviate vomiting; it enters the stomach and spleen where its hot acrid properties dry damp, and enters the liver to disperse knotted liver qi. Thus it is effective in treating disharmony of the liver and spleen associated with cold which manifests as acid reflux or vomiting. It enters the kidney and leads fire downwards to warm the lower jiao and is indicated to treat abdominal and hernial pain. The combination of Wu Zhu Yu and Sheng Jiang warms the stomach and transforms accumulated fluids. The clear wine is added to the decoction for its penetrating property, which opens the channels and promotes the flow of qi, thus facilitating the action of the other herbs in dispelling cold and restoring yang.

Differential Treatment of Cold Extremities

Cold extremities are a feature of both Shao Yin and Jue Yin patterns. In Shao Yin the treatment is Si Ni Tang (Fu Zi, Gan Jiang and Zhi Gan Cao); in Jue Yin, there are two patterns. The first is where the cold limbs are due to blood deficiency with cold congealing the blood and the indicated formula is Dang Gui Si Ni Tang (Dang Gui, Shao Yao, Gui Zhi, Xi Xin, Tong Cao, Zhi Gan Cao, Da Zao). The second is where the cold has penetrated the liver and stomach and the formula is Dang Gui Si Ni jia Wu Zhu Yu Sheng Jiang Tang (Dang Gui, Shao Yao, Gui Zhi, Xi Xin, Tong Cao, Zhi Gan Cao, Da Zao, Sheng Jiang, Wu Zhu Yu). The chief differences between the three formulas are as follows. The Shao Yin formula, Si Ni Tang, contains Fu Zi and Gan Jiang, which are not in the two Jue Yin formulas; Wu Zhu Yu and Sheng Jiang are in the second Jue Yin formula but not in Si Ni Tang or Dang Gui Si Ni Tang.

COMPARISON OF SI NI TANG AND DANG GUI SI NI TANG: In Shao Yin, cold extremities are attributed to interior yin cold and the devastation of yang qi. Shao Yin is associated with the kidney, the organ of water, which suffers when yang is deficient and there is insufficient fire within the water. In the Shao Yin pattern, Gan Jiang and Fu Zi are needed to warm the fire and resuscitate the yang. In Jue Yin, cold extremities are due to deficient blood which is congealed by cold. Jue Yin pertains to the liver which stores blood and is nourished by yin. Hot acrid herbs such as Gan Jiang and Fu Zi will consume yin and deplete blood, and so Dang Gui and Shao Yao are used to nourish yin and blood and soften the liver. In brief, in Shao Yin disease, the focus is to warm the yang with such herbs as Gan Jiang and Fu Zi, while in Jue Yin disease, the focus is on nourishing the liver blood by using Dang Gui and Shao Yao. Because hot acrid herbs such as Gan Jiang and Fu Zi are drying and can injure yin and blood, they are used sparingly and with caution in patterns of blood or yin deficiency.

COMPARISON OF DANG GUI SI NI TANG AND DANG GUI SI NI JIA WU ZHU YU SHENG JIANG TANG: Both Dang Gui Si Ni Tang and its modified version contain the herbs Gui Zhi and Xi Xin to penetrate and warm the channels. Dang Gui Si Ni Tang is used for a pattern of blood deficiency where cold has congealed the blood and the inclusion of those two warm and acrid herbs is sufficient. To also include the hot and acrid Fu Zi and Gan Jiang would create a harsh and drying effect.

COMPARISON OF SI NI TANG AND DANG GUI SI NI JIA WU ZHU YU SHENG JIANG TANG: In the second Jue Yin pattern not only is there deficient blood with congealed cold, but the cold has penetrated the liver and stomach, causing a more serious condition with the additional symptoms of vomiting, excessive salivation, and pain in the stomach and the lower abdomen. The cold is more severe than in the Dang Gui Si Ni Tang pattern, and has affected the zang. Therefore the inclusion of more warming herbs is warranted. However, Fu Zi and Gan Jiang of the original Si Ni Tang, from which this formula is derived, are still too harsh. Instead of Gan Jiang, Sheng Jiang is used, and instead of Fu Zi, Wu Zhu Yu is used.

The rationale for this is that Sheng Jiang is not hot but warm; it is more moderate than Gan Jiang and therefore can warm the middle without injuring yin and blood. Secondly, Sheng Jiang is lighter and moves outwards, and is thus better to disperse cold, while Gan Jiang targets the interior and tends to move inwards and stay there. Thirdly, Sheng Jiang is better to treat vomiting. Wu Zhu Yu, whilst still hot and acrid, is also bitter; it is draining and descending, as opposed to Fu Zi which is dispersing and ascending. Moreover, Wu Zhu Yu enters the stomach and liver as well as the kidney and therefore not only supplements the fire of the kidneys, but also warms the liver and stomach. It moves the liver qi and its descending action redirects rebellious qi, thus alleviating vomiting. It is specific for excess salivation and hernial pain, or other abdominal pain caused by cold stagnating in the liver channel.

Ancient Application of Dang Gui Si Ni jia Wu Zhu Yu Tang Formulas

- *Yi Xue Ru Men:* For the treatment of Jue Yin disease characterised by cold extremities, lower abdominal pain, or vomiting or retracted testes or blood deficiency with a pulse verging on expiry, use Dang Gui Si Ni Tang. If there is severe coldness, add Wu Zhu Yu, Sheng Jiang; and if the pulse does not surface, add Ren Shen.
- *Lei Ju Fang Guang Yi:* For the treatment of retained lochia characterised by fever, headache, cold in the abdomen, vomiting, a soft or loose stool, and numbness or swelling in the lower limbs, use Dang Gui Si Ni jia Wu Zhu Yu and Sheng Jiang Tang.

Modern Application of Dang Gui Si Ni jia Wu Zhu Yu Tang Formulas

Zhao et al used Dang Gui Si Ni jia Wu Zhu Yu Sheng Jiang Tang with complete success in the treatment of two cases of retracted testes. One case occurred 30 minutes after exposure to cold. Apart from feeling very cold, there was acute abdominal pain accompanied by cold extremities, nausea and vomiting. His pulse was faint and thready and he had a moist white tongue coat. The second case occurred following sexual intercourse. He experienced a pulling pain in the lower abdomen, followed by the retraction of his testes. His limbs were cold, and he suffered from occasional cold sweat, dizziness, fatigue, a thready and faint pulse and a moist tongue. Dang Gui Si Ni jia Wu Zhu Yu Sheng Jiang Tang was used to treat both cases. They recovered after three packs (*Guang Dong Zhong Yi* 1960; 6:305).

Case Study

Acrocyanosis or Raynaud's Sign

Extracted from Xin Zhong Yi 1983; (4)

A female patient had suffered from peripheral cyanosis due to arterial spasm for many years. The fingers were numb, immersion in hot water caused pain and her right index finger had chronic ulceration. Acupuncture had not been effective. Her pulse was even, weak and thready and the tip of her tongue was red. She was prescribed Dang Gui Si Ni Tang to unblock the yang and harmonise the ying, with Wu Zhu Yu and Sheng Jiang added to purge the excess cold. After 16 packs, there was a significant improvement in the cyanosis and the ulcerated index finger healed.

Cold Bind in the Urinary Bladder

Clause 340

病者手足厥冷，言我不结胸，小腹满，按之痛者，此冷结在膀胱关元也。

The patient has desertion cold of the hands and feet, one says it is not chest bind, if the lower abdomen is full, and there is pain on palpation, this is cold bind in the urinary bladder at Guan Yuan.

DISCUSSION: Cold extremities can be associated with yin, yang, heat, cold, deficiency or excess; accompanying symptoms must be analysed before coming to a differential diagnosis. The statement that there is no chest bind eliminates the upper and middle jiao as possible locations of the disease; distension in the lower abdomen, where pain is elicited by pressure, confirms that it is, in fact, a lower jiao disorder. The lower abdomen pertains to the Jue Yin channel. *Ling Shu: Jing Mai Pian (Chapter 10: The Channels)* says: "The foot Jue Yin channel originates at the big toe and runs upwards traversing the instep, and the shin, an inch from the inner ankle, and eight inches above the ankle, after connecting with Tai Yin, it follows the inner leg to the groin, crossing the genitals to the lower abdomen". Because the Ren vessel passes over the urinary bladder, and the liver channel intersects with Guan Yuan (Ren 4) in the lower abdomen, cold in the liver channel can transfer to the bladder via this point.

Clause 340 describes the diagnostic features of cold extremities, absence of chest bind, and distension in the lower abdomen with pain on palpation, and concludes that there is cold bind in the urinary bladder at Guan Yuan. In the clinical situation, further identifying symptoms would be sought and found, such as aversion to cold, a preference for warmth and clear urination. Lower abdominal fullness is not specific for cold bind in the urinary bladder, and further differentiation must be made to distinguish this pattern from Tai Yang water amassment or blood amassment, both of which are lower jiao disorders characterised by fullness in the lower abdomen. Water amassment is characterised by inhibited urination; blood amassment is characterised by manic behaviour. *Yi Zong Jin Jian* states: "Uninhibited urination with lower abdominal fullness is due to blood amassment in the urinary bladder; inhibited urination is due to water amassment in the urinary bladder; warm extremities with dark urination are due to heat in the urinary bladder; cold extremities with clear urination are due to cold bind in the urinary bladder".

Although *Shang Han Lun* proposed no specific formula, suggestions have been made by past scholars. Zhu Gong recommended Dang Gui Si Ni jia Wu Zhu Yu Sheng Jiang Tang; and You Zai Jing suggested Si Ni Tang or Bai Tong Tang to resuscitate the yang and eliminate pathogenic yin cold. This is a pattern of cold in the liver channel. Moxa can be used on Guan Yuan (Ren 4), and Dang Gui Si Ni Tang with the addition of Wu Zhu Yu and Sheng Jiang can be prescribed to warm the channels and dissipate cold.

Cold Turbidity with Vomiting

Wu Zhu Yu Tang Pattern

Clause 378

干呕，吐涎沫，头痛者，吴茱萸汤主之。

If there is dry retching, drooling and a headache, Wu Zhu Yu Tang governs.

DISCUSSION: Clause 378 describes a pattern of cold in the liver attacking the stomach. The Jue Yin liver channel connects to the stomach before crossing the diaphragm into the chest and upper jiao and finally ascending via the throat to the vertex of the head. The yin cold accumulation in the liver assails the stomach, preventing the proper descent of qi, so there is counterflow and dry retching.

The turbid yin then ascends to the throat and mouth, manifesting as excessive salivation and drooling. If the turbid yin continues its upward movement there will be headache. Wu Zhu Yu Tang warms the liver and stomach and redirects rebellious qi downward.

In *Shang Han Lun*, Wu Zhu Yu Tang is used to treat a Yang Ming pattern of deficiency cold manifesting with vomiting, where there is epigastric distension and discomfort alleviated by warmth and pressure. This pattern is characterised by a thin white tongue coat and a wiry pulse. Wu Zhu Yu Tang is also used to treat patterns of Shao Yin yang deficiency when exuberant yin cold results in the counterflow of turbid yin, manifesting with the symptoms of vomiting, cold limbs, and severe agitation with a feeling that one is about to die. Wu Zhu Yu Tang warms cold in the liver channel and descends the rebellious upsurge of turbid yin. Similarly, in a Jue Yin pattern of cold in the liver and stomach, manifesting with dry retching, excessive salivation and headache, Wu Zhu Yu Tang is prescribed to warm the liver channel and the middle jiao, and to redirect qi downwards in order to stop the dry retching and drooling. These three patterns are all characterised by vomiting due to cold, and so Wu Zhu Yu Tang is indicated.

The key symptoms of this pattern are dry retching and drooling. From this, it is understood that in addition to dry retching, there is stomach reflux with a sour taste. There is possibly a small amount of green fluid ejected with the dry retching, and increased production of clear saliva from the mouth, which is copious, sticky and frothy. Clear saliva is the result of cold in the stomach, and is produced as a result of the disordered stomach qi and the retching and nausea; the retching is accompanied by a cold sensation. This parallels what is commonly called a 'bilious attack'. A headache at the vertex of the head is pathognomonic for a headache associated with the foot Jue Yin liver channel. Headaches associated with the Tai Yang channel are located in the occiput; those associated with Yang Ming are located on the forehead; and those associated with Shao Yang are often unilateral and are located in the parietal region and the temple, while Jue Yin headaches are located at the vertex.

The indication of Wu Zhu Yu Tang for headache is conditional on the following. (1) The location of the headache at the vertex; (2) The nature of the pain as an intense pulling sensation; (3) The absence of signs of an exterior pattern or of heat, and the accompanying symptoms of vomiting and retching or drooling; (4) The presentation of a pale, lack-lustre complexion, a submerged and wiry or tight pulse, a dull red tongue with a thin, white and possibly greasy tongue coat. Wu Zhu Yu Tang can be modified as follows.

- For severe vomiting, add Ban Xia, Fu Ling, Zhu Ru and Ding Xiang.
- For a particularly intense headache, add Gao Ben, Chuan Xiong, Bai Zhi, Chuan Niu Xi.
- Where it is accompanied by stomach pain due to cold, add Gao Liang Jiang, Xiang Fu.
- For turbid dampness characterised by a greasy tongue coat, add Huo Xiang, Pei Lan.
- For qi deficiency, add Huang Qi and Bai Zhu.
- For abdominal fullness, add Bai Kou Ren, Fo Shou.
- For acid reflux, add Wu Zei Gu and Wa Leng Zi.

Case Study

Stomach Pain

Extracted from Greta Young's case studies

A 41-year-old male patient presented with stomach pain and with vomiting of a clear liquid which worsened in cold weather. He was dizzy and had no appetite; his tongue was pale and the tongue coat moist and slippery. The pulse was thready and wiry. He had been suffering from a duodenal ulcer for two years. The diagnosis was liver cold harassing the stomach. The treatment principle was to warm the liver and disperse cold, suppress counterflow and ease pain. Three packs of Wu Zhu Yu Tang were prescribed: Wu Zhu Yu 9g, Dang Shen 15g, Sheng Jiang 12g, Da Zao 5 pieces, Fa Ban Xia 10g, Mu Xiang 6g.

After three packs of the above medication, he attended for a second consultation. The stomach pain and vomiting had stopped, the vertigo had subsided and there was a feeling of warmth in the stomach. His pulse was thready and moderate and the tongue was white and moist. Five packs of a modification of Liu Jun Zi Tang were prescribed: Dang Shen 15g, Bai Zhu 10g, Fu Ling 15g, Wu Zhu Yu 5g, Fa Ban Xia 10g, Zhi Gan Cao 5g, Sheng Jiang 3 pieces, Chen Pi 10g, Mu Xiang 10g. After these five packs, his appetite improved and his bowel and urination returned to normal. The formula was repeated, omitting Wu Zhu Yu and adding Huang Qi 15g for ten more packs.

Discussion: In a pattern of liver cold harassing the stomach, the liver disharmony is the root and the stomach disharmony is the branch. Wu Zhu Yu warms the liver and stomach and is thus indicated in a pattern of liver cold harassing the stomach. The patient was suffering from spleen and stomach insufficiency with the liver exploiting the deficiency. Mu Xiang and Ban Xia were added to suppress the rebellious counterflow.

Water Jue

Fu Ling Gan Cao Tang Pattern

Clause 356

伤寒，厥而心下悸，宜先治水，当服茯苓甘草汤，却治其厥，不尔，水渍入胃，必作利也。

Shang han, there is jue and palpitations below the heart, it is appropriate to treat the water first, one should take Fu Ling Gan Cao Tang, but if one treats the jue by another method, the water will enter right into the stomach, there will be diarrhoea.

DISCUSSION: The term 'jue' refers to a pattern of cold limbs due to desertion of yang qi; contributing factors include cold, heat, blood deficiency with cold accumulation, and phlegm. In dealing with a desertion pattern, it is essential to identify the causative factors in order to give appropriate treatment. Clause 356 describes a pattern of cold extremities accompanied by palpitations in the epigastric area, thus indicating water accumulation in the stomach. In this pattern, it is the accumulated water which obstructs the yang qi and results in jue or cold extremities. Treatment must therefore be focused on eliminating water as the cause of the jue, and so Fu Ling Gan Cao Tang is used to free the yang and transform qi. Once excess water is eliminated, the distribution of yang qi will be normal and the cold extremities will be warmed. Here, the word 'stomach' is intended to include the concept of the intestines as well. If, however, in treating the jue, this principle is not followed, and some other method is used to try and treat the cold extremities without first eliminating the water, the excess water will find its way into the stomach and intestines and cause diarrhoea.

The patterns described here by Clause 356 and Clause 355, which appears in Chapter 2 Tai Yang Disease, share some similarities. They are both characterised by cold extremities caused by the obstruction of yang qi, however, the pathogenesis differs. In Clause 355, the cause of the obstruction is excess phlegm in the chest and diaphragm (also known as phlegm jue), and Gua Di San is used to induce vomiting to eliminate the phlegm. The cold extremities of the water jue pattern described in Clause 356, are however, as the pattern name suggests, caused by accumulated water in the stomach obstructing the proper flow of yang qi. The indicated formula is Fu Ling Gan Cao Tang to free the yang, transform fluids and promote urination.

Clause 356 serves as a guide in the treatment of palpitations occurring simultaneously with cold extremities, the focus being first to eliminate water. It also serves as a reminder of the importance of sound diagnosis based on identifying the 'root' or underlying cause in order to choose the most appropriate treatment. Past scholars explained that once the water accumulation is resolved, the distribution of yang qi would be restored and so the coldness of the extremities would be eliminated. Disorders relating to water accumulation are generally rooted in yang deficiency, where deficient yang is unable to support transformation, and so the appropriate strategy is to unblock the yang and transform water. The pattern described in this clause can coincide with the modern diagnosis of cardiac and renal failure, where there are palpitations and oedema as a result of decreased urinary output.

Desertion Patterns and Moxibustion

Clause 349

伤寒脉促，手足厥逆，可灸之。

Shang han, the pulse is skipping, there is desertion reversal of the hands and feet, moxibustion may be used.

DISCUSSION: A skipping pulse is a rapid pulse with an interrupted beat and a tripping, uneven rhythm. The rapidity usually indicates heat, and the interruption to the rhythm indicates constraint or obstruction. When a skipping pulse occurs simultaneously with cold hands and feet in shang han disease, it is indicative of yang deficiency where it is exuberant yin which impedes the flow, and so warming therapy is appropriate. In this case, the accelerated pulse is a reflection of the struggle of deficient yang against the yin pathogen, and the obstructive nature of the yin pathogen causes the rhythm to trip and stumble unevenly. Moxibustion not only warms the channels and scatters yin cold, but also unblocks obstruction and promotes the flow of qi and blood.

There are two aspects to a skipping pulse: its speed, which is rapid, and its rhythm, which is uneven, and in the past there has been some discussion as to what a skipping pulse indicates. Zhang Xu Gu said: "A rapid pulse with intermission is known as a skipping pulse. This is due to the pathogenic constraint of yang qi. The cold extremities can be treated with moxibustion to unblock the network vessels so that the movement of qi can bring recovery." You Zai Jing said: "Yang exuberance is characterised by a skipping pulse while yin exuberance is characterised by a knotted pulse. The cold extremities and skipping pulse are not indications of yang deficiency but are due to yang constraint and moxibustion can cause the yang to be vented outward" (*Shang Han Guan Zhu Ji*). This interpretation is based on the Jue Yin channel's relationship with the liver, which regulates the flow of qi. You Zai Jing's reasoning was that when a pathogen has affected the liver, its function of spreading qi is impaired; thus there will be cold extremities and a skipping pulse.

Neither of these interpretations explains how yang deficiency might result in a rapid or skipping pulse. The first speaks of constraint of yang and the second makes no mention of yang deficiency. However, in various circumstances, a rapid pulse can be due to heat, cold, excess or deficiency. If the pulse is rapid and forceful, it indicates yang excess and heat; if it is rapid and forceless, it indicates yang deficiency and cold. Qian Tian Lai said: "Where yin is exuberant, yang can not establish a foothold, and hence the pulse is deficient, rapid, short and swift" (*Shang Han Shuo Yuan Ji*). In view of this, and in view of the recommendation to use moxibustion, this pattern is one of deficiency cold. It should be noted that moxibustion is contraindicated for heat patterns, whether due to excess or deficiency, and Clause 115 is a reminder of the transmuted pattern which can arise because of inappropriate moxibustion therapy. No specific location is suggested for moxibustion, but Tai Chong (Liv 3), Guan Yuan (Ren 4) and Qi Hai (Ren 6) can be used.

Cold Diarrhoea and Hiccough Patterns

Clause 358

伤寒四五日，腹中痛，若转气下趣少腹者，此欲自利也。

Shang han for four or five days, there is pain in the abdomen, if the migratory qi tends to descend to the lesser abdomen, this means imminent spontaneous diarrhoea.

DISCUSSION: In shang han disease which has lasted for four or five days, there is a probabililty of transmission. Roaming abdominal pain of no fixed location reflects the changing movement of qi. If it tends to descend to the lower abdomen, it is because of the yin cold accumulation which has arisen as a result of deficient spleen yang. There is then a situation of deficiency cold with yin accumulation having migrated or transferred to the lower jiao. The arrival of this cold sensation in the lower abdomen means that there will be diarrhoea.

The phenomenon of abdominal pain and the descent of qi into the lower abdomen is a feature of many patterns and is not confined to yang deficiency with yin cold accumulation. It is important not to make such an assumption but to analyse the pattern in terms of the eight principles before reaching a diagnosis. Patterns of cold and deficiency abound, as can be seen in diseases of the yin channels, such as the cold patterns of Tai Yin, where abdominal pain accompanied by the descent of cold qi to the lower jiao also results in diarrhoea. Yang Ming fu excess can also present with abdominal pain followed by the descent of qi into the lower jiao, the difference being that in that case, it is not followed by a bowel movement.

Clause 358 continues the discussion of Clauses 353 and 354 which predict the looming of yin cold diarrhoea, and where the pathogenesis is yang deficiency and yin exuberance resulting in the descent of cold qi. The description of the descent of qi here in Clause 358 can be compared with the line in Clause 356 where the transfer of water into the stomach and intestines precedes diarrhoea. From the modern medicine perspective, the pattern of sensing descent of qi which can precede diarrhoea relates directly to increased urgency of peristaltic movement and the coincident transport of faeces to the rectum.

Clause 380

伤寒，大吐、大下之，极虚，复极汗者，其人外气怫郁，复与之水以发其汗，因得哕。所以然者，胃中寒冷故也。

Shang han, if there is severe vomiting and severe purgation, causing extreme deficiency, following which there is extreme sweating, the person has glowering constraint of exterior qi, water then is given to enable sweating, causing hiccough. The reason for this being, there is coldness in the stomach.

DISCUSSION: If shang han disease is incorrectly treated with harsh emetics and purgatives, the qi of all three jiao suffers damage, particularly the yang of the spleen and stomach; zheng qi is also depleted and this extreme deficiency means there is no recovery. The adverse treatments have resulted in both exterior and interior cold, characterised by aversion to cold with the absence of sweat. Mistaking this for an unresolved exterior pattern, heavy sweating was then promoted. However, the promotion of sweat is contraindicated in a deficiency condition and it constitutes a further assault on the yang of the middle jiao. The repeated loss of fluids gives rise to constraint of severe heat in the exterior, causing the sweating to stop, so the patient is given water to help with the continued production of sweat. The damage to the yang qi has affected the spleen's function of transformation and resulted in the accumulation of fluids in the stomach which, in turn, impairs the stomach's descending function. The accumulation of fluids and yin cold in the stomach obstructs the descent of qi, giving rise to rebellious qi which manifests as hiccoughing.

In *Shang Han Lun*, hiccough, known as *e ni* (呃逆), can be associated with heat, cold, excess or deficiency. As explained in the discussion on Xuan Fu Dai Zhe Tang (Clause 161), hiccough can also be the result of phlegm. In Clause 380, however, the underlying cause is yang deficiency with cold accumulation, and so the clause states that the reason for the hiccoughs is cold in the stomach.

Hiccoughs are generally self-limiting and resolve spontaneously, but at times they are a manifestation of a pattern which requires identification and treatment, and sometimes are a manifestation of a serious or chronic disease where depletion of the spleen and stomach is severe and prognosis is poor. For a pattern of spleen yang deficiency and cold, Li Zhong Wan can be used with the addition of Ding Xiang and Wu Zhu Yu; for a pattern of deficiency heat, Zhu Ye Shi Gao Tang can be used; and for excess heat, Xiao Cheng Qi Tang is suitable. For treatment of hiccough resulting from qi constraint, Si Ni San can be used with the addition of Shi Di and Zhu Ru; where there is phlegm obstruction, Xuan Fu Dai Zhe Tang is the indicated formula.

> **Clause 381**
>
> 伤寒哕而腹满，视其前后，知何部不利，利之即愈。
>
> Shang han with hiccoughing and abdominal fullness, observe the anterior and posterior, know which part is not free, freeing will bring recovery.

DISCUSSION: Hiccough and abdominal fullness are differentiated according to whether they are the result of an excess or a deficiency pattern. However, the statement "freeing will bring recovery" refers to disinhibiting constraint or obstruction, and from that it can be understood that the hiccoughs are due to obstructional excess.

If the pattern is associated with intestinal obstruction, then it can be understood that stomach qi is not descending, and this is the cause of the abdominal fullness and hiccoughs; in this case, there will also be constipation. If, on the other hand, the abdominal fullness is a result of water accumulation, with resulting hiccough, then there will be inhibited urination.

The point of differentiation is in knowing whether the restriction is in urination or in defaecation, hence the advice to 'observe the anterior and posterior', referring to the anterior and posterior yin orifices. Only by identifying whether the obstruction is due to constipation or to water accumulation can the underlying disharmony be addressed.

Clause 381 describes the method of diagnosis and treatment of a hiccough which is a manifestation of an excess pattern. Because it is caused by excess, the implication is that the prognosis is good. Appropriate formulas to treat inhibited urination are Wu Ling San, Zhu Ling Tang and Mu Li Ze Xie San; for inhibited bowel movement, the three Cheng Qi Tang can be used. This pattern differs from Clause 232, which reads: "If there is only a floating pulse, no other sign, give Ma Huang Tang. If there is no urination, and abdominal distension with hiccoughing, it is not treatable". That clause describes a pattern of devastated stomach qi characterised by inhibited urination, abdominal fullness and hiccough, and the pathogenesis is quite different.

Summary of Cold Patterns in Jue Yin

Jue Yin cold patterns are attributed either to cold in the channel or cold in the zang. Cold in the channel with blood deficiency is characterised by a thready pulse verging on expiry and cold extremities; the indicated formula is Dang Gui Si Ni Tang. Patterns associated with cold in the zang are attributed to yang deficiency with exuberant yin cold; the guiding formula is Dang Gui Si Ni jia Wu Zhu Yu Sheng Jiang Tang. For cold in the the liver and stomach with turbid counterflow manifesting as dry retching and drooling, Wu Zhu Yu Tang is indicated. For cold bind in the urinary bladder characterised by cold extremities and lower abdominal fullness with pain on palpation, moxibustion can be used to warm the channels, and Si Ni Tang can be given to resuscitate the yang. For yang deficiency with water retention characterised by cold extremities and palpitations in the epigastrium, Fu Ling Gan Cao Tang is the indicated formula. For yang deficiency with exuberant yin characterised by a swift skipping pulse and cold extremities, moxibustion is recommended.

7.3.3 Heat Patterns in Jue Yin

Heat Jue or Desertion Due to Heat

Jue refers to coldness of the limbs caused by yang failing to reach the extremities. There are two possible reasons: deficiency of yang qi and obstruction of yang qi. In either case, the flow of yang does not reach these distal branches of the body, but in the first case it is because of essential insufficiency, and in the second, the flow can not reach the extremities because of some obstruction. Obstruction can take the form of cold (cold jue), roundworms (roundworm jue), water (water jue), phlegm (phlegm jue) and heat (heat jue). Where the flow is not seriously affected, the condition is mild, but Jue Yin patterns are associated with such a disruption to the flow that yin and yang can no longer interact, and it is this situation which is referred to as desertion. Heat jue, therefore, does not refer to a standard pattern of heat, but to one which is caused by heat and where heat is a major element of its pathogenesis and symptomatology. In heat jue, there are still cold extremities.

Clause 335

伤寒一二日至四五日，厥者，必发热。前热者，后必厥。厥深者热亦深，厥微者热亦微。厥应下之，而反发汗者，必口伤烂赤。

Shang han for one or two days or even four or five days, if there is jue, there will be fever. If first there is heat, afterwards there will be jue. If the jue is severe, the fever is also severe, if the jue is mild the fever is also mild. For jue one should purge, but if instead sweat is promoted, the mouth will be injured with ulceration and redness.

DISCUSSION: The reference to shang han disease informs the reader that the aetiology of this pattern is an externally contracted pathogenic cold which, with the passage of time, has transformed into heat. If the heat is such that it obstructs the flow of qi, then it must be severe, in which case the jue would be preceded by fever. The fever is a manifestation of deep-seated heat which obstructs the flow of yang qi, constraining it deep within the body. The yang qi can not flow freely; it can not communicate with yin and can not flow to the extremities to warm them, thus the limbs are cold.

This is a pattern of true heat and false cold where, despite exuberant heat locked in the interior, the patient's skin is cold and the hands and feet are cold. This is because the yang qi constrained in the interior has transformed into heat and obstructs the flow of yang qi. In heat jue, the obstruction caused by this pathogenic heat results in desertion cold, which refers to cold in the extremities due to the non-distribution of yang qi and its inability to reach the four limbs. The peculiarity of true heat false cold patterns is the misleading manifestation of cold signs which occur in the presence of true heat, and so a conscientious approach to diagnosis is required. This phenomenon is referred to as 'severe heat with severe desertion' (热深厥深), which derives from the fact that the deeper in the body the heat pathogen lies, the more pronounced is the desertion cold of the extremities. This is because heat jue is attributed to the constraint of yang generating pathogenic heat, which obstructs the flow of yang qi, and so there is a directly proportional relationship between the severity of the cold limbs and the severity of the interior heat which presents as fever. This is expressed in the phrase: "If the jue is severe, the fever is also severe, if the jue is mild the fever is also mild". In addition to the fever and cold extremities mentioned in the clause, there are fever, a thirst for cold drinks, a red tongue with a yellow coat, dark urination, and constipation where there is a hard stool with the discharge of foul fluid. This is known as *re jie pang liu* (热结旁流), for which a direct translation is 'knotting of heat with collateral flow'.

A pattern of heat jue is a pattern of exuberant interior heat, and so, in the absence of an exterior pattern, the strategy is to purge. If sweating were promoted, the loss of fluids would exacerbate the interior heat, which would flare upwards and sear the mouth, causing redness and ulceration.

Providing there is evidence of bowel excess, clearing heat by purgation is a fundamental premise of treatment and Cheng Qi Tang is the guiding formula. Where there is no evidence of bowel excess, Bai Hu Tang is indicated to clear qi level heat.

To summarise the treatment strategies for jue: Si Ni Tang is indicated to resuscitate the yang in cold jue; Bai Hu Tang or Cheng Qi Tang is indicated to clear heat in heat jue; Fu Ling Gan Cao Tang is indicated to unblock the yang and promote urination in water jue; Wu Mei Wan is the indicated formula for roundworm jue; Dang Gui Si Ni Tang is used for jue due to blood deficiency with congealed cold; and Si Ni San is the formula used to disperse constrained liver qi in jue caused by qi constraint. In *Shang Han Lun*, there is a range of treatments for the various jue patterns and it is essential to differentiate the pattern and treat accordingly.

Clause 339

伤寒热少微厥，指头寒，嘿嘿不欲食，烦躁．数日，小便利，色白者，此热除也，欲得食，其病为愈；若厥而呕，胸胁烦满者，其后必便血。

Shang han disease, there is a slight fever and mild jue, cold fingers, untalkativeness with no desire for food, vexation. After several days, if the urination is free, and the colour is clear, this means the heat is eliminated, if there is a desire to eat, there will be recovery from the disease; if there is jue and vomiting, and there is vexation and fullness in the chest and hypochondrium, later, there will be blood in the stool.

DISCUSSION: In a Jue Yin pattern associated with shang han or cold injury, if the jue, or coldness of the extremities, is accompanied by fever, then this marks a pattern of heat jue, which refers to cold extremities caused by heat. In Clause 335, discussed previously, a situation of severe heat and severe jue was described and explained in terms of the direct relationship of the severity of heat to the severity of jue. Here in Clause 339, there is a slight fever and mild jue, describing a situation at the other end of the scale where the constrained heat is less severe, and therefore the symptom of jue or cold extremities is mild. This is borne out by the fact that the jue affects only the fingers, and not the hands and feet, or arms and legs. However, although the yang constraint is milder than that in Clause 335, it is still sufficient to cause vexation and dark urination. The untalkativeness is a reflection of the constraint, and the lack of appetite is due to heat constraint affecting the descent of stomach qi.

After the course of illness runs for several days, there can be recovery or deterioration. If there is clear and uninhibited urination signalling the abatement of heat, and a return of the appetite demonstrating harmony of stomach qi, then recovery will take place. However, if the jue becomes severe, with vomiting, vexation, and fullness in the chest and hypochondrium, this signals significant deterioration. The vomiting shows that the stomach is more seriously affected, and the pain and distension in the chest and hypochondrium show that the constrained heat has intensified and is harassing the channels. This severe heat will then scorch the network vessels, causing the blood to flow recklessly, leaving the vessels and giving rise to blood in the stool. Si Ni San can be modified with heat clearing herbs to release constraint and clear the knotted heat.

Clause 350

伤寒脉滑而厥者，里有热，白虎汤主之。

Shang han, if the pulse is slippery and there is jue, there is heat in the interior, Bai Hu Tang governs.

DISCUSSION: The jue or cold extremities can be due to heat or to cold. Cold jue is attributed to yang deficiency with exuberant yin; the pulse is submerged and faint, or rapid and forceless. If cold extremities are accompanied by a slippery pulse the pattern is not one of deficiency and cold but of interior heat, because a slippery pulse is a yang pulse, and is largely associated with a yang excess pattern. The phrase "there is heat in the interior" confirms that this understanding of the pathogenesis is correct, and the indicated formula is Bai Hu Tang, which will relieve the jue or cold extremities by clearing the constrained heat.

Clause 350 diagnoses the interior heat not on the basis of a rapid pulse, but on the basis of one which is slippery, because a slippery pulse is a yang pulse which is related to heat. The key points of diagnosis for heat jue are: (1) cold extremities with fever and scorching heat in the chest and abdomen; (2) cold extremities with vexing thirst, sweating, dark urination and a red tongue with a yellow tongue coat; (3) if the heat transforms into bowel excess, there will be constipation with a dry stool, sometimes with a foul watery discharge; (4) a pulse which is slippery and rapid or submerged, excess and forceful.

Diarrhoea with Blood and Pus in the Stool

Clause 363

下利，寸脉反浮数，尺中自涩者，必清脓血。

If there is diarrhoea, the cun pulse is nonetheless floating and rapid, it is choppy in the chi position, there will be pus and blood in the stool.

DISCUSSION: The typical pulse of Jue Yin yang deficiency diarrhoea is submerged and slow. A cun pulse pertains to yang, and a pulse which is floating and rapid is also a yang pulse. So a rapid floating pulse in the cun position indicates the return of yang qi and, therefore, also indicates imminent recovery. However, a choppy pulse in the chi or cubit position is indicative of an impediment in the flow of blood. This means that the return of yang was unmoderated, and that yin and blood were injured by the excessive yang heat. Thus the rapid and floating cun pulse is a reflection of exuberance of yang, and the choppy chi pulse indicates damage to yin blood. The hyperactive yang in the presence of deficient yin results in injury to the network vessels, which eventuates in bleeding and a purulent exudate. The Jue Yin liver channel pertains to the lower jiao and so the network vessels affected are those in the lower jiao, and the blood and pus appear in the stool.

Chen Xiu Yuan said: "Clause 362 is about exuberant yin with damage to yang, while Clause 363 is about exuberant yang with injury to yin". The injury to yin by the exuberant yang causes diarrhoea attributed to heat with blood and pus in the stool. Tang Rong Chuan said: "Diarrhoea with blood and pus in the stool is dysentery". Clause 363 describes heat diarrhoea, which would be accompanied by abdominal pain and tenesmus, even though those symptoms are not mentioned in the clause. No formula is specified for this disorder, but *Gu Ben Shang Han Za Bing Lun* suggests Bai Ye E Jiao Tang (Bai Ye 3 liang; E Jiao 2 liang; Gan Jiang (dry fried) 2 liang; Mu Dan Pi 3 liang). Ke Yun Bo suggests Bai Tou Weng Tang, while Wang Ling You suggests Huang Qin Tang.

Clause 367

下利脉数而渴者，今自愈；设不差，必清脓血，以有热故也。

If there is diarrhoea, a rapid pulse and thirst, now there will be spontaneous recovery; if there is no despatch, there will be blood and pus in the stool, this is because there is heat.

DISCUSSION: In Jue Yin, if a rapid pulse and thirst manifest in a pattern of yang deficiency diarrhoea, there are two possible explanations. (1) The rapid pulse and thirst are a sign of the return of yang and the subsequent recession or 'despatch' of yin, and thus herald recovery. This is similar to the situation described in Clause 361 where diarrhoea is accompanied by mild fever, sweating and a rapid pulse, which together signal imminent spontaneous recovery. (2) There has been an excessive return of yang, where yang heat has scorched the yin network vessels and resulted in diarrhoea with blood and pus in the stool.

Bai Tou Weng Tang Pattern

Clause 371

热利下重者，白头翁汤主之。

Heat diarrhoea with heaviness below, Bai Tou Weng Tang governs.

BAI TOU WENG TANG: Bai Tou Weng 2 liang; Huang Bai 3 liang; Huang Lian 2 liang; Qin Pi 3 liang.

DIRECTIONS: Boil these four ingredients in 7 sheng of water, reducing to 2 sheng. Strain and take 1 sheng warm. If there is no recovery, take another sheng.

DISCUSSION: Jue Yin heat diarrhoea is characterised by abdominal pain, thirst and a heavy sensation in the rectum, which may equate to tenesmus in contemporary terms;

the tongue is red with a yellow tongue coat. The diarrhoea is attributed to the downpour of heat in the liver channel harassing the large intestine, obstructing the flow of qi and causing the accumulation of turbidity. Therefore, the heavy sensation in the rectum is not only a key feature of damp heat diarrhoea, but is specific as a diagnostic feature of Jue Yin heat diarrhoea. The blood and pus in the stool are due to the harassment of heat in the blood, and the indicated treatment formula is Bai Tou Weng Tang, which stops diarrhoea by clearing toxic heat, drying damp and cooling blood.

Bai Tou Weng is bitter and cold; it clears damp heat from the intestines, relieves toxicity, disperses constrained liver qi and cools blood. It is specific for damp heat dysentery characterised by blood and pus in the stool. Qin Pi is bitter and cold, it clears damp heat from the liver, gallbladder and large intestine and, when combined with Bai Tou Weng, relieves toxic heat, cools blood and stops diarrhoea. Huang Lian and Huang Bai clear toxic damp heat from the lower jiao; in addition, by draining fire and parching damp, Huang Lian relieves stagnation caused by the accumulation of damp heat and stops bleeding caused by fire.

Differentiation of Diarrhoea Patterns and their Treatment

Bai Tou Weng Tang and Tao Hua Tang are both indicated for diarrhoea with blood and pus in the stool; the difference is in the pathogenesis.

- Bai Tou Weng Tang is indicated for heat diarrhoea in Jue Yin where damp heat excess in the liver channel harasses the large intestine, giving rise to blood and pus in the stool. Accompanying symptoms are abdominal pain, thirst, and a red tongue with a yellow tongue coat. The strategy is to clear heat, cool the liver and stop diarrhoea.
- Tao Hua Tang is indicated for a deficiency of spleen and kidney yang where insecurity of the lower jiao results in diarrhoea with blood and pus in the stool. It is accompanied by a dull complexion and an aching abdomen. There is no thirst and the strategy is to warm the middle, dispel cold, astringe the intestines and stop diarrhoea.

Huang Qin Tang and Ge Gen Qin Lian Tang are both associated with heat diarrhoea but differ in their clinical features.

- Huang Qin Tang is indicated for Shao Yang gallbladder heat characterised by diarrhoea, abdominal pain, fever and a bitter taste in the mouth. The treatment principle is to clear heat from the Shao Yang.
- Ge Gen Qin Lian Tang is indicated for a Yang Ming fu pattern associated with heat and is characterised by diarrhoea, fever, wheezing, spontaneous sweating, a parched throat and a strong thirst. The strategy is to clear Yang Ming heat.

Clause 373

下利欲饮水者，以有热故也，白头翁汤主之。

If there is diarrhoea with a desire to drink, this is because there is heat, Bai Tou Weng Tang governs.

DISCUSSION: The key diagnostic features of Jue Yin heat diarrhoea are: (1) diarrhoea with blood and pus in the stool; (2) a heavy sensation in the rectum; (3) fever and thirst. Clause 373 reiterates the key symptom of thirst in Jue Yin damp heat diarrhoea, already mentioned in Clause 367. The thirst is attributed to interior heat which has damaged fluids, and Bai Tou Weng Tang is indicated. Diarrhoea with thirst can further be differentiated according to whether it is associated with heat, cold, deficiency or excess. In general, diarrhoea due to cold and deficiency is not accompanied by thirst or, if so, the fluid intake is negligible. An example of this can be found in Clause 282, which mentions that spontaneous diarrhoea and thirst are associated with Shao Yin. This alludes to the fact that yang deficiency diarrhoea can be accompanied by thirst which is not due to heat damaging the fluids, but to deficient yang being unable to transform and distribute the fluids. In this type of thirst there is a preference for warm drinks.

Ancient Application of Bai Tou Weng Tang

- *San Yin Fang:* For the treatment of protracted and unremitting heat dysentery.

- *Shang Han Lun Yi Shi:* For the treatment of bleeding haemorrhoids or *chang feng* (肠风).

Modern Application of Bai Tou Weng Tang

- *Bacterial dysentery.* Luo et al treated 249 cases of bacterial dysentery with Bai Tou Weng Tang at the Hangzhou Infectious Diseases Hospital. This clinical trial compared the results of Chinese and Western medicine. The outcome showed a shortened recovery time using Chinese medicine, with an average time for complete recovery of one week (*Zhejiang Zhong Yi Za Zhi* 1957 6:242).
- *Amoebic dysentery.* Yang et al used a modified version of Bai Tou Weng Tang to treat 25 cases of amoebic dysentery. The formula used was: Bai Tou Weng 15g, Qin Pi 15g, Di Yu 15g, Huang Bai 10g, Ku Shen 10g. The subjects took an average of 5–10 packs. The result was: fully recovered = 22; satisfactory = 3. (*Zhejiang Zhong Yi Za Zhi* 1960 6:269.)

Case Study

Damp Heat Diarrhoea

Extracted from the lecture notes of Professor Fu Yanling

Pearls of Wisdom Seminar, October 2007

A 49-year-old male patient had complained of recurrent fever and abdominal pain which had started four years previously and occurred once a month. The Western diagnosis was Crohn's disease. Amoxycillin was not effective. He had also been treated by Chinese medicine but that was not effective either. He presented with vexation, insomnia, irritability, a red complexion, a subjective sense of palpitations, a bitter taste in the mouth, aversion to greasy food, a dry stool, dark urination, a red tongue with a thick yellow tongue coat and a flooding, slippery pulse. The diagnosis was damp heat in the large intestine and the treatment principle was to clear heat, drain fire, dry damp and cool blood. He was prescribed Bai Tou Weng Tang modified: Bai Tou Weng 12g, Huang Lian 5g, Huang Bai 9g, Qin Pi 9g, Lian Qiao 15g, Zhi Zi 12g, Jiu Da Huang 6g, Gan Cao 5g, Da Zao 15g. After three packs, his symptoms improved substantially and the same formula was repeated in a smaller dosage for another four packs. At the third consultation he was given a modification of Huang Qin Tang and at the fourth, fourteen packs of a modified version of Ban Xia Xie Xin Tang was prescribed. All symptoms resolved and Liu Jun Zi Tang was then given to consolidate the treatment.

Discussion: This case is a pattern of excess heat demonstrated by symptoms such as vexation, insomnia and irritability. Cold and bitter herbs were needed to clear heat, with Gan Cao and Da Zao added to regulate and tonify the spleen and stomach.

The Relationship Between Heat Jue and Diarrhoea

Clause 374

下利谵语者，有燥屎也，宜小承气汤。

If there is diarrhoea with delirious speech, and there is a hard stool, Xiao Cheng Qi Tang is appropriate.

DISCUSSION: A hard stool or constipation with a foul watery discharge from the bowel, which is accompanied by delirious speech, is a symptom of Yang Ming fu excess. The leakage is water which has bypassed the stool, giving rise to a foul watery discharge, and is not what is usually referred to as diarrhoea. Ke Yun Bo explained the delirious speech as evidence of interior excess heat thus: "A hard stool is the root of delirious speech which is attributed to Yang Ming Bowel excess; congestion obstructs the qi dynamic and the heat flares upwards to harass the heart." The pathogenesis of this pattern is the obstruction of knotted heat manifesting as a hard stool accompanied by something resembling diarrhoea in the form of a foul watery discharge. This is known as *re jie pang liu* (热结旁流), for which a direct translation is 'knotting of heat with collateral flow'. The strategy is to eliminate the obstruction with Xiao Cheng Qi Tang.

This type of diarrhoea has much in common with the Shao Yin diarrhoea described in

Clause 321, which is also characterised by the discharge of faecal fluid. In Shao Yin, however, there is no delirious speech, but there is epigastric pain and a parched mouth. The Shao Yin pattern represents a more serious pattern and Da Cheng Qi Tang is the appropriate formula. Although the pathomechanism is similar, the condition described here in Clause 374 is milder, and once the interior excess is eliminated, both the delirious speech and the diarrhoea will be resolved.

The significance of Clause 374 appearing in the Jue Yin chapter is firstly, that it serves to continue the discussion of diarrhoea in Clauses 371 and 373 and serves to supplement the treatment strategies for Jue Yin heat diarrhoea. Secondly, it demonstrates that the phenomenon of a hard stool with foul watery discharge in Jue Yin must be differentiated according to whether there is blood and pus in the stool and heaviness in the rectum, or whether there is a hard stool with a foul watery discharge and delirious speech. Thirdly, the foul watery discharge is more typical of a Yang Ming pattern of heat bind and fu excess. The significance of this in the Jue Yin chapter is that it represents an excessive return of yang qi, where the yang heat has consumed the yin fluids and transformed into dryness, and on the basis of this pathogenesis, the two patterns are unexpectedly linked together.

It must be noted, however, that the foul watery discharge of re jie pang liu is not the same thing as what is normally referred to as heat diarrhoea. Diarrhoea due to excess heat is characterised by spasmodic abdominal pain eased by a bowel motion, and the abdomen is generally soft, with no palpable hard masses. The watery discharge of re jie pang liu is subsidiary to the knotted bind of the hard stool. The hard stool, which may not be passed at all or only passed in small pieces, is the main testament to knotted heat bind; the foul watery discharge does not represent the passing of a stool, and therefore offers no relief.

A distinction must also be made between the foul watery discharge associated with excess heat, and a watery stool with undigested food particles attributed to deficiency cold. Excess heat diarrhoea is malodorous and accompanied by such symptoms as thirst and warmth of the body and extremities; deficiency cold diarrhoea is not strongly malodorous, the associated abdominal pain is relieved by warmth and pressure, and is accompanied by cold extremities.

Clause 375

下利后更烦，按之心下濡者，为虚烦也，宜栀子豉汤。

Following diarrhoea if there is more vexation, and softness below the heart on palpation, this is empty vexation, Zhi Zi Chi Tang is appropriate.

DISCUSSION: If heat diarrhoea is treated correctly, the heat symptoms, which consist of vexation as well as the diarrhoea itself, will be resolved; their resolution shows that the heat has been cleared. Clause 375 describes a case where the diarrhoea has been resolved, but not the residual heat constrained in the chest. The softness below the heart which is found on palpation indicates that turbid qi is being properly eliminated and there is no accumulation of a substance such as water or phlegm. Therefore, it is known that the vexation is due to formless heat, in other words, heat which is not knotted with a substance such as water or phlegm. It is this formless heat which harasses the heart. Zhong Jing's reference to "empty vexation" or *xu fan* (虚烦) does not refer to vexation caused by deficiency, but to the formlessness of the heat pathogen which is causing the vexation. The use of the word 'insubstantial' in this context may be compared to its use in the term 'insubstantial phlegm'. Insubstantial vexation is discussed with the Zhi Zi Chi Tang patterns in Chapter 2, section 2.7.1 in relation to Clause 76, and is defined in the glossary.

Because the vexation is an expression of constrained heat, the indicated formula is Zhi Zi Chi Tang, which vents constrained heat outward. A Zhi Zi Chi Tang pattern is characterised by insubstantial vexation, which is discussed in both the Tai Yang and Yang Ming chapters, where formless heat gives rise to the symptoms of vexation, insomnia and anguish in the heart.

Softness in the epigastric area found on palpation is an additional sign of insubstantial vexation. If there is fullness and hardness below the heart, then the pathogen is not formless, but has formed a hard and palpable mass. It is the result of an unresolved excess pathogen which has bound with a material substance such as phlegm, blood stasis, water or food, or there may be a knotting of heat and dryness in the intestines, manifesting as a hard stool. In such cases, the vexation is described as excess vexation, on account of the excess and substantial nature of a formed and knotted bind.

In *Shang Han Lun* there are many references to abdominal diagnosis, and of the 397 clauses, there are more than one-hundred clauses which address this subject. For example, in blood amassment, the lower abdomen is described as hard and full or as having knotted bind; in major chest bind, there is pain below the heart which is soft on palpation, or alternatively, there is hardness, fullness and pain extending from below the heart to the lower abdomen; and in minor chest bind, the hardness is below the heart and there is pain on palpation. From this it can be seen that abdominal palpation plays a significant role as a diagnostic technique in *Shang Han Lun*.

There are five main objectives of abdominal diagnosis: (1) to identify the pathogenesis; (2) to differentiate between excess and deficiency, heat and cold; (3) to determine the treatment principle for the dispensing of appropriate herbs; (4) to understand the seriousness of the condition so as to prescribe the appropriate dosage and to avoid contraindicated therapies; (5) to understand the progress and the prognosis of the disease.

Summary of Heat Patterns in Jue Yin

Jue Yin heat diarrhoea can be part of a pattern of heat jue or a pattern of heat diarrhoea. Heat jue is attributed to the constraint of pathogenic heat which obstructs the dispersal of yang qi, as explained in Clause 335: "First there is heat, afterwards there will be jue"; this statement also explains the direct relationship between the degree of coldness in the limbs and the heat which caused it: "If the jue is severe, the fever is also severe, if the jue is mild the fever is also mild". Based on this principle, where the heat constraint is mild, there will be a mild pattern of heat jue characterised by a slight fever and mild jue, and cold in the fingers only (Clause 339). The appropriate treatment for heat jue is to clear or purge heat, and the use of acrid warm herbs to promote sweating is contraindicated.

Jue Yin heat diarrhoea is attributed to the downpour of heat in the liver channel harassing the large intestine, obstructing the flow of qi and causing the accumulation of turbidity. It is treated with Bai Tou Weng Tang to eliminate the stagnation of damp heat in the large intestine. The symptoms are diarrhoea with blood and pus in the stool, abdominal pain, a heavy sensation in the rectum, and fever and thirst. If the heat diarrhoea is accompanied also by speech, it can be treated with Xiao Cheng Qi Tang.

Section Four

7.4 ABATEMENT AND ADVANCEMENT OF JUE YIN DISEASE

Clause 331

伤寒先厥后发热而利者，必自止；见厥复利。

Shang han, if first there is jue and then fever and diarrhoea, it will cease spontaneously; if jue is seen, there will be diarrhoea again.

DISCUSSION: The abatement and advancement of fever and jue do not represent separate disease states, but are a reflection of the waxing and waning of yin and yang in the course of Jue Yin disease. This phenomenon indicates the status of zheng qi: its relative strength and thus its ability to combat the pathogenic qi. Clause 331 describes the alternation of jue, or cold extremities, with fever, where the cold extremities represent the predominance of yin qi and the fever marks the return of yang qi. If the jue is followed by fever, even though there is diarrhoea, then yang qi is returning and the diarrhoea will soon stop. If, however, jue is seen without fever, the yang qi has receded, and there will be a recurrence of diarrhoea.

The reference to jue in this clause is to cold jue, which is attributed to exuberant yin with deficient yang, and is typically accompanied by diarrhoea. This signifies that yin is prevailing and the disease is advancing. If fever then appears, it is because yang qi is returning, yin will soon be defeated, and hence the diarrhoea will soon stop. If, after the diarrhoea stops, cold extremities appear again, then the return of yang qi was insufficient and unstable, and has allowed the yin cold to prevail again, as evidenced by the recurrence of diarrhoea. In this way, the relative status of yin and yang can be determined by evaluating the symptoms of cold extremities, fever and diarrhoea.

Clause 334

伤寒，先厥后发热，下利必自止。而反汗出，咽中痛者，其喉为痹。发热无汗，而利必自止；若不止，必便脓血。便脓血者，其喉不痹。

Shang han, first there is jue and afterwards there is fever, diarrhoea will spontaneously cease. And on the contrary if there is sweating, and pain in the throat, the throat is impeded. Fever with no sweating, the diarrhoea will stop spontaneously; if the diarrhoea does not stop, there will be blood and pus in the stool. If there is blood and pus in the stool, the throat is not impeded.

DISCUSSION: In shang han the cold extremities are a reflection of exuberant yin cold; the fever which follows represents the return of yang. Thus the situation where cold extremities are followed by fever is a sign of the return of yang qi and the corresponding abatement of yin cold. If the return of yang qi is moderate and appropriate, yang deficiency diarrhoea will be resolved. However, if the return of yang is excessive and immoderate, it will transform into excess heat giving rise to a transmuted pattern. Manifestations vary depending on the movement of the excess pathogenic heat and on which zang is affected. If the yang heat surges upward causing fluids to be vented outward, then there is sweating; if the excessive yang heat flares to the upper jiao scorching the throat, then the throat will be sore. Conversely, if the heat descends and is constrained in the interior, there will be fever but no sweating; if the heat damages the network vessels in the lower jiao, blood will be chaotic and there will be blood and pus in the stool but no sore throat, as the heat is not affecting the upper jiao.

Zhong Jing did not specify a formula but various formulas have since been recommended by *Shang Han Lun* scholars. Wang Ling You suggested Huang Qin Tang to clear toxic heat and parch damp; Zhang Lu suggested Bai Tou Weng Tang to address the blood and pus in the stool. The general consensus of opinion is that the blood and pus in the stool is a direct result of excessive return of yang heat which injures the network vessels. Both Huang Qin Tang and Bai Tou Weng Tang are appropriate. If there is a sore throat, Jie Geng Tang can be used to clear heat and relieve toxicity.

Clause 336

伤寒病，厥五日，热亦五日，设六日当复厥；不厥者自愈。厥终不过五日，以热五日，故知自愈。

Shang han disease, there is jue for five days, and fever also for five days, if there is a sixth day, there should be jue again; if there is no jue, there will be spontaneous recovery. The cycle of jue will not exceed five days, because the fever lasts five days, so it is known there will be spontaneous recovery.

DISCUSSION: In Jue Yin disease, fever and its abatement are a reflection of the contention of the zheng qi against the pathogenic qi, and the waxing and waning of yin and yang can be seen in the alternation of jue and fever. Zhong Jing therefore used the symptoms of fever and jue to determine the advancement or abatement of disease. The five day alternating cycles of jue and fever are purely nominal and should not be taken literally. The critical point is that the two phases are identical, showing that the relative status of zheng qi and pathogenic qi is equal and predictable. Therefore, following five days of fever, one may expect jue to manifest again, and if not, then it can be understood that the zheng qi has finally prevailed over the pathogen and so there will be recovery. The phrase, "The cycle of jue will not exceed five days" demonstrates not only that the yang return is predictable, but also that it is moderate and not excessive. The five day cycle of both the yin phase and the yang phase is even and balanced; if yin and yang are in equilibrium, recovery will ensue.

Clause 341

伤寒发热四日，厥反三日，复热四日。厥少热多者，其病当愈；四日至七日，热不除者，必便脓血。

Shang han with fever for four days, but jue for three days, then again fever for four days. If there is less jue than fever, there will be recovery from the disease; if from the fourth to the seventh day, the fever is not eliminated, there will be blood and pus in the stool.

DISCUSSION: Clause 341 describes a pattern where four days of fever precede three days of jue with cold limbs, thus showing that the yang phase of the cycle is of longer duration than the yin phase. This represents the advance of yang and the abatement of yin, and thus shows that the prognosis is good and recovery will take place. If, however, this pattern is broken, and the fever does not recede from the fourth to the seventh day (in other words, there is no yin phase at all), then the return of yang is excessive, the network vessels will be assaulted by the yang heat, and the damage will result in blood and pus in the stool.

Clause 342

伤寒厥四日，热反三日，复厥五日，其病为进。寒多热少，阳气退，故为进也。

Shang han with jue for four days, but fever for three days, then again jue for five days, the disease is advancing. There is more cold and less heat, yang qi is retreating, this is why it is advancing.

DISCUSSION: Earlier in this section, Clause 336 described how the moderate return of yang qi bodes well for recovery. Here, Clause 342 describes the converse situation where the recession of yang qi is a sign of disease advancement. By describing the manifestations of the waxing and waning of yin and yang, Zhong Jing is able to explain and predict the outcome. Fluctuations in their relative balance manifest either as cold extremities, reflecting the preponderance of yin, or as fever, reflecting the advance of yang. The predominance of fever over jue or cold extremities shows that yang is prevailing and is strong enough to defeat the yin cold: as yin abates, so the disease abates, and recovery will therefore take place. This clause describes the converse situation, where the manifestation of jue or cold extremities is of longer duration than the fever. This represents a predominance of yin cold with a corresponding abatement of yang; yang qi is inadequate and unable to overcome the yin cold. The final statement, "this is why it is advancing" refers to the advancement of the disease. This method of prognosis is ingenious in its inception, the more so for its simplicity.

Clause 332

（一）伤寒，始发热六日，厥反九日而利。凡厥利者，当不能食；今反能食者，恐为除中（一云消中)。食以索饼，不发热者，知胃气尚在，必愈。恐暴热来出而复去也。后日脉之，其热续在者，期之旦日夜半愈。（二）所以然者，本发热六日，厥反九日，复发热三日，并前六日，亦为九日，与厥相应，故期之旦日夜半愈。（三）后三日脉之，而脉数，其热不罢者，此为热气有余，必发痈脓也。

(1) Shang han, starting with fever for six days, but there is jue for nine days and diarrhoea. Wherever there is jue and diarrhoea, there should be an inability to eat; if now however there is an ability to eat, it is feared to be chu zhong *(which some call* xiao zhong*). If the person is fed noodles, and there is no fever, it is known that there is good stomach qi, there will be recovery. One fears that sudden heat may come but then go. If the next day observation shows the fever persists, one can*

expect recovery the next day at midnight. (2) The reason for this being, originally there was fever for six days, jue then for nine days, then fever for three days again, which, adding the first six days, is a total of nine days, and is equal to the jue and so one can expect recovery the next day at midnight. (3) If three days later, observation shows that the pulse is rapid and the fever has not abated, this means there is an excess of heat, there will be suppurating ulcers.

DISCUSSION: This rather long and complex clause has been divided into three sections for easier analysis and explanation. The discussion revolves around the ability to eat and the fluctuating cycle of fever and jue, or cold extremities, which are used to determine a prognosis. The ability to eat is an indication of the status of stomach qi, and the cycle of alternating fever and jue is a reflection of the relative balance of yin and yang.

The first section describes the situation of nine days of jue alternating with only six days of fever. This shows that yin cold is prevailing and yang qi is weak, and indicates that the disease is advancing. Under these circumstances, one expects that with the jue, there will be diarrhoea and a poor appetite due to inadequate yang qi. The ability to eat is generally associated with the restoration of the middle qi ascribed to the return of yang qi. However, there is more than one interpretation. This clause explains that if, paradoxically, in the absence of the return of yang, the person is able to eat, then deterioration is suspected, heralding *chu zhong* (除中), which is the devastation and ultimate expiry of the middle qi. The parenthesised comment gives it the alternative name of *xiao zhong*, which refers to *xiao ke* meaning insatiable thirst and is usually thought to parallel diabetes. This interpretation of the appearance of improvement as a sign of non-recovery is explained as being the sudden surge of false energy which can appear prior to death, the final flicker of the candle before it is extinguished.

To test whether the ability to eat bodes for a good or bad prognosis, the person is given noodles. (Note: *suo bing* (索饼) may be translated as 'string pastry', i.e. flour dough which has been formed into string-like noodles.) If, after eating the noodles, there is no feverish reaction, then it shows the stomach's function is good and that yang qi is prevailing, and so there will be recovery at midnight of the next day. If, on the contrary, after eating the noodles there is a sudden fever which fades and is replaced by a drastic reduction of temperature, then the stomach qi has expired, the yang qi is devastated and the renewed appetite was a false sign, representing the last flare of vitality before death. A third development is where, after eating the noodles, there arises a fever which persists for three days. This persistence of fever represents the resurfacing of the yang qi; so in this case also, recovery can be expected at midnight of the next day.

The second section assesses the relative balance of the cycles of jue and fever. It explains that although initially there were six days of fever and nine days of cold extremities, the occurrence of fever for three days after eating the noodles results in a total of nine days of fever, and so the balance is equal. This represents the corresponding balance of yin and yang, and so there will be recovery. The third paragraph describes a situation where the fever has persisted beyond those three days and continued for a further three days. This describes a situation of excessive yang return, which damages the network vessels of the lower jiao and results in suppurating ulcers. Thus Clause 332 covers the various possible developments in the recovery phase of Jue Yin disease, including the less favourable outcomes.

Clause 333

伤寒脉迟六七日，而反与黄芩汤彻其热。脉迟为寒，今与黄芩汤复除其热，腹中应冷，当不能食；今反能食，此名除中，必死。

Shang han, the pulse was slow for six or seven days, but nevertheless, Huang Qin Tang was given to eliminate the fever. A pulse which is slow relates to cold, now Huang Qin Tang is given to eliminate the fever, there must be cold in the abdomen, the person should not be able to eat; but now the person can eat. This is *chu zhong*, the person will die.

DISCUSSION: A slow pulse is a reflection of cold where warm herbs should be used. In this case, the presence of fever has resulted in the erroneous administration of Huang Qin Tang, which is a cold formula. Jue Yin disease is often characterised by true cold and false heat and it is essential to distinguish the true signs from the false, to differentiate heat from cold and deficiency from excess, and also to understand which is the branch and which the root. In this case, the presence of fever has led to a mistaken diagnosis of a concurrent pattern of Tai Yang and Shao Yang, and Huang Qin Tang was given to treat the fever. Because a pattern of deficiency and cold was treated with cold herbs, there was further damage to the already deficient yang, and so there is cold in the abdomen and an inability to eat. If the person is unexpectedly able to eat, this is not a positive sign, but indicates the seriousness of the devastation to stomach qi, where it is close to expiry and is known as chu zhong. The imminent expiry of the middle qi means that prognosis is poor and the person will die.

The imminent expiry of middle qi, or chu zhong, has been precipitated by incorrect treatment, where cold herbs were used to treat a cold pattern. In this, the chu zhong differs from that described in Clause 332, which is a natural progression of the disease. In Chinese medicine, the phenomenon of temporary vitality prior to death is referred to as false shen or *jia shen* (假神) of which chu zhong is but one manifestation. The sudden brightness of demeanor and improvement in appetite is a common phenomenon and should not be mistaken for a sign of recovery.

Summary of Abatement and Advancement of Jue Yin Disease

The determination of the advancement or abatement of disease is based on fluctuations in fever and jue or cold extremities. These symptoms represent the waxing and waning of yin and yang, which in turn indicate the status of zheng qi in relation to the pathogenic qi. Cold extremities are a reflection of the preponderance of yin, and fever reflects the advance of yang. If fever manifests, then yang prevails and is able to defeat the yin cold, thus the disease will abate. Conversely, if cold extremities due to jue are the predominant feature, then yin prevails and yang has retreated. Yang is unable to defeat yin and so the disease advances. Predominance of one over the other is determined by comparing the duration of jue and fever in their alternating cycles. This is summarised as follows.

1. Equal duration of fever and jue shows that yin and yang are balanced and the prognosis is good.
2. A longer duration of fever than jue indicates the return of yang qi and signals recovery.
3. More jue than fever indicates a preponderance of yin and inadequate yang, thus representing advancement of the disease.
4. Jue alone with no fever is a reflection of exuberant yin in the interior where yang is devastated. The situation is critical.
5. Persistence of fever after the abatement of jue represents an excessive return of yang qi which, depending on the area affected, may manifest as a sore throat or blood and pus in the stool.

Section Five

7.5 CONTRAINDICATED TREATMENTS IN JUE YIN DISEASE

Clause 330

诸四逆厥者，不可下之；虚家亦然。

Whenever there is a case of four reversal jue, one should not purge; this also applies to cases of deficiency.

DISCUSSION: Cold extremities are associated with jue patterns, which are, for the main part, attributed to an underlying pattern of cold and deficiency. Clause 330 states that purging is contraindicated in patients who are suffering from cold extremities and also in those who are deficient. In such cases, the appropriate strategy is to warm and tonify, and that strategy applies even in the absence of cold extremities. Purgation can, however, be used where cold extremities are attributed not to cold, but to heat. For example, in heat jue, where constrained heat impedes the dispersal of yang qi, as described in Clause 335. In that case, purgation is used to eliminate the heat which is the cause of the cold extremities.

Clause 347

伤寒五六日，不结胸，腹濡，脉虚，复厥者，不可下；此亡血，下之死。

Shang han for five or six days, if there is no chest bind, the abdomen is soft, the pulse is deficient, and jue occurs again, one must not purge; this is devastation of blood, purgation will cause death.

DISCUSSION: If shang han has not been resolved by the fifth or sixth day, then by this time, the pathogen is likely to have entered the interior causing a transmuted pattern of disease. Having entered the interior, the pathogenic heat can knot with phlegm and water in the chest and diaphragm causing chest bind. If this happens, the pulse will be submerged and tight, and there will be hardness, fullness and pain below the heart; this is chest bind. However, we are told that it is not chest bind, and the abdomen is soft. If the pathogenic heat transmits into Yang Ming and transforms into a pattern of dryness and excess, there will be abdominal fullness and pain aggravated by pressure, constipation and a submerged, excess and forceful pulse; but we are told that the abdomen is soft, and so we are led to the conclusion that it is not a Yang Ming pattern. The clause goes on to describe a deficient pulse and cold extremities, pronouncing that there is devastation of blood and therefore one can not purge. The presence of jue shows that this is a pattern of yang deficiency with yin cold, manifesting as cold limbs, and the deficient pulse indicates not only deficiency of yang but also deficiency of blood. If there is constipation, it is directly linked to a deficiency of blood and yin. It must not be mistaken for constipation caused by heat, because the use of purgatives will further injure both yin fluids and yang qi. These are already so depleted that further damage may endanger life. No formula is recommended to treat the pattern of devastated blood, but Gui Qi Jian Zhong Tang, which is Xiao Jian Zhong Tang adding Dang Gui and Huang Qi, is suitable.

This is similar to the pattern described in Clause 385, which reads: "Aversion to cold, the pulse is faint and there is recurrent diarrhoea, the diarrhoea ceases, there is blood collapse". Both diarrhoea patterns are associated with yang deficiency, where exhaustion of yin fluids has led to blood collapse.

Clause 364

下利清谷，不可攻表，汗出必胀满。

There is diarrhoea with undigested food particles, one should not attack the exterior, if sweat issues, there will be distension and fullness.

DISCUSSION: Diarrhoea with undigested food particles is attributed to spleen and kidney yang deficiency with exuberant yin cold in the interior; deficient spleen yang is unable to transform food and grain or transport the refined food essences. The strategy is to address the interior deficiency by warming the interior, dissipating cold and resuscitating yang; Si Ni Tang is an appropriate formula. The reference to not attacking or resolving the exterior if there is diarrhoea with undigested food particles complies with the principle of treating interior deficiency before addressing an exterior condition. The reference to distension and fullness following the issue of sweat refers to the departure from that principle, where incorrect promotion of sweat would result in a transmuted pattern.

Sweat is sourced from the transformation and evaporation of fluids which is fuelled by yang qi. Loss of sweat can therefore drain yang qi as well as deplete fluids. By depleting yang, the inappropriate promotion of sweat can cause diarrhoea and abdominal fullness. It is therefore essential to comply with the principle of tonifying interior deficiency before treating the exterior. Clause 364 is better understood when read with Clauses 91 and 372, which together explain that the ben and biao, or root and branch, must be correctly prioritised for good results and to avoid transmutation. There is no recommended formula for this pattern, but Gui Zhi Ren Shen Tang, which is a formula that both warms the interior and releases the exterior, is generally accepted as suitable. If there is abdominal fullness, formulas based on Si Ni Tang or Huang Qi Jian Zhong Tang can be used.

Clause 376

呕家有痈脓者，不可治呕；脓尽自愈。

If a patient who suffers from vomiting has ulcers, one should not treat the vomiting; when the suppuration stops, there will be spontaneous recovery.

DISCUSSION: If someone who suffers from vomiting also has ulcers, this suggests a patten of constrained yang with stagnation of qi and blood and toxic heat accumulating in the interior. It is the underlying toxicity which causes both the emesis and the ulceration. Vomiting is the body's way of expelling the toxins. Anti-emetic therapy should therefore not be used because it would cause the toxicity to be retained in the interior. The strategy must instead be directed at relieving the interior toxicity and discharging pus, thus addressing the underlying pattern.

Clause 376 does not specify which zang is affected, but based on theories pertaining to purulent lesions, it is generally accepted that ulceration is located in the lungs or stomach. There is no recommended formula but the *Jin Gui Yao Lue* formula Pai Nong Tang or Discharge Pus Decoction can be used (Sheng Gan Cao 2 liang, Jie Geng 3 liang, Sheng Jiang 1 liang, Da Zao 10 pieces), or another formula from *Yi Xue Xin Wu,* Jia Wei Jie Geng Tang (Jie Geng, Gan Cao, Bei Mu, Ju Hong, Jin Yin Hua, Yi Yi Ren, Ting Li Zi, Bai Ji) is also effective.

Differential Treatment of Vomiting

The aetiological factors in vomiting include cold, heat, the accumulation of water or phlegm, food stagnation, qi stagnation, and toxic heat manifesting as ulceration. Accurate diagnosis to identify the root cause is essential, and differential diagnosis results in differential strategies. For example, Wu Zhu Yu Tang is suitable for vomiting caused by cold turbidity in the liver and stomach characterised by dry retching and drooling; Si Ni Tang is indicated for the treatment of vomiting where there is uninhibited urination, a slight fever, cold extremities, and a faint pulse, all of which indicate a deficiency of yang with yin cold accumulation resulting in the counterflow of turbidity; Xiao Chai Hu Tang is indicated for vomiting with fever in Jue Yin resulting from the restoration of yang qi, and the subsequent return of the disease to the Shao Yang channel, where the gallbladder fire harasses the stomach. Clause 379 says: "If there is vomiting and fever, Xiao Chai Hu Tang governs". Here, Clause 376 describes vomiting which is associated with suppurating sores or ulcers, which are the result of toxic heat, most commonly occurring in the lung and stomach.

Summary of Contraindicated Treatments in Jue Yin Disease

Purgation is contraindicated in Jue Yin disease which is characterised by cold extremities, deficiency or the devastation of blood; sweat promotion is contraindicated where yang deficiency is accompanied by diarrhoea due to interior cold, because sweating tends to damage yang qi further, and also causes loss of fluids, and so will exacerbate the condition. Therapies aimed at stopping vomiting directly should not be used for a person with ulcerative lesions, as this may lead to the accumulation of toxicity and cause the ulcer to suppurate into the interior.

Section Six

7.6 PROGNOSIS AND RECOVERY IN JUE YIN DISEASE

7.6.1 Prognosis in Jue Yin Disease

Jue Yin Zhong Feng

Clause 327

厥阴中风，脉微浮为欲愈；不浮为未愈。

Jue Yin zhong feng, a pulse which is faint and floating means imminent recovery; not floating indicates no recovery.

DISCUSSION: Disease of the Jue Yin channel falls into the category of a yin pattern, and yet, a floating pulse is a yang pulse. A Jue Yin pattern with a floating pulse is a yin pattern where the emerging yang pulse heralds the return of yang qi. To quote *Bian Mai Fa*: "In yin disease with a yang pulse, the person will live; in yang disease with a yin pulse, the person will die". Clause 327 is an example of a yin disease with a floating or yang pulse, and explains that if the pulse remains sunken, the prognosis is poor. This is because a floating pulse indicates the return of yang, but a pulse which can not rise to the surface is a reflection of inadequate wei yang unable to contend with the yin pathogen. Nevertheless, a distinction must be made between a pulse which floats due to the emergence of yang, and a pulse which floats due to the separation of yin and yang, which may occur as a result of excess yin or dual devastation of yin and yang. Where the floating pulse indicates the restoration of yang, there is a gradual change from submerged to superficial, and the pulse has root, showing the strengthening of yang. Where there is imminent separation of yin and yang, the change is sudden and unexpected, and there is no root, which is indicative of the desertion of yang and a poor prognosis.

Jue Yin Cold Patterns and their Prognosis

Clause 329

厥阴病、渴欲饮水者，少少与之愈。

Jue Yin disease, if there is thirst with a desire to drink water, giving a little will bring recovery.

DISCUSSION: Thirst is not typical of a cold pattern in Jue Yin, so if there is a desire to drink water, and particularly if the thirst is satisfied with just a little water, then this does not represent excessive heat, but represents the retreat of yin and a moderate return of yang qi. Because it represents a spontaneous return of yang qi, no treatment is required other than to give the person a small amount of water to drink. The rationale for not giving more is that a large amount would inhibit the yang qi; all that is needed is a small amount to supplement the stomach yin, thus harmonising yin and yang to facilitate recovery.

Thirst in Jue Yin Disease

Although thirst is not a characteristic feature of Jue Yin disease, there are three scenarios where it presents.

1. Jue Yin complex heat and cold pattern with heat in the upper jiao and cold in the lower jiao which is characterised by insatiable thirst.
2. Jue Yin disease with an excessive return of yang qi characterised by thirst caused by yang heat consuming fluids.
3. Jue Yin disease where the yin pathogen has retreated but the return of yang is as yet insufficient to distribute fluids in the upper jiao and so there is a mild thirst.

Zhong Jing is emphatic about the significance of thirst both in diagnosis and treatment. In *Shang Han Lun*, there are forty clauses where thirst is mentioned, covering a range of patterns, each with a different pathogenesis. The patterns are as follows.

1. Pathogenic warmth constraining the exterior as in Tai Yang wen bing (warm disease) where the strategy is to use acrid cool herbs to release the exterior.
2. Exuberant heat in the interior where the indicated formulas are Bai Hu Tang and Bai Hu jia Ren Shen Tang to clear heat and generate fluids.
3. Heat knotting with water, as in chest bind, where the indicated formulas are Da Xian Xiong Tang to drain heat and dispel water, or Zhu Ling Tang to nourish yin, clear heat and promote urination.
4. Damp heat constraint where the indicated formula is Yin Chen Hao Tang to clear heat and drain damp to eliminate yellowing in a jaundice pattern, or Bai Tou Weng Tang to treat dysentery due to damp heat.
5. Tai Yang disease where yin fluids are depleted following the promotion of sweat, and a little water is given to harmonise the stomach.
6. Water accumulation obstructing the interior where the indicated formula is Wu Ling San to transform qi and move water in the lower jiao, and Xiao Qing Long Tang to release the exterior and transform phlegm fluid in the lungs.
7. Gallbladder heat impairing the pivot mechanism of qi, where the indicated formulas are Xiao Chai Hu Tang or Chai Hu Gui Zhi Gan Jiang Tang.
8. Heat and cold complex where the indicated formula is Wu Mei Wan to clear heat from the upper jiao and warm the lower jiao.
9. Yang deficiency with exuberant yin where the formula is Si Ni Tang to warm the yang and transform qi.
10. The excessive return of yang in recovery from Jue Yin disease, where the indicated formula is Huang Qin Tang.

Clause 360

下利有微热而渴，脉弱者，今自愈。

Diarrhoea with slight fever and thirst, if the pulse is weak, spontaneous recovery is imminent.

DISCUSSION: Disease development is strongly influenced by the relative balance of zheng qi and pathogenic qi, with recovery dependent on the strength and predominance of zheng qi. In Jue Yin disease, diarrhoea occurring with cold extremities due to jue is ascribed to yang deficiency with exuberant yin cold. If diarrhoea presents with an excess pulse, the excess nature of the pulse is a reflection of the abundance of the yin pathogen, thus signifying that zheng qi is weak and yang qi deficient. In Clause 360, diarrhoea presents with a weak pulse, indicating a reduction in pathogenic yin cold; the slight fever and thirst indicate the return of yang qi, and so it is expected that the diarrhoea will be resolved and recovery will take place.

The fact that the fever is slight is highly significant, because it indicates the moderate return of yang, as opposed to an excessive return, as already discussed in regard to Clauses 334 and 341. Vigorous fever and strong thirst would be a sign of excess heat in the interior. A pulse which was submerged and excess, or flooding and big, would also indicate the presence of vigorous pathogenic qi; therefore the weak pulse is an indicator not of deficient zheng qi, but of the abatement of the pathogenic qi. Other signs of recovery would be the gradual cessation of diarrhoea and warmth returning to the limbs.

Clause 361

下利脉数，有微热汗出，今自愈；设复紧，为未解。

There is diarrhoea and the pulse is rapid, there is a mild fever and sweating, spontaneous recovery is imminent; if the pulse is then tight, there is no resolution.

DISCUSSION: This clause is a sequel to Clause 360, just discussed, where a weak pulse is shown to signify the abatement of pathogenic qi. Here, in Clause 361, Jue Yin disease presenting with diarrhoea associated with yang deficiency and cold suddenly presents with a rapid pulse accompanied by mild fever and sweating. The rapid yang pulse in a Jue Yin cold pattern is a sign of transformation from yin to yang, and is a reflection of the yang qi prevailing over the yin pathogen; the mildness of the fever indicates that the yang is not excessive, and the sweating demonstrates the resumption of the movement and function of yang qi.

This clause has a similar thrust to Clause 331 which states: "Shang han, if first there is jue and then fever and diarrhoea, it will cease spontaneously; if jue is seen, there will be diarrhoea again". Thus it describes the arrival of fever following cold extremities as a harbinger of recovery, whilst contrasting this with the return of cold extremities and diarrhoea, the significance being that the return of the diarrhoea is a sign of the return of yin cold, and so recovery has not taken place. Here, in Clause 361, there is also diarrhoea, and fever is also seen as predicting recovery. Similarly, a statement is made that if the pulse becomes tight, the disease will not be resolved. In comparing the two clauses, it can be seen that the tight pulse of this clause is a manifestation of yin cold constraining qi, just as the cold extremities were in the earlier clause. The change of the pulse from rapid, representing yang, to tight, representing yin, demonstrates that yang is retreating; yin prevails, and so recovery can not take place.

Impending Death in Deficiency Cold Patterns of Jue Yin

Clause 343

伤寒六七日，脉微、手足厥冷、烦躁，灸厥阴。厥不还者，死。

Shang han for six or seven days, the pulse is faint, there is desertion cold of the hands and feet, and vexation and agitation, moxa Jue Yin. If the desertion is not returned, the person will die.

DISCUSSION: In shang han disease which has lasted for six or seven days, there is a faint pulse and cold extremities due to desertion resulting from yang deficiency. This pattern is characterised by exuberant yin and weak yang. The yang struggles to prevail but is repelled by the excess yin in the interior and floats upwards causing vexation and agitation. The vexation is therefore a manifestation of false heat in a pattern of true cold, and so the treatment is to warm and resuscitate the yang by using moxibustion on the Jue Yin channel. Following this, there are two possible developments: (1) warmth returns to the extremities, demonstrating the return of yang; (2) the limbs remain cold, demonstrating the persistence of cold jue; there is no return of yang, no recovery, and death is imminent.

In *Shang Han Lun,* vexation is associated with yang while agitation is associated with yin. Vexation or *fan* (烦) is a feeling, whilst agitation or *zao* (躁) describes the restless, involuntary and often repetitive movement of the limbs made by a patient who is seriously ill. There are three patterns associated with agitation. (1) Pathogenic heat in the exterior, where the correct treatment of appropriate sweat promotion was not used, giving rise to the constraint of yang qi (Clauses 110 and 114). (2) Incorrect sweat promotion with damage to fluid as described in Clause 221. (3) Exuberant yin and deficient yang as in Clauses 298, 338, 343 and 344. In this instance, the patient is critically ill, and agitation may be considered the dominant feature. The original text recommends moxibustion; no specific acupuncture points are mentioned in the clause, but some have been proposed by scholars at different times since. Because the Jue Yin channel pertains to the liver, Tai Chong (Liv 3) and Xing Jian (Liv 2) are deemed suitable based on their respective roles as the source point and the fire point of the liver channel. Zhang Xu Gu suggested that moxa should be applied to Guan Yuan (Ren 4) and Qi Hai (Ren 6). Clinical experience has shown that moxa on Guan Yuan and Qi Hai can warm the yang, and that moxibustion on Bai Hui (Du 20) and Shen Que (Ren 8) can restore and resuscitate yang qi.

Clause 344

伤寒发热，下利、厥逆、躁不得卧者，死。

Shang han with fever, there is diarrhoea and reversal due to desertion, if the person is too agitated to sleep, the person will die.

DISCUSSION: In shang han disease, fever which accompanies diarrhoea and cold extremities (referred to here as jue ni or 'reversal due to desertion') can signal the return of yang in a Jue Yin pattern; there is corresponding abatement of yin and prospective recovery. If yang returns, then the diarrhoea would cease and the extremities become warm. However, in Clause 344, although there is fever, the diarrhoea and cold extremities persist, demonstrating that yin still predominates. In this case, the fever does not signal the return of yang but is a false sign in a pattern of true cold, where exuberant yin has repelled the true yang. The agitation and restlessness are signs of looming yang desertion where death will be the outcome. The significance of interior cold as a sign of critical disease is also mentioned in Clause 338.

Fever in Jue Yin can be interpreted as either a sign of yang return or a sign of yang desertion. If it is indeed associated with the return of yang, there will be spontaneous resolution of cold extremities and diarrhoea. However, when fever presents in a pattern of yang desertion, there will be an exacerbation of diarrhoea and jue, or cold extremities, signalling not the return of yang, but deterioration in the condition. This is because the fever in this case is, in fact, a false sign. It is the result of exuberant interior yin cold repelling the deficient yang and as such, heralds the imminent desertion of yang, the separation of yin and yang, and therefore, death.

Analysis of Vexation and Agitation

A distinction must be made between the vexation and insomnia found in a Zhi Zi Chi Tang pattern, and the agitation and inability to sleep described here in Clause 344. Vexation refers to a subjective feeling of restlessness caused by heat harassing the heart shen; the heat also causes difficulty in sleeping or disturbs the sleep. In contrast, agitation refers to an altered state of consciousness, where there are physical signs of agitation manifesting as involuntary, restless movements of which the patient is generally unaware, and it is this agitation which disturbs the sleep.

Clause 345

伤寒发热，下利至甚，厥不止者，死。

Shang han with fever, the diarrhoea is extreme, if the jue does not cease, the person will die.

DISCUSSION: Fever in shang han with diarrhoea which is severe and incessant where there are also cold extremities or jue, is a reflection of the desertion of true yang; deficient yang is unanchored by yin and so floats upwards and outwards, manifesting as fever. The prognosis of death in Clause 345 is based on the fact that there is not only fever, but also the persistence of severe diarrhoea and unremitting coldness in the extremities. These two factors are crucial in the diagnosis. Although, as discussed already in Clause 360, the presence of fever can signal a return of yang qi, and the cessation of diarrhoea combined with the return of warmth to the limbs bodes for a good outcome even if there is no fever. Here, the converse situation presents itself, and the extreme diarrhoea combined with cold extremities or jue indicates the inevitability of death.

Clause 346

伤寒六七日不利，便发热而利，其人汗出不止者，死，有阴无阳故也。

Shang han for six or seven days with no diarrhoea, if by chance there is fever and diarrhoea, and the person sweats incessantly, the person will die, because there is yin without yang.

DISCUSSION: Where shang han is prolonged, as suggested here by the nominal period of six to seven days, and uncharacteristically, there is no diarrhoea, then this simply indicates that the condition is mild. But after that time, if fever, diarrhoea and incessant sweating suddenly occur, this indicates a critical change in the development of the disease and careful scrutiny is warranted. If the fever is associated with the return of yang, it will be followed by the cessation of diarrhoea. However, this clause describes a pattern where diarrhoea occurs with the fever, even where there was no diarrhoea before. This demonstrates the exacerbation of disease, not the return of yang. If there is no sweating, then the disease is still treatable, but incessant sweating is testament to devastated yang, and of itself ensures further depletion of both yang qi and yin fluids. Thus it signals inevitable collapse and is considered to be a sign of imminent death.

Other clauses describing fever in Jue Yin as a sign of imminent death are: (1) Clause 344, which describes yin exuberance with agitation and an inability to sleep; (2) Clause 345, which describes yang deficiency with continuous diarrhoea and cold extremities; and (3) Clause 346 which describes incessant sweating leading to the devastation of yang.

Clause 362

下利、手足厥冷、无脉者，灸之。不温，若脉不还，反微喘者，死；少阴负趺阳者，为顺也。

If there is diarrhoea, desertion cold of the hands and feet and no pulse, one should use moxa. There is no warmth, if the pulse does not return, on the contrary, there is mild panting, the person will die; if Shao Yin is less than fu yang, it is favourable.

DISCUSSION: Occurring together, diarrhoea, cold extremities and a pulse which can not be palpated are indicative of yang deficiency with exuberant yin. Thus they represent a critical condition and are the same symptoms as those found in Clause 315 which describes a desertion pattern in Shao Yin. Here in Clause 362, it is feared that the administration of herbs alone will be inadequate, and so moxibustion is recommended as an immediate and supplementary measure to support the restoration of yang. Subsequent to the moxibustion treatment, if warmth returns to the limbs, and the pulse becomes palpable, then yang is returning, the pathogen is in retreat, and recovery is possible. However, if, as described in the clause, warmth does not return and the pulse remains hidden, then clearly there is no improvement. Further to this, if there is shortness of breath, then kidney yang is exhausted; it can not grasp qi and the breath has no root. Because the kidneys fail to hold the qi, it escapes via the expired breath from the upper jiao, leading to further exhaustion of true yang. In all, this pattern is one where the kidney yang has been depleted to the point where it is close to expiry and thus portends death.

The last statement refers to the pulse, comparing that of the Shao Yin or kidney pulse with that of the instep pulse, known as fu yang. When a disease has reached a critical point in its development, and the pulse is not palpable in any of the three positions at the wrist, then the practitioner can palpate the pulse on the Shao Yin channel at Tai Xi (K3) or the pedal pulse on the Yang Ming channel at Chong Yang (St 42). This pulse is also known as fu yang or instep yang, because of its location on a yang channel on the instep. The absence of either of these pulses predicts a poor outcome.

Tai Xi is the source point of the kidneys and represents the root of the pulse, while Chong Yang is on the stomach channel and indicates the strength of the stomach qi. A pulse should have root, stomach and spirit. The importance of the kidney pulse at Tai Xi being weaker than the instep pulse is that, despite devastation of kidney yang, there is still stomach qi, and so the pulse will survive and the person will live. This is borne out by the saying "If stomach qi is present, there is life". The qi of the stomach represents postheaven qi and that of the kidneys represents preheaven qi. The two are mutually supportive and their status serves as a guide in determining prognosis in critical conditions. As the source of qi and blood, the stomach provides the blood vessels with these vital substances, without which there would be no pulse. Therefore, if the stomach qi has not expired, there will be a pulse and the prognosis is favourable. For this reason, Zhong Jing says that the outcome is favourable as long as there is a pulse at the instep.

Clause 368

下之后，脉绝，手足厥冷，晬时脉还，手足温者生；脉不还者死。

Following diarrhoea, the pulse has expired, there is desertion cold of the hands and feet, if within one day the pulse returns, and the hands and feet are warm the person will live; if the pulse does not return the person will die.

DISCUSSION: After diarrhoea, expiry of the pulse accompanied by cold extremities indicates devastated yang affecting the function of the heart and kidney. If within the period of one day, the pulse returns, and the hands and feet become warm, then the person will live; if the pulse fails to return then the person will die.

There are two possible interpretations of an expired pulse with cold extremities following diarrhoea. The first interpretation is that it represents a sudden acute attack of pathogenic cold which has caused severe diarrhoea and resulted in damage to fluids and a temporary interruption to the flow of yang qi. The second is that it represents chronic long-term disease where source qi is depleted and true yang is exhausted. In both cases the recommended treatment is moxibustion.

Clause 369

伤寒下利日十余行，脉反实者，死。

Shang han with diarrhoea in excess of ten times a day, if the pulse is nonetheless excess, the person will die.

DISCUSSION: In shang han, if there is diarrhoea occurring over ten times a day, the pulse should be submerged and slow, or faint and weak, as befitting the pattern of deficiency cold and devastation of zheng qi. Such a pulse, being true to the pattern, is known as *zhen zang mai* (真脏脉) or true zang pulse. However, if the pulse is not true to the pattern of repeated episodes of diarrhoea, representing a deficiency pattern, but is excess, then death is imminent. This is stated in the *Ling Shu: Wu Jin Pian (Chapter 61: The Five Prohibitions)* which says: "Disease with diarrhoea, with a pulse which is flooding and big, this is the second adverse condition."

Summary of Impending Death in Deficiency Cold Patterns of Jue Yin

There are various manifestations which signal a poor prognosis in Jue Yin patterns of deficiency cold. (1) A faint pulse, cold extremities, vexation and agitation, where it is recommended to moxa points on the Jue Yin channel; if the cold extremities persist, then yang is exhausted. (2) Fever, diarrhoea and cold extremities with agitation and an inability to sleep indicating exuberance of yin and desertion of yang. (3) Fever, exacerbation of diarrhoea and no pulse; the patient does not respond to moxibustion but starts to pant or have a mild wheeze; then there is yin cold in the lower jiao, yang is devastated and unable to hold qi, and true yang expires via the upper jiao. (4) After diarrhoea there are cold extremities and an expired pulse; if the pulse does not return within twenty-four hours, then yang is exhausted. (5) If there is diarrhoea but an excess pulse, then the condition is critical and death is imminent.

Outcomes in Jue Yin Deficiency Cold Diarrhoea

Clause 365

下利，脉沉而弦者，下重也；脉大者，为未止；脉微弱数者，为欲自止，虽发热不死。

If there is diarrhoea, the pulse is submerged and wiry, then there is heaviness below; if the pulse is big, the diarrhoea will not cease; if the pulse is faint, weak and rapid, it is about to cease spontaneously, although there is fever, the person will not die.

DISCUSSION: A submerged pulse pertains to an interior disharmony and a wiry pulse pertains to the liver, to stagnation, and to pain. In Jue Yin, diarrhoea can be associated with either heat or cold, and this clause describes Jue Yin heat diarrhoea. The Jue Yin channel is related to the liver which rules the free flow of qi and abhors constraint. If the pathogen in the Jue Yin channel affects the liver and impairs its function of dispersing qi, the resulting qi stagnation can lead to the generation of heat and the accumulation of damp. The liver damp heat descends to the lower jiao and manifests as damp heat in the intestines. Damp gives rise to a heavy sensation in the rectum whilst the heat gives rise to faecal urgency and diarrhoea.

The damp heat is in the interior, hence the submerged pulse, and it is related to the liver, hence the pulse is wiry. A change in the pulse from submerged and wiry to big indicates advancement of the disease. This is based on the *Su Wen*: *Mai Yao Jing Wei Lun Pian* (*Chapter 17: Discourse on the Essentials of the Pulse*) which says: "A big pulse indicates that the impetus of the disease is on the advance". The increase in volume indicated by a big pulse represents a corresponding increase in pathogenic qi. When a big pulse occurs in a diarrhoea pattern, the strength of the pathogen means the diarrhoea will not stop because the disease is continuing to progress; the implication of the non-cessation of diarrhoea in Clause 365 is that the condition is deteriorating. However, if the pulse changes either from a submerged, wiry pulse, or from a big pulse to one which is faint, weak and rapid, this is a sign of retreat of the pathogen with subsequent recovery. The change from submerged and wiry indicates that the liver disharmony and stagnation have been resolved, and the change from a big pulse reflects the abatement of the pathogenic qi. The fever and rapid pulse could be a reflection of residual heat in the intestines, or equally, interior cold with a return of yang qi. In either case, it will be temporary, and there is no indication at that particular stage that the condition will worsen or that the person will die.

The pulse is an important tool of diagnosis; it can inform as to the progress or advancement of disease. A pulse which is faint, weak and rapid indicates retreat of the pathogenic qi and the presence of fever is immaterial. A pulse which is rapid, big and forceful will be accompanied by exacerbation of fever and diarrhoea, and the prognosis is poor. This Jue Yin diarrhoea pattern characterised by a heavy sensation in the rectum is a pattern of heat diarrhoea which can parallel the modern diagnosis of dysentery.

Clause 366

下利脉沉而迟，其人面少赤、身有微热、下利清谷者，必郁冒汗出而解，病人必微厥，所以然者，其面戴阳，下虚故也。

Diarrhoea with a pulse which is submerged and slow, if the person's face is a little red, there is a mild fever, and diarrhoea with undigested food particles, there will be oppressed dizziness and sweating with resolution, the patient will have mild jue, the reason for this being, the face bears the sign of yang, and the lower jiao is deficient.

DISCUSSION: Diarrhoea and a pulse which is slow and submerged are a manifestation of yang deficiency with exuberant yin. The deficient yang is unable to transform food and so there are undigested food particles in the stool. *Su Wen: Zhi Zhen Yao Da Lu Pian (Su Wen Chapter 74: Essential Great Discourse to Reach the Truth)*: "Every disease with watery fluids which are clear, pure and cold, all pertain to cold"

The diarrhoea with undigested food particles, the submerged, slow pulse and the cold extremities show the true pattern to be one of interior cold; however, in spite of this, the face is a little red and there is a mild fever. These are signs of false heat, although it is important to note that the symptoms are mild and therefore the pattern is not severe, meaning that the zheng qi is adequate to contend with the pathogenic qi. The term *yu mao* 郁冒refers to a sense of faintness with blurred vision and chest oppression. The pathogenesis is the waxing and waning of yang qi as the yang qi vies with the yin cold, where the stirring of the yang qi in its battle to vanquish yin gives rise to a foggy sensation in the head, dizziness and an oppressed sensation in the chest.

An episode of sweating following the manifestation of yu mao is a sign of imminent recovery, because it represents the strength of the zheng qi as it overcomes the pathogenic cold; conversely, if the pathogenic qi prevails, there will be no sweating, because yang is devastated. The reference to mild jue, or mild cold in the hands and feet, shows that warmth is returning and the interior cold pattern is in retreat. The statement 'the face bears the sign of yang' simply refers to the redness of the face, red being the colour of yang heat. The flushed face and the mild fever are the result of deficient yang being cast upward as it is repelled by the interior yin cold; as such, both are manifestations of false heat.

In *Shang Han Lun*, formulas commonly used to treat a pattern of upcast yang are Bai Tong Tang and Tong Mai Si Ni Tang. However the pattern described here in Clause 366 is a mild one and will resolve spontaneously after an episode of yu mao and sweating. Yu mao is a sign of the contention between the zheng qi and the pathogenic qi and is differentiated according to whether it relates to excess or deficiency. An excess pattern of yu mao is a sign of disease resolution. If there is pathogenic excess, the appropriate strategy is to purge heat. In general, the prognosis is good. A deficiency pattern of yu mao can also bring recovery, as exemplified in Clause 366, but careful diagnosis is required to identify the pattern and ensure a good outcome. A favourable outcome is dependent on the return of yang, which is demonstrated by an episode of yu mao followed by sweating, warmth gradually returning to the extremities, and a general improvement in the other symptoms. Conversely, if there is no sweating after yu mao, and there is further deterioration of the symptoms, such as incessant sweating, the exacerbation of jue and a faint pulse, then these all point to the devastation of yang and the outcome is unfavourable.

Clause 377

呕而脉弱，小便复利，身有微热，见厥者，难治，四逆汤主之。

If there is vomiting and the pulse is weak, the urination is again free, there is slight fever, and jue can be seen, it is difficult to treat, Si Ni Tang governs.

DISCUSSION: Vomiting associated with deficiency, as indicated by a weak pulse, is attributed to devastated stomach yang which has resulted in the counterflow of yin cold. The weak pulse and clear, copious urination reflect the exuberance of yin cold in the interior; not only is deficient yang unable to warm and promote the flow of qi and blood, but cold retards, congeals and obstructs the flow. The mechanism behind the uninhibited urination is similar to that described in Clause 282, where deficiency and cold in the lower jiao results in clear urination and an inability to control water. If, as well as fever, there is a gradual warming of the four limbs, then yang has returned and the outcome is favourable. However, the presence of fever when the extremities are cold is evidence of severe yin cold in the interior repelling yang, with the possible desertion of yang. Si Ni Tang can be used to restore yang.

Summary of Prognosis in Jue Yin Disease

The discussion of prognosis in Jue Yin disease is quite detailed; the Jue Yin deficiency cold pattern and its prognosis can be summarised as follows.

- *Yang return with recovery.* The return of yang qi results in the cessation of vomiting and diarrhoea and the gradual warming of the four limbs. The pulse is harmonised and the prognosis is good. Key points of diagnosis: thirst (Clause 329); a slight fever with a rapid pulse (Clause 360); slight fever with sweating (Clause 361).
- *Yang desertion with impending death.* The devastated yang qi is further damaged by worsening and persistent vomiting and diarrhoea. The extremities are cold, the pulse is faint verging on expiry, and the prognosis is poor. Key points of diagnosis: diarrhoea with an excess pulse (Clause 369); agitation with an inability to sleep (Clause 344); incessant sweating (Clause 346).
- *Excessive return of yang and its transformation to heat.* Fever, rapid pulse, thirst and, if the heat damages the network vessels, there will be either blood in the stool, a sore throat or throat impediment. These represent the transformation of a yin pattern into a yang pattern. The key features are: diarrhoea with blood and pus in the stool (Clause 363, 367); diarrhoea with a big pulse (Clause 365).

7.6.2 Jue Yin Recovery Period

Clause 328

厥阴病欲解时，从丑至卯上。

The time that Jue Yin disease is about to resolve, is from chou to mao.

DISCUSSION: Jue Yin stands in an exterior–interior relationship with Shao Yang, whose recovery period is from 3am to 9am, while the recovery period for Jue Yin is between the hours of 1am to 7am which represents the axis of transformation from yin to yang, where yin ends and yang returns.

Section Seven

7.7 SUMMARY OF THE JUE YIN CHAPTER

Jue Yin disease is the terminal stage of the six channel patterns and is attributed to exuberant yin cold and yang deficiency. It is characterised by patterns of heat and cold complex, where extreme cold may herald the return of yang. Jue Yin disease also features the waxing and waning of yin and yang which mirror the fluctuations in the struggle of the zheng qi against the pathogenic qi. If zheng qi prevails, there will be yang return and if pathogenic qi prevails, there will be yang desertion and death. Some special features of Jue Yin patterns are an insatiable thirst, an upsurge of qi harassing the heart, searing heat and pain in the heart, hunger with no desire for food, and vomiting of roundworms after eating. These symptoms are the mark of heat and cold complex patterns in Jue Yin disease.

There are five categories of Jue Yin disease based on the clinical manifestations.

1. Patterns of heat and cold complex.
2. Jue or desertion patterns.
3. Vomiting and hiccough patterns.
4. Diarrhoea patterns.
5. Patterns of the advancement or abatement of jue and fever.

HEAT AND COLD COMPLEX: There are three patterns, as follows.

(i) *Wu Mei Wan Pattern:* a pattern of heat and cold complex where roundworms may be vomited; it is characterised by abdominal pain, a faint pulse and cold extremities.

(ii) *Gan Jiang Huang Qin Huang Liang Ren Shen Tang Pattern:* a pattern of deficiency cold diarrhoea which has been treated with purgation and emesis resulting in the pathogenic heat sinking inward; this is characterised by the vomiting of food immediately after eating, and by diarrhoea.

(iii) *Ma Huang Sheng Ma Tang pattern:* this pattern represents heat in the upper jiao and cold in the lower jiao; it is characterised by cold extremities, a sore throat, the spitting of blood and pus, incessant diarrhoea and a pulse which is slow and submerged in the cun position.

JUE OR DESERTION PATTERN: The term jue refers to cold extremities caused by the non-interaction of yin and yang. In *Shang Han Lun*, there are ten jue patterns, differentiated according to aetiology.

(i) *Heat jue:* exuberant heat constrained in the interior obstructs the proper flow of yang qi; it is characterised by fever, thirst, sweating, and a slippery, forceful pulse. The indicated formulas are Bai Hu Tang or Cheng Qi Tang.

(ii) *Cold jue:* yang deficiency with exuberant yin cold; it is characterised by cold extremities, diarrhoea with undigested food particles, and a faint pulse verging on expiry. The indicated formula is Si Ni Tang.

(iii) *Blood deficiency with congealed cold:* characterised by cold extremities and a thready pulse verging on expiry. The formula is Dang Gui Si Ni Tang.

(iv) *Roundworm jue:* interior harassment and obstruction caused by roundworms obstructing the dispersal of yang qi; it is characterised by occasional vexation, vomiting and cold extremities; the formula is Wu Mei Wan.

(v) *Water jue:* stomach yang deficiency with the accumulation of water in the interior; it is characterised by palpitations below the heart and an absence of thirst. The formula is Fu Ling Gan Cao Tang.

(vi) *Phlegm jue:* phlegm obstruction in the chest and diaphragm obstructing the dispersal of yang qi; it is characterised by cold extremities, vexation and fullness below the heart, hunger with no desire for food, an urge to vomit but an abilty to do so and a tight pulse. The formula indicated is Gua Di San to promote emesis, which is discussed in Clause 355.

(vii) *Zang jue:* interior yang deficiency with yang insufficient to reach and warm the extremities; it is characterised by a faint pulse, cold extremities, agitation and constant restlessness. The indicated formula is Si Ni Tang.

(viii) *Qi constraint jue:* constrained yang qi unable to disperse; it is characterised by varying symptoms such as cough, palpitations, inhibited urination, abdominal pain or diarrhoea with rectal heaviness. The formula is Si Ni San.

(ix) *Turbid cold harassing the stomach:* this is a pattern of yang deficiency with exuberant yin cold; it is characterised by nausea, vomiting, vexation and agitation. The formula is Wu Zhu Yu Tang.

(x) *Cold bind in the urinary bladder:* deficiency of yang qi with pathogenic cold bind in the urinary bladder; it is characterised by cold extremities, fullness of the lower abdomen and pain on pressure. The formula is Si Ni Tang or Dang Gui Si Ni Tang.

VOMITING AND HICCOUGH PATTERNS: The Jue Yin channel is associated with the liver which governs the free flow of qi. The normal qi dynamic is dependent on the dispersing function of the liver. If impaired, there will be vomiting and hiccough. Vomiting and hiccough are attributed to cold in the liver harassing the stomach; this pattern is characterised by turbid counterflow, which may manifest as vomiting, dry retching, hiccoughing, drooling or headache. The formulas are Wu Zhu Yu Tang or Si Ni Tang.

DIARRHOEA PATTERNS: Jue Yin heat diarrhoea is the result of liver damp heat descending to the lower jiao; it is characterised by heat diarrhoea and rectal heaviness and a strong thirst. The formula is Bai Tou Weng Tang. If there is a bind of dryness and heat in the intestines characterised by a foul watery discharge, delirious speech and abdominal fullness, the formula is Xiao Cheng Qi Tang. If, following diarrhoea, there is vexation due to residual heat harassing the chest and diaphragm, the formula is Zhi Zi Chi Tang to vent the constrained heat. Cold diarrhoea is attributed to exuberant yin repelling the yang; it is characterised by diarrhoea with undigested food particles, sweating and cold extremities. The formula is Tong Mai Si Ni Tang.

ABATEMENT AND ADVANCEMENT OF JUE YIN DISEASE: The advancement or retreat of disease in Jue Yin is subject to the waxing and waning of yin and yang. This is reflected in jue, or cold extremities, which is associated with the retreat of yang and the advance of disease, while fever is associated with the return of yang. Assessment is made by comparing the duration of the fever phase with that of the jue phase.

Jue Yin Recovery Period

The Jue Yin channel qi peaks between the hours of chou and mao (1am to 7am) and so this is the optimal time for recovery.

霍亂
Huo Luan 8

Section One

8.1 OUTLINE OF HUO LUAN

Definition of Huo Luan

Huo luan (霍乱) is a disease characterised by the sudden manifestation of alternating episodes of vomiting and diarrhoea. Because of the sudden onset of such disruptive symptoms and the disordered nature of the pattern, the name huo luan is given, which can be translated as 'sudden upheaval'; other translations include 'sudden rebellion' and 'sudden turmoil'. The disorder known as huo luan in Chinese medicine can refer to a range of acute stomach and intestinal disorders such as food poisoning or gastroenteritis; all can be treated using a similar strategy. It must not be confused with the contemporary Chinese name for cholera.

Aetiology and Pathogenesis of Huo Luan

Huo luan can be caused by the ingestion of contaminated food or drink, or the invasion of any of the six excesses. This results in a combined exterior and interior pattern and manifests as heat and cold complex affecting the qi dynamic of the middle jiao.

In describing five kinds of upheaval, *Ling Shu: Wu Luan Pian* (*Ling Shu Chapter 34 The Five Upheavals*) reads: "Huang Di asks: What is counterflow and upheaval? Qi Bo says: Clear qi is in the yin, turbid qi is in the yang, ying qi moves with the yang, wei qi moves against the yin, the clear and the turbid attack each other, there is upheaval and harassment in the chest, this is called great oppression ... if the upheaval is in the intestines and stomach, then it is called sudden upheaval ...". These are not just causes, but are factors in the development of huo luan, its manifestations and its clinical features. Because huo luan is generally associated with an exterior pathogen, it can also be characterised by headache, fever, aversion to cold and body pain, reminiscent of a Tai Yang shang han pattern.

Classification of Huo Luan

Discussion of huo luan originated in the *Huang Di Nei Jing* with further development taking place in the Sui (581-618) and Tang (618-907) dynasties. *Cao Yuan Fang*, from that era, says: "Dry huo luan is attributed to the contraction of cold harassing the stomach and intestine causing indigestion, abdominal fullness, vexation, severe pain and shortness of breath. The absence of vomiting and diarrhoea is attributed to the presence of excess in the bowel. This is known as dry huo luan". *Wai Tai Mi Yao* (792 AD) says: "Disease characterised by vomiting and diarrhoea is known as damp huo luan".

Huo luan patterns are classified according to their clinical features: damp huo luan is characterised by alternating vomiting and diarrhoea associated with damp; dry huo luan is characterised by a desire to vomit with no vomitus, an absence of diarrhoea, vexation and restlessness, acute abdominal pain, shortness of breath and sweating. This chapter deals with damp huo luan, which can be further categorised according to whether it is a cold pattern, attributed to cold damp, or a heat pattern, attributed to summerheat. Apart from the key symptoms of vomiting and diarrhoea, the initial stage is marked by exterior symptoms.

Section Two

8.2 PRINCIPAL FEATURES OF HUO LUAN

Symptoms of Huo Luan

Clause 382

问曰：病有霍乱者何？答曰：呕吐而利，此名霍乱。

Question: What is huo luan disease? Answer: Vomiting and diarrhoea, this is huo luan.

DISCUSSION: The principal characteristics of huo luan disease are vomiting and diarrhoea, which are manifestations of a serious disharmony of the stomach and intestines, affecting the digestion, the transformation of fluids, and the transportation of turbidity. These are all a reflection of damp accumulation, and a huo luan damp pattern is further differentiated according to whether it is associated with heat or cold.

The onset of a cold pattern is characterised by vomiting and diarrhoea. The diarrhoea is initially sloppy; this can develop into a foul-smelling watery diarrhoea which can even appear to be just a turbid watery substance. There are glomus and an oppressed sensation in the chest, abdominal pain, cold extremities, cramps, a pale tongue with a thin white tongue coat and a submerged, thready and faint pulse. The treatment is to warm the middle and transform dampness. At the initial stage, it can be treated with Huo Xiang Zheng Qi San modified. When it becomes chronic, and is more serious, Fu Zi Li Zhong Wan or Si Ni Ren Shen Tang can be used. If there is incessant sweating, cold extremities, a hoarse voice, cramps and a faint pulse verging on expiry, all of which indicate yang desertion, Tong Mai Si Ni jia Zhu Dan Zhi can be given to regulate the yin and yang.

A huo luan heat pattern is ascribed to an attack of summerheat and is characterised by sudden vomiting and diarrhoea, a foul-smelling stool, headache, fever, thirst, an oppressed sensation in the chest, vexation, dark urination, abdominal pain, cramps, a greasy, yellow tongue coat, and a rapid, soggy pulse. The treatment is to clear heat and transform damp with the formula Wang Shi Lian Pu Yin (Hou Po, Huang Lian, Shi Chang Pu, Ban Xia, Xiang Chi, Shan Zhi Zi, Lu Gen) or Re Zhao Tang (Dou Chi, Jiao Zhi Zi, Huang Qin, Pei Lan, Hou Po, Ban Xia, Bai Dou Kou). If there are cold extremities, abdominal pain, spontaneous sweating, thirst, cyanosed lips and nails, vomiting of a sour substance, diarrhoea, dark urination and a hidden pulse attributed to severe constrained heat in the interior, use Zhu Ye Shi Gao Tang, with an increased dose of Shi Gao to clear heat and generate fluids. Hot, acrid or parching herbs must not be prescribed.

Clause 383

问曰：病发热、头痛、身疼、恶寒、吐利者，此属何病？答曰：此名霍乱。霍乱自吐下，又利止，复更发热也。

Question: If the disease has fever, headache, body pain, aversion to cold and vomiting and diarrhoea, what disease does this pertain to? Answer: This is huo luan. Huo luan is spontaneous vomiting and diarrhoea, and when the diarrhoea ceases, there will be fever once again.

DISCUSSION: Clause 383 distinguishes between huo luan and shan han. Huo luan disease is attributed to the contraction of an exterior pathogen and is characterised by exterior symptoms such as fever, aversion to cold. The constrained exterior pathogen blocks the channel qi and manifests as headache and body pain with aversion to cold; the contention between the zheng qi and pathogenic qi manifests as fever. If this were a Tai Yang shang han pattern, there would be no interior symptoms unless the pathogen had fallen inward, when it could disrupt the qi dynamic of the spleen and stomach giving rise to vomiting and diarrhoea. The pattern described in Clause 383, however, is characterised by vomiting and diarrhoea right from the onset, as well as fever, aversion to cold, headache and body pain. The interior symptoms are acute; they are an essential part of the pattern and not the result of transmutation or of combination. Therefore, it is not a shang han exterior pattern.

In huo luan, unlike a pattern of Tai Yang shang han, it is the interior signs of vomiting and diarrhoea which take precedence. The simultaneous presence of exterior signs makes it similar to some concurrent patterns of shang han disease. For instance, the concurrent pattern of Tai Yang and Yang Ming is also characterised by vomiting and diarrhoea, resembling huo luan. It also has both exterior and interior signs; Ge Gen Tang is used to release the exterior, and once the exterior pattern is resolved there should be spontaneous harmony of the interior, and the vomiting and diarrhoea should resolve.

The pathology of huo luan is mainly attributed to disharmony of the spleen and stomach with disruption in the metabolism of the clear and the turbid. In a concurrent pattern of Tai Yang and Yang Ming once the exterior is resolved, the interior is harmonised. However, in huo luan, the focus is on harmonising the interior, after which the exterior may remain unresolved. Huo Xiang Zheng Qi Tang can be used in the initial stage. This is explained in the clause when it says: "when the diarrhoea ceases, there will be fever once again". There is no nominated formula for this condition, but reference can be made to the application of Gui Zhi Tang as discussed with Clause 387, where it could be used to mildly harmonise the exterior when the vomiting and diarrhoea are resolved.

Treatment of Huo Luan

Clause 384

（一）伤寒，其脉微涩者，本是霍乱，今是伤寒，却四五日，至阴经上，转入阴必利。本呕下利者，不可治也；（二）欲似大便，而反矢气，仍不利者，此属阳明也，便必硬，十三日愈。所以然者，经尽故也。下利后，当便硬，硬则能食者愈。今反不能食，到后经中，颇能食，复过一经能食，过之一日当愈；不愈者，不属阳明也。

(1) Shang han, if the pulse is faint and choppy, it was originally huo luan, now it is shang han, but on the fourth or fifth day, it reaches the yin channels, transferring to yin means there will be diarrhoea. If there was vomiting and diarrhoea in the beginning, it is untreatable; (2) if the person feels as if he wants to pass a stool, but instead there is faecal qi and still no diarrhoea, this pertains to Yang Ming, the stool is hard, on the thirteenth day there will be recovery. The reason for this being, it has passed right through the channel. After the diarrhoea, the stool will be hard, if it is hard then the person can eat, there will be recovery. Now however there is no ability to eat, when the pathogen reaches the next channel, the person can eat a little, after passing one more channel the person can eat, after one day there will be recovery; if there is no recovery, it does not pertain to Yang Ming.

DISCUSSION: The first section of Clause 384 describes the difference between huo luan with exterior symptoms and a shang han pattern with transmission to the yin channel, which is characterised by vomiting and diarrhoea. If, in the shang han pattern, the exterior is unresolved and there is subsequent transmission to the yin channels, there will be fever, aversion to cold, vomiting and diarrhoea. This presentation closely resembles huo luan with exterior symptoms. The difference is in the pulse, which is floating in an unresolved shang han pattern, but faint and choppy in a huo luan pattern with exterior symptoms. This is because repeated vomiting and diarrhoea damage qi, blood and fluids, giving rise to a pulse that is faint, choppy and forceless. Furthermore, an exterior shang han pattern can take four or five days before the pathogen transmits to the interior, represented by the yin channels, causing vomiting and diarrhoea. By contrast, the vomiting and diarrhoea of huo luan occur as part of the initial acute symptomatology. Although the statement that it can not be treated by any means implies that the prognosis is poor, it is however an allusion to the fact that it can not be treated like a shang han pattern, where sweating is used to release the exterior.

If, after the episode of vomiting and diarrhoea, the person feels the need to pass a stool but can only pass wind, referred to here as faecal qi, this is because intestinal fluids have dried up after the vomiting and diarrhoea; the stool is actually dry, hence, it is said that it pertains to Yang Ming. The dry stool is evidence that the pathogen has not fallen into the yin channels. It is therefore appropriate to regulate the stomach or, alternatively, there will be spontaneous recovery after thirteen days. Note in *Shang Han Lun* it takes six days to go through the three yang and three yin channels and the period of thirteen days represents two cycles plus one day. Although the diarrhoea and vomiting have caused significant fluid loss, there is no abdominal fullness, no pain which resists pressure, and no tidal fever; by this we know it is not a Yang Ming stomach excess pattern.

The second section of Clause 384 analyses the changes which take place following the vomiting and diarrhoea, where the ability to eat can testify to the state of the stomach qi. Even if the stool is hard, if the person can eat, this shows there is no intestinal obstruction, and so there will be recovery. In the case of the person not being able to eat at first, but then gradually regaining an appetite, this shows that the pathogen is passing out of the channel and in about seven days, the return of stomach qi will be complete and there will be full recovery the next day. Finally, the clause explains that if the person's recovery does not follow that course, then the pattern is not one of fluid damage affecting the Yang Ming and the stomach. A review of the diagnosis would then be warranted.

Channel Passage: Jing Jin & Guo Jing

Jing jin (经尽) translated literally means 'at the channels' end' and refers to the passage of the pathogen through all the channels. In *Shang Han Lun*, the time taken for this to occur is six days. Clause 8 states: "Tai Yang disease, where there is headache for over seven days with spontaneous recovery, it is because the pathogen has passed through the channels". *Guo jing* (过经) can be translated as 'passing through the channel' and refers to disease transmission and the subsequent pathological changes as it passes from one channel to another. The inference is that the course of disease has exceeded the time when channel transmission might be expected to take place (see Clauses 105, 217, 384). In *Shang Han Lun Bian Zheng Guang Zhu,* Wang Hu said: "*Guo jing* (or passing through the channel), refers to the complete passage of the six channels".

Si Ni jia Ren Shen Tang in the Treatment of Huo Luan

Clause 385

恶寒、脉微而复利，利止，亡血也。四逆加人参汤主之。

Aversion to cold, the pulse is faint and there is recurrent diarrhoea, the diarrhoea ceases, there is devastation of blood. Si Ni jia Ren Shen Tang governs.

SI NI JIA REN SHEN TANG: Zhi Gan Cao 2 liang; Fu Zi (raw, skin removed) 1 piece broken into eight; Gan Jiang 1½ liang; Ren Shen 1 liang.

DIRECTIONS: Boil all four ingredients in 3 sheng of water, reducing to 1 sheng 2 ge. Strain and take warm twice a day.

DISCUSSION: An exterior pattern is characterised by aversion to cold and a floating pulse. A faint pulse in the presence of aversion to cold is indicative of yang deficiency. Here, the yang deficiency is attributed to a huo luan pattern where vomiting and diarrhoea have damaged both yang qi and fluids. The recurrent diarrhoea is a sign of yang deficiency unable to transform water and grain, and qi deficiency unable to secure and astringe fluids. When the diarrhoea stops, it is not necessarily a sign of the return of yang qi and imminent recovery. In huo luan, the cessation of diarrhoea is more likely to be a sign of deficient yang being unable to transform and produce fluids, so the absence of diarrhoea is evidence of spleen dysfunction, not of spleen health. The cessation of diarrhoea accompanied by aversion to cold and a faint pulse is a sign of yang desertion and fluid exhaustion; if yang and yin are both insufficient, there is no source for blood and no fire for its production; therefore the clause pronounces that there is devastation of blood.

Fu Zi, Gan Jiang and Zhi Gan Cao are the ingredients of Si Ni Tang, whose principal function is to resuscitate deserted yang. The addition of Ren Shen augments qi, generates fluids, and supports the source to rescue collapse; thus it can prevent desertion. Zhang Lu said: "It is not appropriate to treat blood collapse with Gan Jiang and Fu Zi as these may damage the yin". However, after diarrhoea with strong aversion to cold associated with the desertion of yang, Si Ni Tang is used to resuscitate the yang. The use of Ren Shen not only augments qi and generates fluids, but also supports the functions of Fu Zi and Gan Jiang.

The cessation of diarrhoea can be attributed either to the return of spleen yang and its function of transformation and transportation, or to blood collapse. Where spleen yang has been restored, there will be revitalised energy, and alleviation of abdominal fullness and pain. However, where there is blood collapse there is no revitalisation of energy; on the contrary, there are cold extremities, fatigue and aversion to cold, showing the non-return of yang, and parched skin and a submerged and thready pulse reflecting the depletion of blood. Si Ni jia Ren Shen Tang is therefore appropriate.

Ancient Application of Si Ni jia Ren Shen Tang

- *Jing Yue Quan Shu:* Si Wei Hui Yang Yin, which is an alternative name for Si Ni jia Ren Shen Tang, is advocated for the treatment of source yang desertion.
- *Wei Sheng Bao Jian Shi Yi:* For treatment of a shang han yin pattern characterised by pervasive coldness and cold sweat on the forehead and back of the hands.

Modern Application of Si Ni jia Ren Shen Tang

- Chronic enteritis or colitis characterised by a pale, lack-lustre complexion, aversion to cold, cold extremities, a poor appetite, abdominal fullness after eating, a sloppy stool, pain and a sense of cold in the stomach, undigested food particles in the stool, a pale tongue with a greasy white tongue coat and a pulse which is submerged and faint. This is a pattern of cold and deficiency of the spleen and kidneys and can be treated with Si Ni jia Ren Shen Tang modified. If there is incessant diarrhoea, replace Gan Jiang with Pao Jiang and add Wu Wei Zi. For nausea and regurgitation of fluids, add Jiang Ban Xia, Duan Mu Li; for abdominal fullness with a preference for warmth and pressure, add Gao Liang Jiang and Zhi Xiang Fu.
- Tachycardia: when the presentation of tachycardia fits a Chinese medicine pattern of qi and yang deficiency, characterised by cold extremities, aversion to cold, an oppressed sensation in the chest, shortness of breath, fatigue, a pale tongue and a pulse which is submerged and slow, or faint and weak, Si Ni Tang jia Ren Shen can be used with the addition of Gui Zhi and Dan Shen.

Wu Ling San and Li Zhong Wan in the Treatment of Huo Luan

Clause 386

霍乱，头痛、发热、身疼痛，热多欲饮水者，五苓散主之；寒多不用水者，理中丸主之。

Huo luan with headache, fever and body pain, if heat predominates and there is a desire to drink water, Wu Ling San governs; if cold predominates and there is no need for water, Li Zhong Wan governs.

WU LING SAN: Zhu Ling (skin removed) 18 zhu; Ze Xie 1 liang 6 zhu; Bai Zhu 18 zhu; Fu Ling 18 zhu; Gui Zhi (bark removed) ½ liang.

DIRECTIONS: Grind all five ingredients into a powder and mix well. Take one square spoon (approx 6–9g) of the mixture with rice water (water taken from the pot as the rice is cooking) three times per day. Drink plenty of warm water and follow the same directions for Gui Zhi Tang in order to promote a sweat, and recovery will follow.

LI ZHONG WAN: Ren Shen 3 liang; Gan Jiang 3 liang; Zhi Gan Cao 3 liang; Bai Zhu 3 liang.

DIRECTIONS: Grind and sieve the ingredients, then mix with honey to make pills about the size of the yolk of a hen's egg. Add one pill to several ge of boiling water, crush and take the mixture warm. Take one pill in the same manner three or four times a day and twice at night. If there is no heat in the abdomen, take up to three or four more pills crushed in boiling water in the same fashion. Note: this method is not as effective as a decoction. To decoct the formula, slice the four ingredients, each in the same dose, and boil in 8 sheng of water until reduced to 3 sheng. Strain and take 1 sheng warm, three times a day. If a tremor is felt above the umbilicus, the kidney qi has been stirred; omit Bai Zhu and add 4 liang of Gui Zhi. For excessive vomiting, omit Bai Zhu and add 3 liang of Sheng Jiang. For excessive diarrhoea, retain Bai Zhu; for palpitations, add 2 liang of Fu Ling; for thirst with a desire to drink water, increase Bai Zhu from 3 liang to 4.5 liang. For abdominal pain, increase Ren Shen from 3 liang to 4.5 liang. For abdominal fullness, omit Bai Zhu and add 1 piece of Fu Zi. After taking the decoction, wait about the time it takes to eat a meal, then have about 1 sheng of hot gruel to slightly warm the body. Do not remove the clothes or bedclothes.

DISCUSSION: Huo luan which presents with headache, fever and body pain is a dual exterior and interior disorder and the treatment must accord with the relative degree of heat and cold. If an exterior yang pattern predominates, there will be more heat and a thirst for water. In this case, the pattern represents the concurrence of the pathogen in both the channel and the fu of Tai Yang; the headache, fever and body pain reflect the exterior channel disorder, and the fu disorder manifests with water accumulation in the stomach and intestines due to non-transformation of qi in the urinary bladder. If the water is in the intestines, there is diarrhoea; if there is stomach qi counterflow, there is vomiting; if there is non-transformation of qi and non-dispersion of fluids, there is thirst. If the pathogen is constrained between the exterior and the muscle layer, obstructing the flow of channel qi, there is headache and body pain; the dual exterior and interior disorder results in the non-transformation of qi giving rise to inhibited urination. The indicated formula is Wu Ling San. If there is more cold than heat, then it is a Tai Yin pattern which is characterised by spontaneous diarrhoea and no thirst. The indicated formula is Li Zhong Wan to warm and transform cold damp in the middle jiao.

The chief herb of Li Zhong Wan is Ren Shen, which augments qi and warms yang; Gan Jiang warms the middle and disperses cold; Gan Cao and Bai Zhu strengthen the spleen, and Bai Zhu dries damp. This is a key formula in the treatment of a Tai Yin deficiency cold pattern, where its function is to regulate the middle, hence its name Li Zhong Wan, which means 'regulate the middle pill'. Although it can be used in pill form, it is commonly prepared as a decoction. If given as a decoction, after administration there should be a feeling of warmth in the abdomen as testimony to its efficacy. If the abdomen does not feel warm, the dosage can be increased from one to three or four pills per dose or, if the pill method was used, the formula can be decocted to increase the therapeutic effect. About half an hour or so after administration (the time it takes to eat a meal), some hot gruel should be consumed to keep the body warm and the patient should be covered with warm clothing and a blanket.

Modifications

Modifications of Li Zhong Wan include the following. (1) For tremor in the umbilicus indicating kidney deficiency resulting in the upsurge of qi, also known as *ben tun*, omit Bai

Zhu and add Gui Zhi to warm the kidney and calm the counterflow. (2) For excessive vomiting indicating water retention in the stomach with counterflow stomach qi, omit Bai Zhu and add Sheng Jiang to warm yang and transform water to ease vomiting. (3) For incessant diarrhoea indicating the sinking of spleen qi and the impaired transformation and transportation function of spleen yang, retain Bai Zhu to tonify the spleen and parch dampness. (4) For palpitations due to water qi harassing the heart, add Fu Ling to disinhibit water and calm the shen. (5) For thirst arising from the failure of the spleen to distribute essences and fluid, increase the dosage of Bai Zhu to tonify the spleen and augment qi. (6) For abdominal pain due to weakness of the middle qi, increase the dosage of Ren Shen to 4.5 liang. (7) For interior coldness manifesting as abdominal coldness, increase the dosage of Gan Jiang. (8) For abdominal fullness due to cold qi stagnation, omit Bai Zhu and add Fu Zi to warm and unblock the yang, dissipate coldness and alleviate the fullness.

Clause 386 describes two key strategies in the treatment of huo luan. If there is exterior and interior disharmony, the treatment addresses both the exterior and interior by using Wu Ling San to release the exterior and to promote urination in order to treat the diarrhoea. If, however, the disorder is characterised by interior cold, the indicated formula is Li Zhong Wan to warm the interior and strengthen the spleen. The principal features indicating Li Zhong Wan are diarrhoea, abdominal fullness with occasional abdominal pain, an absence of thirst, a poor appetite, a thin white tongue coat and a submerged, slow and forceless pulse. A severe sense of cold in the abdomen or diarrhoea with undigested food particles represents a more serious condition.

Ancient Application of Li Zhong Wan

- *Qian Jin Fang:* For treatment of huo luan with vomiting and diarrhoea, abdominal fullness, indigestion and heart and abdominal pain, if there is cramp add 3 liang of Shi Gao.
- *Sheng Ji Zong Lu:* For treatment of infantile crying due to coldness of the spleen and stomach, abdominal coldness, wind in the abdomen, nausea and vomiting.
- *Zhi Zhi Fang:* For treatment of cough due to lung coldness, add E Jiao, Wu Wei Zi.
- *Yin Zheng Lue Li:* For treatment of coldness and inability to eat, use half of Li Zhong Tang mixed with half of Xiao Jian Zhong Tang.
- *Zhang Shi Yi Tong:* Lian Li Tang add Huang Lian and Fu Ling for treatment of interior cold due to cold injury or externally contracted summerheat with heat in the upper jiao and coldness in the lower jiao characterised by vomiting, acid reflux and watery diarrhoea.

According to ancient texts, Li Zhong Wan can be used to treat a range of disorders such as a cold huo luan pattern with no thirst; haemoptysis with oedema in the four limbs due to spleen deficiency and damp accumulation; mildly cold extremities and fatigue due to spleen qi deficiency; spermatorrhoea due to spleen deficiency; restless foetus or threatened abortion when caused by cold and deficiency in the middle jiao; and stomach reflux due to cold and deficiency in the middle jiao.

Modern Application of Li Zhong Wan

- Gastric ulcers or chronic gastritis when there is an underlying pattern of cold and deficiency in the middle jiao, characterised by a bland taste in the mouth, a preference for warmth and pressure, exacerbation of the symptoms by cold, a thin white or greasy white tongue coat, and a submerged and thready or submerged and slow pulse. The Chinese Liberation Army Air Force Hospital treated 40 cases of chronic gastritis with 21 cases of full recovery and 16 cases where the outcome was deemed effective. Huang et al used Li Zhong Wan modified (Dang Shen, Bai Zhu, Pao Jiang, Gan Cao, Chen Pi, Mu Xiang, Bai Ji, San Qi, Pu Huang, Wu Yao) to treat 46 cases of duodenal ulcers due to deficient cold where the outcome was 32 cases of full recovery, 13 cases of effective improvement and 2 cases deemed ineffective (*Xin Yi Yao Xue Za Zhi* 1977; 7:30).
- Infantile convulsions where the pattern is characterised by emaciation, fatigue, a sallow complexion, an absence of thirst, a sloppy stool which is green and watery, cold extremities and occasional convulsions, a pale tongue with a thin white coat and a submerged and

weak pulse or fingers which have turned white. Li Zhong Tang can be used with the addition of Bai Shao, Gou Teng, Tian Ma and Jiang Can.

Case Study

Irritable Bowel Syndrome

Extracted from Fu Yan Ling's case studies:

Pearls of Wisdom Seminar, Melbourne, 2007

A 38-year-old woman presented with recurrent diarrhoea from which she had suffered for five years. The diarrhoea could be triggered by a gust of cold wind or, at times, even sitting on a cold seat. The Western diagnosis was irritable bowel syndrome. From the Chinese medicine perspective, the patient exhibited a range of cold signs: she was averse to cold, with a preference for warmth; the abdomen felt cold, she had no thirst and her appetite was poor. Her complexion was pale, the tongue coat was white, and the pulse was thready. These observations led to a diagnosis of deficiency cold of the spleen and stomach. The treatment principle was to warm the middle and dissipate cold. She was told to refrain from cold or raw food and seven packs of Li Zhong Tang were prescribed: Dang Shen 18g, Chao Bai Zhu 15g, Zhi Gan Cao 12g, Gan Jiang 12g. After several doses of this medication, the symptoms reduced substantially and the abdomen no longer felt cold. At the end of the seven packs, there was no diarrhoea. The formula was repeated with the addition of Fu Ling and Huang Qi, and occasionally with the addition of Chuan Lian Zi. This regimen was continued for two months and she recovered.

Discussion: The patient's prominent cold signs included aversion to cold, a sense of cold in the abdomen, a preference for warmth, a pale complexion, white tongue coat and thready pulse. The diagnosis was insufficiency of spleen and stomach yang which was severely affected by the environmental qi (cold wind). A famous Chinese medicine adage states: "30 percent is due to treatment and 70 percent is dietary". Therefore during the course of treatment, proper diet plays an important role and cold or raw foods should be avoided. The dose of some ingredients was increased because in the clinical situation, dosage can be adjusted according to the individual. If the condition is more serious, the patient's response can be slow and the medication can be increased to two packs per day.

Case Study

Infantile Diarrhoea and Abdominal Pain

Extracted from Fu Yan Ling's case studies:

Pearls of Wisdom Seminar, Melbourne, 2007

A nine-year-old boy had suffered from abdominal pain and frequent diarrhoea for two years. He was emaciated, had a lack-lustre and pale complexion, a poor appetite with occasional nausea, an absence of thirst, a pale tongue with a white, moist tongue coat and a pulse that was thready and rapid. The diagnosis was spleen and stomach deficient and cold. The treatment principle was to warm the middle and dissipate cold. The formula used was a modification of Li Zhong Tang: Dang Shen 10g, Bai Zhu 10g, Zhi Gan Cao 6g, Gan Jiang 8g, Gui Zhi 8g, Cao Dou Kou 8g. Seven packs were prescribed and the patient was instructed to refrain from cold food and ice cream. After three days of medication, the patient's abdominal pain and diarrhoea stopped and his appetite increased.

Case Study

Vomiting Due to Spleen Yang Deficiency and Cold

Extracted from Fu Yan Ling's case studies

Pearls of Wisdom Seminar, Melbourne, 2007

A 40-year-old female had suffered from vomiting for one week following the drinking of very cold water. The vomiting had been constant during the previous week. Her other symptoms included a poor appetite, no desire to drink, a pale complexion, a moist white tongue coat and a soft pulse. The diagnosis was spleen yang deficiency. She was given two packs of a modified version of

Li Zhong Tang: Dang Shen 10g, Bai Zhu 8g, Zhi Gan Cao 6g, Gan Jiang 8g, Ding Xiang 8g, black pepper 0.5g. The directions were to decoct the herbs in 400 mL of water, then to strain and take 200 mL warm, adding 0.5g of black pepper.

After one pack, the vomiting stopped and at the end of the two packs, her vomiting was resolved.

Discussion: Li Zhong Tang is a formula which is aimed at warming the stomach; however, it has little effect on the descent of stomach qi and so Ding Xiang and black pepper are added to descend qi and redirect the counterflow. The black pepper should be added last, after straining the decoction, because subjecting it to cooking will weaken its acrid flavour. Clinical experience has shown that Bai Dou Kou should be treated in the same way to ensure a good therapeutic effect.

The Significance of Vomiting and Diarrhoea

Clause 387

吐利止而身痛不休者，当消息和解其外，宜桂枝汤小和之。

If the vomiting and diarrhoea stop but the body pain remains, one should pause for breath and harmonise the exterior, Gui Zhi Tang is appropriate to harmonise mildly.

DISCUSSION: The cessation of vomiting and diarrhoea indicates that the interior qi is harmonised. The persistence of the body pain, however, shows that ying and wei are in disharmony, and that there is an unresolved residual pathogen harassing the exterior. This is a pattern where the zheng qi is deficient and the promotion of heavy sweating is prohibited. Therefore a small dose of Gui Zhi Tang to harmonise the exterior and also to regulate the spleen and stomach, thus simultaneously facilitating the recovery of stomach qi, and addressing the body pain, is appropriate.

In practice, it is unusual to see an unresolved exterior pattern with a history of vomiting and diarrhoea which has already ceased. However, patterns which mimic this situation, but have no history of vomiting and diarrhoea, are often encountered. These include such presentations as fever with blood in the stool or post-partum deficiency with an attack of pathogenic wind-cold causing body aches and pains, and can be treated with Gui Zhi Tang or Gui Zhi Xin Jia Tang.

Clause 388

吐利汗出，发热恶寒，四肢拘急，手足厥冷者，四逆汤主之。

If there is diarrhoea and sweating, fever and aversion to cold, cramping in the four limbs, and desertion cold in the hands and feet, Si Ni Tang governs.

DISCUSSION: The key symptoms of huo luan are vomiting and diarrhoea. Incessant vomiting and diarrhoea damage the spleen and stomach from the beginning, and if prolonged, kidney yang will also be damaged, and there arises a pattern of spleen and kidney yang deficiency characterised by sweating, aversion to cold and cold extremities. The diarrhoea and sweating are the result of devastated yang, and the fever is attributed to true yang being repelled by exuberant yin cold. Thus it is seen that the vomiting and diarrhoea have not only damaged yin fluids, but have devastated yang, and the formula is Si Ni Tang to resuscitate the devastated yang. Once the yang desertion is reversed, the other symptoms will be resolved spontaneously.

Clause 389

既吐且利，小便复利而大汗出，下利清谷，内寒外热，脉微欲绝者，四逆汤主之。

If as well as vomiting and diarrhoea, the urination is then free and there is profuse sweat, diarrhoea with undigested food particles, interior cold and exterior heat, the pulse is faint and verging on expiry, Si Ni Tang governs.

DISCUSSION: A huo luan pattern characterised by vomiting and diarrhoea might be expected to be characterised by scant urination due to fluid depletion. However, the urination is described as being free, which means it is frequent and copious, here reflecting a critical degree of yang desertion. The clear, copious urination is the result of cold in the lower jiao, with deficient yang unable to control water; deficient yang affects the defence yang, which is unable to secure the exterior, and so there is profuse and incessant sweating. Yang deficiency in the Shao Yin means that the spleen earth is not warmed; the spleen can then not support the rotting and ripening of grain, and so there are undigested food particles in the stool, which is loose and watery. This is a pattern of severe yang deficiency where exuberant yin is forcing the yang to depart.

The treatment strategy for huo luan can serve as a clinical guide for modern gastrointestinal disorders involving diarrhoea and vomiting. However, the following differentiations must be made.

Because huo luan patterns are associated with severe vomiting and diarrhoea, if inadequate or incorrect treatment is given, there can be serious ramifications. They must be differentiated according to whether they are associated with heat or cold, and whether a symptom such as fever is true or false. The urination, stool and the pulse sign are the key clinical features relied on to determine whether it is true or false heat or cold. For true cold with false heat, Si Ni Tang is indicated. If the vomiting and diarrhoea are accompanied by thirst, a foul-smelling stool and a submerged, hidden and forceful pulse, these are indicative of constrained heat and stagnation, and Wang Shi Lian Pu Yin (Hou Po, Huang Liang fried in ginger juice, Shi Chang Pu, Ban Xia, Dan Dou Chi, Chao Shan Zhi) is the appropriate formula.

For a pattern of dual yin and yang deficiency, it is essential first to resuscitate the yang. In its initial stage, a huo luan disorder is characterised by vomiting and diarrhoea, which damages both yin and yang. However, if yin nourishing herbs were used first, when yang was deficient, they would not be easily digested, and their cloying nature would tend to cause stagnation and obstruct the return of yang qi.

Case Study

Infantile Diarrhoea

Extracted from Zhe Jiang Zhong Yi Za Zhi 1964; 8:14

A seven-month-old baby boy had been fed on thin rice gruel because his mother had no milk. Two months previously, after being overfed, he had a bloated and distended abdomen, as well as vomiting, frequent diarrhoea, and a high fever. After Western medical treatment, the fever receded and the episodes of diarrhoea were reduced to 4 to 5 times a day. Two days prior to the consultation, he had caught a cold, and the diarrhoea had become worse, with episodes up to eight times a day. His hands and feet were cold and the tongue coat was white and lacked moisture. The diagnosis was deficiency and cold of the spleen and kidneys. The formula given was a modification of Si Ni Tang: Fu Zi 1.5g, Gan Jiang 9g, Gan Cao 9g were boiled in 350 mL of water, reducing to 150 mL, then Huang Lian 9g was added and the decoction was boiled until reduced to 80 mL. It was then strained and sweetened with sugar. The dose was 8 mL every four hours. The next day, his diarrhoea had eased and his limbs were warm. The same formula was administered for a further three days and he recovered.

Tong Mai Si Ni jia Zhu Dan Zhi Tang Pattern

Clause 390

吐已下断，汗出而厥，四肢拘急不解，脉微欲绝者，通脉四逆加猪胆汁汤主之。

Vomiting has ceased and diarrhoea has halted, if there is sweating and jue with unresolved cramping in the four limbs, and the pulse is faint and verging on expiry, Tong Mai Si Ni jia Zhu Dan Zhi Tang governs.

TONG MAI SI NI JIA ZHU DAN ZHI TANG: Zhi Gan Cao 2 liang; Gan Jiang 3 liang (4 liang for a robust person); Fu Zi (raw, skin removed) 1 piece broken into eight; Zhu Dan Zhi ½ ge.

DIRECTIONS: Boil all four ingredients in 3 sheng of water until reduced to 1 sheng 2 ge. Strain and add Zhu Dan Zhi (pig's bile). Take warm twice a day and the pulse will return. The pig's bile can be substituted with goat's bile.

DISCUSSION: The cessation of vomiting and diarrhoea should signal the return of yang, with the limbs becoming warm. Here, when the vomiting and diarrhoea stop, the extremities are cold and the pulse is faint, verging on expiry. This is not a sign of the return of yang, but is, in fact, a sign of the desertion of yang and the exhaustion of yin. This is because the cessation of diarrhoea is the result of severe depletion of yin fluids. The yang desertion gives rise to incessant sweating, and exhausted yin results in cramping in the limbs. Thus Clause 390 describes a pattern of devastated yang and the exhaustion of yin fluids.

If a potent yang tonic is given, the yang herbs may be rejected and repelled by the interior yin cold, resulting in upcast yang. If a yin tonic is given, it is feared that the cloying nature of yin herbs may obstruct the yang. Therefore, Tong Mai Si Ni jia Zhu Dan Zhi Tang is given to resuscitate the yang and augment the yin. The pig's bile is bitter, cold and moistening, and can serve as a guide for Fu Zi and Gan Jiang, leading them to the yin, and precluding the rejection of acrid and hot herbs by the exuberant interior yin cold. The cold moistening properties of the bile counter the heat and dryness of Fu Zi, thus preventing further damage to yin, and also assist in replenishing the damaged yin.

The above pattern and the Si Ni jia Ren Shen pattern, described earlier in this chapter in Clause 385, are both associated with yang desertion and yin exhaustion; the difference is in the severity of the condition. The Si Ni jia Ren Shen Tang pattern is milder; there is aversion to cold, a faint pulse, cold extremities and cessation of diarrhoea attributed to blood collapse. The Tong Mai Si Ni jia Zhu Dan Zhi Tang pattern represents a more critical condition where yin is repelling yang, and there is a possibility of yang expiry. It is characterised by an absence of both vomiting and diarrhoea, and by incessant sweating, cold extremities, cramping in the limbs and a faint pulse verging in expiry.

Clause 391

吐、利、发汗，脉平，小烦者，以新虚不胜谷气故也。

Vomiting, diarrhoea, the promotion of sweat, if the pulse is normal, and there is slight vexation, this is because the new deficiency is not able to deal with the grain qi.

DISCUSSION: When the vomiting and diarrhoea stop and the pulse is normal, this indicates that the disease is resolved and there will be recovery. The slight vexation is a result of the struggle of the spleen and stomach to function in their deficient state. They are referred to as the new deficiency because of the recent damage sustained as a result of the vomiting, diarrhoea and improper promotion of sweat. They are unable to transform food, or grain qi, giving rise to food stagnation and mild vexation.

The implication of Clause 391 is that during the recovery period it is better to avoid straining the deficient middle jiao by overeating, eating heavy meals or hard-to-digest food. The intake of food should be adequate but moderate. If the mild vexation persists, Bao He Wan can be given to help with digestion.

Summary of Huo Luan

This chapter covers four issues relevant in the diagnosis and treatment of huo luan, and includes five patterns as well as aftercare in the recovery phase.

- *The concept of huo luan.* Huo luan is defined as a disorder characterised by vomiting and diarrhoea of sudden onset.
- *Differentiation between huo luan and shang han.* Huo luan is an acute gastrointestinal disease with vomiting and diarrhoea at onset; a shang han exterior pattern is characterised by fever, aversion to cold and other exterior symptoms at onset, and vomiting and diarrhoea only occur much later, when the disease has progressed for four or five days or more, in response to the pathogen sinking inward.
- *Treatment of huo luan.* (1) If the disease is characterised by fever, headache, body pain and inhibited urination, Wu Ling San is

indicated. If interior cold predominates with cold extremities, Li Zhong Wan or Tang is indicated. (2) True and false patterns must be identified: if the vomiting and diarrhoea are accompanied by fever, cold extremities, diarrhoea with undigested food particles and a faint pulse verging on expiry, this is a pattern of true cold and false heat, and the treatment is Si Ni Tang. (3) Excess must be distinguished from deficiency, and a mild condition from a serious one: if there is aversion to cold, a faint pulse and the recurrence of diarrhoea which then stops, this indicates devastation of blood, where exhaustion of yang has led to desertion of yin; the treatment is Si Ni jia Ren Shen Tang; if the vomiting and diarrhoea stop and there is sweating, cramping in the limbs, and a faint pulse verging on expiry, it is a pattern of yang desertion with yin exhaustion and the treatment is Tong Mai Si Ni jia Zhu Dan Zhi Tang.

- *Aftercare during the recuperative period of huo luan.* If the vomiting and diarrhoea stop, and there is body pain, a small dose of Gui Zhi Tang is recommended. If there is mild vexation after the vomiting and diarrhoea, dietary precautions are necessary.

陰陽易差後勞復病

9 Yin Yang Exchange and Taxation Relapse

Section One

9.1 DEFINITION OF YIN YANG EXCHANGE

Yin Yang exchange and taxation relapse refer to disease arising out of cross-infection or taxation fatigue, and more particularly to disease contracted during convalescence when the zheng qi is not primed. Lifestyle choices are discussed in relation to diet, sexual activity and excessive exertion or taxation on physical resources, which is also known as taxation fatigue. Even when the health is robust, the struggle of the zheng qi against pathogenic qi is a drain on physical resources. When physical resources are at a low ebb, in particular when recovery is incomplete in the convalescent period, the depleted state of zheng qi increases the likelihood of relapse and also increases the likelihood of the convalescent patient succumbing to any new pathogenic attack.

Yin Yang exchange in general refers to disease caused by toxic cross-infection between male (yang) and female (yin). Following shang han febrile disease, yin and yang are not yet balanced, qi and blood are not fully restored, and residual heat is not fully resolved. At this stage, sexual intercourse can lead to toxicity from the male being transferred to the female, known as yang exchange. When female disease infects the male, it is known as yin exchange.

In the convalescent period immediately following contraction of a major shang han illness, the zheng qi is not fully restored, and the deficiency lays the person open to contracting pathogens. If normal daily work is resumed too early, and further to this, a healthy diet is ignored, the likelihood of relapse is increased. This is known as taxation relapse, which implies relapse due to inappropriate exertion, or over-taxation.

Section Two

9.2 YIN YANG EXCHANGE PATTERN

Shao Ku San

Clause 392

伤寒阴阳易之为病，其人身体重、少气、少腹里急，或引阴中拘挛，热上冲胸，头重不欲举，眼中生花，膝胫拘急者，烧裈散主之。

Shang han yin yang exchange disease, if the person feels heavy in the body, there is shortness of breath, and interior urgency in the lesser abdomen, or cramping in the genitals, heat surges upward to the chest, the head feels heavy and there is an unwillingness to raise it, there is blurred vision, cramps in the knees and lower leg, Shao Ku San governs.

SHAO KUN SAN: The crotch of a woman's pants scorched and charred.

DIRECTIONS: Take a square-inch spoonful of the ashes with water, three times daily. When urination is uninhibited and the glans penis is slightly swollen, this indicates recovery. When a woman has this disease, use the charred crotch of men's pants.

DISCUSSION: Clause 392 describes a person (either man or woman) who, during their convalescence from an illness with residual heat, has had sexual intercourse and become infected by a toxic pathogen. According to the theory of Chinese medicine, sexual intercourse has the potential to exhaust the kidney essence. The heaviness in the body and shortness of breath is the result of damage to qi and essence. The depleted essence is unable to nourish the sinews, and there is abdominal urgency, accompanied by genital cramping.

Toxic damp heat has entered via the lower yin orifice, and has not only affected the lower jiao, but has surged upward to harass the chest and manifest as heaviness in the head and blurred vision. The root of this disorder is deficiency of qi and essence, combined with an attack of toxic damp heat. The treatment for this disorder is to descend and expel the pathogen. *Yi Zong Jin Jian* explained: the part of pants closest to the genital area is associated with turbidity and if this is charred and turned to ashes, it can be used to dissipate and disperse. After taking this, there is sweating, urine is passed, and there is recovery. The swelling of the glans penis is a manifestation of the toxic heat being vented outward.

There is little information in literary records on the disorder of yin yang exchange; however, it generally is thought to refer to infection resulting from sexual contact. It could be a sexually transmitted disease, or it could be a localised infection caused by friction and subsequent micro-fissures. In either case, in the convalescent stage, the poor state of the zheng qi has not been strong enough to overcome the pathogen, and residual heat has laid a foundation for the generation of toxic heat.

Section Three

9.3 TAXATION RELAPSE

Zhi Shi Zhi Zi Chi Tang

Clause 393

大病差后劳复者，枳实栀子豉汤主之。

If after dispatch of major disease there is taxation relapse, Zhi Shi Zhi Zi Chi Tang governs.

ZHI SHI ZHI ZI CHI TANG: Zhi Shi (mix-fried) 3 pieces; Zhi Zi (broken) 14 pieces; Xiang Chi 1 sheng (wrapped in gauze).

DIRECTIONS: Boil Zhi Shi and Xiang Chi in 7 sheng of clear starch water (water in which grain has been left to ferment), reducing by 4 sheng. Then add Zhi Zi, boiling until reduced to 2 sheng. Strain and take warm twice a day. Cover the patient with a blanket to obtain a mild sweat. If there is food stagnation, add five or six pieces of Da Huang the size of bo qi zi. Recovery will follow. Note: bo qi zi (博棋子) are stones used traditionally as a chess piece, measuring approximately 1 square inch and about 2 inches high.

DISCUSSION: In the early convalescent phase, when recovering from major illness, restitution of qi, blood and zheng qi has not taken place; heavy work and sexual activity should be avoided in order to rest the body and allow full recuperation. If this practice is not observed, then there is a risk of further depleting the vital substances, even to the point where kidney essence is also damaged. Clause 393 does not specify the nature of the disease, but from the prescribed formula, it can be deduced that there is fever and abdominal fullness.

Zhi Shi loosens the blocked qi in the chest; Zhi Zi clears the head and alleviates vexation; the clear starch water is cool and regulates the stomach to assist digestion. The aim of this formula is to clear heat and supplement the spleen earth in order to eliminate food stagnation. If there is constipation, Da Huang can be added to purge the stagnation. Xiang Chi is used to vent constrained heat outward.

Xiao Chai Hu Tang

Clause 394

伤寒差以后更发热，小柴胡汤主之。脉浮者，以汗解之；脉沉实者，以下解之。

After despatch of shang han there is more fever, Xiao Chai Hu Tang governs. If the pulse is floating, resolution is by sweating; if the pulse is deep and excess, resolution is by purgation.

DISCUSSION: Fever which recurs after the apparent recovery from illness can be due to residual heat, where the pathogen has not been fully resolved and has flared up, or it can be due to a renewed pathogenic attack that has taken advantage of the deficiency. The pulse is used to determine whether the disease is external or internal. If there are neither exterior nor interior signs, then the fever is due to residual pathogenic heat and Xiao Chai Hu Tang can be given to support the zheng qi and expel the residual pathogen. If the pulse is floating, indicating an exterior attack, sweating should be promoted to release the exterior; if the pulse is submerged and excess, indicating interior stagnation, purgation should be used.

Relapse of disease in the period immediately following illness, when zheng qi has not been fully restituted and the health is not yet robust, is common. Clause 394 describes three main developments, each with their treatment strategy.

1. *Residual heat.* The heat pathogen has not been fully expelled This latent heat lingers after the patient seems to have recovered from the illness, only to resurface a short time later, taking advantage of the deficiency and flaring up, causing a recurrence of the fever. Where there is a deficiency of zheng qi with residual heat, Xiao Chai Hu Tang can be used; where there is a dual deficiency of qi and yin with residual heat manifesting with thirst, vexation and fever Zhu Ye Shi Gao Tang can be used; if there is yin deficiency with residual heat characterised by dry retching, vexation, thirst, a red tongue with a scant tongue coat and a thready and rapid pulse, Zhu Ye Yu Nu Jian (Shi Gao, Sheng Di, Mai Dong, Zhi Mu, Niu Xi, Zhu Ye) can be used; if there is qi deficiency with a poor appetite, a sloppy stool, fatigue, a pale tongue with a white tongue coat, Xiao Chai Hu Tang with a large dose of Ren Shen can be used.
2. *Food stagnation.* If during the recovery phase, there is food stagnation, constipation and fever, Xiao Cheng Qi Tang can be used to purge heat from the bowel and eliminate food stagnation. Alternatively, if there is yin deficiency, Zeng Ye Cheng Qi Tang can be used to replenish the yin and purge accumulation.
3. Clause 394 advocates "sweat promotion" or "purgation" but does not indicate which formulas should be used. Past scholars have proposed different theories: Zhong Hong from the Song dynasty said: "a floating pulse with fever should be treated with Chai Hu Gui Zhi Tang". Yu Jia Yan from the Qing dynasty said: "For sweat promotion, Zhi Shi

Zhi Zi Chi Tang can be used; if the pulse is submerged, indicating an interior pattern, Zhi Shi Zhi Zi Da Huang Tang can be used to purge; if there is neither an exterior nor an interior pattern, Xiao Chai Hu Tang can be used to harmonise.

Mu Li Ze Xie San

Clause 395

大病差后，从腰以下有水气者，牡蛎泽泻散主之。

After despatch of major disease, if there is water qi from the waist down, Mu Li Ze Xie San governs.

MU LI ZE XIE SAN: Equal parts of: Mu Li (dry-fried); Ze Xie; Shu Qi (washed in warm water to eliminate the fishy smell); Ting Li Zi (dry-fried); Shang Lu Gen (dry-fried); Hai Zao (washed to eliminate the salt); Gua Lou Gen (Tian Hua Fen).

DIRECTIONS: Pulverise each herb separately and pass through a sieve. Place the powder in a mortar and blend with cooled white rice water (bai yin). Take 1 square-inch spoonful three times a day. If urination becomes uninhibited, stop the medication.

DISCUSSION: In the phase immediately following recovery from major illness, if spleen qi has not been restored, the qi transformation function will be impaired, and this will give rise to the stagnation of damp heat and the accumulation of water, which manifests as swelling below the waist. Other symptoms would be inhibited urination, a sluggish bowel movement, and a pulse which is submerged, excess and forceful. Mu Li Ze Xie San eliminates water and promotes urination. Hai Zao and Mu Li soften and disperse accumulations and so help to reduce the water swelling; Ting Li Zi clears heat and moves water; Shang Lu Gen dissipates water bind and drives out water; Shu Qi dissipates knotted phlegm bind. Mu Li Ze Xie San can thus reduce glomus, soften knotted bind and dissolve accumulation. Gua Lou Gen drains heat and generates fluids; by conserving yin and fluids it counters the potent diuretic effect of the other herbs; it also invigorates blood and resolves toxicity. This is a potent formula which is useful in the treatment of ascites due to liver cirrhosis.

Fluid retention or water swelling in the immediate post-recovery phase is generally associated with deficiency rather than excess. The deficiency is principally a deficiency of yin resulting from unresolved residual heat and the non-transformation of urinary bladder qi, which gives rise to inhibited urination and the retention of water. Accompanying symptoms include thirst, a parched throat, tidal fever, night sweating, a red tongue with a scant tongue coat, and a thready and rapid pulse. The indicated formula is Zhu Ling Tang modified. Qi deficiency is the result of pathogenic heat exhausting the qi. Subsequently, the impaired transformation and transportation function of the spleen gives rise to water accumulation; the primary symptoms are inhibited urination, a poor appetite, a sloppy stool, fatigue, spontaneous sweating, exertional dyspnoea, a slippery, white tongue coat and a slow pulse. The indicated formula is Shen Ling Bai Zhu San combined with Wu Pi Yin modified. If there is oedema in the lower limbs accompanied by a bitter taste in the mouth, epigastric fullness, glomus, dark urination and a yellow and greasy tongue coat, the formula is Mu Li Ze Xie San. The preferred administration method is to blend the powdered herbs in warm rice water. The object of this is to preserve fluids and support the stomach qi. Because this is a powerful diuretic formula, the directions exhort discontinuance once the urination is free and profuse, because prolonged use will be too draining and will damage the zheng qi.

Li Zhong Wan

Clause 396

大病差后，喜唾，久不了了，胸上有寒，当以丸药温之，宜理中丸。

After despatch of major disease, there is a tendency to spit, for a long time without clearing, there is cold in the chest, one should warm with pills, Li Zhong Wan is appropriate.

DISCUSSION: Excessive salivation and spitting is attributed to deficiency cold of the spleen and lungs. The lungs descend and disperse, and regulate the waterways to transport water to the urinary bladder. Cold in the lungs affects the descending function, which carries water to the lower jiao. Cold in the spleen affects the transformation and transportation of fluids, resulting in an accumulation of damp or of fluids in the middle jiao, where damp can transform into phlegm. Yang deficiency of the lungs and spleen affects the transformation of qi, giving rise to excessive salivation and spitting. The treatment strategy is to warm and tonify spleen yang. Based on the five phase theory of earth generating metal, warming and tonifying the spleen will flow on to tonification and warming of the lungs. Clause 396 therefore suggests Li Zhong Wan. In *Jin Gui Yao Lue: Treatment of Lung Wilting, Welling Abscess and Cough* the same principle is reinforced using a different formula: "If there is cold in the lungs there will be vertigo and excessive spitting, Gan Cao Gan Jiang Tang is used to warm."

In practice, for yang deficiency of the lungs and spleen where there is constant spitting of watery sputum, accompanied by an aversion to cold and clear urination, herbs such as Shan Yao, Bian Dou, Chen Pi, Jiang Ban Xia, which transform phlegm and harmonise the stomach, should be added to Li Zhong Wan.

Zhu Ye Shi Gao Tang

Clause 397

伤寒解后，虚羸少气，气逆欲吐，竹叶石膏汤主之。

After shang han resolves, there is deficiency, emaciation and shortness of breath, qi counterflow and a desire to vomit, Zhu Ye Shi Gao Tang governs.

ZHU YE SHI GAO TANG: Zhu Ye 2 bundles; Shi Gao 1 sheng; Ban Xia (washed) ½ jin; Mai Dong (hearts removed) 1 sheng; Ren Shen 2 liang; Zhi Gan Cao 2 liang; Jing Mi (short-grain rice) ½ jin.

DIRECTIONS: Boil the ingredients in 1 dou of water, reducing to 6 sheng. Strain and add the rice. Continue boiling until the rice is cooked and then strain to remove the rice. Take 1 sheng warm three times a day.

DISCUSSION: In the initial recovery phase when the zheng qi is not fully restored, the person is emaciated, fatigued and out of breath, even on slight exertion. This is because both qi and yin are deficient. The desire to vomit is a reflection of stomach disharmony caused by this yin and qi deficiency, where the yin deficient heat has been aggravated by the residual pathogenic heat. Other manifestations of this heat would be vexation, thirst, a parched throat, disturbed sleep, a red tongue with scant tongue coat, and a deficient and rapid pulse.

Zhu Ye Shi Gao Tang clears heat, augments qi, nourishes yin and harmonises the stomach. Zhu Ye clears heat from the heart and stomach and relieves irritability. Shi Gao drains fire and clears residual heat; Ban Xia eases the urge to vomit by redirecting the counterflow; Ren Shen tonifies the deficiency; Mai Dong nourishes the yin of the heart, lungs and stomach; Gan Cao and Jing Mi harmonise the stomach qi and protect the middle qi from the coldness of Shi Gao. This is a formula designed to address deficiency of yin and qi where there is residual heat following a major illness. It simultaneously dispels the residual pathogenic heat and supports the zheng qi by nourishing the yin of the stomach and lungs.

Clauses 396 and 397 both describe symptoms which appear during the recovery period. Clause 396 describes a pattern attributed to residual cold in the spleen exhibiting excessive salivation, where the formula is Li Zhong Wan, and Clause 397 is attributed to residual heat in the stomach, where the indicated formula is Zhu Ye Shi Gao Tang.

Ancient Application of Zhu Ye Shi Gao Tang

- *Wai Tai Mi Yao:* For the treatment of a dual exterior and interior disorder characterised by insubstantial vexation arising from yin deficiency.
- *Huo Ren Shu:* For treatment of the recovery period in the wake of shang han disease characterised by vomiting due to residual

heat in the stomach, Zhu Ye Shi Gao Tang is modified by the addition of Sheng Jiang.

- *Yi Fang Ji Jie:* A modified version of Zhu Ye Shi Gao Tang (Zhu Ye, Shi Gao, Mu Tong, Bo He, Jie Geng, Gan Cao) for the treatment of excess fire in the stomach characterised by insatiable thirst.
- *Zhang Shi Yi Tong:* Ji Ji Tang, which is Zhu Ye Shi Gao Tang modified by adding 3 to 5 fen of Shu Fu Pian, for the treatment of heat in the upper jiao and cold in the lower jiao.

Modern Application of Zhu Ye Shi Gao Tang

- Zhu Ye Shi Gao Tang was used in the treatment of 15 cases of measles with pneumonia. For severe cough, Huang Qin and Pi Pa Ye were added; for tidal fever in the afternoon, Yin Chai Hu and Qing Hao were added; for sore throat, Xuan Shen and Chi Shao were added; for qi deficiency with spontaneous sweating, Huang Qi and Mu Li were added. No antibiotics were used during the course of treatment. The average number of days taken before the fever was resolved was 4 days with full recovery in 7 days (*Liao Ning Zhong Yi Za Zhi* 1980; (3):22).
- Zhu Ye Shi Gao Tang was used in 32 cases of haemorrhagic fever. The average number of days for disease resolution ranged between 7 and 18 days (*He Nan Zhong Yi* 1983; (3):33).
- A modified version of Zhu Ye Shi Gao Tang was used to treat 96 cases of toothache. The formula used was Sheng Shi Gao 40g, Zhu Ye 15g, Zhi Mu 12g, Shan Zhi 12g, Sheng Ma 12g, Xuan Shen 10g. The ingredients were soaked for 30 minutes; 20g of glutinous rice was added and the mixture was boiled until the rice was cooked. One pack was taken each day in two doses. The average course of treatment lasted 3 to 6 days. The results were: 90 cases fully recovered; 5 cases improved, and 1 case not effective (*Sichuan Zhong Yi* 1994; (10):52).
- This formula can be used to treat many deficiency heat or steaming bone patterns characterised by low grade fever, emaciation, fatigue, a thready, rapid and forceless pulse, a red tongue with a scant or thin tongue coat. The effect can be enhanced with the addition of such herbs as Di Gu Pi, Qin Jiao and Yin Chai Hu.

Case Study

Infantile Summerheat

Extracted from Jiangsu Zhong Yi 1996; (7):33

The patient was a 3-year-old boy. His mother reported that during the past month, the child had suffered from a fever which worsened in the afternoon, and also occasionally peaked in the morning. He had a temperature of 39.7°C, was thirsty, had a poor appetite, a sloppy stool, and clear urination. The child was lucid but had a blank expression. His skin was dry and his abdomen was soft. His tongue was red and the tongue coat was greasy and slightly pale. His pulse was soggy and rapid. The formula given was a modification of Zhu Ye Shi Gao Tang: Sheng Shi Gao 15g, Dang Shen 6g, Mai Dong 6g, Ban Xia 3g, Gan Cao 2.4g, Jing Mi 9g (wrapped in a lotus leaf), Mai Ya 6g, Shen Qu 9g, Zhu Ye 12 pieces. After one pack, his fever dropped to 37.8°C and the other symptoms eased; however, his appetite was still poor. He was given a further two packs with 6g Ji Nei Jin added and recovered.

Case Study

Breast Abscess

Extracted from Shang Han Shi Si Jiang

A 23-year-old female patient suffered from a fever of 38.5–39.5°C following surgery to drain an abscess of the breast. Post-operative infection was suspected and she was given an intramuscular injection of antibiotics, but it was not effective. She presented with nausea, vomiting, no appetite, irritability, thirst, dizziness, and hand tremor. Her pulse was rapid and forceful and her tongue was pale red with a thin, yellow coat. She told the Chinese medicine practitioner that she had been diagnosed with septicaemia. The Chinese medicine diagnosis was deficiency of qi and yin, particularly the yin of the stomach. The formula given was a modification of Zhu Ye Shi Gao Tang: Sheng Shi Gao 30g, Mai Dong 24g, Dang Shen 10g, Zhi Gan Cao 10g, Jing Mi one handful, Zhu Ye 10g. After four packs, her fever receded and there was no more vomiting.

Recovery in Taxation Relapse

Clause 398

病人脉已解，而日暮微烦，以病新差，人强与谷，脾胃气尚弱，不能消谷，故令微烦，损谷则愈。

The patient's pulse is already resolved, and in the evening there is mild vexation, this is because the disease is newly despatched, the person is forced to eat, the spleen and stomach qi is still weak, the person can not digest food, leading to mild vexation, reduce food and there will be recovery.

DISCUSSION: The patient's pulse is harmonious, showing that the major illness has been resolved. The mild vexation is the result of the improper and excessive intake of food at a time when the qi of the spleen and stomach is still weak and can not process the food, leading to food stagnation. Heat is then generated, which flares upward harassing the shen. The significance of this occurring in the evening relates to the mutual response between man and heaven. Cosmic yang qi peaks at midday and gradually diminishes towards dusk, with its final recession in the evening, when there is no environmental yang to bolster the yang of the spleen and stomach, which is insufficient to perform its function of digesting the food. The implication is that without the support of the environmental yang, the middle qi is at its lowest in the evening, and problems are more likely to arise at this time, particularly as the person was forced to eat, placing greater demands on the middle qi. The solution therefore is to reduce the intake of food.

Clause 398 should be read with Clause 391 as they both express the notion of the digestive function being weak in the period immediately following illness. During this period, therefore, meals should be small and light, and should be easily digestible in order to avoid placing a strain on the digestive system. This is particularly pertinent in the case of infants and small children or the elderly, whose digestive systems are typically weak. This final clause of *Shang Han Lun* emphasises the importance of paying attention to the protection of the spleen and stomach qi during recovery from illness. The preservation and support of stomach qi as the basis of zheng qi and good health is a recurring theme throughout *Shang Han Lun,* beginning in the chapter on Gui Zhi Tang with the direction to take hot gruel to support the stomach qi and enhance sweat promotion, and ending here, in the final clause, with the admonition to avoid heavy meals when the stomach qi is at a low point.

Summary of Yin Yang Exchange and Taxation Relapse

This chapter deals with the four main patterns of yin yang exchange and taxation relapse disorders, and also emphasises the importance of regulating the spleen and stomach qi in the recovery period immediately following illness. They are summarised as follows.

1. *Aetiology and pathogenesis.* After an episode of major illness, when yin and yang are not fully restored, and qi and blood are still deficient, on a background of unresolved residual heat, good aftercare is essential, and relates to diet, as well as resumption of physical work and sexual activity. If advice to pay attention to these lifestyle factors is not heeded, there can be a relapse of disease.
2. *Pattern and treatment for taxation relapse.*
   (i) Fever: If, in the recovery period, there is excessive exertion before the complete restoration of zheng qi, this may cause relapse characterised by fever, vexation, anguish and abdominal fullness; the indicated formula is Zhi Shi Zhi Zi Chi Tang. If during the early stage of recovery from shang han disease, or when there is taxation relapse or newly contracted disease characterised by fever, the treatment is determined on the basis of the pulse sign: a floating pulse indicates an exterior pattern and sweat promotion is used; a submerged, excess pulse indicates interior pathogenic bind and purgation is used; in a Shao Yang pattern affecting the pivot mechanism, where it is neither exterior nor interior, Xiao Chai Hu Tang is used.
   (ii) Food stagnation during recovery: During the initial recovery phase, when

there is unresolved residual heat, hard-to-digest or heavy meals can result in food stagnation; heat will flare upward harassing the chest and diaphragm and manifest as abdominal fullness with fever and anguish. The formula is Zhi Shi Zhi Zi Chi Tang with the addition of Da Huang. Where food is not digested in the evening because the yang qi of the middle jiao is not supported by environmental yang, the treatment is to reduce food intake.

(iii) Stomach deficiency and cold: After a major illness, if there is deficiency cold in the middle, and the spleen's function of transformation and transportation is impaired, and the lung's function of descending and dispersing is also impaired, there will be excessive salivation and frequent spitting; the indicated formula is Li Zhong Wan to warm the cold.

(iv) Accumulation of damp-heat in the lower jiao: where water accumulates from the waist down, manifesting with inhibited urination and oedema, the formula is Mu Li Ze Xie San.

(v) In the initial recovery phase when the zheng qi is not fully restored, both qi and yin are deficient; there is residual pathogenic heat as well as deficiency and a desire to vomit. The formula is Zhu Ye Shi Gao Tang.

3. *Aftercare following illness.* Relapse of illness is mainly attributed to overexertion, premature resumption of physical work, recurrent contraction of exterior disease, improper diet causing indigestion, or immoderate sexual activity. Moderation in diet and physical activities is advised.

Appendix 1

Additional Clauses

Shang Han Lun has appeared in a number of editions. Many clauses are disputed as to their meaning, their clinical significance, and even as to whether they were part of the original text or have been added later by editors and annotators. For these various reasons, there are some clauses not included in the main body of the text, but which have been included here for the reader's interest and information.

Clause 75

未持脉时，病人手叉自冒心，师因教试令咳，而不咳者，此必两耳聋无闻也。所以然者，以重发汗，虚故如此。发汗后，饮水多必喘；以水灌之亦喘。

When the pulse has not yet been felt, if the person clasps their hands to their heart, and the master therefore instructs the person to try to cough, but he does not cough, this must be because both ears are deaf and do not hear. The reason for this being, because of repeated sweat promotion, there is this kind of deficiency. After the promotion of sweat, drinking a lot of water will cause panting; forcing the ingestion of water will also cause panting.

DISCUSSION Sweat is the fluid of the heart: excessive promotion of sweat damages the heart yin which fails to anchor yang, allowing it to escape, resulting in depletion of heart yang. The clasping of the hands to the chest is intended to indicate that the patient suffers from palpitations, with the pressure of the hands being an attempt to suppress the palpitations. The heart and kidney are linked via the Shao Yin. Because they are interactive, the deficiency of one can affect the other, and thus heart deficiency may lead to kidney deficiency. When the patient fails to respond to the physician's request to cough, it is because his hearing is impaired. This is because heart deficiency can lead to kidney deficiency, and because the kidneys open into the ears; deficiency of the heart has resulted in deafness. Thus the clause shows that repeated sweat promotion can damage not only the heart but also the kidneys. Apart from damaging the heart and kidney yang, incorrect sweat promotion can also damage the stomach fluids, causing dryness and thirst. If there is dry heat in the stomach, the ingestion of water will moisten the dryness; however, if there is no excess heat in the stomach, ingested water will accumulate and manifest as a water qi disorder. The stomach is located below the diaphragm and the upsurge of water qi will harass the lungs causing wheezing. This serves as a warning for patients recently recovered from shang han disease who were treated with repeated promotion of sweat: because of the damage to yang qi caused by the excessive sweating, it is best to avoid water by bathing, and also better to avoid exposure to drafts. This is because the skin pores and interstices are insecure and susceptible to the invasion of pathogenic wind or cold. Furthermore, a nourishing diet is required to replenish the spleen and stomach qi.

Clause 105

伤寒十三日，过经，谵语者，以有热也，当以汤下之。若小便利者，大便当硬，而反下利，脉调和者，知医以丸药下之，非其治也。若自下利者，脉当微厥。今反和者，此为内实也，调胃承气汤主之。

Shang han for thirteen days, if it has passed through the channel and there is delirious speech, it is because there is heat, one should purge with a decoction. If the urination is free, the stool should be hard, but there is diarrhoea, and the pulse is harmonious, one knows the physician used a herbal pill to purge, and this is not the treatment. If there is spontaneous diarrhoea, the pulse should be faint and there will be desertion cold. If now however there is harmony, this is interior excess, Tiao Wei Cheng Qi Tang governs.

DISCUSSION When shang han disease has lasted for some time, the pathogen then passes into the next channel, resulting in a pattern of Yang Ming intestinal heat bind, where the turbid heat surges upward and harasses the heart shen, manifesting as delirious speech. The Cheng Qi Tang group of formulas can be used to purge the heat bind. It would be expected that the urination would be uninhibited and the stool hard, but instead of the hard stool there is diarrhoea. If there is diarrhoea, considering that the disease has persisted for more than ten days, this is likely to be because it has transmitted to a yin channel, giving rise to a concurrent pattern of Tai Yang and Shao Yin, characterised by a faint and submerged pulse and cold extremities. Contrary to the expected, however, the pulse is harmonious and there are no cold extremities, and so it is not a pattern of exuberant yin. Further, when a purgative pill is given to purge the heat, it is too mild: the interior excess bind is not fully eliminated. The spontaneous diarrhoea which follows is not due to effective purging, but is the result of heat retained in the interior. Tiao Wei Cheng Qi Tang is the appropriate formula to purge the heat and harmonise the stomach. This is because of the three Cheng Qi Tang; Tiao Wei Cheng Qi Tang is the one with Gan Cao, which has the dual function of harmonising the stomach qi and moderating the harsh effects of Da Huang and Mang Xiao.

Clause 108

伤寒，腹满、谵语、寸口脉浮而紧，此肝乘脾也，名曰纵，刺期门。

Shang han, with abdominal fullness and delirious speech, the cun kou pulse is floating and tight, this is the liver overacting on the spleen, known as restraint, needle Qi Men.

DISCUSSION Abdominal fullness and delirious speech is generally associated with a Yang Ming bowel excess pattern, when the pulse is submerged and excess, but a pulse which is floating and tight in the cun position shows it is not a Yang Ming pattern. A tight or wiry pulse pertains to the interior and is a yin pulse, associated with the liver. A floating pulse is yang and represents pathogenic heat. The floating tight pulse is a reflection of liver heat harassing the heart, which manifests as delirious speech. The abdominal fullness is a result of liver excess impairing the function of the spleen which, in five phase theory, is referred to as the liver wood overacting on the spleen earth. The treatment strategy is to purge the liver heat by needling Qi Men (Liv 14) which is the front mu point (募穴), or collecting point, of the liver.

Clause 109

伤寒发热，啬啬恶寒，大渴欲饮水，其腹必满，自汗出；小便利，其病欲解。此肝乘肺也，名曰横，刺期门。

Shang han disease with fever, there is huddled aversion to cold and strong thirst with a desire to drink water, the abdomen will be full, and there is spontaneous sweating; the urination is free, the disease is about to resolve. This is the liver overacting on the lungs, it is called rebellion, needle Qi Men.

DISCUSSION Shang Han disease with fever and huddled aversion to cold is associated with a Tai Yang pattern; strong thirst and abdominal fullness are the result of the non-dispersion of fluids; the spontaneous sweating is the manifestation of an unresolved exterior pattern. It could be mistaken for a Tai Yang fu pattern with an unresolved exterior, but the abdominal fullness of a Tai Yang fu pattern is limited to the lesser abdomen. The pattern is actually one of 'wood insulting metal', where the liver overacts on the lungs, referred to in the clause as 'rebellion'. The assault on the lungs has affected their ability to rule the exterior, causing a disharmony of ying and wei; thus there is fever, aversion to cold and sweating. The lungs' function of dispersing fluids and regulating the water passages is also adversely affected, giving rise to thirst and abdominal fullness. Because the lungs regulate the waterways, if this function is impaired, there will be inhibited urination. Conversely, if the urination is free and uninhibited, then the lung qi is in harmony and recovery is imminent. Since the root of the disease is not in the lungs but in exuberant liver qi, the advice is to needle Qi Men (Liv 14), to drain the liver.

Clause 119

太阳伤寒者，加温针必惊也。

If there is Tai Yang shang han, and warm needling is used, there will be fright.

DISCUSSION The correct treatment for Tai Yang shang han is Ma Huang Tang. The use of warm needling to promote sweat results in excessive sweating which not only depletes yin fluids and ying blood, but also scatters the qi of the heart and gallbladder, resulting in palpitations, restlessness and fright, with a potential also to lead to ben tun and derangement. The warm needling mentioned here, is not the same as the warm needle techniques used by modern practitioners of Chinese medicine, but is believed to refer to 'hot needle' or 'fire needle', which had a much stronger effect, inducing sweat and giving rise to restlessness and fright. Fire therapy was prevalent during the Eastern Han period and was used to treat many illnesses, but is no longer in use today. Nevertheless, it is interesting to draw a parallel between the adverse effects of fire therapy and those of radiotherapy, which are associated with a burning sensation, consume yin and often cause haemorrhage.

Clause 192

阳明病，初欲食，小便反不利，大便自调，其人骨节疼，翕翕如有热状，奄然发狂，濈然汗出而解者，此水不胜谷气，与汗共并，脉紧则愈。

Yang Ming disease, initially there is a desire to eat, nevertheless the urination is not free, the stool is naturally regular, the person has joint pain, feather warmth as if there is a fever, if there is sudden derangement, streaming sweat and resolution, this is water unable to overcome the grain qi, combining with the sweat, a tight pulse means recovery.

DISCUSSION Yang Ming shang han is characterised by an inability to eat. Clause 192 describes a Yang Ming pattern with a desire to eat, demonstrating that yang has returned and there is no longer a pattern of deficiency cold in the middle jiao. If the yang return is excessive and the pathogen has transformed into dryness, the stool would be dry and hard, and the urination copious. Here, however, the urination is inhibited and the stool normal, thus demonstrating that the condition has not transformed into dryness, and the joint pain is a reflection of damp having accumulated in the interior. This pathogenic damp constrains the yang qi giving rise to a slight fever. If zheng qi is strong and the qi of the spleen and stomach is promoted, they are not affected by the damp, and so the damp is expelled together with the sweat. The invigoration of the yang qi makes the body warm, similar to fever, and the suddenness of its return can result in manic behaviour. However this, together with the sweating, is a result of the stimulated yang qi and thus heralds recovery. The implication of the tight pulse is that it is strong, as opposed to the moderate and forceless pulse of a Yang Ming shang han pattern.

Clause 198

阳明病，但头眩，不恶寒，故能食而咳，其人咽必痛。若不咳者，咽不痛。

Yang Ming disease, there is only dizziness, no aversion to cold, and the person is able to eat and coughs, and the person's throat should be sore. If there is no cough, there is no sore throat.

DISCUSSION Yang Ming disease with no aversion to cold, with fever, and the ability to eat is called zhong feng or wind strike, and represents a Yang Ming wind heat pattern. The pathogenic wind heat harasses the head causing dizziness; if it harasses the lung there is cough. The throat is the gateway of the lungs and stomach and so, when the wind heat assails the lungs, the throat is also affected. If there is no cough, then the lungs are not harassed by wind heat, and so, the throat is not sore.

Clause 201

阳明病，脉浮而紧者，必潮热，发作有时。但浮者，必盗汗出。

Yang Ming disease, if the pulse is floating and tight, there must be tidal fever, occurring periodically. If it is floating only, there will be night sweats.

DISCUSSION A floating pulse in Yang Ming disease indicates an unresolved channel pattern, whilst the tight pulse indicates interior excess. Hence there should be tidal fever occurring at regular intervals. Based on the pulse sign and the tidal fever, this is a Yang Ming channel pattern and a fu pattern occurring simultaneously. If the pulse is floating and not tight, and there is no tidal fever, then the pathogen is still at the channel level and has not transmitted to the fu. In Chinese medicine, sleeping is explained as yang entering yin, at which time the defence yang is deficient and the exterior is unsecured. If pathogenic heat exploits the deficiency, there will be night sweats.

Clause 218

伤寒四五日，脉沉而喘满，沉为在里，而反发其汗，津液越出，大便为难，表虚里实，久则谵语。

Shang han for four or five days, the pulse is submerged and there is panting and fullness, submerged means the disease is in the interior, however, sweating is promoted, body fluids vent outward, defaecation is difficult, the exterior is deficient and the interior is excess, if this endures, there will be delirious speech.

DISCUSSION Clause 218 describes shang han disease which after four or five days then presents with panting, fullness and a submerged pulse. From the pulse, it is seen to be an interior pattern; the fullness is a reflection of qi congestion in the interior, and the panting a result of that congestion obstructing the diffusion of lung qi. Sweat promotion is not the correct treatment, and the inappropriate loss of sweat has damaged the exterior, causing exterior deficiency, and has depleted fluids, resulting in a dry stool. It is this which is referred to in the clause as interior excess. If the condition persists the dryness can generate heat, which will harass the heart shen, giving rise to delirious speech. If there is an unresolved exterior pathogen, the correct strategy would be to promote sweating before purging. This is done to avoid the possibility of the unresolved pathogen falling inwards after purgation. However, if the exterior is fully resolved, and there is interior excess only, one should not attack the exterior as further fluid damage will exacerbate the interior excess.

Clause 225

脉浮而迟，表热里寒，下利清谷者，四逆汤主之。

When the pulse is floating and slow, there is heat in the exterior and cold in the interior, and diarrhoea with undigested food particles, Si Ni Tang governs.

DISCUSSION The loose stool with undigested food particles is generally associated with the debilitation of yang qi, where the kidney yang is insufficient and unable to support the function of transformation and transportation; kidney fire fails to warm the earth, and damp and cold sink and accumulate in the lower jiao. The floating pulse is a reflection of the exterior heat, which alludes to the fever of an exterior pattern; the slow pulse is a reflection of the interior cold, which relates to the diarrhoea. In accordance with Chinese medicine theory, where a patient exhibits interior deficiency and cold, the strategy is to tonify the yang, warm the interior and disperse the cold. The guiding formula is Si Ni Tang.

Clause 244

太阳病，寸缓关浮尺弱，其人发热汗出，复恶寒，不呕，但心下痞者，此以医下之也。如其不下者，病人不恶寒而渴者，此转属阳明也。小便数者，大便必硬，不更衣十日，无所苦也。渴欲饮水，少少与之，但以法救之。渴者，宜五苓散。

Tai Yang disease, if the cun is moderate, the guan is floating and cubit is weak, the person has fever and sweating, followed by aversion to cold, no retching, but glomus below the heart, this is because the physician used purgation. If no purgation was used, the patient has no aversion to cold and is thirsty, it has shifted to the Yang Ming. If urination is frequent, the stool will be hard, with no change of clothes for ten days, without any discomfort. There is thirst with a desire to drink water, give a little, only by this method will there be recovery. If there is thirst, Wu Ling San is appropriate.

DISCUSSION The moderate cun pulse is a reflection of exterior cold; the floating guan pulse relates to the pathogenic wind; the weak cubit pulse indicates interior deficiency. The pulse thus describes an exterior pattern of Tai yang zhong feng or Tai yang wind strike exterior pattern, as reflected further in the symptoms of fever and aversion to cold. The weak pulse indicates interior deficiency which may have pre-existed or may have been caused by the purgation. The absence of retching indicates that there has been no transmission to the Shao Yang. Purgation is contraindicated in an exterior pattern, and the physician's adverse treatment has damaged the stomach qi and given rise to glomus below the heart.

If there has been no purgation and the patient has fever and sweating with no aversion to cold, and is also thirsty, this means that no other appropriate treatment was given to release the exterior and resolve the pathogen, and it has subsequently transmitted to the Yang Ming. A Yang Ming pattern represents heat with fluid damage. Because the heat obstructs the proper distribution of fluids, with fluids being diverted to the urinary bladder, there is further loss of fluids due to frequent urination, the stool will be dry and there will be constipation. The phrase "no change of clothes" is a euphemistic expression for going to the lavatory to pass a stool. However, there is no discomfort: no tidal fever, no delirious speech, and no abdominal fullness. In this case, Ma Zi Ren Wan or Mi Jian Dao can be used to moisten the intestines. If, on the other hand, there is thirst, and a desire to drink, then this is not due to the non-distribution of fluids, but is due to heat having consumed fluids. Therefore, a small amount of water should be given to moisten the stomach. A larger amount is not given, because it could result in water accumulation. If the simple therapy of drinking a small amount of water is not effective, Bai Hu Tang or Bai Hu jia Ren Shen Tang can be considered. The third scenario is where the thirst is associated with the pathogen affecting qi transformation in the urinary bladder. In this case, fluids are not transformed and are retained in the urinary bladder, and so Wu Ling San is appropriate to promote urination in order to eliminate the water.

Although the clause nominates Wu Ling San, there are in fact various strategies available to the practitioner, depending on the presenting pattern and its manifestations. This clause thus serves as a reminder that disease does not always follow a set pathway and it is essential to adhere to the teaching: "observe the pulse and signs to determine what error was committed and treat accordingly".

Clause 348

发热而厥，七日下利者，为难治。

When there is fever and jue, with diarrhoea for seven days, this is difficult to treat.

DISCUSSION Symptoms of fever and jue, or cold extremities due to desertion of yang, are the manifestation of a true cold and false heat pattern, with exuberant interior yin and the up-casting of yang qi. Diarrhoea which has lasted for seven days reflects further deterioration, with devastation of yang and exuberance of yin. You Yi suggested that fever accompanied by jue, or cold extremities, is a reflection of a yang pattern following interior deficiency. If, after seven days, the zheng qi gradually returns and the pathogenic cold retreats, then there will be cold extremities followed by the abatement of fever; if the fever and cold extremities both persist, and there is also diarrhoea, then the zheng qi has not returned, and the diarrhoea is a mark of further deterioration.

One explanation for the phrase "this is difficult to treat" is that, because this is not purely a yin cold pattern, acrid sweet and warm herbs can not be used to warm and tonify the interior and treat the jue. Because of the jue and the diarrhoea, bitter cold herbs can not be used to treat the fever, as they would further damage yang qi. This paradox makes the pattern hard to treat (*Shang Han Guan Zhu Ji*). This clause follows on from Clause 346 articulating a pattern of fever and *jue* which is accompanied by diarrhoea and has persisted for seven days. Even though the patient may not die, it is nevertheless a disease which is difficult to treat (*Shang Han Lun Ji Zhu*).

Appendix 2

Outline of Clauses in the Sequence of the Zhao Edition

The original text, called *Shang Han Za Bing Lun, (Discourse on Cold Injury and Miscellaneous Disease)* was lost soon after it was written but not, fortunately, before another version was edited in the Western Jin period (265–316 AD) by Wang Shu He. He compiled the sections relating to externally contracted disease into a separate work, which is what has come down to us as the *Shang Han Lun*. Subsequently, in the Song dynasty (1127–1279 AD), the sections of *Shang Han Za Bing Lun* relating to other diseases of internal medicine, termed miscellaneous diseases, were reorganised to form the book now known as *Jin Gui Yao Lue* (*Essential Prescriptions of the Golden Cabinet*). There is no longer an extant text of the original Song dynasty edition in China, and today there are two editions of *Shang Han Lun* which are relied upon. The earlier of these is *Zhu Jie Shang Han Lun (Annotations to Shang Han Lun)* by Cheng Wu Ji from the Jin-Yuan period, which appeared in about 1144 AD and was the earliest annotated edition. The second version of *Shang Han Lun* used today has come to be referred to as the Song edition, simply because the original Song edition no longer exists. It is, in fact, the Zhao Kai Mei edition from the Ming dynasty (1368–1644).

Shang Han Lun is formatted as a series of clauses; the Zhao edition consists of ten fascicles, twenty-two chapters, and in excess of 800 clauses. Most *Shang Han Lun* texts provide ten chapters with a total of 398 clauses. Since *Shang Han Lun* was written some one-thousand eight-hundred years ago and has been subject to successive compilation and editing, the text which comes to us today may not be an exact replica of the original as written by Zhong Jing. Nevertheless, the readers should be aware that the intrinsic links between clauses remain. In keeping with the classical nature of that edition, the original clauses are reproduced here with traditional characters.

CLAUSES 1–178: TAI YANG CHAPTER

Clause 1

太陽之為病，脈浮，頭項強痛而惡寒。

Tai Yang is diseased, the pulse is floating, the head and neck are stiff and painful and there is aversion to cold.

NOTE: Principal features of Tai Yang disease.

Clause 2

太陽病，發熱汗出，惡風，脈緩者，名為中風。

Tai Yang disease, there is fever and sweating, aversion to wind, where the pulse is moderate, it is called wind strike.

Clause 3

太陽病，或已發熱，或未發熱，必惡寒，體痛，嘔逆，脈陰陽俱緊者，名為傷寒。

Tai Yang disease, whether there is fever, or there is no fever, there must be aversion to cold, body ache, vomiting, where the yin and yang of the pulse are both tight, it is called shang han.

NOTE: Pattern differentiation between Tai Yang zhong feng (wind strike) and Tai Yang shang han (cold injury) based on the pulse.

Clause 4

傷寒一日，太陽受之，脈若靜者，為不傳；頗欲吐，若躁煩，脈數急者，為傳也。

Shang han for one day, Tai Yang is affected, where the pulse is calm, it means no transmission; there is an urge to vomit, if there is agitation and vexation, where the pulse is rapid and urgent, there is transmission.

Clause 5

傷寒二三日，陽明、少陽證不見者，為不傳也。

Shang han for two or three days, there is no sign of a Yang Ming or Shao Yang pattern, there is no transmission.

NOTE: Differentiation between transmission and non-transmission of Tai Yang disease.

Clause 6

太陽病，發熱而渴，不惡寒者，為溫病。若發汗已，身灼熱者，名風溫。風溫為病，脈陰陽俱浮，自汗出，身重，多眠睡，鼻息必鼾，語言難出。若被下者，小便不利，直視失溲；若被火者，微發黃色，劇則如驚癇，時瘛瘲，若火熏之；一逆尚引日，再逆促命期。

Tai Yang disease, if there is fever and thirst, with no aversion to cold, it is wen bing. If sweat has already been promoted, with the body scorching hot, it is called feng wen. In feng wen, the yin and yang pulses are both floating, there is spontaneous sweating, the body is heavy, there is somnolence, stertorous breathing, difficulty speaking. If there was purging, the urination will not be free, there will be a fixed gaze and loss of continence; if there was fire therapy, there will be slight yellowing, if severe there will be convulsions, periodic spasmodic jerking, as if fumed by fire; one adverse treatment will prolong it, further adverse treatment will hasten the expiry of life.

NOTE: A comparison of wen bing and feng wen (warm disease and wind warmth) and contraindications in a pattern of wind cold.

Clause 7

病有發熱惡寒者，發于陽也；無熱惡寒者，發于陰也。發于陽，七日愈。發于陰，六日愈。以陽數七、陰數六也。

If the disease has fever and aversion to cold, it stems from yang; if there is no fever and aversion to cold, it stems from yin. That which stems from yang, recovery is in seven days. That which stems from yin, recovery is in six days. This is because yang numbers seven and yin numbers six.

NOTE: The difference between disease according to whether it stems from yin or yang, based on symptoms at onset.

Clause 8

太陽病，頭痛至七日以上自愈者，以行其經盡故也。若欲作再經者，針足陽明，使經不傳則愈。

Tai Yang disease, where there is headache for over seven days with spontaneous recovery, it is because the pathogen has passed through the channels. If it is about to transmit to another channel, needling foot Yang Ming will cause it not to transmit and there will be recovery.

NOTE: After seven days of Tai Yang disease there may be spontaneous recovery. This should be cross-referenced to Clauses 4 and 5 describing the possible transmission of Tai Yang disease irrespective of the number of days it has endured.

Clause 9

太陽病欲解時，從巳至未上。

The time that Tai Yang disease is ready to resolve, is from si to wei.

Clause 10

風家，表解而不了了者，十二日愈。

Patients suffering from wind, where the exterior is resolved but not thoroughly, will recover in twelve days.

NOTE: Clauses 9 and 10 discuss recovery from Tai Yang disease in terms of cosmic influence.

Clause 11

病人身大熱，反欲得衣者，熱在皮膚，寒在骨髓也；身大寒，反不欲近衣者，寒在皮膚，熱在骨髓也。

Where the patient's body has great heat, nevertheless he wants more clothing, the heat is in the skin, the cold is in the bone marrow; where the body has great cold, nevertheless he does not want more clothing, the cold is in the skin, the heat is in the bone marrow.

NOTE: Differentiation of true or false heat and cold.

Clause 12

太陽病中風，陽浮而陰弱，陽浮者，熱自發，陰弱者，汗自出。嗇嗇惡寒，淅淅惡風，翕翕發熱，鼻鳴干嘔者，桂枝湯主之。

Tai Yang zhong feng, yang is floating and yin is weak, where yang is floating, there is spontaneous fever, where yin is weak, there is spontaneous sweating. Huddled aversion to cold, wetted aversion to wind, feather-warm fever, with a snuffly nose and dry retching, Gui Zhi Tang governs.

Clause 13

太陽病，頭痛，發熱，汗出，惡風，桂枝湯主之。

Tai Yang disease, the head aches, there is fever, sweating, aversion to wind, Gui Zhi Tang governs.

NOTE: Additional symptoms of Gui Zhi Tang.

Clause 14

太陽病，項背強幾幾，反汗出惡風者，桂枝加葛根湯主之。

Tai Yang disease, the neck and back are stiff and taut, however where there is sweating and aversion to wind, Gui Zhi jia Ge Gen Tang governs.

NOTE: Description of a Gui Zhi Tang pattern with additional symptoms, and the appropriate modification.

Clause 15

太陽病，下之後，其氣上沖者，可與桂枝湯，方用前法。若不上沖者，不得與之。

Tai Yang disease, after purgation, where the qi surges upward, one can give Gui Zhi Tang, in accordance with the earlier method. If there is no upsurge, it must not be given.

Clause 16A

太陽病三日，已發汗，若吐、若下、若溫針，仍不解者，此為壞病，桂枝不中與之也。觀其脈證，知犯何逆，隨證治之。

Tai Yang disease for three days, sweating has already been promoted, if there is vomiting, if there is purging, if there is warm needling, and there is still no resolution, this is transmuted disease, Gui Zhi is not appropriate. Observe the pulse and signs, know the error committed, treat according to the pattern.

Clause 16B

桂枝本為解肌，若其人脈浮緊，發熱汗不出者，不可與之也。常須識此勿令誤也。

Gui Zhi Tang is basically to resolve the muscle layer, if the patient's pulse is floating and tight, where there is fever and no sweat, it can not be given. One must bear this in mind to avoid making a mistake.

Clause 17

若酒客病，不可與桂枝湯，得之則嘔，以酒客不喜甘故也。

If there is drinker's disease, one should not give Gui Zhi Tang, doing so will cause vomiting, this is because drinkers do not tolerate sweetness.

Clause 18

喘家作桂枝汤，加厚朴，杏子佳。

Wheezing patients presenting with Gui Zhi Tang, adding Hou Po and Xing Ren is good.

NOTE: Description of a Gui Zhi Tang pattern with additional symptoms and the appropriate modification.

Clause 19

凡服桂枝湯吐者，其後必吐膿血也。

Whenever Gui Zhi Tang is taken there is vomiting, following which there is vomiting of pus and blood.

NOTE: Contraindications for the use of Gui Zhi Tang.

Clause 20

太陽病，發汗，遂漏不止，其人惡風，小便難，四肢微急，難以屈伸者，桂枝加附子湯主之。

Tai Yang disease, sweating is promoted, followed by incessant leaking, the person is averse to wind, has difficult urination, where the four limbs are slightly tense, there is difficulty bending and stretching, Gui Zhi jia Fu Zi Tang governs.

Clause 21

太陽病，下之後，脈促，胸滿者，桂枝去芍藥湯主之。

Tai Yang disease, after purgation, the pulse is hasty, where there is fullness in the chest, Gui Zhi qu Shao Yao Tang governs.

Clause 22

若微寒者，桂枝去芍藥加附子湯主之。

If there is slight cold, Gui Zhi qu Shao Yao jia Fu Zi Tang governs.

Clause 23

太陽病，得之八九日，如虐狀，發熱惡寒，熱多寒少，其人不嘔，清便欲自可，一日二三度發。脈微緩者，為欲愈也；而脈微而惡寒者，此陰陽俱虛，不可更發汗、更下、更吐也；面色反有熱色者，未欲解也，以其不能得小汗出，身必癢，宜桂枝麻黃各半湯。

Tai Yang disease, for eight or nine days, malaria-like symptoms, fever and aversion to cold, more fever less cold, the person does not vomit, urine and stool are normal, occurring two or three times in a day. Where the pulse is slightly moderate, this is imminent recovery; and where the pulse is faint with aversion to cold, this is deficiency of both yin and yang, one should not further promote sweating, nor purging, nor vomiting; and where the complexion is a hot colour, there is no imminent recovery, this is because the patient cannot raise a mild sweat, the body will itch, Gui Zhi Ma Huang Ge Ban Tang is appropriate.

Clause 24

太陽病，初服桂枝湯，反煩不解者，先刺風池、風府，卻與桂枝湯則愈。

Tai Yang disease, initially having administered Gui Zhi Tang, but there is vexation with no resolution, first needle Feng Chi and Feng Fu, then give Gui Zhi Tang and there will be recovery.

Clause 25

服桂枝湯，大汗出，脈洪大者，與桂枝湯，如前法。若形似虐，一日再發者，汗出必解，宜桂枝二麻黃一湯。

Having taken Gui Zhi Tang, there is copious sweat, if the pulse is flooding and big, give Gui Zhi Tang as before. If the disease resembles malaria, occurring again during the day, sweating will resolve it, Gui Zhi Er Ma Huang Yi Tang is appropriate.

Clause 26

服桂枝湯，大汗出後，大煩渴不解，脈洪大者，白虎加人參湯主之。

Having taken Gui Zhi Tang, after profuse sweating, there is severe vexation and unresolved thirst, if the pulse is flooding and big, Bai Hu jia Ren Shen Tang governs.

Clause 27

太陽病，發熱惡寒，熱多寒少，脈微弱者，此無陽也，不可發汗，宜桂枝二越婢一湯。

Tai Yang disease, there is fever and aversion to cold, there is more fever and less cold, where the pulse is faint and weak, this is an absence of yang, one should not promote sweat, Gui Zhi Er Yue Bi Yi Tang is appropriate.

Clause 28

服桂枝湯，或下者，仍頭項強痛，翕翕發熱，無汗，心下滿微痛，小便不利者，桂枝去桂加茯苓白術湯主之。

Having administered Gui Zhi Tang, or if there was purgation, the head and neck are still stiff and painful, feather-warm fever, absence of sweating, fullness and slight pain below the heart, where the urination is not free, then Gui Zhi qu Gui jia Fu Ling Bai Zhu Tang governs.

NOTE: Clauses 20–28 should be read in conjunction with Clause 16, which outlines the treatment principle for huai bing (transmuted disease), i.e. observe the symptoms and signs and treat accordingly. Clause 28 describes the treatment for Tai Yang inhibited channel qi: Gui Zhi Tang is used to resolve a Tai Yang exterior pattern by promoting sweat; however, Gui Zhi qu Gui jia Fu Ling Bai Zhu Tang is used to promote urination. This illustrates the difference between the treatment strategies of Tai Yang channel and fu patterns.

Clause 29

傷寒脈浮，自汗出，小便數，心煩，微惡寒、腳攣急，反與桂枝欲攻其表，此誤也。得之便厥、咽中干、煩躁吐逆者，作甘草干姜湯與之，以復其陽。若厥愈足溫者，更作芍藥甘草湯與之，其腳即伸。若胃氣不和，譫語者，少與調胃承氣湯。若重發汗，復加燒針者，四逆湯主之。

Shang han the pulse is floating, there is spontaneous sweating, frequent urination, there will be heart vexation, a slight aversion to cold, and cramps in the feet, but Gui Zhi Tang is given to attack the exterior, this is a mistake. Having given it, there is jue, the throat is dry, and if there is vexation and agitation with vomiting due to reversal, administer Gan Cao Gan Jiang Tang to restore the yang. If the jue recovers and the feet become warm, then after administering Shao Yao Gan Cao Tang, the feet will then stretch. Where the stomach qi is disharmonious, if the speech is delirious, give a little Tiao Wei Cheng Qi Tang. Where heavy sweating was promoted, if then there is repeated hot needling, Si Ni Tang governs.

Clause 30

問曰：證象陽旦，按法治之而增劇，厥逆，咽中干，兩脛拘急而譫語。師曰：言夜半手足當溫，兩腳當伸，後如師言。何以知此？答曰：寸口脈浮而大，浮為風，大為虛，風則生微熱，虛則兩脛攣，病形象桂枝，因加附子參其間；增桂令汗出，附子溫經，亡陽故也。厥逆，咽中干，煩躁，陽明內結，譫語煩亂；更飲甘草干姜湯。夜半陽氣還，兩足當熱，脛尚微拘急，重與芍藥甘草湯，爾乃脛伸。以承氣湯微溏，則止其譫語，故知病可愈。

Question: A pattern similar to Yang Dan, treated according to the rule, but it is more severe, there is desertion reversal, dryness in the throat, arresting spasm in both calves and delirious speech. The master said: Now, in the middle of the night the hands and feet will be warm, both feet will stretch, and later it was as the master said. How did he know? (2) Answer: The cun pulse is floating and big, floating indicates wind, big indicates deficiency, the wind generates a mild fever, the deficiency causes cramps in both calves. The disease resembles Gui Zhi, so Fu Zi should be added in; increasing Gui causes sweating, but Fu Zi warms the channels, this is because there is devastation of yang. Where there is desertion reversal, a dry throat, vexation and agitation, there is Yang Ming interior bind, delirious speech and derangement; it is better to drink Gan Cao Gan Jiang Tang. In the middle of the night, yang qi returns, the two feet must be warm, if the legs have mild cramps, give a large dose of Shao Yao Gan Cao Tang, then the legs will stretch. Because of Cheng Qi Tang there is slight sloppiness, then the delirious speech will stop, so we know the disease is recovering.

NOTE: The understanding of this clause is linked to Clause 16's admonition to "observe the symptoms and signs and treat accordingly". Clause 30 describes the outcome of an incorrect treatment using Gui Zhi Tang, the subsequent correct treatment of the adverse outcomes, and the need to differentiate correct treatment as either warming yang, resuscitating devastated yang, augmenting yin, or purging heat. It is essential to understand the original error and address the condition based on the symptoms and pulse sign.

Clause 31

太陽病，項背強幾幾，無汗惡風，葛根湯主之。

Tai Yang disease, the neck and back are stiff and taut, absence of sweat and aversion to wind, Ge Gen Tang governs.

Clause 32

太陽與陽明合病者，必自下利，葛根湯主之。

If there is Tai Yang and Yang Ming concurrent disease, there will be diarrhoea, Ge Gen Tang governs.

Clause 33

太陽與陽明合病，不下利，但嘔者，葛根加半夏湯主之。

Tai Yang and Yang Ming concurrent disease, there is no diarrhoea, there is just vomiting, Ge Gen jia Ban Xia Tang governs.

Clause 34

太陽病，桂枝證，醫反下之，利遂不止，脈促者，表未解也；喘而汗出者，葛根黄芩黄連湯主之。

Tai Yang disease, Gui Zhi Tang pattern, but the physician has purged, there is incessant diarrhoea, if the pulse is skipping, the exterior is unresolved; if there is wheezing and sweating, Ge Gen Qin Lian Tang governs.

NOTE: Differentiation between Ge Gen Tang and one of its modifications.

Clause 35

太陽病，頭痛發熱，身疼腰痛，骨節疼痛，惡風,無汗而喘者，麻黃湯主之。

Tai Yang disease, there is headache, fever, body pain and back ache, the joints are aching and painful, where there is aversion to wind, no sweat and wheezing, Ma Huang Tang governs.

Clause 36

太陽與陽明合病，喘而胸滿者，不可下，宜麻黃湯。

Tai Yang and Yang Ming concurrent disease, if there is wheezing and fullness in the chest, one should not purge, Ma Huang Tang is appropriate.

Clause 37

太陽病，十日已去，脈浮細而嗜臥者，外已解也。設胸滿脅痛者，與小柴胡湯；脈但浮者，與麻黃湯。

Tai Yang disease, ten days have passed, where the pulse is floating and fine and the patient is sleepy, the exterior pattern has resolved. In the event of chest fullness and pain in the hypochondrium, give Xiao Chai Hu Tang; where there is only a floating pulse, give Ma Huang Tang.

NOTE: Clauses 35, 36 and 37 describe additional symptoms of Tai Yang shang han in order to differentiate between the symptoms and signs, pathogenesis and treatment of Tai Yang shang han and those of Tai Yang zhong feng, thus expanding the scope of Ma Huang Tang.

Clause 38

太陽中風，脈浮緊，發熱惡寒，身疼痛，不汗出而煩躁者，大青龍湯主之。若脈微弱，汗出惡風者，不可服者。服者則厥逆，筋惕肉瞤，此為逆也。

Tai Yang zhong feng, the pulse is floating and tight, there is fever and aversion to cold, body aches and pains, with no sweat but with vexation, Da Qing Long Tang governs. If the pulse is faint and weak, where there is sweating and aversion to wind, one should not take medication. Medication will cause desertion reversal, the muscles will jerk and the flesh will twitch, it is an adverse treatment.

Clause 39

傷寒脈浮緩，身不疼，但重，乍有輕時，無少陰證者，大青龍湯發之。

Shang han with a pulse which is floating and moderate, the body does not ache, there is only heaviness, from time to time there is a sense of relief, in the absence of a Shao Yin pattern, Da Qing Long Tang promotes.

Clause 40

傷寒表不解，心下有水氣，干嘔發熱而咳，或渴，或利，或噎，或小便不利，少腹滿，或喘者，小青龍湯主之。

Shang han with an unresolved exterior, water qi below the heart, dry retching, fever and cough, or thirst, or diarrhoea, or dysphagia, or the urination is not free, lesser abdominal distension, or wheezing, Xiao Qing Long Tang governs.

Clause 41

傷寒心下有水氣，咳而微喘，發熱不渴；服湯已，渴者，此寒去、欲解也；小青龍湯主之。

Shang han, there is water qi below the heart, cough and a slight wheeze, fever without thirst; having taken the decoction, if there is thirst, the cold is going and is about to resolve; Xiao Qing Long Tang governs.

NOTE: Clauses 38, 39, 40 and 41 describe Tai Yang shang han patterns which are accompanied by additional symptoms: Da Qing Long Tang is indicated for exterior cold with interior heat; Xiao Qing Long Tang is indicated for exterior cold with retention of phlegm fluids in the interior.

Clause 42

太陽病，外證未解，脈浮弱者，當以汗解，宜桂枝湯。

Tai Yang disease, where the exterior pattern is unresolved, with the pulse floating and weak, it must be resolved by sweating, Gui Zhi Tang is appropriate.

Clause 43

太陽病，下之微喘者，表未解故也，桂枝加厚樸杏子湯主之。

Tai Yang disease, where there is mild wheezing after purgation, then the exterior is not resolved, Gui Zhi jia Hou Po Xing Zi Tang governs.

Clause 44

太陽病，外證未解，不可下也，下之為逆，欲解外者，宜桂枝湯。

Tai Yang disease, the exterior pattern is unresolved, one should not purge, purging would be adverse, if you wish to resolve the exterior, Gui Zhi Tang is appropriate.

Clause 45

太陽病，先發汗不解，而復下者，脈浮者不愈。浮為在外，而反下者，故令不愈，今脈浮，故在外，當須解外則愈，宜桂枝湯。

Tai Yang disease, initial sweating does not resolve, and where there is then purgation, the pulse will be floating and there is no recovery. Floating means it is in the exterior, but contrarily, there was purgation, so it does not bring recovery, currently the pulse is floating, then it is in the exterior, one must resolve the exterior then there will be recovery, Gui Zhi Tang is appropriate.

NOTE: Clauses 42, 43, 44 and 45 describe the use of Gui Zhi Tang following sweat promotion with Ma Huang Tang.

Clause 46

太陽病，脈浮緊，無汗發熱，身疼痛，八九日不解，表證仍在，此當發其汗。服藥已，微除，其人發煩目瞑，劇者必衄，衄乃解。所以然者，陽氣重故也。麻黃湯主之。

Tai Yang disease, the pulse is floating and tight, no sweat, fever, body aches and pains, unresolved after eight or nine days, the exterior pattern is still present, then one should promote sweat. After having taken the herbs, there is slight relief, the patient is vexed and the eyes closed, if it is serious, there will be spontaneous bleeding, only through bleeding is there resolution. The reason for this being, the yang qi is heavy. Ma Huang Tang governs.

Clause 47

太陽病，脈浮緊，發熱，身無汗，自衄者愈。

Tai Yang disease, the pulse is floating and tight, fever, there is no sweating, spontaneous nose bleed will bring recovery.

NOTE: Tai Yang shang han (cold injury) can be resolved by nosebleed.

Clause 48

二陽并病，太陽初得病時，發其汗，汗先出不徹，因轉屬陽明，續自微汗出，不惡寒。若太陽病證不罷者，不可下，下之為逆，如此可小發汗。設面色緣緣正赤者，陽氣怫郁在表，當解之、熏之。若發汗不徹，不足言，陽氣怫郁不得越，當汗不汗，其人躁煩，不知痛處，乍在腹中，乍在四肢，按之不可得，其人短氣但坐，以汗出不徹故也，更發汗則愈。何以知汗出不徹？以脈濇故知也。

Lagover disease of the two yang, when Tai Yang first contracts disease, sweating is promoted, the sweating at first is incomplete, so it will transmit to Yang Ming, there will be continued slight spontaneous sweating, with no aversion to cold. If the Tai Yang disease pattern is not finished, one should not purge, purging is adverse, in this case one may mildly promote sweat. If the facial complexion is constantly really crimson, then yang qi is gloweringly constrained in the exterior, one should resolve it, by fuming. If the promotion of sweat is not complete, then needless to say, the yang qi is gloweringly constrained and unable to escape; when there should be sweat there is none, the person is agitated and vexed, and does not know the location of the pain, whether it is in the abdomen, or in the four limbs, palpation can not find it, the person is short of breath and can only sit, it is because the promotion of sweat was incomplete, further sweat promotion will result in recovery. How can one know if there is incomplete promotion of sweat? It is because the pulse is choppy.

NOTE: Aetiology of a concurrent pattern of Tai Yang and Yang Ming and its treatment. Description of how the inappropriate treatment of Tai Yang disease may cause transmission to Yang Ming.

Clause 49

脈浮數者，法當汗出而愈。若下之，身重心悸者，不可發汗，當自汗出乃解。所以然者，尺中脈微，此里虛，須表里實，津液自和，便自汗出愈。

Where the pulse is floating and rapid, there should be sweating with recovery. If there is purgation, with heaviness in the body and palpitations; one should not promote sweat, there will be spontaneous sweating then resolution.

The reason for this being, the cubit pulse is faint, this is interior deficiency, the exterior and the interior must be replete, the body fluids harmonise spontaneously, so that spontaneous sweating will bring about recovery.

Clause 50

脈浮緊者，法當身疼痛，宜以汗解之。假令尺中遲者，不可發汗。何以知然？以榮氣不足，血少故也。

Where the pulse is floating and tight, there should be body aches and pains, it is appropriate to promote sweat for resolution. Should the cubit pulse now be slow, one should not promote sweat. How do we know the reason? It is because the nutrient qi is insufficient, blood is scarce.

Clause 51

脈浮者，病在表，可發汗，宜麻黃湯。

Where the pulse is floating, the disease is in the exterior, one may promote sweat, Ma Huang Tang is appropriate.

Clause 52

脈浮而數者，可發汗，宜麻黃湯。

Where the pulse is floating and rapid, one may promote sweat, Ma Huang Tang is appropriate.

NOTE: Clauses 49, 50, 51 and 52 discuss the pulse sign and the appropriate use of Ma Huang Tang. Clauses 49 and 50 describe a pulse that is floating or floating and tight, where Ma Huang Tang can be used; however, if the chi pulse is slow or faint, Ma Huang Tang is contraindicated. Clauses 51 and 52 describe a pulse that is either floating, or floating and rapid, where Ma Huang Tang can be used to promote sweating. It is essential to choose the formula according to the indicated symptoms and not rely on the pulse sign alone.

Clause 53

病常自汗出者，此為榮氣和，榮氣和者，外不諧，以衛氣不共榮氣諧和故爾。以榮行脈中，衛行脈外，復發其汗，榮衛和則愈，宜桂枝湯。

Where the disease has constant spontaneous sweat, this means that nutrient qi is harmonious, when the nutrient qi is harmonious, the exterior is in discord, because the defence qi is not in concord with the nutrient qi. Because nutrient qi moves within the vessels, defence qi moves outside the vessels, further promotion of sweating, the nutrient and defence will harmonise then there will be recovery, Gui Zhi Tang is appropriate.

Clause 54

病人藏無他病，時發熱自汗出而不愈者，此衛氣不和也，先其時發汗則愈，宜桂枝湯。

The patient's zang have no disease, where there is occasional fever and spontaneous sweating but without recovery, it means defence qi is disharmonious, promoting sweat in advance will bring recovery, Gui Zhi Tang is appropriate.

NOTE: Gui Zhi Tang can be used to treat spontaneous sweating if the pathogenesis is attributed to disharmony of ying and wei.

Clause 55

傷寒脈浮緊，不發汗，因致衄者，麻黃湯主之。

Shang han, the pulse is floating and tight, sweat is not promoted, resulting in nose bleed, Ma Huang Tang governs.

Clause 56

傷寒不大便六七日，頭痛有熱者，與承氣湯。其小便清者，知不在里，仍在表也，當須發汗；若頭痛者，必衄，宜桂枝湯。

Shang han with no stool for six or seven days, where there is headache and fever, give Cheng Qi Tang. When the urine is clear, we know it is not in the interior, it is still in the exterior, one must promote sweating; if there is headache, there will be nose bleed, Gui Zhi Tang is appropriate.

Clause 57

傷寒發汗已解，半日許復煩，脈浮數者，可更發汗，宜桂枝湯。

Shang han already resolved by sweating, after about half a day, there is again vexation, where the pulse is floating and rapid, one may promote sweat, Gui Zhi Tang is appropriate.

NOTE: Clauses 55, 56 and 57 discuss the different development of Tai Yang shang han diseases; Clause 56 is a sequel to Clause 55, describing shang han disease where there is a constrained pathogen and a potential for nose bleed. The conclusion that can be drawn from these clauses is that the scope of Gui Zhi Tang is far greater than that of Ma Huang Tang, as Gui Zhi Tang is not only indicated for Tai Yang zhong feng (wind strike) but is also suitable for a range of Tai Yang disorders.

Clause 58

凡病，若發汗、若吐、若下、若亡血、亡津液，陰陽自和者，必自愈。

In all illness, where sweating is promoted, where there is vomiting, where there is purging, where there is devastation of blood or devastation of fluid, if yin and yang harmonise spontaneously, there will be spontaneous recovery.

NOTE: This clause should be read in conjunction with Clauses 7 and 16, which explain that the harmonisation of yin and yang is the foundation of recovery, and therefore the fundamental principle of treatment. This is a guiding principle in the treatment of huai bing (transmuted disease) resulting from incorrect treatment.

Clause 59

大下之後，復發汗，小便不利者，亡津液故也。勿治之，得小便利，必自愈。

After potent purging, sweating is then promoted, where the urination is not free, it is because body fluids are devastated. Do not treat, once the urination is free, there will be spontaneous recovery.

Clause 60

下之後，復發汗，必振寒，脈微細。所以然者，以內外俱虛故也。

After purgation, sweat is again promoted, there will be shivering cold, the pulse is faint and thready. The reason for this being, the interior and exterior are both deficient.

Clause 61

下之後，復發汗，晝日煩躁不得眠，夜而安靜，不嘔不渴，無表證，脈沉微，身無大熱者，干姜附子湯主之。

After purging, sweating is again promoted, in the daytime the patient is vexed, agitated and unable to sleep, in the night-time, however, quiet and peaceful, there is no vomiting and no thirst, an absence of exterior symptoms, a pulse which is submerged and faint, if no vigorous fever, Gan Jiang Fu Zi Tang governs.

NOTE: Clauses 59, 60 and 61 describe the potential for transmutation of disease as a consequence of initial incorrect purgation followed by sweat promotion, with particular emphasis on the significance of the pulse sign.

Clause 62

發汗後，身疼痛，脈沉遲者，桂枝加芍藥生姜各一兩人參三兩新加湯主之。

After promoting sweat, there is aching and pain in the body, where the pulse is submerged and slow, Gui Zhi jia Shao Yao Sheng Jiang Ge Yi Liang Ren Shen San Liang Xin jia Tang governs.

Clause 63

發汗後，不可更行桂枝湯，汗出而喘，無大熱者，可與麻黃杏仁甘草石膏湯。

After the promotion of sweat, one should not repeat Gui Zhi Tang, if there is sweating and wheezing, no severe fever, one may give Ma Huang Xing Ren Gan Cao Shi Gao Tang.

Clause 64

發汗過多，其人叉手自冒心，心下悸，欲得按者，桂枝甘草湯主之。

After promoting sweat excessively, if the person clasps their hands to their heart, there are palpitations below the heart, a desire for pressure, Gui Zhi Gan Cao Tang governs.

Clause 65

發汗後，其人臍下悸者，欲作奔豚，茯苓桂枝甘草大棗湯主之。

After the promotion of sweat, the person feels palpitations below the umbilicus, this is about to manifest as ben tun, Fu Ling Gui Zhi Gan Cao Da Zao Tang governs.

Clause 66

發汗後，腹脹者，厚樸生姜甘草人參湯主之。

After promoting sweat, the abdomen is distended, Hou Po Sheng Jiang Ban Xia Gan Cao Ren Shen Tang governs.

Clause 67

傷寒若吐、若下後，心下逆滿，氣上沖胸，起則頭眩，脈沉緊，發汗則動經，身為振振搖者，茯苓桂枝白術甘草湯主之。

If there is vomiting in shang han, and if after purging there is fullness below the heart due to reversal, an upsurge of qi to the chest, on standing there is dizziness, the pulse is submerged and tight, and if the promotion of sweat causes stirring in the channels, with the body quivering and trembling, Fu Ling Gui Zhi Bai Zhu Gan Cao Tang governs.

Clause 68

發汗，病不解，反惡寒者，虛故也，芍藥甘草附子湯主之。

After promoting sweat, if the disease is not resolved, instead there is aversion to cold, it is due to deficiency, Shao Yao Gan Cao Fu Zi Tang governs.

Clause 69

發汗，若下之，病仍不解，煩躁者，茯苓四逆湯主之。

Having promoted sweat, where there was purging, if the disease is still not resolved, and there is vexation, Fu Ling Si Ni Tang governs.

Clause 70

發汗後，惡寒者，虛故也；不惡寒，但熱者，實也，當和胃氣，與調胃承氣湯。

Following the promotion of sweat, if there is aversion to cold, it is due to deficiency; if there is no aversion to cold but there is heat, it is due to excess, one must harmonise the stomach qi, give Tiao Wei Cheng Qi Tang.

NOTE: Sweat promotion is the indicated treatment for Tai Yang disease, but if it is inappropriate or inadequate, it still constitutes incorrect treatment. Clauses 62–70 describe transmutation due to incorrect sweat promotion.

Clause 71

太陽病，發汗後，大汗出，胃中干，煩躁不得眠，欲得飲水者，少少與飲之，令胃氣和則愈。若脈浮，小便不利，微熱消渴者，五苓散主之。

Tai Yang disease, after the promotion of sweat, there is profuse sweating, the stomach is dry, there is vexation and an inability to sleep, if there is a desire to drink, give a small amount of water, it will cause the stomach qi to harmonise then there will be recovery. If the pulse is floating, the urination is not free, with a slight fever and insatiable thirst, Wu Ling San governs.

Clause 72

發汗已，脈浮數，煩渴者，五苓散主之。

Having promoted sweat, the pulse is floating and rapid, with vexation and thirst, Wu Ling San governs.

Clause 73

傷寒汗出而渴者，五苓散主之；不渴者，茯苓甘草湯主之。

Shang han with sweating and thirst, Wu Ling San governs; with no thirst, Fu Ling Gan Cao Tang governs.

Clause 74

中風發熱，六七日不解而煩，有表里證，渴欲飲水，水入則吐者，名曰水逆，五苓散主之。

Zhong feng with fever, for six or seven days is unresolved and there is vexation, there are exterior and interior patterns, thirst with a desire to drink, if drinking causes vomiting, it is called water reversal, Wu Ling San governs.

NOTE: Clauses 71–74 describe an unresolved exterior pattern which has resulted in water amassment in the lower jiao and inhibited urination. Inhibited urination can be attributed to depletion of fluid or to non-transformation of qi and the pathology and treatment differ.

Clause 75

未持脈時，病人手叉自冒心，師因教試令咳，而不咳者，此必兩耳聾無聞也。所以然者，以重發汗，虛故如此。發汗后，飲水多必喘；以水灌之亦喘。

When the pulse has not yet been felt, if the person clasps their hands to their heart, and the master therefore instructs the person to try to cough, but he does not cough, this must be because both ears are deaf and do not hear. The reason for this being, because of repeated sweat promotion, there is this kind of deficiency. After the promotion of sweat, drinking a lot of water will cause panting; forcing the ingestion of water will also cause panting.

NOTE: This clause describes a transmuted pattern following repeated sweat promotion. The pathology is similar to that of the pattern described in Clause 64 but differs in the degree of severity.

Clause 76

發汗吐下後，虛煩不得眠，若劇者，必反覆顛倒，心中懊憹，梔子豉湯主之；若少氣者，梔子甘草豉湯主之；若嘔者，梔子生姜豉湯主之。

After sweating, vomiting or purging, there is insubstantial vexation and an inability to sleep, if it is severe, there will be tossing and turning, anguish in the heart, Zhi Zi Chi Tang governs; if there is shortness of breath, Zhi Zi Gan Cao Chi Tang governs; if there is retching, Zhi Zi Sheng Jiang Chi Tang governs.

Clause 77

發汗，若下者，而煩熱，胸中窒者，梔子豉湯主之。

After sweating, if there is purging, and vexation and fever, a stifled sensation in the chest, Zhi Zi Chi Tang governs.

Clause 78

傷寒五六日，大下之後，身熱不去，心中結痛者，未欲解也，梔子豉湯主之。

Shang han for five or six days, after potent purging, the fever does not abate, if there is a knotted pain in the heart, there is no imminent resolution, Zhi Zi Chi Tang governs.

Clause 79

傷寒下後，心煩腹滿，臥起不安者，梔子厚樸湯主之。

Shang han after purging, there is heart vexation and abdominal fullness, restlessness lying and sitting, Zhi Zi Hou Po Tang governs.

Clause 80

傷寒，醫以丸藥大下之，身熱不去，微煩者，梔子干姜湯主之。

Shang han, it is treated with a great purging pill, if the fever does not abate, there is slight vexation, Zhi Zi Gan Jiang Tang governs.

Clause 81

凡用梔子湯，病人舊微溏者，不可與服之。

Whenever Zhi Zi Tang is used, if the patient has only a sloppy stool, one should not give this formula.

NOTE: Clauses 76–81 are associated with constrained heat in the diaphragm. The treatment strategy must differentiate between fire constraint and damp accumulation in the lower jiao. Fire flares upwards and so manifests in the upper jiao; damp sinks downwards and so manifests in the lower jiao.

Clause 82

太陽病發汗，汗出不解，其人仍發熱，心下悸、頭眩、身瞤動，振振欲擗地者，真武湯主之。

Tai Yang disease, sweat is promoted, there is sweating with no resolution, if the person still has fever, palpitations below the heart, dizziness, the body is twitching, trembling and about to fall down, Zhen Wu Tang governs.

NOTE: This clause describes a pattern of yang deficiency following sweat promotion and shows that water accumulation can be attributed either to non-transformation of qi or to yang deficiency.

Clause 83

咽喉干燥者，不可發汗。

Where the throat is parched and dry, one should not promote sweating.

Clause 84

淋家，不可發汗，發汗必便血。

In patients with dysuria, one should not promote sweat, the promotion of sweat will cause bloody urination.

Clause 85

瘡家，雖身疼痛，不可發汗，汗出則痓。

Patients suffering from sores, even if there are body aches and pains, one should not promote sweat, if sweat is promoted there will be tetany.

Clause 86

衄家，不可發汗，汗出必額上陷、脈急緊，直視不能眴，不得眠。

In patients with nose bleed, one should not promote sweat, if there is sweating the forehead will be sunken, the pulse will be urgent and tense, the gaze will be straight and fixed, unable to sleep.

Clause 87

亡血家，不可發汗，發汗則寒栗而振。

Patients with desertion of blood, one should not promote sweat, the promotion of sweat will cause cold shivering and shaking.

Clause 88

汗家，重發汗，必恍惚心亂，小便已陰疼，與禹余糧丸。

In patients with sweating, sweat is again promoted, there will be absentmindedness and derangement, yin pain after urination, give Yu Yu Liang Wan.

Clause 89

病人有寒，復發汗，胃中冷，必吐蛔。

A patient has cold, promotion of sweat is repeated, the stomach will be cold, there will be vomiting of roundworms.

NOTE: Clauses 83–89 explain the contraindications for the use of Ma Huang Tang.

Clause 90

本發汗，而復下者，此為逆也；若先發汗，治不為逆。 本先下之，而反汗之，為逆；若先下之，治不為逆。

Where there should be sweating, but instead there is purgation, this is adverse; if sweating is promoted first, the treatment is not adverse. Where there should be purgation first, but instead there is sweating, it is adverse; if purging is used first, the treatment is not adverse.

Clause 91

傷寒,醫下之，續得下利，清谷不止，身疼痛者，急當救里。後身疼痛，清便自調者，急當救表。救里宜四逆湯，救表宜桂枝湯。

Shang han, the treatment is purging, followed by diarrhoea, unremitting with undigested food particles, the body is aching, one must hasten to rescue the interior. Afterwards there is body pain, the watery stool has righted itself, one must hasten to rescue the exterior. Si Ni Tang is appropriate to rescue the interior, Gui Zhi Tang is appropriate to rescue the exterior.

Clause 92

病發熱頭痛，脈反沉，若不差，身體疼痛，當救其里。四逆湯方。

The disease has fever and headache, the pulse is submerged, if there is no recovery and there are body aches and pains, one must treat the interior. The formula is Si Ni Tang.

NOTE: Clauses 90, 91 and 92 describe the sequence of treatment for combined exterior and interior patterns, stating that the standard strategy is to first release the exterior before treating the interior, but where there is interior deficiency, the deficiency should be first supplemented before treating the exterior pattern.

Clause 93

太陽病，先下而不愈，因復發汗，以此表里俱虛，其人因致冒。冒家汗出自愈。所以然者，汗出表和故也。里未和，然後復下者。

Tai Yang disease, first there is purging but there is no recovery, and so sweating is then promoted, because of this both exterior and interior are deficient, the person will then be faint. Patients who feel faint will sweat and recover spontaneously. The reason for this being, sweating harmonises the exterior. Where the interior is not harmonised, one should purge later.

Clause 94

太陽病未解，脈陰陽俱停，必先振栗汗出而解。但陽脈微者，先汗出而解；但陰脈微者，下之而解。若欲下者，宜調胃承氣湯。

Yang disease is not resolved, the pulses at yin and yang both stop, first there will be shivering and sweat then resolution. Where the yang pulse alone is faint, first there will be sweat then resolution; where the yin pulse alone is faint, purging will bring resolution. If purging is desired, Tiao Wei Cheng Qi Tang is appropriate.

Clause 95

太陽病，發熱出汗者，此為榮弱衛強，故使汗出，欲救邪風者，宜桂枝湯。

Tai Yang disease, there is fever and sweating, this is because the nutrient is weak and the defence is strong, so by causing sweat, there will be relief of evil wind, Gui Zhi Tang is appropriate.

NOTE: Clauses 93, 94 and 95 read in sequence describe transmuted patterns caused by incorrect treatment and three different scenarios of spontaneous recovery without medication.

Clause 96

傷寒五六日中風，往來寒熱，胸脅苦滿、默默不欲飲食、心煩喜嘔，或胸中煩而不嘔，或渴，或腹中痛，或脅下痞硬，或心下悸、小便不利，或不渴、身有微熱，或咳者，小柴胡湯主之。

Shang han zhong feng for five or six days, alternating chills and fever, if there is pain and fullness in the chest and ribs, the patient is untalkative with no desire for food or drink, vexation and nausea, or vexation in the chest with no vomiting, or thirst, or pain in the abdomen, or hard glomus beneath the ribs, or palpitations below the heart and urination which is not free, or no thirst and a slight fever, or a cough, Xiao Chai Hu Tang governs.

Clause 97

血弱氣盡，腠理開，邪氣因入，與正氣相搏，結於脅下。正邪分爭，往來寒熱，休作有時，默默不欲飲食。臟腑相連，其痛必下，邪高痛下，故使嘔也，小柴胡湯主之。服柴胡湯已，渴者屬陽明，以法治之。

Blood is weak and qi exhausted, the interstices are open, evil qi enters, it vies with the zheng qi, knotting below the ribs. The upright battles the evil, chills and fever come and go, off and on periodically, the patient is untalkative with no desire to eat or drink. The zang fu are interconnected, the pain will be below, the evil is high and the pain is low, hence causing vomiting, Xiao Chai Hu Tang governs. If, having taken Chai Hu Tang, there is thirst pertaining to Yang Ming, treat according to the rule.

Clause 98

得病六七日，脈遲浮弱、惡風寒、手足溫，醫二三下之，不能食而脅下滿痛，面目及身黃、頸項強、小便難者，與柴胡湯，后必下重。本渴飲水而嘔者，柴胡湯不中與也，食谷者噦。

Ill for six or seven days, the pulse is slow, floating and weak, there is aversion to wind and cold, the hands and feet are warm, the physician purged two or three times, if there is an inability to eat and fullness and pain under the ribs, the face, eyes and skin are yellow, the neck is stiff, and urination is difficult, give Xiao Chai Hu Tang, later there is heaviness below. If originally there was thirst and after drinking water there was vomiting, Chai Hu Tang should not be given, if the patient eats, he will vomit.

Clause 99

傷寒四五日，身熱、惡風、頸項強、脅下滿，手足溫而渴者，小柴胡湯主之。

Shang han for four or five days, if there is fever, aversion to wind, stiffness of the neck, fullness under the ribs, warm hands and feet and thirst, Xiao Chai Hu Tang governs.

Clause 100

傷寒，陽脈澀，陰脈弦，法當腹中急痛，先與小建中湯；不差者，小柴胡湯主之。

Shang han, the yang pulse is choppy, the yin pulse is wiry, there must be acute pain in the abdomen, first give Xiao Jian Zhong Tang; if it is not despatched, Xiao Chai Hu Tang governs.

Clause 101

傷寒中風，有柴胡証，但見一証便是，不必悉具。凡柴胡湯病証而下之，若柴胡証不罷者，復與柴胡湯，必蒸蒸而振，卻復發熱汗出而解。

Shang han zhong feng, with Chai Hu signs, observing just one sign will do, there is no need for all to be present. Where there is purgation in a Chai Hu Tang pattern, if the Chai Hu pattern is not finished, give Chai Hu Tang again, there will be steaming and shivering, followed by fever and sweating then recovery.

Clause 102

傷寒二三日,心中悸而煩者，小建中湯主之。

Shang han for two or three days, if there are palpitations in the heart and vexation, Xiao Jian Zhong Tang governs.

Clause 103

太陽病，過經十余日，反二三下之。後四五日，柴胡証仍在者，先與小柴胡湯。嘔不止、心下急、郁郁微煩者，為未解也，與大柴胡湯下之則愈。

Tai Yang disease, having passed through the channel for more than ten days, nevertheless purgation was used two to three times. Four or five days later, if a Chai Hu pattern is still present, first give Xiao Chai Hu Tang. Vomiting is ceaseless, there is urgency below the heart, depression and mild vexation, this means there is no resolution, give Da Chai Hu Tang and purging will bring recovery.

Clause 104

傷寒十三日不解，胸脅滿而嘔，日晡所發潮熱，已而微利。此本柴胡証，下之以不得利；今反利者，知醫以丸藥下之，此非其治也。潮熱者，實也。先宜服小柴胡湯以解外，后以柴胡加芒硝湯主之。

Shang han for thirteen days with no resolution, the chest and ribs are full and there is vomiting, late afternoon tidal fever, then mild diarrhoea. This is actually a Chai Hu pattern, purgation should not cause diarrhoea; but now there is diarrhoea, know it is because the physician used a pill to purge, this is not the treatment. If there is tidal fever, it is excess. First it is appropriate to take Xiao Chai Hu Tang to release the exterior, afterwards Chai Hu jia Mang Xiao Tang governs.

Clause 105

傷寒十三日，過經譫語者，以有熱也，當以湯下之。若小便利者，大便當硬，而反下利，脈調和者，知醫以丸藥下之，非其治也。若自下利者，脈當微厥。今反和者，此為內實也，調胃承氣湯主之。

Shang han for thirteen days, if it has passed through the channel and there is delirious speech, it is because there is heat, one should purge with a decoction. If the urination is free, the stool should be hard, but there is diarrhoea, and the pulse is harmonious, one knows the physician used a herbal pill to purge, and this is not the treatment. If there is spontaneous diarrhoea, the pulse should be faint and there will be desertion cold. If now however there is harmony, this is interior excess, Tiao Wei Cheng Qi Tang governs.

Clause 106

太陽病不解，熱結膀胱，其人如狂，血自下，下者愈。其外不解者，尚未可攻，當先解其外。外解已，但少腹急結者，乃可攻者，宜桃核承氣湯。

Tai Yang disease is not resolved, heat knots in the urinary bladder, the person seems deranged, blood descends spontaneously, descent brings recovery. Where the exterior is not resolved, one should not attack yet, one must first resolve the exterior. Having resolved the exterior, but there is tense knotting in the lesser abdomen, then one should attack, Tao He Cheng Qi Tang is appropriate.

Clause 107

傷寒八九日，下之，胸滿、煩驚、小便不利、譫語、一身盡重，不可轉側者，柴胡加龍骨牡蠣湯主之。

Shang han for eight or nine days, with purgation, if the chest is full, there is vexation and fright, the urination is not free, there is delirious speech, the whole body feels heavy, so that the patient can not turn over, Chai Hu jia Long Gu Mu Li Tang governs.

NOTE: Clauses 96–107 describe a Xiao Chai Hu Tang pattern in Shao Yang, and its modifications and contraindications. It draws the reader's attention to the use of Xiao Jian Zhong Tang, Tiao Wei Cheng Qi Tang and Tao He Cheng Qi Tang, and by so doing, contrasts these patterns for the purpose of differentiation. For example, Xiao Chai Hu Tang is indicated for hypochondriac fullness; pain below the heart is treated with Da Chai Hu Tang; lesser abdominal pain is treated with Tao He Cheng Qi Tang. Thus the differential treatments are given for the various patterns of hypochondriac qi constraint, heat bind in the middle jiao and blood stasis bind in the lower jiao. Clauses 100 and 102 explain that Shao Yang disease with deficiency can be treated first with Xiao Jian Zhong Tang before using Xiao Chai Hu Tang, while Tai Yang disease with deficiency can be treated with Xiao Jian Zhong Tang as the principle treatment. Other references to this strategy are found in Clauses 49 and 50.

Clause 108

傷寒，腹滿、譫語、寸口脈浮而緊，此肝乘脾也，名曰縱，刺期門。

Shang han, with abdominal fullness and delirious speech, the cun kou pulse is floating and tight, this is the liver overacting on the spleen, known as restraint, needle Qi Men.

Clause 109

傷寒發熱，嗇嗇惡寒，大渴欲飲水，其腹必滿，自汗出；小便利，其病欲解。此肝乘肺也，名曰橫，刺期門。

Shang han disease with fever, there is huddled aversion to cold and strong thirst with a desire to drink water, the abdomen will be full, and there is spontaneous sweating; the urination is free, the disease is about to resolve. This is the liver overacting on the lungs, it is called rebellion, needle Qi Men.

NOTE: Clauses 108 and 109 are associated with patterns of the liver and gallbladder harassing the spleen and the lung. These come under the scope of Xiao Chai Hu Tang and its modifications.

Clause 110

太陽病二日，反躁，凡熨其背而大汗出，大熱入胃，胃中水竭，躁煩必發譫語。十余日振栗自下利者，此為欲解也。故其汗從腰以下不得汗，欲小便不得，反嘔、欲失溲、足下惡風、大便硬、小便當數，而反不數及不多；大便已，頭卓然而痛，其人足心必熱，谷氣下流故也。

Tai Yang disease for two days, but there is agitation, whenever a hot poultice is applied to the back and there is profuse sweating, severe heat will enter the stomach, exhausting the stomach fluids, there will be agitation and vexation with delirious speech. If more than ten days have passed and there is shivering and spontaneous diarrhoea, this means it is about to resolve. And so the sweat will not issue from the waist down, the patient tries to pass urine but can not, instead there is vomiting and almost a loss of continence, the bottoms of the feet are averse to wind, the stool is hard and, although urination should be frequent, it is infrequent and scant; once a stool is passed, there is an extraordinary headache, and the soles of the patient's feet will be hot, this being due to the downward flow of the grain qi.

Clause 111

太陽病中風，以火劫發汗。邪風被火熱，血氣流溢，失其常度，兩陽相熏灼，其身發黃。陽盛則欲衄，陰虛小便難。陰陽皆虛竭，身體則枯燥，但頭汗出，劑頸而還。腹滿、微喘、口干、咽爛，或不大便，久則譫語，甚者至噦、手足躁擾、捻衣摸床。小便利者，其人可治。

Tai Yang zhong feng, fire was used to force sweating. Evil wind was fuelled by the fire, blood and qi flow and spill over, losing normality, these two yang fume and scorch each other, the body turns yellow. Yang exuberance results in a tendency to nose bleed, yin deficiency and inhibited urination. Both yin and yang are deficient and exhausted and the body is withered and dried, sweat pours from the head alone, stopping at the neck. There is abdominal distension, slight wheezing, a dry mouth, ulceration of the throat, or there is no stool, if it persists there will be delirious speech, even to the point of vomiting, the arms and legs are agitated and restless, the patient twists their clothing and plucks at the bedding. If urination is free, the patient can be treated.

Clause 112

傷寒脈浮，醫以火迫劫之，亡陽必驚狂、臥起不安者，桂枝去芍藥加蜀漆牡蠣龍骨救逆湯主之。

Shang han with a floating pulse, because the physician has used fire to force, if there is devastation of yang there will be manic behaviour, and restlessness both lying down or getting up, Gui Zhi qu ShaoYao jia Shu Qi Mu Li Long Gu Jiu Ni Tang governs.

Clause 113

形作傷寒，其脈不弦緊而弱，弱者必渴，被火必譫語，弱者發熱，脈浮，解之當汗出愈。

Resembling shang han, the pulse is not wiry or taut but weak, if weak there will be thirst, if treated with fire there will be delirious speech, if with the weakness there is fever, the pulse is floating, resolution by sweating should bring recovery.

Clause 114

太陽病，以火熏之，不得汗，其人必躁；到經不解，必清血，名為火邪。

Tai Yang disease, because of fuming by fire, sweating is not obtained, the person will be agitated; if it reaches the channel and does not resolve, there will be blood in the stool , it is called fire evil.

Clause 115

脈浮、熱甚，而反灸之，此為實。實以虛治，因火而動，必咽燥、吐血。

The pulse is floating, the fever is extreme, despite this moxibustion is used, this is excess. Excess has been treated as deficiency, because of the fire there is activity, the throat will be parched, and there will be vomiting of blood.

Clause 116

微數之脈，慎不可灸。因火為邪，則為煩逆，追虛逐實，血散脈中，火氣雖微，內攻有力，焦骨傷筋，血難復也。脈浮，宜以汗解，用火灸之，邪無從出，因火而盛；病從腰以下，必重而痺，名火逆也。欲自解者，必當先煩，煩乃有汗而解，何以知之？脈浮，故知汗出解。

A faint and rapid pulse, be warned one should not use moxibustion. Because fire is an evil, it will cause vexation and counterflow, by targeting deficiency and pursuing excess, blood will be dissipated in the vessels, even if the fire evil is mild, it will attack the interior vigorously, scorching the bones and injuring the sinews, the blood will be difficult to restore. If the pulse is floating, it is appropriate to resolve with sweating, using fire or moxibustion, the evil has no place to exit, because the fire is superabundant; the disease is from the waist down, there will be heaviness and impediment, this is called fire counterflow. If there is about to be spontaneous resolution, there must first be vexation, only after vexation will there be sweating and resolution, how does one know this? The pulse is floating, so it is known that sweating brings resolution.

Clause 117

燒針令其汗，針處被寒，核起而赤者，必發奔豚。氣從少腹上沖心者，灸其核上各一壯，與桂枝加桂湯，更加桂二兩也。

Hot needling caused sweating, the needle site is attacked by cold, if a nodule erupts which is red, there will be running piglet. If qi from the lesser abdomen surges upward to the heart, place one cone of moxa on each nodule, give Gui Zhi jia Gui Tang, with the addition of 2 liang of Gui Zhi.

Clause 118

火逆下之，因燒針煩躁者，桂枝甘草龍骨牡蠣湯主之。

Adverse fire therapy and purgation, if, due to hot needling, there is vexation and agitation, Gui Zhi Gan Cao Long Gu Mu Li Tang governs.

Clause 119

太阳伤寒者，加温针必惊也。

If there is Tai Yang shang han, and warm needling is used, there will be fright.

NOTE: Clauses 110–119 are associated with transmutations resulting from incorrect treatment with fire therapy. Fire therapy was commonly employed in the Han era, and included such therapies as hot needling, moxibustion, fuming therapy and hot compress. The use of any of those therapies in the treatment of an exterior pattern has the potential to cause transmutation, and underlines the adverse effects of such therapies.

Clause 120

太陽病，當惡寒、發熱，今自汗出，　反不惡寒、發熱、關上脈細數者，以醫吐之過也。一二日吐之者，腹中饑、口不能食；三四日吐之者，不喜糜粥，欲食冷食，朝食暮吐，以醫吐之所致也，此為小逆。

TaiYang disease, there should be aversion to cold and fever, now there is spontaneous sweating, but if there is no aversion to cold or fever and the guan pulse is thready and rapid, it is because the physician has wrongly induced vomiting. If there is vomiting for one or two days, there is hunger in the abdomen but the mouth is unable to eat; if there is vomiting for three or four days, the patient doesn't want gruel, he wants to eat cold food, food eaten in the morning is vomited in the evening, it is because of the physician inducing vomiting, this is a minor adverse treatment.

Clause 121

太陽病，　吐之，　但太陽病當惡寒，　今反不惡寒，不欲近衣，此為吐之內煩也。

Tai Yang disease, there is vomiting, but Tai Yang disease should have aversion to cold, now however there is no aversion to cold, no desire to wear more clothing, this means the vomiting has caused interior vexation.

Clause 122

病人脈數，數為熱，當消谷引食。而反吐者，此以發汗，令陽氣微，膈氣虛，脈乃數也。數為客熱，不能消谷；以胃中虛冷，故吐也。

The patient's pulse is rapid, rapid relates to heat, and there should be insatiable hunger with huge consumption. If instead there vomiting, this is due to the promotion of sweat, causing yang qi to be faint, diaphragm qi is deficient, the pulse is still rapid. Rapid relates to visitant heat, an inability to digest food; because there is deficiency cold in the stomach and so there is vomiting.

Clause 123

太陽病，過經十余日，心下溫溫欲吐而胸中痛，大便反溏，腹微滿，郁郁微煩。先此時自極吐下者，與調胃承氣湯；若不爾者，不可與。但欲嘔、胸中痛、微溏者，此非柴胡證，以嘔故知極吐下也。調胃承氣湯。

Tai Yang disease, having passed through the channel for ten days or more, there is discomfort below the heart with a desire to vomit and pain in the chest, the stool however is loose, the abdomen slightly full, there is constraint with mild vexation. If prior to this time, there was severe emesis and purgation, give Tiao Wei Cheng Qi Tang; if it is not so, it should not be given. But even if there is a desire to vomit, pain in the chest and slight looseness, this is not a Xiao Chai Hu Tang pattern, because the vomiting is known to be due to severe emesis and purgation.

NOTE: Clauses 120–123 describe transmutation following the incorrect administration of emetics, sweat promotion and purgation, which has resulted in vomiting. Clauses 120 and 122 describe cold vomiting as being the result of the damage to fluids and stomach yang caused by incorrect use of sweat promotion and emetics. Clauses 121 and 123 cite fluid damage and stomach dryness caused by incorrect emesis and purgation as the reason.

Clause 124

太陽病六七日，表證仍在，脈微而沉，反不結胸，其人發狂者，以熱在下焦，少腹當硬滿，小便自利者，下血乃愈。所以然者，以太陽隨經，瘀熱在里故也，抵當湯主之。

Tai Yang disease for six or seven days, the exterior pattern is still present, the pulse is faint and submerged, but there is no chest bind, where the person is deranged, due to heat in the lower jiao, the lesser abdomen will have hard distension, where the urination is spontaneously free, the descent of blood will bring recovery. The reason for this being, having followed the Tai Yang channel, the stasis heat is in the interior, Di Dang Tang governs.

Clause 125

太陽病，身黃，脈沉結，少腹硬，小便不利者，為無血也。小便自利，其人如狂者，血證諦也，抵當湯主之。

Tai Yang disease, the body is yellow, the pulse deep and knotted, the lesser abdomen is hard, where urination is not free, it is not blood. The urination is spontaneously free, where the person seems deranged, it is certainly a blood pattern, Di Dang Tang governs.

Clause 126

傷寒有熱，少腹滿，應小便不利，今反利者，為有血也，當下之，不可余藥，宜抵當丸。

Shang han with heat, lesser abdominal fullness, it should be that the urination is not free, where now on the contrary it is free, this is blood, it should be purged, one should not add herbs, Di Dang Wan is appropriate.

Clause 127

太陽病，小便利者，以飲水多，必心下悸；小便少者，必苦里急也。

Tai Yang disease, where urination is free, because of drinking much water, there will be palpitations below the heart; where urination is scant, there will be discomfort and urgency in the interior.

NOTE: Clauses 124–127 differentiate between blood amassment and water amassment patterns. The key difference between these two patterns is whether the urination is inhibited or uninhibited. A comparison can be made with the water amassment patterns described in Clauses 71, 73 and 74.

Clause 128

問曰：病有結胸、有藏結，其狀何如？

答曰：按之痛，寸脈浮，關脈沉，名曰結胸也。

Question: A disease with chest bind and zang bind, what are the symptoms?
Answer: Pain on pressure, the cun pulse is floating, guan pulse is submerged, it is called chest bind.

Clause 129

何謂臟結？

答曰：如結胸狀，飲食如故、時時下利，寸脈浮、關脈小細沉緊，名曰臟結。舌上白胎滑者，難治。

Question: What is zang bind?
Answer: It is like chest bind, the intake of food and drink are as usual, there is frequent diarrhoea, the cun pulse is floating, the guan

pulse is small, fine, submerged and tight, it is called zang bind. If the tongue coat is white and slippery, it is difficult to treat.

Clause 130

藏結無陽證，不往來寒熱，其人反靜，舌上胎滑者，不可攻也。

Zang bind, with no yang pattern, no alternating chills and fever, if the person is nonetheless calm, and the tongue coat is slippery, one should not attack.

NOTE: Clauses 128, 129 and 130 differentiate between chest bind and zang bind, and their prognosis and contraindications. Chest bind is an excess pattern associated with heat; zang bind is a deficiency pattern associated with cold. Although the patterns are similar in some respects, their pathology is different.

Clause 131A

病發于陽，而反下之，熱入因作結胸；病發于陰，而反下之，因作痞也。所以成結胸者，以下之太早故也。

In disease stemming from yang, there is adverse purgation, heat enters and so chest bind forms; in disease stemming from yin, there is adverse purgation, and so glomus forms. The reason for chest bind is that purgation was used too early.

Clause 131B

結胸者，項亦強，如柔痉狀，下之則和，宜大陷胸丸。

If there is chest bind, the neck is stiff, as in soft tetany, purgation will bring harmony, Da Xian Xiong Wan is appropriate.

Clause 132

結胸證，其脈浮大者，不可下，下之則死。

Chest bind pattern, if the pulse is floating and big, one should not purge, purging will cause death.

Clause 133

結胸證悉俱, 煩躁者亦死。

Chest bind signs are all present, if there is vexation and agitation, the patient will die.

Clause 134

太陽病，脈浮而動數，浮則為風，數則為熱，動則為痛，數則為虛。頭痛、發熱、微盜汗出，而反惡寒者，表未解也。醫反下之，動數變遲，膈內拒痛，胃中空虛，客氣動膈，短氣躁煩，心中懊憹，陽氣內陷，心下因硬，則為結胸，大陷胸湯主之。若不結胸，但頭汗出，余處無汗，劑頸而還，小便不利，身必發黃。大陷胸湯方。

Tai Yang disease, the pulse is floating but stirring and rapid, floating indicates wind, rapid indicates heat, stirring indicates pain, rapid indicates deficiency. There is headache, fever and mild night sweats, but if there is aversion to cold, the exterior is not resolved. However, the physician uses adverse purgation, stirring and rapid change to slow, there is pain in the diaphragm which resists pressure, emptiness and deficiency in the stomach, the visitant qi stirs the diaphragm, there is shortness of breath, agitation and vexation, anguish in the heart, yang qi fills the interior, causing hardness below the heart, which is chest bind, Da Xian Xiong Tang governs. If there is no chest bind, but sweat issues from the head, there is no sweat elsewhere, it stops at the neck, the urination is not free, the body will turn yellow. Da Xian Xiong Tang formula.

Clause 135

傷寒六七日，結胸熱實，脈沉而緊，心下痛，按之石硬者，大陷胸湯主之。

Shan han for six or seven days, chest bind with heat excess, the pulse is submerged and tight, if there is pain below the heart, stone-hard upon palpation, Da Xian Xiong Tang governs.

Clause 136

傷寒十余日，熱結在里，復往來寒熱者，與大柴胡湯；但結胸，無大熱者，此為水結在胸脅也，但頭微汗出者，大陷胸湯主之。

Shang han for more than ten days, if there is heat bind in the interior, with alternating chills and fever, give Da Chai Hu Tang; if there is only chest bind, without vigorous fever, this is water knotted in the chest and ribs, if a slight sweat issues only from the head, Da Xian Xiong Tang governs.

Clause 137

太陽病，重發汗而復下之，不大便五六日，舌上燥而渴、日晡所小有潮熱，從心下至少腹硬滿而痛，不可近者，大陷胸湯主之。

Tai Yang disease, repeated sweat promotion then purging, no stool for five or six days, the tongue surface is dry and there is thirst, in the late afternoon there is mild tidal fever, if from below the heart to the lesser abdomen there is hard distension and pain such that the patient will not allow anyone near, Da Xian Xiong Tang governs.

NOTE: Clauses 131–137 describe the pattern of major chest bind, which is the knotting of heat and water, and also contrast chest bind and glomus.

Clause 138

小結胸病，正在心下，按之則痛，脈浮滑者，小陷胸湯主之。

Minor chest bind disease, just below the heart, if there is pain on palpation, the pulse is floating and slippery, Xiao Xian Xiong Tang governs.

NOTE: Clause 138 describes the difference between major chest bind and minor chest bind.

Clause 139

太陽病，二三日，不能臥，但欲起，心下必結，脈微弱者，此本有寒分也。反下之，若利止，必作結胸；未止者，四日復下之，此作協熱利也。

Tai Yang disease, on the second or third day, the person can not lie down, but wants to get up, there will be knotting below the heart, if the pulse is faint and weak, there was originally coldness. Nevertheless, purgation is used, when the diarrhoea stops, there will be knotting in the chest; if there is no cessation, on the fourth day there is again purgation, this will cause a complex of fever and diarrhoea.

NOTE: Clause 138 describes Tai Yang disease with pre-existing accumulation of water and cold. Incorrect treatment may result either in chest bind or in concurrent fever and diarrhoea.

Clause 140

太陽病，下之，其脈促，不結胸者，此為欲解也；脈浮者，必結胸；脈緊者，必咽痛；脈弦者，必兩脅拘急；脈細數者，頭痛未止；脈沉緊者，必欲嘔；脈沉滑者，協熱利；脈浮滑者，必下血。

Tai Yang disease, after purgation, if the pulse is skipping, and there is no chest bind, this means recovery is imminent; if the pulse is floating, there will be chest bind; if the pulse is taut, the throat will be sore; if the pulse is wiry, there will be constrained tightness in both sides of the chest; if the pulse is thready and rapid, there will be constant headache; if the pulse is submerged and taut, there will be nausea; if the pulse is submerged and slippery, there will be a complex of fever and diarrhoea; if the pulse is floating and slippery, blood will descend.

NOTE: Clause 140 describes the possible outcomes resulting from incorrect purgation in Tai Yang disease. 1) Return of zheng qi with subsequent retreat of the pathogen and spontaneous recovery. 2) Transmission to the Shao Yin channel with a sore throat. 3) Transmission to the Shao Yang channel with fullness in the hypochondrium. 4) No transmission with the Tai Yang pattern remaining, manifesting with headache; 5) transmission to the Shao Yang manifesting with nausea. 6) An unresolved exterior pattern with concurrent fever and diarrhoea. 7) Heat in the blood aspect with haemorrhage. This clause serves to remind the reader that incorrect purgation of Tai Yang disease does not result in chest bind alone.

Clause 141

寒實結胸，無熱證者，與三物白散。

Cold excess chest bind, with no heat signs, give San Wu Bai San.

NOTE: Clause 141 compares a pattern of chest bind due to excess cold, with a chest bind pattern dues to excess heat.

Clause 142

太陽與少陽并病，頭項強痛，或眩冒，時如結胸，心下痞硬者，當刺大椎第一間、肺俞、肝俞，慎不可發汗，發汗則譫語，脈弦，五日譫語不止，當刺期門。

In Tai Yang and Shao Yang lagover disease, where there is stiffness and pain of the head and neck, dizziness, and sometimes something which resembles chest bind with hard glomus below the heart; one should needle Da Zhui (Du 14), Fei Shu (UB 13), and Gan Shu (UB 18);

caution must be taken not to promote sweat, as sweating will cause delirious speech and a wiry pulse; and if after five days, the delirious speech persists, one should needle Qi Men (Liv 14).

Clause 143

婦人中風，發熱惡寒，經水適來，得之七八日，熱除而脈遲、身涼、胸脅下滿，如結胸狀、譫語者，此為熱入血室也，當刺期門，隨其實而取之。

A woman has zhong feng, there is fever and aversion to cold, coinciding with the arrival of the menstrual flow, having been sick for seven or eight days, if the fever is resolved and the pulse is slow, the body is cool, there is fullness beneath the chest and the ribs, it is like chest bind, with delirious speech, this means the heat is entering the chamber of blood, one must needle qi men, selecting it to suit the excess.

NOTE: Clause 143 describes a pattern of heat entering the blood chamber which is characterised by distension in the chest and hypochondrium resembling chest bind.

Clause 144

婦人中風，七八日續得寒熱，發作有時，經水適斷者，此為熱入血室，其血必結，故使如瘧狀，發作有時，小柴胡湯主之。

A woman has zhong feng, for seven or eight days it continues with chills and fever, occurring periodically, coinciding with the cessation of the menstrual flow, this is heat entering the chamber of blood, the blood will become knotted, thus causing malaria-like symptoms, occurring periodically, Xiao Chai Hu Tang governs.

Clause 145

婦人傷寒，發熱，經水適來。晝日明了，暮則譫語，如見鬼狀者，此為熱入血室。無犯胃氣，及上二焦，必自愈。

A woman has shang han, there is fever, coinciding with the arrival of the menstrual flow, if in the daylight hours she is lucid, and in the evening there is delirious speech, as if seeing ghosts, this is heat entering the chamber of blood. Without attacking the stomach and the upper two jiao, there will be spontaneous recovery.

Clause 146

傷寒六七日，發熱微惡寒、支節煩痛、微嘔、心下支結，外証未去者，柴胡桂枝湯主之。

Shang han for six or seven days, there is fever and a slight aversion to cold, vexing joint pain in the limbs, mild vomiting, a sustained knot below the heart, the exterior pattern has not been resolved, Chai Hu Gui Zhi Tang governs.

Clause 147

傷寒五六日，已發汗而復下之，胸脅滿微結、小便不利、渴而不嘔、但頭汗出、往來寒熱、心煩者，此為未解也，柴胡桂枝干姜湯主之。

Shang han for five or six days, following the promotion of sweat, there has then been purgation, if the chest and ribs are full with a slight bind, urination is not free, there is thirst but no vomiting, sweating only from the head, alternating chills and fever, and vexation, this means there is no resolution, Chai Hu Gui Zhi Gan Jiang Tang governs.

Clause 148

傷寒五六日，頭汗出、微惡寒、手足冷、心下滿、口不欲食、大便硬、脈細者，此為陽微結，必有表，復有裡也。脈沉，亦在裡也。汗出，為陽微；假令純陰結，不得復有外証，悉入在裡，此為半在裡半在外也。脈雖沉緊，不得為少陰病。所以然者，陰不得有汗，今頭汗出，故知非少陰也，可與小柴胡湯；設不了了者，得屎而解。

Shang han for five or six days, if there is sweating from the head, mild aversion to cold, cold hands and feet, fullness below the heart, no desire to eat, a hard stool and a thready pulse, this is a mild yang bind, there will be both exterior and interior signs. A submerged pulse, it is also in the interior. Sweating indicates the mild yang; if it were pure yin bind, there would be no more exterior signs, it would have entirely entered the interior; this is half in the exterior and half in the interior. Although the pulse is submerged and tight, it does not mean a Shao Yin disease. The reason being, yin has no sweat, here there is sweating from the head, and so we know it is not Shao Yin, one may give Xiao Chai Hu Tang; if it is not fully cleared, once a stool is passed, it will resolve.

NOTE: Clauses 142–148 describe pattern identification in disorders similar to chest bind.

Clause 149

傷寒五六日，嘔而發熱者，柴胡湯證具，而以他藥下之，柴胡證仍在者，復與柴胡湯。此雖已下之，不為逆，必蒸蒸而振，卻發熱汗出而解。若心下滿而硬痛者，此為結胸也，大陷胸湯主之。但滿而不痛，此為痞，柴胡不中與之，宜半夏瀉心湯。

Shang han for five or six days, with vomiting and fever, Xiao Chai Hu Tang signs are present, but other herbs have been used to purge, if the Chai Hu signs are still present, give Xiao Chai Hu Tang again. Even though purgation has been used, it is not adverse, there will be steaming and quivering, followed by fever and sweating and resolution. If there is fullness with hard pain below the heart, it is chest bind, Da Xian Xiong Tang governs. If there is only fullness with no pain, it is glomus, it is not suitable to give Chai Hu, Ban Xia Xie Xin Tang is appropriate.

NOTE: Clause 149 describes three different outcomes of incorrect purgation of Shao Yang disease. The transmuted pattern of chest bind is described in Clauses 128–138.

Clause 150

太陽、少陽并病，而反下之，成結胸；心下硬、下利不止，水漿不下，其人心煩。

Tai Yang Shao Yang lagover disease, but nonetheless there is purgation, it will turn into chest bind; hardness below the heart, incessant diarrhoea, an inability to get fluid down, the person is vexed.

NOTE: In Clauses 128–150, Zhong Jing explained chest bind in terms of aetiology, pathogenesis, key symptoms, classifications, treatment, formulas and prognosis.

Clause 151

脈浮而緊，而復下之，緊反入里，則作痞，按之自濡，但氣痞耳。

The pulse is floating and tight, but again there is purging, the tightness instead enters the interior, causing a glomus, it is soft when pressed, it is only a qi glomus.

Clause 152

太陽中風，下利嘔逆，表解者，乃可攻之。其人漐漐汗出，發作有時，頭痛、心下痞硬滿、引脅下痛、干嘔、短氣、汗出不惡寒者，此表解里未和也。十棗湯主之。

Tai Yang zhong feng, there is diarrhoea and counterflow vomiting, if the exterior is resolved, one may still purge. If the person has continuous sweating, occurring at a set time, headache, hard glomus and hard distension below the heart, pain which extends under the ribs, dry retching, shortness of breath, sweating with no aversion to cold, then the exterior is resolved but the interior is not harmonised. Shi Zao Tang governs.

Clause 153

太陽病，醫發汗，遂發熱、惡寒；因復下之，心下痞。表里俱虛，陰陽氣并竭，無陽則陰獨。復加燒針，因胸煩、面色青黃、膚瞤者，難治；今色微黃，手足溫者，易愈。

Tai Yang disease, the physician has promoted sweat, it is followed by fever and aversion to cold; because purgation was repeated, there is glomus below the heart. The exterior and interior are both deficient, yin, yang and qi are also exhausted, there is no yang but yin alone. Hot needling is then used, causing chest vexation, if the facial complexion is greenish yellow, and the skin twitches, it is difficult to treat; now the complexion is slightly yellow, if the hands and feet are warm, recovery is easy.

NOTE: Clauses 151–153 describe glomus occurring as a result of incorrect purgation in Tai Yang disease.

Clause 154

心下痞，按之濡，其脈關上浮者，大黃黃連瀉心湯主之。

Glomus below the heart, soft upon palpation, the pulse is floating on the guan position, Da Huang Huang Lian Xie Xin Tang governs.

Clause 155

心下痞，而復惡寒、汗出者，附子瀉心湯主之。

There is glomus below the heart, if there is also aversion to cold and sweating, Fu Zi Xie Xin Tang governs.

Clause 156

本以下之，故心下痞，與瀉心湯。痞不解，其人渴而口燥煩，小便不利者，五苓散主之。

Due to purging, there is glomus below the heart, give Xie Xin Tang. The glomus is not resolved, the person is thirsty and there is a dry mouth and vexation, where urination is not free, Wu Ling San governs.

NOTE: Clauses 155 and 156 describe heat glomus and heat glomus with exterior yang deficiency, and treatment. Clause 156 describes the treatment for water glomus where incorrect purgation has resulted in glomus associated with water accumulation in the interior with disruption of the qi dynamic. The implication is that glomus can be attributed to heat or cold as well as qi and water.

Clause 157

傷寒汗出解之後，胃中不和，心下痞硬，干噫食臭，脅下有水氣，腹中雷鳴，下利者，生姜瀉心湯主之。

Shang han after resolution by sweating, if there is no harmony in the stomach, there is hard glomus below the heart, dry belching with a foul food odour, water qi under the ribs, intestinal rumbling, diarrhoea, Sheng Jiang Xie Xin Tang governs.

Clause 158

傷寒中風，醫反下之，其人下利，日數十行，谷不化，腹中雷鳴，心下痞硬而滿，干嘔、心煩不得安。醫見心下痞，謂病不盡，復下之，其痞益甚。此非結熱，但以胃中虛，客氣上逆，故使硬也。甘草瀉心湯主之。

Shang han or zhong feng, the physician has nonetheless purged, the person has diarrhoea, ten or more times in one day, with untransformed food, rumbling in the abdomen, hard glomus and fullness below the heart, and dry retching and inconsolable vexation. The physician sees the glomus below the heart, thinking the disease is not ended, again purges, making the glomus more severe. This is not knotted heat, but is due to deficiency in the stomach, visitant qi ascends in reverse, thus causing the hardness. Gan Cao Xie Xin Tang governs.

NOTE: Clause 158 is a continuation of the discussion of glomus initiated in Clause 149. It expands the patterns of heat and cold complex, showing that they can be accompanied by phlegm, water or deficiency. Treatment must be based on the pathogenesis.

Clause 159

傷寒服湯藥，下利不止，心下痞硬。服瀉心湯已，復以他藥下之，利不止，醫以理中與之，利益甚。理中者，理中焦，此利在下焦，赤石脂禹余糧湯主之。復不止者，當利其小使。

Shang han having taken herbs, there is incessant diarrhoea, hard glomus below the heart. Xie Xin Tang was already taken, then because other purgatives were used, the diarrhoea cannot be stopped, the physician gives Li Zhong, but the diarrhoea is more severe. Li Zhong is to regulate the middle jiao, but this diarrhoea is in the lower jiao, Chi Shi Zhi Yu Yu Liang Tang governs. If the diarrhoea still persists, one should promote urination.

NOTE: Clause 159 explains that the treatment of glomus caused by incorrect purgation is not confined to the administration of Xie Xin Tang; Li Zhong Wan can be used to treat diarrhoea attributed to interior cold in the middle jiao; Chi Shi Zhi Yu Yu Liang Tang is appropriate for uncontrollable diarrhoea; Wu Ling San is indicated for diarrhoea associated with accumulation of damp.

Clause 160

傷寒吐下後，發汗、虛煩，脈甚微，八九日心下痞硬，脇下痛、氣上沖咽喉、眩冒、經脈動惕者，久而成痿。

Shang han after emetics and purgation, there is sweat promotion insubstantial vexation, the pulse is extremely faint, after eight or nine days there is a hard glomus below the heart, if there is pain under the ribs, an upsurge of qi to the throat, dizziness and twitchiness in the channel vessels, if it persists, there will be flaccidity.

NOTE: This is an illustration of yet another glomus pattern with a different pathology.

Clause 161

傷寒發汗，若吐、若下，解後，心下痞硬，噫氣不除者，旋復代赭湯主之。

Shang han there is promotion of sweat, if there is vomiting, if there is purgation, after resolution, there is a hard glomus below the heart, unremitting belching, Xuan Fu Dai Zhe Tang governs.

NOTE: This is phlegm glomus.

Clause 162

下後，不可更行桂枝湯，若汗出而喘，無大熱者，可與麻黃杏仁甘草石膏湯。

After purgation, one should not repeat Gui Zhi Tang, if there is sweating and wheezing, no severe fever, one may give Ma Huang Xing Ren Gan Cao Shi Gao Tang.

NOTE: The reason for Clause 162 being included in the section on glomus patterns is unknown. It relates more closely to Clause 63 and describes the potential for heat congestion in the lungs following sweat promotion and purgation.

Clause 163

太陽病，外證未除，而數下之，遂協熱而利，利下不止，心下痞硬，表里不解者，桂枝人參湯主之。

Tai Yang disease, the exterior pattern is not eliminated, and there has been multiple purging, pursuant to this a complex of fever and diarrhoea, the diarrhoea is incessant, there is hard glomus below the heart, if the exterior and interior are not resolved, Gui Zhi Ren Shen Tang governs.

NOTE: This is a pattern of concurrent fever and diarrhoea characterised by hard glomus below the heart.

Clause 164

傷寒大下後，復發汗，心下痞、惡寒者，表未解也。不可攻痞，當先解表，表解乃可攻痞。解表宜桂枝湯，攻痞宜大黃黃連瀉心湯。

Shang han after severe purgation, sweating is then promoted, if there is glomus below the heart, aversion to cold, the exterior is unresolved. One should not attack the glomus, one must first resolve the exterior, once the exterior is resolved, then one may attack the glomus. To resolve the exterior, Gui Zhi Tang is appropriate, to attack the glomus, Da Huang Huang Lian Xie Xin Tang is appropriate.

NOTE: Clause 164 describes heat glomus with an exterior pattern and is better read with Clause 163, which also describes glomus with an unresolved exterior pattern, the difference being that the pattern in Clause 163 is marked by diarrhoea while that in Clause 164 is not.

Clause 165

傷寒發熱，汗出不解，心中痞硬，嘔吐而下利者，大柴胡湯主之。

Shang han with fever, sweating with no resolution, hard glomus in the heart, vomiting and diarrhoea, Da Chai Hu Tang governs.

NOTE: Clause 165 describes glomus in a Shao Yang pattern accompanied by Yang Ming interior excess as well as glomus. Clauses 103 and 136 should also be referenced in order to understand the symptoms and pathogenesis of Da Chai Hu Tang.

Clause 166

病如桂枝證，頭不痛、項不強、寸脈微浮、胸中痞硬、氣上沖喉咽不得息者，此為胸有寒也，當吐之，宜瓜蒂散。

The disease resembles a Gui Zhi Tang pattern, there is no headache, no stiffness in the neck, the cun pulse is slightly floating, there is hard glomus in the chest, qi surges up to the throat making it difficult to breathe, it is due to cold in the chest, one should induce vomiting, Gua Di San is appropriate.

NOTE: Clause 166 describes obstruction in the chest and epigastrium caused by phlegm and food stagnation; the formula is Gua Di San; this clause should be read with Clause 355.

Clause 167

病脅下素有痞，連在臍旁，痛引少腹入陰筋者，此名藏結，死。

The disease normally has glomus under the ribs, extending to the side of the umbilicus, if the pain goes to the lesser abdomen and enters the yin tendon, it is called zang bind, the person will die.

NOTE: This is a continuation of the discussion of zang bind in Clauses 128, 129 and 130; because it is attributed to exuberant yin cold, it is a difficult-to-treat disorder and the prognosis is poor with possible death.

Clause 168

傷寒若吐若下后，七八日不解，熱結在裡，表裡俱熱，時時惡風、大渴、舌上干燥而煩、欲飲水數升者，白虎加人參湯主之。

Shang han following emesis and purgation, is not resolved in seven or eight days, heat is knotted in the interior, if there is heat in both the exterior and interior, with constant aversion to wind, severe thirst, the surface of the tongue is dry, there is agitation and vexation, a desire to drink several sheng of water, Bai Hu jia Ren Shen Tang governs.

Clause 169

傷寒無大熱、口燥渴、心煩、背微惡寒者，白虎加人參湯主之。

Shang han without vigorous fever, if there is a parched mouth and thirst, vexation, the back has a slight aversion to cold, Bai Hu jia Ren Shen Tang governs.

Clause 170

傷寒脈浮、發熱、無汗，其表不解，不可與白虎湯。渴欲飲水，無表証者，白虎人參湯主之。

Shang han with a floating pulse, there is fever with no sweating, the exterior is not resolved, one should not give Bai Hu Tang. If there is thirst with a desire to drink water, no exterior pattern, Bai Hu jia Ren Shen Tang governs.

NOTE: This represents the consequences of incorrect treatment of Tai Yang disease, with transmission to Yang Min, manifesting with exuberant heat and fluid damage.

Clause 171

太陽、少陽并病，心下硬、頸項強而眩者，當刺大椎、肺俞、肝俞，慎勿下之。

Tai Yang Shao Yang lagover disease, if there is hardness below the heart, stiffness of the neck and dizziness, one should needle Da Zhui (Du 14), Fei Shu (UB 13) and Gan Shu (UB 18), taking caution not to purge.

Clause 172

太陰與少陽合病，自下利者，與黃芩湯；若嘔者，黃芩加半夏生姜湯主之。

Tai Yang and Shao Yang concurrent disease, if there is spontaneous diarrhoea, give Huang Qin Tang; if there is vomiting, Huang Qin jia Ban Xia Sheng Jiang Tang governs.

NOTE: Clauses 171 and 172 are associated with a Tai Yang and Shao Yang lagover pattern presenting as a concurrent pattern. It serves as a guideline for pattern and treatment differentiation, and should be read with Clauses 32, 33, 36, 48, 142, 150, 219, 220, 256 and 268 relating to concurrent patterns. In particular, Clause 171 should be read with Clauses 142 and 150, and Clause 172 should be read with Clauses 32 and 33.

Clause 173

傷寒，胸中有熱，胃中有邪氣，腹中痛，欲嘔吐者，黃連湯主之。

Shang han if there is heat in the chest, evil qi in the stomach, pain in the abdomen and nausea and vomiting, Huang Lian Tang governs.

NOTE: Clause 173 discusses a pattern of heat and cold complex characterised by abdominal pain and vomiting. It is better read in conjunction with Clauses 149, 157 and 158. The pattern described above differs from the heat and cold complex patterns of Xie Xin Tang, as it is a pattern of heat which has been repelled by the cold in the lower jiao surging to the upper jiao. The aetiology is similar but the pathogenesis is different.

Clause 174

傷寒八九日，風濕相搏，身體疼煩，不能自轉側，不嘔、不渴、脈浮虛而澀者，桂枝附子湯主之。若其人大便硬，小便自利者，去桂加白術湯主之。

Shang han for eight or nine days, the wind and damp vie with each other, the body aches vexatiously, the person can not turn over, if there is neither vomiting nor thirst, the pulse is floating, deficient and choppy, then Gui Zhi Fu Zi Tang governs. If the person has a hard stool, and urination is free, Qu Gui jia Bai Zhu Tang governs.

Clause 175

風濕相搏，骨節疼煩，掣痛不得屈伸，近之則痛劇，汗出短氣，小便不利，惡風不欲去衣，或身微腫者，甘草附子湯主之。

The wind and damp vie with each other, there is vexatious joint pain, there is pulling pain and an inability to bend and stretch, the pain is worse with contact, if there is sweating and shortness of breath, urination which is not free, aversion to wind with reluctance to remove clothing, or slight oedema, Gan Cao Fu Zi Tang governs.

NOTE: Clauses 174 and 175 are associated with treatment of a wind cold damp bi pattern which bears similarity to a Tai Yang exterior pattern.

Clause 176

傷寒脈浮滑，此以表有熱，裡有寒，白虎湯主之。

Shang han, the pulse is floating and slippery, this is heat in the exterior and cold in the interior, and Bai Hu Tang governs.

NOTE: This is an example of the Tai Yang pathogen having transmitted to Yang Ming.

Clause 177

傷寒脈結代，心動悸，炙甘草湯主之。

Shang han, the pulse is knotted and intermittent, there are throbbing palpitations, Zhi Gan Cao Tang governs.

Clause 178

脈按之來緩, 時一止復來者, 名曰結。又脈來動而中止，更來小數，中有還者反動，名曰結，陰也；脈來動而中止，不能自還，因而復動者，名日代，陰也。得此脈，必難治。

If the pulse is moderate on palpation, occasionally stopping and then starting again, it is called knotted. Also, a pulse which is stirring but is interrupted, then on returning is small and rapid, occasionally returning to normal but stirring again, it is called knotted, this is yin; a pulse which is stirring but is interrupted, if unable to return, it is because when it returns it is stirring, it is called intermittent, this is yin. If this is the pulse, it will be difficult to treat.

NOTE: Clauses 177 and 178 describe shang han disease with heart deficiency, and its treatment. Clause 178 describes in detail the knotted and intermittent pulse images. This pattern implicates the Shao Yin heart, thus demonstrating the exterior–interior relationship of Tai Yang and Shao Yin.

CLAUSES 179–262: YANG MING CHAPTER

Clause 179

問曰：病有太陽陽明，有正陽陽明，有少陽陽明，何謂也？答曰：太陽陽明者，脾約是也；正陽陽明者，胃家實是也；少陽陽明者，發汗、利小便已，胃中燥、煩、實、大便難也。

Question: There are the diseases of Tai Yang Yang Ming, Zheng Yang Yang Ming and Shao Yang Yang Ming, what is meant by this? Answer: Tai Yang Yang Ming, is spleen restraint; Zheng Yang Yang Ming is excess in the domain of the stomach; Shao Yang Yang Ming is where, after the promotion of sweat and urination, there is dryness in the stomach, vexation, excess and difficult defaecation.

Clause 180

陽明之為病，胃家實是也。

Yang Ming is diseased, the stomach's domain is excess.

NOTE: Clause 180 describes the aetiology, classification, location and pathogenesis of Yang Ming disease, chiefly characterised as being patterns of excess heat in the stomach and intestines.

Clause 181

問曰：何緣得陽明病？答曰：太陽病，若發汗、若下、若利小便，此亡津液，胃中干燥，因轉屬陽明。不更衣，內實大便難者，此名陽明也。

Question: What is the cause of Yang Ming disease? Answer: Tai Yang disease, if there is sweat promotion, if there is purgation, if there is promotion of urination, this devastates fluids, there is dryness in the stomach, and so it transmitted to the Yang Ming. If there is no change of clothes, internal excess with a difficult bowel movement, this is Yang Ming.

Clause 182

問曰：陽明病外証雲何？答曰：身熱，汗自出，不惡寒反惡熱也。

Question: What are the exterior symptoms of Yang Ming disease? Answer: Fever, spontaneous sweating, no aversion to cold but aversion to heat.

Clause 183

問曰：病有得之一日，不發熱而惡寒者，何也？答曰：雖得之一日，惡寒將自罷，即汗出而惡熱也。

Question: The disease that has lasted for one day, if there is no fever but there is aversion to cold, why is this? Answer: Although it has lasted one day, the aversion to cold will cease spontaneously, then there will be sweating and aversion to heat.

Clause 184

問曰：惡寒何故自罷？答曰：陽明居中，主土也。萬物所歸，無所復傳，始雖惡寒，二日自止，此為陽明病也。

Question: Why does aversion to cold cease spontaneously? Answer: Yang Ming resides in the middle, it governs earth. A myriad things converge, without passing further, although it starts with aversion to cold, in two days it finishes spontaneously, this is Yang Ming disease.

Clause 185

本太陽初得病時，發其汗，汗先出不徹，因轉屬陽明也。傷寒發熱、無汗、嘔不能食，而反汗出濈濈然者，是轉屬陽明也。

Originally, when Tai Yang first contracted disease, sweating was promoted, sweating at first was incomplete, so it transmitted to Yang Ming. If there is fever in shang han, no sweating, vomiting and an inability to eat, nonetheless sweat is streaming forth, it has transmitted to Yang Ming.

Clause 186

傷寒三日，陽明脈大。

Shang han for three days, the Yang Ming pulse is big.

Clause 187

傷寒，脈浮而緩，手足自溫者，是為系在太陰。太陰者，身當發黃。若小便自利者，不能發黃；至七八日大便硬者，為陽明病也。

Shang han, the pulse is floating and moderate, if the hands and feet are spontaneously warm, it is then in the Tai Yin. If it is Tai Yin, the body should become yellow. If urination is spontaneously free, there can be no yellowing; if on the seventh or eighth day the stool is hard, this is Yang Ming disease.

Clause 188

傷寒轉系陽明者，其人濈然微汗出也。

If shang han has transferred to Yang Ming, the person will have a slight streaming sweat.

NOTE: Clauses 181–188 further expand the aetiology and symptomatology of Yang Ming disease.

Clause 189

陽明中風，口苦、咽干、腹滿、微喘、發熱、惡寒、脈浮而緊，若下之，則腹滿小便難也。

Yang Ming zhong feng, a bitter taste in the mouth, a parched throat, abdominal fullness, slight panting, fever, aversion to cold, and a pulse that is floating and tight, if there is purgation, then the abdomen will be full and urination difficult.

Clause 190

陽明病，若能食，名中風；不能食，名中寒。

Yang Ming disease, if the person can eat, it is called zhong feng; if the person can not eat, it is called zhong han.

NOTE: Clause 189 describes the difference between Yang Ming zhong feng (wind strike) and zhong han (cold strike). It describes Yang Ming zhong feng (wind strike) with constrained heat characterised by a bitter taste in the mouth, a parched throat, abdominal fullness and mild wheezing. Purging is contraindicated because interior excess has not formed. Clause 190 cites the difference between zhong feng and zhong han based on the ability to eat. This relies on the ability to eat being a sign of the robustness of stomach yang.

Clause 191

陽明病，若中寒者，不能食，小便不利，手足濈然汗出，此欲作固瘕，必大便初硬後溏。所以然者，以胃中冷，水谷不別故也。

Yang Ming disease, if it is zhong han, the person can not eat, the urination is not free, the hands and feet sweat profusely, this means a firm mass is about to form, the stool will be hard at first and sloppy afterwards. The reason for this being, that because of cold in the stomach, there is no separation of water and grain.

Clause 192

陽明病，初欲食，小便反不利，大便自調，其人骨節疼，翕翕如有熱狀，奄然發狂，濈然汗出而解者，此水不勝谷氣，與汗共並，脈緊則愈。

Yang Ming disease, initially there is a desire to eat, nevertheless the urination is not free, the stool is naturally regular, the person has joint pain, feather warmth as if there is a fever, if there is sudden derangement, streaming sweat and resolution, this is water unable to overcome the grain qi, combining with the sweat, a tight pulse means recovery.

Clause 193

陽明病欲解時，從申至戌上。

The time that Yang Ming disease is ready to resolve, is from shen to xu.

Clause 194

陽明病，不能食，攻其熱必噦。所以然者，胃中虛冷故也。以其人本虛，攻其熱必噦。

Yang Ming disease, the person can not eat, attacking the heat will cause hiccoughs. The reason for this being, there is empty cold in the stomach. Because the person was already deficient, attacking heat will cause hiccoughs.

Clause 195

陽明病，脈遲，食難用飽，飽則微煩頭眩，必小便難，此欲作谷癉，雖下之，腹滿如故，所以然者，脈遲故也。

Yang Ming disease, the pulse is slow, it is difficult to eat one's fill, and if full, there is mild vexation and dizziness, urination will be difficult, this means grain jaundice is about to occur, in spite of purging, there is abdominal fullness as before, the reason for this being, that the pulse is slow.

Clause 196

陽明病，法多汗，反無汗，其身如虫行皮中狀者，此以久虛故也。

Yang Ming disease, the rule is profuse sweat, if however there is no sweat and it is as if worms are crawling beneath the skin, it is due to prolonged deficiency.

Clause 197

陽明病，反無汗而小便利，二三日嘔而咳，手足厥者，必苦頭痛；若不咳，不嘔，手足不厥者，頭不痛。

Yang Ming disease, nevertheless there is no sweating and the urination is free, on the second or third day, there is vomiting and cough, there will be a severe headache; if there is no cough, no vomiting, no reversal cold of the hands and feet, then the head will not ache.

NOTE: Clauses 191–197 are associated with Yang Ming deficiency cold patterns.

Clause 198

陽明病，但頭眩，不惡寒，故能食而咳，其人咽必痛。若不咳者，咽不痛。

Yang Ming disease, there is only dizziness, no aversion to cold, and the person is able to eat and coughs, and the person's throat should be sore. If there is no cough, there is no sore throat.

Clause 199

陽明病，無汗，小便不利，心中懊憹者，身必發黃。

Yang Ming disease, there is no sweating, if the urination is not free, and there is anguish in the heart, the body will turn yellow.

Clause 200

陽明病，被火，額上微汗出，而小便不利者，必發黃。

Yang Ming disease, treated with fire, if there is slight sweating on the forehead, and urination is not free, there will be yellowing.

Clause 201

陽明病，脈浮而緊者，必潮熱，發作有時。但浮者，必盜汗出。

Yang Ming disease, if the pulse is floating and tight, there must be tidal fever, occurring periodically. If it is floating only, there will be night sweats.

Clause 202

陽明病，口燥，但欲漱水，不欲咽者，此必衄。

Yang Ming disease, the mouth is dry, there is a desire only to rinse the mouth, there will be external bleeding.

NOTE: Clauses 198–202 describe a Yang Ming heat pattern with varying manifestations. This refines the reader's skills of pattern identification.

Clause 203

陽明病，本自汗出。醫更重發汗，病已差，尚微煩不了了者，此必大便硬故也。以亡津液，胃中干燥，故令大便硬。當問其小便　日幾行，若本小便日三四行，今日再行，故知大便不久出。今為小便數少，以津液當還入胃中，故知不久必大便也。

Yang Ming disease, there was originally spontaneous sweating. The physician promoted further sweating, the disease was already despatched, if there is still mild vexation that is not cleared, this means the stool will be hard. Because of devastated body fluids, dryness in the stomach, making the stool hard. One must ask about the urination, how many times a day it is passed. If urination was being passed three or four times a day, now it is twice a day, then you know a stool will be passed before long. If the urination is currently frequent and scant, it is because the body fluids are returning to the stomach, hence you know before long a stool will be passed.

NOTE: Clause 203 emphasises the fact that Yang Ming disease with no bowel movement is differentiated as either heat bind or fluid damage.

Clause 204

傷寒嘔多，雖有陽明証，不可攻之。

Shang han with frequent vomiting, although it is a Yang Ming pattern, one should not attack.

Clause 205

陽明病，心下硬滿者，不可攻之。攻之，利遂不止者死；利止者愈。

Yang Ming disease, if there is hardness and fullness below the heart, one should not attack. Attacking, if followed by incessant diarrhoea, the person will die; if the diarrhoea stops, the person will recover.

Clause 206

陽明病，面合色赤，不可攻也。必發熱，色黃者，小便不利也。

Yang Ming disease, the whole face is crimson, one should not attack. Then there will be fever, yellowing, the urination will not be free.

NOTE: Clauses 204, 205 and 206 describe the adverse outcomes of purgation when used incorrectly in Yang Ming disease, with the potential for incessant vomiting, hardness and fullness below the heart, and a flushed face, indicating the disease is located in the upper jiao. This emphasises that purging should be used only for Yang Ming bowel excess.

Clause 207

陽明病，不吐、不下、心煩者，可與調胃承氣湯。

Yang Ming disease, if there is no vomiting, no purgation, and vexation, one may give Tiao Wei Cheng Qi Tang

Clause 208

陽明病，脈遲，雖汗出不惡寒者，其身必重，短氣、腹滿而喘，有潮熱者，此外欲解，可攻裡也。手足濈然汗出者，此大便已硬也，大承氣湯主之；若汗多、微發熱惡寒者，外未解也；其熱不潮，未可與承氣湯；若腹大滿不通者，可與小承氣湯，微和胃氣，勿令至大泄下。

Yang Ming disease, if the pulse is slow, even though there is sweating with no aversion to cold, the body will be heavy, if there is shortness of breath, abdominal fullness and wheezing, with tidal fever, this is because the exterior is about to resolve, one may purge the interior. If there is sweating from the hands and feet, the stool is already hard, Da Cheng Qi Tang governs. If sweating is profuse, there is a slight fever and aversion to cold, the exterior is not resolved; the fever is not tidal, one must not give Cheng Qi Tang. If there is severe abdominal fullness with constipation, one may give Xiao Cheng Qi Tang, to mildly harmonise the stomach qi, do not induce potent purging.

Clause 209

陽明病， 潮熱，大便微硬者，可與大承氣湯，不硬者， 不可與之。若不大便六七日，恐有燥屎，欲知之法，少與小承氣湯，湯入腹中，轉矢氣者，,此有燥屎也， 乃可攻之；若不轉矢氣者，此但初頭硬，后必溏，不可攻之，攻之必脹滿不能食也。欲飲水者，與水則噦。其后發熱者，必大便復硬而少也，以小承氣湯和之。不轉矢氣者，慎不可攻也。小承氣湯。

Yang Ming disease, there is tidal fever, if the stool is slightly hard, one can give Da Cheng Qi Tang, if the stool is not hard, one should not give it. If no stool is passed for six or seven days, one fears the stool is dry, the way to find out is, give a little Xiao Cheng Qi Tang, once the decoction enters the abdomen, if faecal qi moves, this means there is a dry stool, so one can attack; if faecal qi does not move, it is hard only at the start, afterwards it will be sloppy, one should not attack, attacking will cause abdominal fullness and an inability to eat. If there is a desire to drink water, giving water will cause regurgitation. If after this there is fever, the stool will again be hard and scant, giving Xiao Cheng Qi Tang will harmonise. If faecal qi does not move, beware that one should not attack. Xiao Cheng Qi Tang.

NOTE: Clauses 207, 208 and 209 supplement Clauses 204, 205 and 206 in their description of Yang Ming patterns where purgation is appropriate; at the same time they explain the differentiation of purgation according to the severity of the pattern, and whether Xiao or Da Cheng Qi Tang is indicated.

Clause 210

夫實則譫語，虛則鄭聲。鄭聲者，重語也；直視、譫語、喘滿者死，下利者亦死。

Thus excess causes delirious speech, deficiency causes muttering. Muttering means repetitive speech; a fixed gaze, delirious speech, panting and fullness mean death; diarrhoea also means death.

Clause 211

發汗多，若重發汗者，亡其陽，譫語，脈短者死；脈自和者不死。

Heavy sweat is promoted, if sweating is promoted again, there will be collapse of yang and delirious speech, if the pulse is short, the person will die; where the pulse is spontaneously harmonised, the person will not die.

Clause 212

傷寒，若吐、若下後不解，不大便五六日，上至十余日，日晡所發潮熱，不惡寒，獨語如見鬼狀；若劇者，發則不識人，循衣摸床，惕而不安，微喘直視，脈弦者生，澀者死。微者，但發熱譫語者，大承氣湯主之。若一服利，則止後服。

Shang han, if, after emesis and purgation, there is no resolution, there is no stool for five or six days, even for more than ten days, in the late afternoon there will then be tidal fever, no aversion to cold, the person will talk to themself as if seeing ghosts; if it is serious, then they will not recognise anyone, will pick at their clothes and pat the bedding, be fearful and restless, will pant slightly and stare straight ahead, if the pulse is wiry, the person will live, if choppy they will die. If mild, where there is only fever with delirious speech, Da Cheng Qi Tang governs. If, having taken one dose, there is diarrhoea, then stop subsequent doses.

Clause 213

陽明病，其人多汗，以津液外出，胃中燥，大便必硬，硬則譫語，小承氣湯主之。若一服譫語止者，更莫復服。

Yang Ming disease, the person sweats profusely, due to body fluids exiting, there is dryness in the stomach, the stool will be hard, the hardness causes delirious speech, Xiao Cheng Qi Tang governs. If after one dose the delirious speech stops, no more should be given.

Clause 214

陽明病，譫語、發潮熱、脈滑而疾者，小承氣湯主之。因與承氣湯一升，腹中轉氣者，更服一升；若不轉氣者，勿更與之。明日又不大便，脈反微澀者，裡虛也，為難治，不可更與承氣湯也。

Yang Ming disease, if there is delirious speech, tidal fever, a pulse which is slippery and swift, Xiao Cheng Qi Tang governs. Because one sheng of Cheng Qi Tang was given, qi moves in the abdomen, then a further one sheng should be taken; if there is no moving of qi, a further dose should not be given. If the next day again there is no stool, moreover the pulse is faint and choppy, the interior is deficient, it is difficult to treat, one should not give any more Cheng Qi Tang.

Clause 215

陽明病，譫語、有潮熱、反不能食者，胃中必有燥屎五六枚也；若能食者，但硬耳。宜大承氣湯下之。

Yang Ming disease, if there is delirious speech, tidal fever but an inability to eat, there will be five or six lumps of dry stool in the stomach; where a person is able to eat, it is just hard. Da Cheng Qi Tang is appropriate.

Clause 216

陽明病，下血、譫語者，此為熱入血室。但頭汗出者，刺期門，隨其實而瀉之，濈然汗出則愈。

In Yang Ming disease, if blood descends and there is delirious speech, it means that heat has entered the chamber of blood. If there is sweating from the head only, needle Qi Men, address the excess by purging, and a continuous sweat will bring recovery.

Clause 217

汗出譫語者，以有燥屎在胃中，此為風也。須下者，過經乃可下之。下之若早，語言必亂，以表虛裡實故也。下之愈，宜大承氣湯。

If there is sweating and delirious speech, it is because of a dry stool in the stomach, this is wind. If one must purge, since it has passed through the channel then one may purge. If one purges early, speech will be deranged, this is because the exterior is deficient and the interior is excess. Purgation will bring recovery, Da Cheng Qi Tang is appropriate.

Clause 218

傷寒四五日，脈沉而喘滿，沉為在裡，而反發其汗，津液越出，大便為難，表虛裡實，久則譫語。

Shang han for four or five days, the pulse is submerged and there is panting and fullness, submerged means the disease is in the interior, however, sweating is promoted, body fluids vent outward, defaecation is difficult, the exterior is deficient and the interior is excess, if this endures, there will be delirious speech.

Clause 219

三陽合病，腹滿、身重，難以轉側，口不仁、面垢、譫語、遺尿。發汗，則譫語；下之則額上生汗、手足逆冷。若自汗出者，白虎湯主之。

Concurrent disease of the three yang, there is abdominal fullness, a sensation of heaviness, difficulty in turning over, the mouth is numb, the face grimy and there is delirious speech and enuresis. If sweat is promoted, there will be delirious speech; if purgation is used, sweat will appear on the forehead, and the hands and feet will be cold. If there is spontaneous sweating, Bai Hu Tang governs.

Clause 220

二陽並病，太陽証罷，但發潮熱，手足漐漐汗出，大便難而譫語者，下之則愈，宜大承氣湯。

Lagover pattern of the two yang, Tai Yang pattern has finished, but there is tidal fever, sweat pouring from the hands and feet, if passing a stool is difficult and there is delirious speech, purging will bring recovery, Da Cheng Qi Tang is appropriate.

NOTE: Clauses 210–220 discuss Yang Ming patterns marked by delirious speech and their prognosis.

Clause 221

陽明病，脈浮而緊、咽燥、口苦、腹滿而喘、發熱汗出、不惡寒反惡熱、身重。若發汗則躁，心憒憒，反譫語；若加溫針，必怵惕煩躁不得眠；若下之，則胃中空虛，客氣動膈，心中懊憹。舌上胎者，梔子豉湯主之。

Yang Ming disease, the pulse is floating and tight, the throat is dry, there is a bitter taste in the mouth, abdominal fullness and wheezing, fever and sweating, no aversion to cold but an aversion to heat, the body feels heavy. If sweating is promoted, there will be agitation, an unsettled heart with delirious speech; if warm needling is added, there will be apprehension, agitation and inability to sleep; if there is purgation, then the stomach will feel empty and hollow, visitant qi will stir the diaphragm, there will be anguish in the heart. If there is a coat on the tongue, Zhi Zi Chi Tang governs.

Clause 222

若渴欲飲水，口干舌燥者，白虎加人參湯主之。

If there is thirst with a desire to drink water, the mouth is dry and the tongue parched, Bai Hu jia Ren Shen Tang governs.

Clause 223

若脈浮、發熱、渴欲飲水、小便不利者，豬苓湯主之。

If the pulse is floating, there is fever, thirst with a desire to drink water, and the urination is not free, Zhu Ling Tang governs.

Clause 224

陽明病，汗出多而渴者，不可與豬苓湯。以汗多胃中燥，豬苓湯復利其小便故也。

Yang Ming disease, if there is profuse sweating and thirst, one should not give Zhu Ling Tang. Because of the profuse sweating, there is dryness in the stomach, Zhu Ling Tang will further promote urination.

NOTE: Clauses 221–224 describe the treatment of Yang Ming heat patterns.

Clause 225

脈浮而遲，表熱裡寒，下利清谷者，四逆湯主之。

When the pulse is floating and slow, there is heat in the exterior and cold in the interior, and diarrhoea with undigested food particles, Si Ni Tang governs.

Clause 226

若胃中冷，不能食者，飲水則噦。

If the stomach is cold, and the person can not eat, drinking will cause hiccoughs.

Clause 227

脈浮、發熱、口干、鼻燥，能食者則衄。

The pulse is floating, there is fever, the mouth is parched, the nose is dry, if the person can eat, then there will be external bleeding.

NOTE: Clauses 226 and 227 cite the ability or inability to eat as a criterion to differentiate between stomach heat and stomach cold.

Clause 228

陽明病下之，其外有熱，手足溫，不結胸，心中懊憹，飢不能食，但頭汗出者，梔子豉湯主之。

Yang Ming disease treated with purgation, there is heat in the exterior, the hands and feet are warm, there is no chest bind, if there is anguish, hunger with no desire to eat, sweating from the head only, Zhi Zi Chi Tang governs.

Clause 229

陽明病，發潮熱、大便溏、小便自可、胸脅滿不去者，與小柴胡湯。

Yang Ming disease, if there is tidal fever, the stool is sloppy, urination is as usual, and fullness in the chest and ribs does not abate, give Xiao Chai Hu Tang.

Clause 230

陽明病，脅下硬滿，不大便而嘔，舌上白胎者，可與小柴胡湯。上焦得通，津液得下，胃氣因和，身濈然汗出而解。

Yang Ming disease, if there is hardness and fullness under the ribs, no stool but vomiting, and a white tongue coat, one may give Xiao Chai Hu Tang. The upper jiao is freed, body fluids descend, the stomach qi is therefore harmonised, there is continuous sweat and recovery.

Clause 231

陽明中風，脈弦浮大，而短氣、腹都滿，脅下及心痛，久按之氣不通，鼻干，不得汗，嗜臥，一身及目悉黃，小便難，有潮熱，時時噦，耳前后腫，刺之小差，外不解。病過十日，脈續浮者，與小柴胡湯。

Yang Ming zhong feng, the pulse is wiry, floating and big, and there is shortness of breath, distension throughout the abdomen, pain under the ribs and in the heart, a sense of qi blockage under prolonged pressure, a dry nose, an absence of sweat, a desire to lie down, the body and eyes are all yellow, urination is difficult, there is tidal fever, constant hiccoughing, swelling in front of and behind the ear, needling gives some relief, the exterior is not resolved. The disease has lasted over ten days, if the pulse is still floating, give Xiao Chai Hu Tang.

Clause 232

脈但浮，無余証者，與麻黃湯。若不尿，腹滿加噦者，不治。

If there is only a floating pulse, no other sign, give Ma Huang Tang. If there is no urination, and abdominal distension with hiccoughing, it is not treatable.

Clause 233

陽明病，自汗出，若發汗，小便自利者，此為津液內竭，雖硬不可攻之；當須自欲大便，宜蜜煎導而通之。若土瓜根及大豬膽汁，皆可為導。

Yang Ming disease, there is spontaneous sweating, if sweating is promoted, if the urination is spontaneously free, this is exhaustion of body fluids in the interior, although there is hardness, one should not attack; there must be a natural urge to pass a stool, Mi Jian Dao is appropriate to lead and unblock. If there is Tu Gua Gen and the bile from a large pig, both can lead.

NOTE: Clauses 228–233 describe various strategies in the treatment of Yang Ming disease.

Clause 234

陽明病，脈遲，汗出多，微惡寒者，表未解也，可發汗，宜桂枝湯。

Yang Ming disease, the pulse is slow, there is copious sweating, if there is a mild aversion to cold, the exterior is not resolved, one may promote sweating, Gui Zhi Tang is appropriate.

Clause 235

陽明病、脈浮、無汗而喘者，發汗則愈，宜麻黃湯。

Yang Ming disease, the pulse is floating, if there is no sweating but there is wheezing, the promotion of sweating will bring recovery, Ma Huang Tang is appropriate.

NOTE: Clause 234 describes a Yang Ming pattern where there is unresolved exterior deficiency, where the indicated formula is Gui Zhi Tang, while Clause 235 describes Yang Ming disease with unresolved exterior excess, where the indicated formula is Ma Huang Tang; nevertheless, Zhong Jing nominates these formulas as being "appropriate", and does not give them the status of "governing" formulas.

Clause 236

陽明病，發熱、汗出者，此為熱越，不能發黃也。但頭汗出，身無汗，劑頸而還，小便不利，渴引水漿者，此為瘀熱在裡，身必發黃，茵陳蒿湯主之。

Yang Ming disease, if there is fever and sweating, this means the heat is passing on, there will be no yellowing. If there is sweat only from the head, no sweat from the body, stopping at the neck, the urination is not free, there is thirst which leads to fluids, this is stasis heat in the interior, the body will turn yellow, Yin Chen Hao Tang governs.

Clause 237

陽明証，其人喜忘者，必有畜血。所以然者，本有久瘀血，故令喜忘；屎雖硬，大便反易，其色必黑者，宜抵當湯下之。

Yang Ming pattern, the person is forgetful, there must be blood amassment. The reason for this being, originally there was prolonged blood stasis, so this caused the forgetfulness. Although the stool is hard, the stool is nevertheless easily passed, since the colour will be black, Di Dang Tang is appropriate.

NOTE: The indicated formula for Yang Ming damp heat jaundice is Yin Chen Hao Tang while treatment for Yang Ming blood heat jaundice is Di Dang Tang.

Clause 238

陽明病，下之，心中懊憹而煩，胃中有燥屎者，可攻。腹微滿，初頭硬，後必溏，不可攻之。若有燥屎者，宜大承氣湯。

Yang Ming disease, there is purgation, if there is anguish and vexation, and a dry stool in the stomach, one may attack. There is mild abdominal fullness, the start of the stool is hard, the end will be sloppy, one should not purge. If there is a dry stool, Da Cheng Qi Tang is appropriate.

Clause 239

病人不大便五六日，繞臍痛、煩躁、發作有時者，此有燥屎，故使不大便也。

The patient has not passed a stool for five or six days, if there is pain around the umbilicus, vexation and agitation, occurring periodically, this is because there is a dry stool, causing constipation.

Clause 240

病人煩熱，汗出則解；又如瘧狀，日晡所發熱者，屬陽明也。脈實者，宜下之；脈浮虛者，宜發汗。下之與大承氣湯，發汗宜桂枝湯。

The patient is vexed and has a fever, sweating brings resolution; then there are malaria-like symptoms, if in the late afternoon there is tidal fever, this pertains to Yang Ming. If the pulse is excess, purgation is appropriate; if the pulse is floating and deficient, sweat promotion is appropriate. For purgation give Da Cheng Qi Tang, to promote sweating Gui Zhi Tang is appropriate.

Clause 241

大下後，六七日不大便，煩不解，腹滿痛者，此有燥屎也。所以然者，本有宿食故也。宜大承氣湯。

After strong purging, if there is no stool for six or seven days, unresolved vexation, the abdomen is full and painful, this means there is a dry stool. The reason for this being, originally there was accumulated food. Da Cheng Qi Tang is appropriate.

Clause 242

病人小便不利，大便乍難乍易，時有微熱，喘冒不能臥者，有燥屎也，宜大承氣湯。

The patient's urination is not free, passing a stool is sometimes difficult and sometimes easy, with an occasional mild fever, if there is wheeze and dizziness with an inability to sleep, there is a dry stool, Da Cheng Qi Tang is appropriate.

Clause 243

食谷欲嘔，屬陽明也，吳茱萸湯主之；得湯反劇者，屬上焦也.

An urge to vomit after eating food pertains to Yang Ming, Wu Zhu Yu Tang governs; if taking the decoction makes the condition worse instead, it pertains to the upper jiao.

NOTE: Clauses 238–243 describe Yang Ming bowel excess and the methods of pattern identification in order to determine whether purgation is appropriate. They should be read with Clauses 208, 209, 212, 215, 217, 220, 238 and 239.

Clause 244

太陽病，寸緩關浮尺弱，其人發熱汗出，復惡寒，不嘔，但心下痞者，此以醫下之也。如其不下者，病人不惡寒而渴者，此轉屬陽明也。小便數者，大便必硬，不更衣十日，無所苦也。渴欲飲水，少少與之，但以法救之。渴者，宜五苓散。

Tai Yang disease, if the cun is moderate, the guan is floating and cubit is weak, the person has fever and sweating, followed by aversion to cold, no retching, but glomus below the heart, this is because the physician purged. If no purgation was used, the patient has no aversion to cold and is thirsty, it has shifted to the Yang Ming. If urination is frequent, the stool will be hard, with no change of clothes for ten days, without any discomfort. There is thirst with a desire to drink water, give a little, only by this method will there be recovery. If there is thirst, Wu Ling San is appropriate.

Clause 245

脈陽微而汗出少者，為自和也；汗出多者，為太過。陽脈實，因發其汗，出多者，亦為太過。 太過者，為陽絕於裡，亡津液， 大便因硬也。

The pulse is yang and faint and there is a mild sweat, this means there is spontaneous harmony; if there is profuse sweating, this is excessive. If the yang pulse is full, because the sweating was profuse, then this is excessive. Excessive means that yang is exhausted in the interior, fluids are devastated, hence the stool is hard.

Clause 246

脈浮而芤， 浮為陽，芤為陰，浮芤相搏，胃氣生熱，其陽則絕。

The pulse is floating and hollow, floating is yang, hollow is yin, the floating contends with the hollow, the stomach qi generates heat, the yang will be devastated.

Clause 247

趺陽脈浮而澀，浮則胃氣強，澀則小便數；浮澀相搏，大便則硬，其脾為約，麻子仁丸主之。

The Fu Yang pulse is floating and choppy, floating denotes strong stomach qi and choppy denotes frequent urination; the floating and choppy pulses contend with each other, the stool is hard, this means the spleen is restrained, Ma Zi Ren Wan governs.

NOTE: Clauses 244–247 describe the pathogenesis and treatment of pi yue or spleen restriction, which is attributed to exuberant heat and fluid damage.

Clause 248

太陽病三日，發汗不解，蒸蒸發熱者，屬胃也，調胃承氣湯主之。

Tai Yang disease for three days, the promotion of sweat does not resolve it, there is steaming heat, it pertains to the stomach, Tiao Wei Cheng Qi Tang governs.

Clause 249

傷寒吐後，腹脹滿者，與調胃承氣湯。

Shang han disease after vomiting, if the abdomen is distended and full, give Tiao Wei Cheng Qi Tang.

Clause 250

太陽病，若吐、若下、若發汗後，微煩，小便數、大便因硬者，與小承氣湯，和之愈。

Tai Yang disease, after vomiting, purgation and sweat promotion, if there is mild vexation, frequent urination, causing the stool to be hard, give Xiao Cheng Qi Tang, to harmonise and bring recovery.

Clause 251

得病二三日，脈弱，無太陽、柴胡証，煩躁、心下硬；至四五日，雖能食，以小承氣湯，少少與，微和之，令小安；至六日，與承氣湯一升。若不大便六七日，小便少者，雖不受食，但初頭硬，後必溏，未定成硬，攻之必溏；須小便利，屎定硬，乃可攻之，宜大承氣湯。

Sickness for two or three days, the pulse is weak, there is no sign of a Tai Yang or Chai Hu pattern, there is vexation and agitation, hardness below the heart; on the fourth or fifth day, even if able to eat, give a very small dose of Xiao Cheng Qi Tang to mildly harmonise, and calm a little; on the sixth day, give one sheng of Cheng Qi Tang. Where there is no stool for six or seven days, if the urination is scant, even if there is an inability to eat, the stool is hard only at the start, afterwards it will be sloppy, there is no formation of hardness, attacking will cause sloppiness; the urination must be free, the stool formed hard, then one may attack, Da Cheng Qi Tang is appropriate.

Clause 252

傷寒六七日，目中不了了，睛不和，無表裡証，大便難，身微熱者，此為實也。急下之，宜大承氣湯。

Shang han for six or seven days, the vision is not clear, there is no harmony in the eyes, there is neither an exterior nor an interior pattern, passing a stool is difficult, the body emits a mild heat, this is excess. Urgent purgation is needed, Da Cheng Qi Tang is appropriate.

Clause 253

陽明病，發熱、汗多者，急下之，宜大承氣湯。

Yang Ming disease, if there is fever and copious sweating, for urgent purgation, Da Cheng Qi Tang is appropriate.

Clause 254

發汗不解，腹滿痛者，急下之，宜大承氣湯。

Promoting sweat does not bring resolution, if there is abdominal fullness and pain, for urgent purgation, Da Cheng Qi Tang is appropriate.

Clause 255

腹滿不減，減不足言，當下之，宜大承氣湯。

Abdominal fullness is not reduced, or reduction is inadequate so to speak, one must purge, Da Cheng Qi Tang is appropriate.

Clause 256

陽明少陽合病，必下利，其脈不負者，為順也；負者，失也，互相克賊，名為負也，脈滑而數者，有宿食也，當下之，宜大承氣湯。

In a concurrent pattern of Yang Ming and Shao Yang, there will be diarrhoea, if the pulse has no deficit, it is favourable; if it has a deficit, this is loss, mutual subjugation and plunder, this is deficit, if the pulse is slippery and rapid, there is accumulated food, one must purge, Da Cheng Qi Tang is appropriate.

NOTE: Clauses 248–256 describe the use of the three Cheng Qi Tang: Clauses 248 and 249 refer to Tiao Wei Cheng Qi Tang; Clause 250 gives the indications for Xiao Cheng Qi Tang; Clause 251 distinguishes between Xiao and Da Cheng Qi Tang on the basis of the ability or inability to eat; Clauses 252, 253 and 254 describe the three urgent purgation patterns of Yang Ming; Clauses 255 and 256 also describe patterns where purging is urgent, but instead of the term "urgent purgation", the phrase "one must purge" is used. The general application of the three Cheng Qi Tang is described earlier in Clauses 207–209; Yang Ming bowel excess with delirious speech and the use of Da and Xiao Cheng Qi Tang is described in Clauses 210–218; and the use of Da Cheng Qi Tang to purge a hard stool is described Clauses 238–242.

Clause 257

病人無表裡証，發熱七八日，雖脈浮數者，可下之。假令已下，脈數不解，合熱則消谷善飢，至六七日，不大便者，有瘀血，宜抵當湯。

The patient has neither an exterior nor an interior pattern, with fever for seven or eight days, although the pulse is floating and rapid, one may purge. If purgation was already used, the pulse is rapid and there is no resolution, there is combined heat causing rapid digestion with insatiable hunger, if for six or seven days there is no stool, there is blood stasis, Di Dang Tang is appropriate.

Clause 258

若脈數不解，而下不止，必協熱便膿血也。

If the pulse is rapid and there is no resolution, and there is incessant diarrhoea, there will be heat combined with pus and blood in the stool.

Clause 259

傷寒發汗已，身目為黃，所以然者，以寒濕在裡不解故也。以為不可下也，於寒濕中求之。

Shang han where sweat was promoted, the body and eyes are yellow, the reason for this being, cold damp is unresolved in the interior. Presumably one should not purge, seek the cold and damp.

Clause 260

傷寒七八日，身黃如橘子色，小便不利，腹微滿者，茵陳蒿湯主之。

Shang han for seven or eight days, if the body is yellow like the colour of a mandarin, the urination is not free, and the abdomen is slightly distended, Yin Chen Hao Tang governs.

Clause 261

傷寒身黃，發熱。梔子柏皮湯主之。

Shang han, the body is yellow, and there is fever. Zhi Zi Bai Pi Tang governs.

Clause 262

傷寒瘀熱在裡，身必黃， 麻黃連軺 赤小豆湯主之。

Shang han with stasis heat in the interior, the body will turn yellow, Ma Huang Lian Qiao Chi Xiao Dou Tang governs.

NOTE: Clauses 259–262 describe Yang Ming jaundice patterns and their differential treatments: Clause 259 describes jaundice due to cold damp; Clause 260 focuses on damp heat in the interior; Clause 261 describes the treatment of damp heat where there is possibly more heat than damp but with no reference to either the exterior or interior; Clause 262 describes the treatment of damp heat with an exterior pattern. Other clauses relating to jaundice are: Clause 195, which describes grain jaundice; Clause 236, which describes a Yin Chen Hao Tang pattern; Clause 231, which describes a concurrent pattern of the three yan, where Xiao Chai Hu Tang is indicated to treat the jaundice; and Clause 200, which describes Yang Ming jaundice resulting from adverse fire therapy. Thus Yang Ming jaundice patterns can be categorised as damp heat, cold damp, jaundice due to fire therapy, and the jaundice of a concurrent pattern of the three yang. The principal pattern is damp heat.

CLAUSES 263–272: SHAO YANG CHAPTER

Clause 263

少陽之為病，口苦、咽干、目眩也。

Shao Yang disease, the mouth has a bitter taste, the throat is dry, the eyes are dizzy.

NOTE: Principal features of Shao Yang disease.

Clause 264

少陽中風，兩耳無所聞、目赤、胸中滿而煩者，不可吐下，吐下則悸而驚。

Shao Yang zhong feng, the two ears can not hear, the eyes are scarlet, if there is fullness in the chest and vexation, one should not induce vomiting or purgation, vomiting and purgation will cause palpitations and fright.

Clause 265

傷寒，脈弦細、頭痛發熱者，屬少陽。少陽不可發汗，發汗則譫語。此屬胃，胃和則愈；胃不和，煩而悸。

Shang han, if the pulse is wiry and fine and there is headache and fever, it pertains to Shao Yang. In Shao Yang, one should not promote sweat, the promotion of sweat can cause delirious speech. This pertains to the stomach, harmony of the stomach will bring recovery; if there is disharmony of the stomach, there will be vexation and palpitations.

NOTE: Clauses 264 and 265 are associated with contraindications in Shao Yang disease, with the implication that the correct treatment for Shao Yang disease is harmonisation.

Clause 266

本太陽病不解，傳入少陽者，脅下硬滿，干嘔不能食，往來寒熱，尚未吐下，脈沉緊者，與小柴胡湯。

Originally Tai Yang disease was not resolved, if it transmits to Shao Yang, there is hardness and fullness under the ribs, dry retching and an inability to eat, alternating chills and fever, and there is neither emetic nor purgation, the pulse is submerged and tight, give Xiao Chai Hu Tang.

Clause 267

若已吐、下、發汗、溫針、譫語，柴胡湯証罷，此為壞病。知犯何逆，以法治之。

If after vomiting, purgation, sweat promotion or warm needling, there is delirious speech, the Chai Hu Tang pattern is finished, this is transmuted disease. Know the error committed, and treat according to the rule.

NOTE: Clause 266 is a description of disease transmission from Tai Yang to Shao Yang as a result of incorrect treatment; Clause 267 describes the treatment principle for a transmuted pattern with delirious speech resulting from the incorrect use of emetics, purgation and sweat promotion. The same principle is expressed in Clause 16.

Clause 268

三陽合病，脈浮大，上關上，但欲眠睡，目合則汗。

Concurrent disease of the three yang, the pulse is floating and big, rising from the guan to the cun position, the person wants only to sleep, when the eyes close there is sweating.

Clause 269

傷寒六七日，無大熱，其人躁煩者，此為陽去入陰故也。

Shang han for six or seven days, without a high fever, if the person is agitated and vexed, this is because the yang is receding and entering yin.

Clause 270

傷寒三日，三陽為盡，三陰當受邪。其人反能食而不嘔，此為三陰不受邪也。

Shang han for three days, the three yang are ended, the three yin must contract the evil. The person can nevertheless eat and there is no vomiting, this is because the three yin do not contract the evil.

Clause 271

傷寒三日，少陽脈小者，欲已也。

Shang han for three days, if the Shao Yang pulse is small, it is about to end.

Clause 272

少陽病欲解時，從寅至辰上。

The time that Shao Yang disease is ready to resolve, is from yin to chen.

NOTE: Clauses 268–272 describe possible changes associated with Shao Yang disease.

CLAUSES 273–280: TAI YIN CHAPTER

Clause 273

太陰之為病，腹滿而吐，食不下，自利益甚，時腹自痛，若下之，必胸下結硬。

Tai Yin is diseased, the abdomen is full and there is vomiting, there is an inability to eat, extreme spontaneous diarrhoea, periodic spontaneous pain in the abdomen, if there is purging, there will be a knotted hardness below the chest.

NOTE: Principal features of Tai Yin disease.

Clause 274

太陰中風，四肢煩疼，陽微陰澀而長者，為欲愈。

Tai Yin zhong feng, there is vexing pain in the four limbs, if yang is faint, yin is choppy but long, it is about to recover.

Clause 275

太陰病欲解時，從亥至丑上。

The time that Tai Yin disease is ready to resolve, recovery is from hai to chou.

Clause 276

太陰病、脈浮者，可發汗，宜桂枝湯。

Tai Yin disease, if the pulse is floating, one may promote sweat, Gui Zhi Tang is appropriate.

NOTE: Clauses 274, 275 and 276 describe factors associated with spontaneous recovery of Tai Yin disease.

Clause 277

自利不渴者，屬太陰，以其臟有寒故也，當溫之。宜服四逆輩。

If there is spontaneous diarrhoea without thirst, is pertains to Tai Yin, because there is cold in the zang organ, and one should warm.

It is appropriate to administer a Si Ni type of formula.

NOTE: Indicated treatment for Tai Yin disease.

Clause 278

傷寒，脈浮而緩，手足自溫者，系在太陰；太陰當發身黃，若小便自利者，不能發黃；至七八日，雖暴煩下利，日十余行，必自止，以脾家實，腐穢去故也。

Shang han, the pulse is floating and moderate, if the hands and feet are spontaneously warm, this is in the Tai Yin; in Tai Yin the body should become yellow, if urination is spontaneously free, there can be no yellowing; on the seventh or eighth day, despite sudden vexation and diarrhoea, occurring over ten times a day, it will stop spontaneously, due to the spleen's domain being in excess, putrid filth is being eliminated.

Clause 279

本太陽病，醫反下之，因爾腹滿時痛者，屬太陰也，桂枝加芍藥湯主之。大實痛者，桂枝加大黃湯主之。

Originally there was Tai Yang disease, the physician nevertheless purges, if because of this the abdomen is full and there is periodic pain, it pertains to Tai Yin, Gui Zhi jia Shao Yao Tang governs. If there is strong excess pain, Gui Zhi jia Da Huang Tang governs.

Clause 280

太陰為病，脈弱，其人續自便利，設當行大黃芍藥者，宜減之，以其人胃氣弱，易動故也。

Tai Yin is diseased, the pulse is weak, the person continues to have spontaneous diarrhoea, if Da Huang and Shao Yao are to be given, it is appropriate to reduce, because the person's stomach qi is weak, so it is easily affected.

NOTE: Clauses 278, 279 and 280 describe the treatment of Tai Yin disease and transmuted patterns.

CLAUSES 281–325: SHAO YIN CHAPTER

Clause 281

少陰之為病，脈微細，但欲寐也。

Shao Yin is diseased, the pulse is faint and thready, the person desires only to sleep.

Clause 282

少陰病，欲吐不吐，心煩但欲寐，五六日自利而渴者，屬少陰也。虛故引水自救；若小便色白者，少陰病形悉具，小便白者，以下焦虛有寒，不能制水，故令色白也。

Shao Yin disease, there is an urge to vomit but no vomiting, the heart is vexed and the person wants only to sleep, if on the fifth or sixth day there is diarrhoea and thirst, this pertains to Shao Yin. There is deficiency so taking water will give spontaneous relief; if the colour of the urine is clear, the signs of Shao Yin are all there, if urine is clear, it is because there is deficiency and cold in the lower jiao, an inability to control water, and so it causes the colour to be clear.

Clause 283

病人脈陰陽俱緊，反汗出者，亡陽也，此屬少陰，法當咽痛而復吐利。

The patient's yin and yang pulse are both tight, nevertheless there is sweating, this is devastation of yang, it pertains to Shao Yin, there will be a sore throat and then vomiting and diarrhoea.

NOTE: Clauses 282 and 283 describe supplementary symptoms of Shao Yin disease which show that a yang deficiency pattern may have some features which resemble a heat pattern.

Clause 284

少陰病，咳而下利、譫語者，被火氣劫故也。小便必難，以強責少陰汗也。

Shao Yin disease, if there is cough and diarrhoea with delirious speech, it is due to being raided by fire. Urination will be difficult, because sweating was wrongly forced in Shao Yin.

Clause 285

少陰病，脈細沉數，病為在裡，不可發汗。

Shao Yin disease, the pulse is thready, submerged and rapid, the disease is in the interior, one should not promote sweating.

NOTE: Clauses 284 and 285 describe a yin deficiency pattern of Shao Yin, drawing the readers' attention to the fact that Shao Yin patterns can be categorised as either cold conversion or heat conversion patterns.

Clause 286

少陰病，脈微，不可發汗，亡陽故也。陽已虛，尺脈弱濇者，復不可下之。

Shao Yin disease, the pulse is faint, one should not promote sweat, because yang will be devastated. If yang is already deficient and the cubit pulse is weak and choppy, one should also not purge.

NOTE: Sweat promotion is contraindicated in both yin deficiency and yang deficiency patterns of Shao Yin. Clause 286 reinforces that neither sweat promotion nor purgation is used in the treatment of Shao Yin disease.

Clause 287

少陰病，脈緊，至七八日自下利，脈暴微，手足反溫，脈緊反去者，為欲解也。雖煩、下利，必自愈。

Shao Yin disease, the pulse is tight, on the seventh or eighth day there is spontaneous diarrhoea, the pulse is suddenly faint, nevertheless the hands and feet are warm, this means it is about to resolve. Even though there is vexation and diarrhoea, there will be spontaneous recovery.

Clause 288

少陰病，下利。若利自止，惡寒而蜷臥，手足溫者，可治。

Shao Yin disease, there is diarrhoea. If the diarrhoea stops spontaneously, there is aversion to cold and a curled up sleeping posture, and the hands and feet are warm, it is treatable.

Clause 289

少陰病，惡寒而蜷，時自煩，欲去衣被者，可治。

Shao Yin disease, there is aversion to cold and a curled up posture, if there is occasional vexation, and a desire to remove the bedclothes, the condition is treatable.

Clause 290

少陰中風，脈陽微陰浮者，為欲愈。

Shao Yin zhong feng, if the pulse is faint in yang and floating in yin, this means there is about to be recovery.

Clause 291

少陰病欲解時，從子至寅上。

The time that Shao Yin disease is ready to resolve, is from zi to yin.

Clause 292

少陰病，吐、利，手足不逆冷，反發熱者，不死。脈不至者，灸少陰七壯。

Shao Yin disease, there is vomiting and diarrhoea, if the hands and feet have no reversal cold, but there is fever, the person will not die. If the pulse does not arrive, use seven cones of moxa on Shao Yin.

NOTE: Clauses 288–292 describe the circumstances associated with spontaneous recovery in Shao Yin disease.

Clause 293

少陰病，八九日，一身手足盡熱者，以熱在膀胱，必便血也。

Shao Yin disease, for eight or nine days, if the whole body and hands and feet are extremely hot, it is because of heat in the urinary bladder, there will be blood in the urine.

NOTE: This describes a pattern of Shao Yin disease associated with the excessive return of yang.

Clause 294

少陰病，但厥、無汗，而強發之，必動其血。未知從何道出，或從口鼻，或從目出者，是名下厥上竭，為難治。

Shao Yin disease, there is only reversal and no sweating, but there has been forced promotion, the blood will stir. It is not known from which passage it will issue, whether from the mouth and nose, or from the eyes, it is known as lower reversal and upper exhaustion, it is difficult to treat.

Clause 295

少陰病，惡寒、身蜷而利、手足逆冷者，不治。

Shao Yin disease, if there is aversion to cold, a curled up posture and diarrhoea, and the hands and feet suffer reversal cold, it is not treatable.

Clause 296

少陰病，吐利躁煩，四逆者，死。

Shao Yin disease, there is vomiting, diarrhoea, agitation and vexation, if the four are reversed, the person will die.

Clause 297

少陰病，下利止而頭眩，時時自冒者，死。

Shao Yin disease, if the diarrhoea ceases and there is dizziness, with periodic loss of lucidity and blurred vision, the person will die.

Clause 298

少陰病，四逆、惡寒而身蜷、脈不至、不煩而躁者，死。

Shao Yin disease, the four are reversed, there is aversion to cold and a curled up posture, if the pulse does not arrive, and there is no vexation but there is agitation, the person will die.

Clause 299

少陰病六七日，息高者，死。

Shao Yin disease for six or seven days, if the breathing is shallow, the person will die.

Clause 300

少陰病，脈微細沉、但欲臥、汗出不煩、自欲吐，至五六日自利，復煩躁不得臥寐者，死。

Shao Yin disease, the pulse is faint, thready and submerged, the person wants to do nothing but sleep, there is sweating without vexation, and an urge to vomit spontaneously, if on the fifth or sixth day there is spontaneous diarrhoea, then vexation and agitation and an inability to sleep, the person will die.

NOTE: Clauses 294–300 are associated with difficult-to-treat disease and terminal disease in Shao Yin.

Clause 301

少陰病，始得之，反發熱、脈沉者，麻黃細辛附子湯主之。

Shao Yin disease, has just started, nevertheless if there is fever and the pulse is submerged, Ma Huang Xi Xin Fu Zi Tang governs.

Clause 302

少陰病，得之二三日，麻黃附子甘草湯微發汗。以二三日無証，故微發汗也。

Shao Yin disease, contracted for two or three days, Ma Huang Fu Zi Gan Cao Tang promotes a mild sweat. Because there were no symptoms for two or three days, a mild sweat must be promoted.

NOTE: Clauses 301 and 302 describe two different concurrent patterns of Tai Yang and Shao Yin.

Clause 303

少陰病，得之二三日以上，心中煩、不得臥，黃連阿膠湯主之。

Shao Yin disease, contracted for more than two or three days, there is vexation in the heart and an inability to sleep, Huang Lian E Jiao Tang governs.

NOTE: Shao Yin heat conversion symptoms and treatment.

Clause 304

少陰病，得之一二曰，口中和，其背惡寒者，當灸之，附子湯主之。

Shao Yin disease, contracted for one or two days, there is harmony in the mouth, the back is averse to cold, moxibustion should be used, Fu Zi Tang governs.

Clause 305

少陰病，身體痛，手足寒，骨節痛，脈沉者，附子湯主之。

Shao Yin disease, if the body is aching, the hands and feet are cold, there is joint pain, and the pulse is deep, Fu Zi Tang governs.

NOTE: Clauses 303 and 304 add to Clauses 301 and 302 by describing yet another Shao Yin exterior cold pattern. However, the yang deficiency is more severe and the cold pathogen more deep-seated than the Ma Huang Fu Zi Xi Xin Tang and Ma Huang Fu Zi Gan Cao Tang patterns described in the earlier clauses.

Clause 306

少陰病，下利便膿血者，桃花湯主之。

Shao Yin disease, if there is diarrhoea with pus and blood in the stool, Tao Hua Tang governs.

Clause 307

少陰病，二三日至四五日，腹痛，小便不利，下利不止，便膿血者，桃花湯主之。

Shao Yin disease, for two, three or even four or five days, if there is abdominal pain, the urination is not free, there is incessant diarrhoea, with pus and blood in the stool, Tao Hua Tang governs.

Clause 308

少陰病, 下利, 便膿血之者, 可刺。

Shao Yin disease, if there is diarrhoea, with pus and blood in the stool, one may needle.

Clause 309

少陰病，吐利，手足逆冷，煩躁欲死者，吳茱萸湯主之。

Shao Yin disease, if there is vomiting and diarrhoea, reversal cold of the hands and feet, vexation and agitation with a feeling one is about to die, Wu Zhu Yu Tang governs.

NOTE: Clauses 306–309 describe different patterns of Shao Yin diarrhoea.

Clause 310

少陰病，下利、咽痛、胸滿、心煩，豬膚湯主之。

Shao Yin disease, there is diarrhoea, the throat is sore, the chest feels full, the heart is vexed, Zhu Fu Tang governs.

Clause 311

少陰病二三日，咽痛者，可與甘草湯；不差，與桔梗湯。

Shao Yin disease for two or three days, if the throat is sore, one may give Gan Cao Tang; if there is no relief, give Jie Geng Tang.

Clause 312

少陰病，咽中傷、生瘡、不能語言、聲不出者，苦酒湯主之。

Shao Yin disease, if there is injury to the throat, an abscess has formed, the person can not speak, or there is no voice, Ku Jiu Tang governs.

Clause 313

少陰病，咽中痛，半夏散及湯主之。

Shao Yin disease, there is pain in the throat, Ban Xia San and Tang govern.

NOTE: Clauses 310–313 describe Shao Yin sore throat patterns.

Clause 314

少陰病，下利，白通湯主之。

Shao Yin disease, there is diarrhoea, Bai Tong Tang governs.

Clause 315

少陰病，下利，脈微者，與白通湯。利不止，厥逆無脈，干嘔，煩者，白通加豬膽汁湯主之。服湯，脈暴出者死，微續者生。

Shao Yin disease, if there is diarrhoea and the pulse is faint, give Bai Tong Tang. If the diarrhoea does not stop, there is desertion reversal and no pulse, dry retching and vexation, Bai Tong jia Zhu Dan Zhi Tang governs. Having taken the decoction, if the pulse suddenly rises the person will die, if a faint pulse continues, they will live.

Clause 316

少陰病，二三日不已，至四五日，腹痛，小便不利，四肢沉重疼痛，自下利者，此為有水氣。其人或咳，或小便利，或下利，或嘔者，真武湯主之。

Shao Yin disease, not finished on the second or third day, if by the fourth or fifth day, there is abdominal pain, the urination is not free, the four limbs are heavy and aching, and there is spontaneous diarrhoea, this is because of water qi. If the person either has a cough, or the urination is free, or there is diarrhoea, or vomiting, Zhen Wu Tang governs.

Clause 317

少陰病，下利清谷，裡寒外熱，手足厥逆，脈微欲絕，身反不惡寒，其人面色赤，或腹滿，或干嘔，或咽痛，或利止脈不出者，通脈四逆湯主之。

Shao Yin disease, there is diarrhoea with undigested food, the interior is cold and the exterior is hot, there is desertion reversal of the hands and feet, the pulse is faint and about to expire, the body is nevertheless not averse to cold, if the person's face is crimson, or there is abdominal distension, or there is dry retching, or the throat is sore, or the diarrhoea ceases and the pulse is not palpable, Tong Mai Si Ni Tang governs.

NOTE: Clauses 314–317 describe Shao Yin cold conversion with diarrhoea as the key symptom.

Clause 318

少陰病，四逆，其人或咳，或悸，或小便不利，或腹中痛，或泄利下重者，四逆散主之。

Shao Yin disease, the four are reversed, if the person has either a cough, or palpitations, or the urination is not free, or there is pain in the abdomen, or diarrhoea with heaviness below, Si Ni San governs.

Clause 319

少陰病，下利六七日，咳而嘔、渴、心煩、不得眠者，豬苓湯主之。

Shao Yin disease, there has been diarrhoea for six or seven days, if there is coughing and vomiting, thirst, heart vexation and an inability to sleep, Zhu Ling Tang governs.

NOTE: This is a yin deficiency pattern of Shao Yin with water and heat bind.

Clause 320

少陰病，得之二三日，口燥咽干者，急下之，宜大承氣湯。

Shao Yin disease, contracted for two or three days, if the mouth is parched and the throat is dry, one should urgently purge, Da Cheng Qi Tang is appropriate.

Clause 321

少陰病，自利清水，色純青，心下必痛，口干燥者，可下之，宜大承氣湯。

Shao Yin disease, spontaneous watery diarrhoea of a greenish colour, there will be pain below the heart, if the mouth is parched, one may purge, Da Cheng Qi Tang is appropriate.

Clause 322

少陰病，六七日，腹脹、不大便者，急下之，宜大承氣湯。

Shao Yin disease, for six or seven days, if the abdomen is distended and there is no stool, one should urgently purge, Da Cheng Qi Tang is appropriate.

NOTE: Clauses 320, 321 and 323 describe the three urgent purgation patterns in Shao Yin.

Clause 323

少陰病，脈沉者，急溫之，宜四逆湯。

Shao Yin disease, if the pulse is submerged, one must urgently warm, Si Ni Tang is appropriate.

Clause 324

少陰病，飲食入口則吐；心中溫溫欲吐，復不能吐。始得之，手足寒，脈弦遲者，此胸中實，不可下也，當吐之。若膈上有寒飲，干嘔者，不可吐也，當溫之，宜四逆湯。

Shao Yin disease, as soon as food and drink are eaten, there is vomiting; there is discomfort in the heart and an urge to vomit, then an inability to vomit. In the beginning if the hands and feet are cold, the pulse is wiry and slow, this is excess in the chest, one should not purge, one must induce vomiting. If there is cold fluid above the diaphragm, and dry retching, one should not induce vomiting, one must warm, Si Ni Tang is appropriate.

Clause 325

少陰病，下利，脈微澀，嘔而汗出，必數更衣，反少者，當溫其上，灸之。

Shao Yin disease, there is diarrhoea, a faint and choppy pulse, vomiting and sweating, and there should be a frequent change of clothes, if instead the stool is infrequent, one should warm the upper jiao, using moxibustion.

NOTE: Clauses 323, 324 and 325 present further discussion of Shao Yin deficiency cold patterns. It can be said that Shao Yin deficiency cold patterns are attributed to deficiency of the heart and kidney.

CLAUSES 326–381: JUE YIN CHAPTER

Clause 326

厥陰之為病，消渴，氣上撞心，心中疼熱，飢而不欲食，食則吐蛔、下之利不止。

Jue Yin is diseased, there is quenchless thirst, qi rushes upward to the heart, there is burning pain in the chest, hunger with no desire to eat, eating causes the vomiting of roundworms and purgation causes incessant diarrhoea.

NOTE: Principal features of Jue Yin heat and cold complex pattern.

Clause 327

厥陰中風，脈微浮為欲愈；不浮為未愈。

Jue Yin zhong feng, a pulse which is faint and floating means imminent recovery; not floating indicates no recovery.

Clause 328

厥陰病欲解時，從丑至卯上。

The time that Jue Yin disease is about to resolve, is from chou to mao.

Clause 329

厥陰病、渴欲飲水者，少少與之愈。

Jue Yin disease, if there is thirst with a desire to drink water, giving a little will bring recovery.

Clause 330

諸四逆厥者，不可下之；虛家亦然。

Whenever there is a case of four reversal jue, one should not purge; this also applies to cases of deficiency.

Clause 331

傷寒先厥后發熱而利者，必自止；見厥復利。

Shang han, if first there is jue and then fever and diarrhoea, it will cease spontaneously; if jue is seen, there will be diarrhoea again.

Clause 332

傷寒，始發熱六日，厥反九日而利。凡厥利者，當不能食；今反能食者，恐為除中（一雲消中）。食以索餅，不發熱者，知胃氣尚在，必愈。恐暴熱來出而復去也。后日脈之，其熱續在者，期之旦日夜半愈。所以然者，本發熱六日，厥反九日，復發熱三日，並前六日，亦為九日，與厥相應，故期之旦日夜半愈。后三日脈之，而脈數，其熱不罷者，此為熱氣有余，必發癰膿也。

Shang han, starting with fever for six days, but there is jue for nine days and diarrhoea. Wherever there is jue and diarrhoea, there should be an inability to eat; if now however there is an ability to eat, it is feared to be *chu zhong* (which some call *xiao zhong*). If the person is fed noodles, and there is no fever, it is known that there is good stomach qi, there will be recovery. One fears that sudden heat may come but then go. If the next day observation shows the fever persists, one can expect recovery the next day at midnight. The reason for this being, originally there was fever for six days, jue then for nine days, then fever for three days again, which, adding the first six days, is a total of nine days, and is equal to the jue and so one can expect recovery the next day at midnight. If three days later, observation shows that the pulse is rapid and the fever has not abated, this means there is an excess of heat, there will be suppurating ulcers.

Clause 333

傷寒脈遲六七日，而反與黃芩湯徹其熱。脈遲為寒，今與黃芩湯復除其熱，腹中應冷，當不能食；今反能食，此名除中，必死。

Shang han, the pulse was slow for six or seven days, but nevertheless, Huang Qin Tang was given to eliminate the fever. A pulse which is slow relates to cold, now Huang Qin Tang is given to eliminate the fever, there must be cold in the abdomen, the person should not be able to eat; but now the person can eat. This is *chu zhong*, the person will die.

NOTE: Clauses 327–333 focus on prognosis in Jue Yin disease inclusive of spontaneous recovery.

Clause 334

傷寒，先厥后發熱，下利必自止。而反汗出，咽中痛者，其喉為痺。發熱無汗，而利必自止；若不止，必便膿血。便膿血者，其喉不痺。

Shang han, first there is jue and afterwards there is fever, diarrhoea will spontaneously cease. And on the contrary if there is sweating, and pain in the throat, the throat is impeded. Fever with no sweating, the diarrhoea will stop spontaneously; if the diarrhoea does not stop, there will be blood and pus in the stool. If there is blood and pus in the stool, the throat is not impeded.

Clause 335

傷寒一二日至四五日，厥者，必發熱。前熱者，后必厥。厥深者熱亦深，厥微者熱亦微。厥應下之，而反發汗者，必口傷爛赤。

Shang han for one or two days or even four or five days, if there is jue, there will be fever. If first there is heat, afterwards there will be jue. If the jue is severe, the fever is also severe, if the jue is mild the fever is also mild. For jue one should purge, but if instead sweat is promoted, the mouth will be injured with ulceration and redness.

Clause 336

傷寒病，厥五日，熱亦五日，設六日當復厥；不厥者自愈。厥終不過五日，以熱五日，故知自愈。

Shang han disease, there is jue for five days, and fever also for five days, if there is a sixth day, there should be jue again; if there is no jue, there will be spontaneous recovery. The cycle of jue will not exceed five days, because the fever lasts five days, so it is known there will be spontaneous recovery.

Clause 337

凡厥者， 陰陽氣不順接， 便為厥. 厥者，手足逆冷者是也.

Whenever the utmost is reached, yin and yang qi do not connect smoothly, so it is called the utmost. At the utmost, it is the hands and feet which suffer reversal cold.

NOTE: Clauses 334–337 describe jue or cold extremities; Clause 335 describes a cold jue pattern with the waxing and waning of yang qi, and the excessive return of yang qi transforming into a heat pattern; Clause 336 is a sequel to Clause 335 describing heat jue and a comparison between cold and heat jue; Clause 337 describes the basic pathogenesis of jue.

Clause 338

傷寒脈微而厥， 至七八日膚冷，其人躁無暫安時者，此為臟厥，非蛔厥也. 蛔厥者， 其人當吐蛔，今病者靜，而復時煩者，此為臟寒. .蛔上入其膈，故煩，須臾復止，得食而嘔，又煩者，蛔聞食臭出，其人常自吐蛔.。蛔厥者，烏梅丸主之. 又主久利.

Shang han with a faint pulse and jue, on the seventh or eighth day, the skin is cold, if the person is agitated without a moment's peace, this is zang jue, it is not roundworm jue. In roundworm jue, the person should vomit roundworms, now the patient is quiet, but if there is repeated vexation, this is cold in the zang. The roundworms go upward and enter the diaphragm, hence the vexation, which all of a sudden stops again. If taking food causes vomiting, and also vexation, the roundworms smell the odour of the food, the person will often spontaneously vomit the roundworms. In roundworm jue, Wu Mei Wan governs, it also governs chronic diarrhoea.

NOTE: Clause 338 describes and differentiates hui jue or roundworm jue from zang jue.

Clause 339

傷寒熱少微厥，指頭寒，嘿嘿不欲食，煩躁.數日，小便利，色白者，此熱除也，欲得食，其病為愈；若厥而嘔，胸脅煩滿者，其後必便血。

Shang han disease, there is a slight fever and mild jue, cold fingers, untalkativeness with no desire for food, vexation. After several days, if the urination is free, and the colour is clear, this means the heat is eliminated, if there is a desire to eat, there will be recovery from the disease; if there is jue and vomiting, and there is vexation and fullness in the chest and hypochondrium, later, there will be blood in the stool.

Clause 340

病者手足厥冷，言我不結胸， 小腹滿，按之痛者， 此冷結在膀胱關元也。

The patient has desertion cold of the hands and feet, one says it is not chest bind, if the lower abdomen is full, and there is pain on palpation, this is cold bind in the urinary bladder at Guan Yuan.

Clause 341

傷寒發熱四日，厥反三日，復熱四日。厥少熱多者，其病當愈；四日至七日，熱不除者，必便膿血。

Shang han with fever for four days, but jue for three days, then again fever for four days. If there is less jue than fever, there will be recovery from the disease; if from the fourth to the seventh day, the fever is not eliminated, there will be blood and pus in the stool.

Clause 342

傷寒厥四日，熱反三日，復厥五日，其病為進。寒多熱少，陽氣退，故為進也。

Shang han with jue for four days, but fever for three days, then again jue for five days, the disease is advancing. There is more cold and less heat, yang qi is retreating, this is why it is advancing.

Clause 343

傷寒六七日，脈微、手足厥冷、煩躁，灸厥陰。厥不還者，死。

Shang han for six or seven days, the pulse is faint, there is desertion cold of the hands and feet, and vexation and agitation, moxa Jue Yin. If the desertion is not returned, the person will die.

Clause 344

傷寒發熱，下利、厥逆、躁不得臥者，死。

Shang han with fever, there is diarrhoea and reversal due to desertion, if the person is too agitated to sleep, the person will die.

Clause 345

傷寒發熱，下利至甚，厥不止者，死。

Shang han with fever, the diarrhoea is extreme, if the jue does not cease, the person will die.

Clause 346

傷寒六七日不利，便發熱而利，其人汗出不止者，死，有陰無陽故也。

Shang han for six or seven days with no diarrhoea, if by chance there is fever and diarrhoea, and the person sweats incessantly, the person will die, because there is yin without yang.

Clause 347

傷寒五六日，不結胸，腹濡，脈虛，復厥者，不可下；此亡血，下之死。

Shang han for five or six days, if there is no chest bind, the abdomen is soft, the pulse is deficient, and jue occurs again, one must not purge; this is devastation of blood, purgation will cause death.

Clause 348

發熱而厥，七日下利者，為難治。

When there is fever and jue, with diarrhoea for seven days, this is difficult to treat.

Clause 349

傷寒脈促，手足厥逆，可灸之。

Shang han, the pulse is skipping, there is desertion reversal of the hands and feet, moxibustion may be used.

NOTE: Clauses 339–349 describe various aspects of Jue Yin disease including the excessive return of yang; yang return with spontaneous recovery; struggle of yin and yang and devastation of yang qi. This gives emphasis to the fact that Jue Yin disease is attributed to the devastation of yang qi and recovery is dependent on the restoration of yang.

Clause 350

傷寒脈滑而厥者，裡有熱，白虎湯主之。

Shang han, if the pulse is slippery and there is jue, there is heat in the interior, Bai Hu Tang governs.

Clause 351

手足厥寒，脈細欲絕者，當歸四逆湯主之。

If there is desertion cold of the hands and feet, and the pulse is thready verging on expiry, Dang Gui Si Ni Tang governs.

Clause 352

若其人內有久寒者，宜當歸四逆加吳茱萸生姜湯。

If the person has long-term interior cold, Dang Gui Si Ni jia Wu Zhu Yu Sheng Jiang Tang is appropriate.

Clause 353

大汗出，熱不去，內拘急，四肢疼。又下利，厥逆而惡寒者，四逆湯主之。

Profuse sweating, the fever does not abate, there is spasm in the interior, pain in the four limbs. If there is also diarrhoea, and desertion reversal and aversion to cold, Si Ni Tang governs.

Clause 354

大汗，若大下利而厥冷者，四逆湯主之。

There is profuse sweating, if there is severe diarrhoea and desertion cold, Si Ni Tang governs.

Clause 355

病人手足厥冷，脈乍緊者，邪結在胸中，心下滿而煩，饑不能食者，病在胸中、當須吐之，宜瓜蒂散。

The patient suffers from cold in the hands and feet, if the pulse is all of a sudden tight, evil is knotted in the chest, there is fullness below the heart and vexation, hunger with no ability to eat, then the disease is in the chest, one should induce vomiting, Gua Di San is appropriate.

Clause 356

傷寒，厥而心下悸，宜先治水，當服茯苓甘草湯，卻治其厥，不爾，水漬入胃，必作利也。

Shang han, there is jue and palpitations below the heart, it is appropriate to treat the water first, one should take Fu Ling Gan Cao Tang, but if one treats the jue by another method, the water will enter right into the stomach, there will be diarrhoea.

Clause 357

傷寒六七日，大下後，寸脈沉而遲，手足厥逆，下部脈不至，喉咽不利，唾膿血，泄利不止者，為難治，麻黃升麻湯主之。

Shang han disease for six or seven days, after heavy purgation, the cun pulse is submerged and slow, there is desertion reversal of the hands and feet, the lower pulse does not arrive, the throat is not free, there is spitting of pus and blood, diarrhoea is incessant, this is difficult to treat, Ma Huang Sheng Ma Tang governs.

NOTE: Clauses 350–357 describe jue due to heat, to cold, to blood deficiency with congealed cold, to phlegm, to water retention, and to heat and cold complex. This is for the purpose of differentiation and is an example of the recurrent *Shang Han Lun* feature of contrasting patterns.

Clause 358

傷寒四五日，腹中痛，若轉氣下趣少腹者，此欲自利也。

Shang han for four or five days, there is pain in the abdomen, if the migratory qi tends to descend to the lesser abdomen, this means imminent spontaneous diarrhoea.

Clause 359

傷寒本自寒下，醫復吐下之，寒格，更逆吐下；若食入口即吐，干姜黃芩黃連人參湯主之。

Shang han disease, originally with spontaneous cold diarrhoea, then the physician induced vomiting and purging, cold repels and there was further adverse vomiting and purgation; if there is vomiting as soon as food enters the mouth, Gan Jiang Huang Qin Huang Lian Ren Shen Tang governs.

NOTE: Clauses 358 and 359 describe diarrhoea in Jue Yin and vomiting due to cold in the stomach. They are better read with Clause 357 relating to incessant diarrhoea.

Clause 360

下利有微熱而渴，脈弱者，今自愈。

Diarrhoea with slight fever and thirst, if the pulse is weak, spontaneous recovery is imminent.

Clause 361

下利脈數，有微熱汗出，今自愈；設復緊，為未解。

There is diarrhoea and the pulse is rapid, there is a mild fever and sweating, spontaneous recovery is imminent; if the pulse is then tight, there is no resolution.

Clause 362

下利、手足厥冷、無脈者，灸之。不溫，若脈不還，反微喘者，死；少陰負趺陽者，為順也。

If there is diarrhoea, desertion cold of the hands and feet and no pulse, one should use moxa. There is no warmth, if the pulse does not return, on the contrary, there is mild panting, the person will die; if Shao Yin is less than fu yang, it is favourable.

Clause 363

下利，寸脈反浮數，尺中自澀者，必清膿血。

If there is diarrhoea, the cun pulse is nonetheless floating and rapid, it is choppy in the chi position, there will be pus and blood in the stool.

Clause 364

下利清谷，不可攻表，汗出必脹滿。

There is diarrhoea with undigested food particles, one should not attack the exterior, if sweat issues, there will be distension and fullness.

Clause 365

下利，脈沉而弦者，下重也；脈大者，為未止；脈微弱數者，為欲自止，雖發熱不死。

If there is diarrhoea, the pulse is submerged and wiry, then there is heaviness below; if the pulse is big, the diarrhoea will not cease; if the pulse is faint, weak and rapid, it is about to cease spontaneously, although there is fever, the person will not die.

Clause 366

下利脈沉而遲，其人面少赤、身有微熱、下利清谷者，必郁冒汗出而解，病人必微厥，所以然者，其面戴陽，下虛故也。

Diarrhoea with a pulse which is submerged and slow, if the person's face is a little red, there is a mild fever, and diarrhoea with undigested food particles, there will be oppressed dizziness and sweating with resolution, the patient will have mild jue, the reason for this being, the face bears the sign of yang, and the lower jiao is deficient.

Clause 367

下利脈數而渴者，今自愈；設不差，必清膿血，以有熱故也。

If there is diarrhoea, a rapid pulse and thirst, now there will be spontaneous recovery; if there is no despatch, there will be blood and pus in the stool, this is because there is heat.

Clause 368

下之後，脈絕，手足厥冷，晬時脈還，手足溫者生；脈不還者死。

Following diarrhoea, the pulse has expired, there is desertion cold of the hands and feet, if within one day the pulse returns, and the hands and feet are warm the person will live; if the pulse does not return the person will die.

Clause 369

傷寒下利日十余行，脈反實者，死。

Shang han with diarrhoea in excess of ten times a day, if the pulse is nonetheless excess, the person will die.

NOTE: Clauses 360–369 mainly describe different types of diarrhoea, possible changes in the course of the disease, and prognosis. It can be seen that Zhong Jing placed particular emphasis on both the pulse sign and the status of the yang qi in order to make a prognosis.

Clause 370

下利清谷，裡寒外熱，汗出而厥者，通脈四逆湯主之。

Diarrhoea with undigested food, the interior is cold and the exterior is hot, if there is sweating and reversal, Tong Mai Si Ni Tang governs.

Clause 371

熱利下重者，白頭翁湯主之。

Heat diarrhoea with heaviness below, Bai Tou Weng Tang governs.

Clause 372

下利腹脹滿，身體疼痛者，先溫其里，乃攻其表，溫里宜四逆湯，攻表宜桂枝湯。

Diarrhoea and abdominal fullness, where the body is aching, first warm the interior, then attack the exterior, Si Ni Tang is appropriate to warm the interior, Gui Zhi Tang to attack the exterior.

Clause 373

下利欲飲水者，以有熱故也，白頭翁湯主之。

If there is diarrhoea with a desire to drink, this is because there is heat, Bai Tou Weng Tang governs.

Clause 374

下利譫語者，有燥屎也，宜小承氣湯。

If there is diarrhoea with delirious speech, and there is a hard stool, Xiao Cheng Qi Tang is appropriate.

Clause 375

下利後更煩，按之心下濡者，為虛煩也，宜梔子豉湯。

Following diarrhoea if there is more vexation, and softness below the heart on palpation, this is empty vexation, Zhi Zi Chi Tang is appropriate.

NOTE: Clauses 370–376 continue the discussion of diarrhoea. Although the sequence may initially appear disordered, the intention is to highlight the possible developments of heat and cold, and deficiency and excess in the course of the disease.

Clause 376

嘔家有痈膿者，不可治嘔；膿盡自愈。

If a patient who suffers from vomiting has ulcers, one should not treat the vomiting; when the suppuration stops, there will be spontaneous recovery.

NOTE: This is a discussion of a vomiting pattern.

Clause 377

嘔而脈弱，小便復利，身有微熱，見厥者，難治，四逆湯主之。

If there is vomiting and the pulse is weak, the urination is again free, there is slight fever, and jue can be seen, it is difficult to treat, Si Ni Tang governs.

Clause 378

干嘔，吐涎沫，頭痛者，吳茱萸湯主之。

If there is dry retching, drooling and a headache, Wu Zhu Yu Tang governs.

Clause 379

嘔而發熱者，小柴胡湯主之。

If there is vomiting and fever, Xiao Chai Hu Tang governs.

NOTE: Clauses 377–379 describe the treatment of vomiting patterns in the order of deficiency, excess, cold pattern then heat, and finally an acute pattern.

Clause 380

傷寒，大吐、大下之，極虛，復極汗者，其人外氣怫郁，復與之水以發其汗，因得噦。所以然者，胃中寒冷故也。

Shang han, if there is severe vomiting and severe purgation, causing extreme deficiency, following which there is extreme sweating, the person has glowering constraint of exterior qi, water then is given to enable sweating, causing hiccough. The reason for this being, there is coldness in the stomach.

Clause 381

傷寒噦而腹滿，視其前後，知何部不利，利之即愈。

Shang han with hiccoughing and abdominal fullness, observe the anterior and posterior, know which part is not free, freeing will bring recovery.

NOTE: Clauses 380 and 381 describe the aetiology and pathogenesis of hiccoughs.

CLAUSES 382–391: HUO LUAN CHAPTER

Clause 382

問曰：病有霍亂者何？答曰：嘔吐而利，此名霍亂。

Question: What is huo luan disease? Answer: Vomiting and diarrhoea, this is huo luan.

Clause 383

問曰：病發熱、頭痛、身疼、惡寒、吐利者，此屬何病？答曰：此名霍亂。霍亂自吐下，又利止，復更發熱也。

Question: If the disease has fever, headache, body pain, aversion to cold and vomiting and diarrhoea, what disease does this pertain to? Answer: This is huo luan. Huo luan is spontaneous vomiting and diarrhoea, and when the diarrhoea ceases, there will be fever once again.

Clause 384

傷寒，其脈微澀者，本是霍亂，今是傷寒，卻四五日，至陰經上，轉入陰必利。本嘔下利者，不可治也；欲似大便，而反矢氣，仍不利者，此屬陽明也，便必硬，十三日愈。所以然者，經盡故也。下利后，當便硬，硬則能食者愈。今反不能食，到后經中，頗能食，復過一經能食，過之一日當愈；不愈者，不屬陽明也。

Shang han, if the pulse is faint and choppy, it was originally huo luan, now it is shang han, but on the fourth or fifth day, it reaches the yin channels, transferring to yin means there will be diarrhoea. If there was vomiting and diarrhoea in the beginning, it is untreatable; if the person feels as if he wants to pass a stool, but instead there is faecal qi and still no diarrhoea, this pertains to Yang Ming, the stool is hard, on the thirteenth day there will be recovery. The reason for this being, it has passed right through the channel. After the diarrhoea, the stool will be hard, if it is hard then the person can eat, there will be recovery. Now however there is no ability to eat, when the pathogen reaches the next channel, the person can eat a little, after passing one more channel the person can eat, after one day there will be recovery; if there is no recovery, it does not pertain to Yang Ming.

NOTE: Clauses 382, 383 and 384 define Huo Luan by describing its key symptoms and pulse sign.

Clause 385

惡寒、脈微而復利，利止，亡血也。四逆加人參湯主之。

Aversion to cold, the pulse is faint and there is recurrent diarrhoea, the diarrhoea ceases, there is devastation of blood. Si Ni jia Ren Shen Tang governs.

Clause 386

霍亂，頭痛、發熱、身疼痛，熱多欲飲水者，五苓散主之；寒多不用水者，理中丸主之。

Huo luan with headache, fever and body pain, if heat predominates and there is a desire to drink water, Wu Ling San governs; if cold predominates and there is no need for water, Li Zhong Wan governs.

Clause 387

吐利止而身痛不休者，當消息和解其外，宜桂枝湯小和之。

If the vomiting and diarrhoea stop but the body pain remains, one should pause for breath and harmonise the exterior, Gui Zhi Tang is appropriate to harmonise mildly.

Clause 388

吐利汗出，發熱惡寒，四肢拘急，手足厥冷者，四逆湯主之。

If there is diarrhoea and sweating, fever and aversion to cold, cramping in the four limbs, and desertion cold in the hands and feet, Si Ni Tang governs.

Clause 389

既吐且利，小便復利而大汗出，下利清谷，內寒外熱，脈微欲絕者，四逆湯主之。

If as well as vomiting and diarrhoea, the urination is then free and there is profuse sweat, diarrhoea with undigested food particles, interior cold and exterior heat, the pulse is faint and verging on expiry, Si Ni Tang governs.

Clause 390

吐已下斷，汗出而厥，四肢拘急不解，脈微欲絕者，通脈四逆加豬膽汁湯主之。

Vomiting has ceased and diarrhoea has halted, if there is sweating and jue with unresolved cramping in the four limbs, and the pulse is faint and verging on expiry, Tong Mai Si Ni jia Zhu Dan Zhi Tang governs.

NOTE: Clauses 385–390 describe the treatment of Huo Luan and cite the use of Wu Ling San and Li Zhong Tang for the purpose of diagnostic differentiation. Clause 387 continues on from Clause 386 to describe an unresolved exterior pattern occurring after the vomiting and diarrhoea stop, and also describes the follow-up management.

Clause 391

吐、利、發汗，脈平，小煩者，以新虛不勝谷氣故也。

Vomiting, diarrhoea, the promotion of sweat, if the pulse is normal, and there is slight vexation, this is because the new deficiency is not able to deal with the grain qi.

NOTE: This is a discussion on the aftercare of Huo Luan in the initial stage of recovery.

CLAUSES 392–398: YIN YANG EXCHANGE CHAPTER

Clause 392

傷寒陰陽易之為病，其人身體重、少氣、少腹裡急，或引陰中拘攣，熱上沖胸，頭重不欲舉，眼中生花，膝脛拘急者，燒褌散主之。

Shang han yin yang exchange disease, if the person feels heavy in the body, there is shortness of breath, and interior urgency in the lesser abdomen, or cramping in the genitals, heat surges upward to the chest, the head feels heavy and there is an unwillingness to raise it, there is blurred vision, cramps in the knees and lower leg, Shao Ku San governs.

NOTE: This clause describes the key symptom and pulse sign of yin yang exchange.

Clause 393

大病差後勞復者，枳實梔子豉湯主之。

If after despatch of major disease there is taxation relapse, Zhi Shi Zhi Zi Chi Tang governs.

Clause 394

傷寒差以後更發熱，小柴胡湯主之。脈浮者，以汗解之；脈沉實者，以下解之。

After despatch of shang han there is more fever, Xiao Chai Hu Tang governs. If the pulse is floating, resolution is by sweating; if the pulse is deep and excess, resolution is by purgation.

Clause 395

大病差後，從腰以下有水氣者，牡蠣澤瀉散主之。

After despatch of major disease, if there is water qi from the waist down, Mu Li Ze Xie San governs.

Clause 396

大病差後，喜唾，久不了了，胸上有寒，當以丸藥溫之，宜理中丸。

After despatch of major disease, there is a tendency to spit, for a long time without clearing, there is cold in the chest, one should warm with pills, Li Zhong Wan is appropriate.

Clause 397

傷寒解後，虛羸少氣，氣逆欲吐，竹葉石膏湯主之。

After shang han resolves, there is deficiency, emaciation and shortness of breath, qi counterflow and a desire to vomit, Zhu Ye Shi Gao Tang governs.

NOTE: Clauses 393–397 describe disease recurrence following resolution of shang han or cold injury, which is attributed to over-taxation, and also to a residual pathogen.

Clause 398

病人脈已解，而日暮微煩，以病新差，人強與谷，脾胃氣尚弱，不能消谷，故令微煩，損谷則愈。

The patient's pulse is already resolved, and in the evening there is mild vexation, this is because the disease is newly despatched, the person is forced to eat, the spleen and stomach qi is still weak, the person can not digest food, leading to mild vexation, reduce food and there will be recovery.

NOTE: Clause 398 describes the aftercare and dietary advice to be followed during recuperation from shang han disease. The objective is to emphasise the importance of combining herbal and dietary therapies in the initial recovery stage of major illness. The message of "reduce food and there will be recovery" highlights the significance of a diet appropriate to the patient's needs without placing a strain on the spleen and stomach qi, which is still weak during this initial recovery phase. Meals should be light and easily digested.

Appendix 3

Clause Index

Appendix 4

Summary of Formulas and Indications

Chapter 2: Tai Yang Disease	
Zhong Feng (Wind Strike)	
Gui Zhi Tang	Exterior deficiency
Gui Zhi jia Ge Gen Tang	Exterior deficiency with inhibited channel qi
Gui Zhi jia Hou Po Xing Zi Tang	Exterior deficiency with wheezing
Gui Zhi jia Fu Zi Tang	Exterior deficiency with damage to yang qi
Gui Zhi qu Shao Yao Tang	Exterior deficiency with fullness in the chest
Gui Zhi qu Shao Yao jia Fu Zi Tang	Exterior deficiency with fullness in the chest and damage to yang qi
Gui Zhi xin jia Tang	Exterior deficiency with damage to ying qi
Gui Zhi qu Gui jia Fu Ling Bai Zhu Tang	Exterior deficiency with inhibited channel qi and water accumulation
Shang Han (Cold Injury)	
Ma Huang Tang	Exterior excess
Ge Gen Tang	Exterior excess with inhibited channel qi
Da Qing Long Tang	Exterior excess with constrained yang qi
Xiao Qing Long Tang	Exterior excess with congested fluids and wheeze
Gui Zhi Ma Huang Ge Ban Tang	Exterior excess with more fever than chills
Gui Zhi Er Ma Huang Yi Tang	Exterior excess with more fever than chills but milder than a Gui Zhi Ma Huang Ge Ban Tang pattern
Gui Zhi Er Yue Bi Yi Tang	Exterior constraint
Tai Yang Fu Patterns	
Wu Ling San	Water amassment with thirst
Fu Ling Gan Cao Tang	Water amassment with no thirst
Tao He Cheng Qi Tang	Blood amassment
Di Dang Tang	Blood amassment (more severe than a Tao He Cheng Qi Tang pattern)
Di Dang Wan	Blood amassment (milder than a Di Dang Tang pattern)

Transmuted Patterns of Tai Yang	
Zhi Zi Chi Tang	Heat constraint in the chest and diaphragm
Zhi Zi Hou Po Tang	Heat constraint in the chest and diaphragm with abdominal fullness
Zhi Zi Gan Jiang Tang	Heat constraint in the chest and diaphragm with cold in the middle jiao
Ma Huang Xing Ren Gan Cao Shi Gao Tang	Heat harassing the lungs
Ge Gen Qin Lian Tang	Heat in the large intestine
Gui Zhi Ren Shen Tang	Unresolved exterior with spleen deficient and cold
Gui Zhi Gan Cao Tang	Heart yang deficiency
Gui Zhi Gan Cao Long Gu Mu Li Tang	Heart yang deficiency with vexation
Gui Zhi qu Shao Yao jia Shu Qi Mu Li Long Gu Jiu Ni Tang	Heart yang deficiency with manic behaviour
Gui Zhi jia Gui Tang	Heart yang deficiency with *ben tun*
Fu Ling Gui Zhi Gan Cao Da Zao Tang	Heart yang deficiency with potential for *ben tun*
Zhi Gan Cao Tang	Heart yin and yang deficiency
Fu Ling Gui Zhi Bai Zhu Gan Cao Tang	Spleen yang deficiency with accumulated water
Hou Po Sheng Jiang Ban Xia Gan Cao Ren Shen Tang	Spleen yang deficiency with phlegm damp accumulation and abdominal fullness
Xiao Jian Zhong Tang	Spleen and heart deficiency
Gan Jiang Fu Zi Tang	Yang deficiency with vexation
Fu Ling Si Ni Tang	Yang deficiency of the heart and kidneys
Zhen Wu Tang	Yang deficiency of the heart and kidneys with unresolved exterior
Gan Cao Gan Jiang Tang	Dual deficiency of yin and yang with exterior deficiency (emphasis on promoting yang)
Shao Yao Gan Cao Tang	Dual deficiency of yin and yang with exterior deficiency (emphasis on promoting yin)
Shao Yao Gan Cao Fu Zi Tang	Deficiency of yin with devastated yang and exterior deficiency
Zang Bind, Chest Bind and Glomus	
Da Xian Xiong Tang	Chest bind with heat excess
Da Xian Xiong Wan	Chest bind with heat excess and neck stiffness
Xiao Xian Xiong Tang	Glomus below the heart
San Wu Bai San	Chest bind with cold excess
Da Huang Huang Lian Xie Xin Tang	Heat glomus
Fu Zi Xie Xin Tang	Heat glomus with exterior yang deficiency
Ban Xia Xie Xin Tang	Glomus due to heat and cold complex with vomiting
Sheng Jiang Xie Xin Tang	Glomus due to heat and cold complex with stomach disharmony and water accumulation
Gan Cao Xie Xin Tang	Glomus due to heat and cold complex with spleen deficiency and diarrhoea
Chi Shi Zhi Yu Yu Liang Tang	Glomus with diarrhoea due to kidney yang deficiency
Xuan Fu Dai Zhe Tang	Glomus with belching
Huang Lian Tang	Heat in the upper jiao and cold in the lower jiao
Patterns Resembling Tai Yang	
Gui Zhi Fu Zi Tang	Wind cold damp bi syndrome
Qu Gui jia Bai Zhu Tang	Wind cold damp bi syndrome with spleen deficiency
Gan Cao Fu Zi Tang	Wind cold damp bi syndrome with restricted movement
Shi Zao Tang	Suspended phlegm fluids
Gua Di San Pattern	Excess phlegm in the diaphragm

He Bing (Concurrent Patterns)	
Ge Gen Tang	Concurrent pattern of Tai Yang and Yang Ming
Ge Gen jia Ban Xia Tang	Concurrent pattern of Tai Yang and Yang Ming with disharmony of the middle jiao
Ma Huang Tang	Concurrent pattern of Tai Yang and Yang Ming with constrained qi in the exterior
Huang Qin Tang	Concurrent pattern of Tai Yang and Shao Yang
Huang Qin jia Ban Xia Sheng Jiang Tang	Concurrent pattern of Tai Yang and Shao Yang with vomiting

Chapter 3: Yang Ming Disease	
Yang Ming Heat Patterns	
Zhi Zi Chi Tang	Constrained heat in the chest and diaphragm
Bai Hu Tang	Interior heat
Bai Hu jia Ren Shen Tang	Interior heat with fluid damage
Zhu Ling Tang	Knotting of heat and water in the lower jiao
Yang Ming Cold Patterns	
Wu Zhu Yu Tang	Stomach yang deficiency with qi reversal
Yang Ming Fu Patterns	
Tiao Wei Cheng Qi Tang	Interior heat with stomach disharmony and a dry stool
Xiao Cheng Qi Tang	Interior heat with abdominal fullness
Da Cheng Qi Tang	Fu excess with knotting of dryness and heat
Ma Zi Ren Wan	Hard dry stool
Mi Jian Dao	Hard dry stool
Tu Gua Gen	Hard dry stool
Pig's Bile	Hard dry stool
Transmuted Patterns of Yang Ming	
Yin Chen Hao Tang	Yellowing due to damp heat (equal heat and damp)
Zhi Zi Bai Pi Tang	Yellowing due to damp heat (more heat than damp)
Ma Huang Lian Qiao Chi Xiao Dou Tang	Yellowing due to damp heat with an unresolved exterior
Di Dang Tang	Heat harassing the blood with a black stool
Acupuncture Qi Men (Liv 14)	Heat entering the chamber of blood

Chapter 4: Shao Yang Disease	
Xiao Chai Hu Tang Patterns	
Xiao Chai Hu Tang	Various manifestations of a half-exterior half-interior pattern
Concurrent Patterns of Shao Yang	
Chai Hu Gui Zhi Tang	Concurrent pattern of Tai Yang and Shao Yang
Da Chai Hu Tang	Concurrent pattern of Yang Ming and Shao Yang
Chai Hu jia Mang Xiao Tang	Concurrent pattern of Yang Ming and Shao Yang to be used once exterior is resolved
Chai Hu Gui Zhi Gan Jiang Tang	Constrained interior heat with alternating chills and fever, fullness in the chest and epigastrium, and inhibited urination
Chai Hu jia Long Gu Mu Li Tang	Constrained interior heat with vexation and delirious speech, fullness in the chest, and inhibited urination

Chapter 5: Tai Yin Disease	
Tai Yin Exterior Pattern	
Gui Zhi Tang	Exterior deficiency
Tai Yin Interior Patterns	
Si Ni Tang Group: **Si Ni Tang** **Li Zhong Wan** **Fu Zi Li Zhong Wan**	Tai Yin cold
Dang Gui Si Ni Tang **Dang Gui Si Ni jia Wu Zhu Yu Shang Jiang Tang**	Blood deficiency with congealed cold
Transmuted Patterns of Tai Yin	
Gui Zhi jia Shao Yao Tang	Abdominal pain
Gui Zhi jia Da Huang Tang	Strong excess abdominal pain

Chapter 6: Shao Yin Disease	
Cold Conversion Patterns	
Si Ni Tang	Kidney yang deficiency with exuberant yin cold
Tong Mai Si Ni Tang	Severe kidney yang deficiency with false heat
Bai Tong Tang	Kidney yang deficiency with diarrhoea
Bai Tong jia Zhu Dan Zhi Tang	Severe kidney yang deficiency with diarrhoea
Zhen Wu Tang	Kidney yang deficiency with diarrhoea and inhibited urination
Fu Zi Tang	Kidney yang deficiency with cold damp accumulation
Wu Zhu Yu Tang	Kidney yang deficiency with vomiting and diarrhoea
Tao Hua Tang	Diarrhoea due to spleen and kidney yang deficiency with blood and pus in the stool
Heat Conversion Patterns	
Huang Lian E Jiao Tang	Disharmony of the heart and kidney with vexation and insomnia
Zhu Ling Tang	Knotting of heat and water in the lower jiao with inhibited urination, vomiting, thirst, vexation and diarrhoea
Concurrent Patterns	
Ma Huang Xi Xin Fu Zi Tang	Concurrent pattern of Shao Yin and Tai Yang where Shao Yin pattern is less advanced
Ma Huang Fu Zi Gan Cao Tang	Concurrent pattern of Shao Yin and Tai Yang where the Shao Yin pattern has progressed
Da Cheng Qi Tang	Concurrent pattern of Shao Yin and Yang Ming
Si Ni San	Concurrent pattern of Shao Yin and Shao Yang
Sore Throat Patterns	
Zhu Fu Tang Pattern	Yin deficiency with fire flaring
Gan Cao Tang	Yin deficiency with toxic fire
Jie Geng Tang	Non-diffusion of lung qi obstructing the throat
Ku Jiu Tang	Toxic phlegm fire injuring the vessels
Ban Xia San or Tang	Cold phlegm inhibiting the throat

Chapter 7: Jue Yin Disease	
Heat and Cold Complex	
Wu Mei Wan	Heat and cold complex with cold extremities
Gan Jiang Huang Qin Huang Lian Ren Shen Tang	Devastation of yang with diarrhoea due to cold in the lower jiao and vomiting due to fluid damage and heat in the upper jiao
Ma Huang Sheng Ma Tang	Pathogenic cold in the exterior and heat in the interior with cold extremities, spitting of blood and pus, and incessant diarrhoea
Cold Patterns	
Si Ni Tang	Yang deficiency with exuberant yin
Dang Gui Si Ni Tang	Blood deficiency with congealed cold
Dang Gui Si Ni jia Wu Zhu Yu Sheng Jiang Tang	Blood deficiency with congealed cold and phlegm fluids with vomiting and drooling
Wu Zhu Yu Tang	Cold in the liver channel with vomiting, drooling and headache
Fu Ling Gan Cao Tang	Cold extremities and palpitations below the heart due to water accumulation
Heat Patterns	
Bai Hu Tang	Cold extremities due to interior heat
Diarrhoea Patterns	
Bai Tou Weng Tang	Heat diarrhoea with a heavy sensation in the rectum

Chapter 8: Huo Luan Patterns	
Huo Luan	
Si Ni jia Ren Shen Tang	Extreme yang deficiency with devastation of blood
Wu Ling San	Dual exterior and interior deficiency with inhibited urination
Li Zhong Wan	Spleen yang deficiency with cold damp in the middle jiao
Tong Mai Si Ni jia Zhu Dan Zhi Tang	Desertion of yang and exhaustion of yin

Chapter 9: Yin Yang Exchange and Taxation Relapse	
Yin Yang Exchange	
Shao Ku San	Toxic damp heat
Taxation Relapse	
Zhi Shi Zhi Zi Chi Tang	Qi exhaustion and taxation relapse
Xiao Chai Hu Tang	Half-interior half-exterior pattern
Mu Li Ze Xie San	Damp heat accumulation in the lower jiao
Li Zhong Wan	Spleen and stomach deficient and cold
Zhu Ye Shi Gao Tang	Unresolved residual heat with qi and yin deficiency and stomach disharmony

Appendix 5

Formula Index

Of the 114 formulas originally contained in *Shang Han Lun*, only 112 remain which detail dosage and preparation, and these are based on a total of 91 herbs. The two missing formulas are Yu Yu Liang Wan禹余粮丸, found in Clause 88, and Li Lu Gan Cao Tang 藜芦甘草汤. No herbal ingredients are specified for Yu Yu Liang Wan, and Wang Ri Xiu 王日休 supplemented this formula with Yu Yu Liang 3 liang, Chi Shi Zhi 3 liang, Sheng Zhi Pi 3 liang and Chi Xiao Dou ½ sheng, directing that the ingredients be ground into powder and mixed with honey. Its modification, Chi Shi Zhu Yu Yu Liang Tang, is mentioned in Clause 159. Li Lu Gan Cao Tang is an emetic formula whose function is to expel phlegm and harmonise the stomach. Some *Shang Han Lun* annotators suggest Li Lu 3–6g and Gan Cao 6–12g.

Environmental and Ethical Considerations

In regard to herbs specified in the traditional formula and their application in the modern day clinic, practitioners are reminded of environmental considerations pertaining to the conservation of protected animal and plant species, and of ethical considerations relating to animal welfare. Cultivated varieties and synthetic substitutes are now often available.

Ma Huang and Fu Zi

Clinically useful herbs affected by prohibition or scheduling include Ma Huang (*ephedrae herba*) and Fu Zi (*aconiti radix lateralis*). In the hands of a qualified herbalist, these herbs are safe and effective, as proven by centuries of clinical evidence. It is unfortunate that in more recent times, instead of being used for one or two days for an acute upper respiratory tract infection, Ma Huang was sold over the counter as a product to help in weight loss. It was consequently taken for extended periods of time by those for whom it was not indicated. Not unexpectedly, adverse effects resulted when Ma Huang was misused in that way and not properly prescribed for the condition for which it is indicated.

Fears about the use of Fu Zi are also held by the Western medical community whose opinion tends to hold great sway. This is a great pity, because it is a valuable item of our materia medica with no satisfactory substitute. When boiled first, and prescribed by a qualified herbalist according to the prescribing principles of Chinese medicine, it is perfectly safe. Apart from centuries of clinical experience (the evidence of which outweighs that of any short-term clinical trial), further trials are currently being conducted in China to determine the level at which the dose may induce adverse side effects (see Appendix 6 for details).

Important Note

In the alphabetical formula index below, underlined **bold** clause numbers refer to those clauses where formula ingredients and directions are described in full. The issue of calculating a modern equivalent of the ancient Han dynasty measures appearing in *Shang Han Lun* is a complex one and is described in Appendix 9. The matter is further clouded by the fact that stipulated doses are not always for a single day, and there is some uncertainty as to whether changes were made by early editors. Dosages have therefore not been converted into grams and for clinical purposes, it is recommended that the practitioner be guided by the standard modern dosage. Often, the more important issue is the ratio of one herb to another, and so where the dose is given in *jin*, the equivalent in *liang* follows in brackets to assist in understanding the ratio of herbs in the formula. To the same end, *zhu* and *fen* have been expressed as a fraction of liang, e.g. 16 *zhu* = ⅔ *liang* or 1 *fen* = ¼ *liang*.

Bai Hu Tang
白虎汤
Clause **176**, 219, 350
Zhi Mu 6 liang
Shi Gao 1 jin (16 liang)
Zhi Gan Cao 2 liang
Jing Mi 6 ge

Bai Hu jia Ren Sheng Tang
白虎加人参汤
Clause 26, 168, 169, **170**, 222
Zhi Mu 6 liang
Shi Gao 1 jin (16 liang)
Zhi Gan Cao 2 liang
Ren Shen 2 liang
Jing Mi 6 ge

Bai Tong Tang
白通汤
Clause **314**
Cong Bai 4 pieces (bulb and stem)
Gan Jiang 1 liang
Fu Zi 1 piece

Bai Tong jia Zhu Dan Zhi Tang
白通汤加猪胆汁汤
Clause **315**
Cong Bai 4 stems
Gan Jiang 1 liang
Fu Zi 1 piece
Human urine 5 ge (approx 100g)
Zhu Dan Zhi (pig's bile) 1 ge

Bai Tou Weng Tang
白头翁汤
Clause **371**, 373
Bai Tou Weng 2 liang
Huang Bai 3 liang
Huang Lian 2 liang
Qin Pi 3 liang

Ban Xia San
半夏散
Clause **313**
Equal amounts of:
Ban Xia
Gui Zhi
Zhi Gan Cao

Ban Xia Tang
半夏汤
Clause **313**
Equal amounts of:
Ban Xia
Gui Zhi
Zhi Gan Cao

Ban Xia Xie Xin Tang
半夏泻心汤
Clause **149**
Ban Xia ½ jin (8 liang)
Huang Qin 3 liang
Gan Jiang 3 liang
Ren Shen 3 liang
Zhi Gan Cao 3 liang
Huang Lian 1 liang
Da Zao 13 pieces

Chai Hu Gui Zhi Gan Jiang Tang
柴胡桂枝干姜汤
Clause **147**
Chai Hu ½ jin (8 liang)
Gui Zhi 3 liang
Gan Jiang 2 liang
Gua Lou Gen 4 liang
Huang Qin 3 liang
Mu Li 2 liang
Zhi Gan Cao 2 liang

Chai Hu Gui Zhi Tang
柴胡桂枝汤
Clause **146**
Chai Hu 4 liang
Gui Zhi 1½ liang
Huang Qin 1½ liang
Ren Shen 1½ liang
Zhi Gan Cao 1 liang
Ban Xia 2½ ge
Shao Yao 1½ liang
Da Zao 6 pieces
Sheng Jiang 1½ liang

Chai Hu jia Long Gu Mu Li Tang
柴胡加龙骨牡蛎汤
Clause **107**
Chai Hu 4 liang
Long Gu 1½ liang
Huang Qin 1½ liang
Sheng Jiang 1½ liang
Qian Dan 1½ liang
Ren Shen 1½ liang
Gui Zhi 1½ liang
Fu Ling 1½ liang
Ban Xia 2½ ge
Da Huang 2 liang
Mu Li 1½ liang
Da Zao 6 pieces

Chai Hu jia Mang Xiao Tang
柴胡加芒硝汤
Clause **104**
Chai Hu 2 liang 16 zhu (2⅔ liang)
Huang Qin 1 liang
Ren Shen 1 liang
Zhi Sheng Jiang 1 liang
Ban Xia 20 zhu (⅚ liang)
Da Zao 4 pieces
Mang Xiao 2 liang
Note: An earlier dose for Ban Xia was 5 pieces

Cheng Qi Tang
承气汤
Clause 30, 56, 208, 214
See Da Cheng Qi Tang

Chi Shi Zhi Yu Yu Liang Tang
赤石脂禹余粮汤
Clause **159**
Chi Shi Zhi 1 jin
Tai Yi Yu Yu Liang 1 jin

Da Chai Hu Tang
大柴胡汤
Clause **103**, 165
Chai Hu ½ jin (8 liang)
Huang Qin 3 liang
Shao Yao 3 liang Paeonia alba)
Ban Xia ½ jin (8 liang)
Sheng Jiang 5 liang
Zhi Shi 4 pieces
Da Zao 12 pieces
Lin Yi's version advocates that 2 liang of Da Huang should be included

Da Cheng Qi Tang
大承气汤
Clause 208, 209, 212, 215, 217, 220, **238**, 240, 241, 242, 251, 252, 253, 254, 255, 256, 320, 321, 322
Da Huang 4 liang
Hou Po ½ jin (8 liang)
Zhi Shi 5 pieces
Mang Xiao 3 ge

Da Huang Huang Lian Xie Xin Tang
大黄黄连泻心汤
Clause **154**, 164
Da Huang 2 liang
Huang Lian 1 liang

Da Qing Long Tang
大青龙汤
Clause **38**, 39
Ma Huang 6 liang
Gui Zhi 2 liang
Zhi Gan Cao 2 liang
Xing Ren 40 pieces
Sheng Jiang 3 liang
Da Zao 10 pieces
Shi Gao the size of a small hen's egg (approx 45g)

Da Xian Xiong Tang
大陷胸汤
Clause **134**, 135, 136, 137, 149
Da Huang 6 liang
Mang Xiao 1 sheng
Gan Sui 1 qian bi (small teaspoon)

Da Xian Xiong Wan
大陷胸丸
Clause **131B**
Da Huang ½ jin
Ting Li Zi ½ jin
Mang Xiao ½ jin
Xing Ren ½ jin

Dang Gui Si Ni Tang
当归四逆汤
Clause **351**
Dang Gui 3 liang
Gui Zhi 3 liang
Shao Yao 3 liang
Xi Xin 3 liang
Zhi Gan Cao 2 liang
Tong Cao 2 liang
Da Zao 25 pieces

Dang Gui Si Ni jia Wu Zhu Yu Sheng Jiang Tang
当归四逆加吴茱萸生姜汤
Clause **352**
Dang Gui 3 liang
Shao Yao 3 liang
Zhi Gan Cao 2 liang
Tong Cao 2 liang
Gui Zhi 3 liang
Xi Xin 3 liang
Sheng Jiang ½ jin (8 liang)
Wu Zhu Yu 2 sheng
Da Zao 25 pieces

Di Dang Tang
抵当汤
Clause **124**, 125, 237, 257
Shui Zhi 30 pieces
Meng Chong 30 pieces
Tao Ren 20 pieces
Da Huang 3 liang

Di Dang Wan
抵当丸
Clause **126**
Shui Zhi 20 pieces
Meng Chong 20 pieces
Tao Ren 25 pieces
Da Huang 3 liang

Mi Jian Dao
蜜煎导
Clause **233**
Honey 7 ge

Fu Ling Gan Cao Tang
茯苓甘草汤
Clause **73**, 356
Fu Ling 2 liang
Gui Zhi 2 liang
Zhi Gan Cao 1 liang
Sheng Jiang 3 liang

Fu Ling Gui Zhi Bai Zhu Gan Cao Tang
茯苓桂枝白术甘草汤
Clause **67**
Fu Ling 4 liang
Gui Zhi 3 liang
Bai Zhu 2 liang
Zhi Gan Cao 2 liang

Fu Ling Gui Zhi Gan Cao Da Zao
茯苓桂枝甘草大枣汤
Clause **65**
Fu Ling ½ jin (8 liang)
Gui Zhi 4 liang
Zhi Gan Cao 3 liang
Da Zao 15 pieces

Fu Ling Si Ni Tang
茯苓四逆汤
Clause **69**
Fu Ling 4 liang
Ren Shen 1 liang
Fu Zi 1 piece
Zhi Gan Cao 2 liang
Gan Jiang 1½ liang

Fu Zi Da Huang Huang Lian Xie Xin Tang
附子大黄黄连泻心汤
See Fu Zi Xie Xin Tang

Fu Zi Tang
附子汤
Clause **304**, 305
Fu Zi 2 pieces
Fu Ling 3 liang
Ren Shen 2 liang
Bai Zhu 4 liang
Shao Yao 3 liang

Fu Zi Xie Xin Tang
附子泻心汤
Clause **155**
Da Huang 2 liang
Huang Lian 1 liang
Huang Qin 1 liang
Fu Zi 1 piece

Gan Cao Fu Zi Tang
甘草附子汤
Clause 175
Zhi Gan Cao 2 liang
Fu Zi 2 pieces
Bai Zhu 2 liang
Gui Zhi 4 liang

Gan Cao Gan Jiang Tang
甘草干姜汤
Clause **29**, 30
Zhi Gan Cao 4 liang
Gan Jiang 2 liang

Gan Cao Tang
甘草汤
Clause **311**
Gao Cao 2 liang

Gan Cao Xie Xin Tang
甘草泻心汤
Clause **158**
Zhi Gan Cao 4 liang
Huang Qin 3 liang
Gan Jiang 3 liang
Ban Xia ½ sheng
Da Zao 12 pieces
Huang Lian 1 liang

Gan Jiang Fu Zi Tang
干姜附子汤
Clause **61**
Gan Jiang 1 liang
Fu Zi 1 piece

Gan Jiang Huang Qin Huang Lian Ren Shen Tang
干姜黄芩黄连人参汤
Clause **359**
Gan Jiang 3 liang
Huang Qin 3 liang
Huang Lian 3 liang
Ren Shen 3 liang

Ge Gen jia Ban Xia Tang
葛根加半夏汤
Clause **33**
Ge Gen 4 liang
Ma Huang 3 liang
Zhi Gan Cao 2 liang
Shao Yao 2 liang
Gui Zhi 2 liang
Sheng Jiang 2 liang
Ban Xia ½ sheng

Ge Gen Qin Lian Tang
葛根黄芩黄连汤
Clause **34**
Ge Gen ½ jin (8 liang)
Zhi Gan Cao 2 liang
Huang Qin 3 liang
Huang Lian 3 liang

Ge Gen Tang
葛根汤
Clause **31**, **32**, 63, 162
Ge Gen 4 liang
Ma Huang 3 liang
Gui Zhi 2 liang
Sheng Jiang 3 liang
Zhi Gan Cao 2 liang
Shao Yao 2 liang
Da Zao 12 pieces

Gua Di San
瓜蒂散
Clause **166**, 355
Gua Di 1 fen (¼ liang)
Chi Xiao Dou 1 fen (¼ liang)

Gui Zhi Er Ma Huang Yi Tang
桂枝二麻黄一汤
Clause **25**
Gui Zhi 1 liang 17 zhu (1⅔ -1¾ liang)
Shao Yao 1 liang 6 zhu (1¼ liang)
Ma Huang 16 zhu (⅔ liang)
Sheng Jiang 1 liang 6 zhu (1¼ liang)
Xing Ren 16 pieces
Zhi Gan Cao 1 liang 2 zhu (1 1/12 liang)
Da Zao 5 pieces

Gui Zhi Er Yue Bi Yi Tang
桂枝二越婢一汤
Clause **27**
18 zhu (¾ liang) each of:
Gui Zhi
Shao Yao
Ma Huang
Zhi Gan Cao
Da Zao 4 pieces
Sheng Jiang 1 liang 2 zhu (1 1/12 liang)
Shi Gao 24 zhu (1 liang)

Gui Zhi Fu Zi Tang
桂枝附子汤
Clause **174**
Gui Zhi 4 liang
Fu Zi 3 pieces
Sheng Jiang 3 liang
Da Zao 12 pieces
Zhi Gan Cao 2 liang

Gui Zhi Gan Cao Long Gu Mu Li Tang
桂枝甘草龙骨牡蛎汤
Clause **118**
Gui Zhi 1 liang
Zhi Gan Cao 2 liang
Mu Li 2 liang
Long Gu 2 liang

Gui Zhi Gan Cao Tang
桂枝甘草汤
Clause **64**
Gui Zhi 4 liang
Zhi Gan Cao 2 liang

Gui Zhi jia Da Huang Tang
桂枝加大黄汤
Clause **279**
Gui Zhi 3 liang
Da Huang 2 liang
Shao Yao 6 liang
Sheng Jiang 3 liang
Zhi Gan Cao 2 liang
Da Zao 12 pieces

Gui Zhi jia Fu Zi Tang
桂枝加附子汤
Clause **20**
Gui Zhi 3 liang
Shao Yao 3 liang
Zhi Gan Cao 3 liang
Sheng Jiang 3 liang
Da Zao 12 pieces
Fu Zi 1 piece

Gui Zhi jia Ge Gen Tang
桂枝加葛根汤
Clause **14**
Ge Gen 4 liang
Shao Yao 3 liang
Gan Cao 2 liang
Sheng Jiang 3 liang
Da Zao 12 pieces
Gui Zhi 2 liang
Ma Huang 3 liang

Gui Zhi jia Gui Tang
桂枝加桂汤
Clause **117**
Gui Zhi 5 liang
Shao Yao 3 liang
Sheng Jiang 3 liang
Zhi Gan Cao 3 liang
Da Zao 12 pieces

Gui Zhi jia Hou Po Xing Zi Tang
桂枝加厚朴杏子汤
Clause **18**, 43
Gui Zhi 3 liang
Zhi Gan Cao 2 liang
Sheng Jiang 3 liang
Shao Yao 3 liang
Da Zao 12 pieces
Hou Po 2 liang
Xing Ren 50 pieces

Gui Zhi jia Shao Yao Tang
桂枝加芍药汤
Clause **279**
Gui Zhi 3 liang
Shao Yao 6 liang
Zhi Gan Cao 2 liang
Da Zao 12 pieces
Sheng Jiang 3 liang

Gui Zhi jia Shao Yao Sheng Jiang Ge Yi Liang Ren Shen San Liang Xin Jia Tang
桂枝加芍药生姜各一两人参三两新加汤
See Gui Zhi Xin Jia Tang

Gui Zhi Ma Huang Ge Ban Tang
桂枝麻黄各半汤
Clause **23**
Gui Zhi 1 liang 16 zhu (1⅔ liang)
1 liang each of:
Shao Yao
Sheng Jiang
Zhi Gan Cao
Ma Huang
Da Zao 4 pieces
Xing Ren 24 pieces

Gui Zhi qu Gui jia Fu Ling Bai Zhu Tang
桂枝去桂加茯苓白术汤
Clause **28**
Shao Yao 3 liang
Zhi Gan Cao 2 liang
Sheng Jiang 3 liang
Bai Zhu 3 liang
Fu Ling 3 liang
Da Zao 12 pieces

Gui Zhi qu Shao Yao Tang
桂枝去芍药汤
Clause **21**
Gui Zhi 3 liang
Zhi Gan Cao 2 liang
Sheng Jiang 3 liang
Da Zao 12 pieces

Gui Zhi qu Shao Yao jia Fu Zi Tang
桂枝去芍药加附子汤
Clause **22**
Gui Zhi 3 liang
Zhi Gan Cao 2 liang
Sheng Jiang 3 liang
Da Zao 12 pieces
Fu Zi 1 piece

Gui Zhi qu Shao Yao jia Shu Qi Mu Li Long Gu Jiu Ni Tang
桂枝去芍药加蜀漆牡蛎龙骨救逆汤
Clause **112**
Gui Zhi 3 liang
Zhi Gan Cao 2 liang
Sheng Jiang 3 liang
Da Zao 12 pieces
Mu Li 5 liang
Shu Qi 3 liang
Long Gu 4 liang

Gui Zhi Ren Shen Tang
桂枝人参汤
Clause **163**
Gui Zhi 4 liang
Zhi Gan Cao 4 liang
Bai Zhu 3 liang
Ren Shen 3 liang
Gan Jiang 2 liang

Gui Zhi Tang
桂枝汤
Clause **12**, 13, 15,16A, 16B, 17, 19, 24, 29, 30, 42, 44, 45, 53, 54, 56, 57, 91, 95, 164, 234, 240, 276, 372, 387
Gui Zhi 3 liang
Shao Yao 3 liang
Zhi Gan Cao 2 liang
Sheng Jiang 3 liang
Da Zao 12 pieces

Gui Zhi Xin Jia Tang
桂枝新加汤
Clause **62**
Gui Zhi 3 liang
Shao Yao 4 liang
Zhi Gan Cao 2 liang
Ren Shen 3 liang
Da Zao 12 pieces
Sheng Jiang 4 liang

Hou Po Sheng Jiang Ban Xia Gan Cao Ren Shen Tang
厚朴生姜甘草人参汤
Clause **66**
Hou Po ½ jin (8 liang)
Sheng Jiang ½ jin (8 liang)
Ban Xia ½ jin (8 liang)
Gan Cao 2 liang
Ren Shen 1 liang

Huang Lian Tang
黄连汤
Clause **173**
Huang Lian 3 liang
Zhi Gan Cao 3 liang
Gan Jiang 3 liang
Gui Zhi 3 liang
Ren Shen 2 liang
Ban Xia ½ sheng
Da Zao 12 pieces

Huang Lian E Jiao Tang
黄连阿胶汤
Clause **303**
Huang Lian 4 liang
Huang Qin 2 liang
Shao Yao 2 liang
Ji Zi Huang (egg yolks) 2
E Jiao 3 liang

Huang Qin Tang
黄芩汤
Clause **172**, 333
Huang Qin 3 liang
Shao Yao 2 liang
Zhi Gan Cao 2 liang
Da Zao 12 pieces

Huang Qin jia Ban Xia Sheng Jiang Tang
黄芩加半夏生姜汤
Clause **172**
Huang Qin 3 liang
Shao Yao 2 liang
Zhi Gan Cao 2 liang
Da Zao 12 pieces
Ban Xia ½ sheng
Sheng Jiang 1½ liang (also recorded as 3 liang)

Jie Geng Tang
桔梗汤
Clause **311**
Jie Geng 1 liang
Gan Cao 2 liang

Ku Jiu Tang
苦酒汤
Clause **312**
Ban Xia 14 pieces
A hen's egg
Rice vinegar

Li Zhong Wan
理中丸
Clause **386**, 396
Ren Shen 3 liang
Gan Jiang 3 liang
Zhi Gan Cao 3 liang
Bai Zhu 3 liang

Ling Gui Zhu Gan Tang
苓桂术甘草汤
See Fu Ling Gui Zhi Bai Zhu Gan Cao Tang

Ma Huang Fu Zi Gan Cao Tang
麻黄附子甘草汤
Clause **302**
Ma Huang 2 liang
Zhi Gan Cao 2 liang
Fu Zi 1 piece

Ma Huang Lian Qiao Chi Xiao Dou Tang
麻黄连轺 赤小豆汤
Clause **262**
Ma Huang 2 liang
Lian Qiao 2 liang
Xing Ren 40 pieces
Chi Xiao Dou 1 sheng
Da Zao 12 pieces
Sheng Zi Bai Pi 1 sheng
Sheng Jiang 2 liang
Zhi Gan Cao 2 liang

Ma Huang Sheng Ma Tang
麻黄升麻汤
Clause **357**
Ma Huang 2½ liang
Sheng Ma 1 liang 1 fen (1¼ liang)
Zhi Mu 18 zhu (¾ liang)
Huang Qin 18 zhu (¾ liang)
Wei Rui (Yu Zhu) 18 zhu (¾ liang)
Shao Yao 6 zhu (¼ liang)
Tian Men Dong 6 zhu (¼ liang)
Gui Zhi 6 zhu (¼ liang)
Zhi Gan Cao 6 zhu (¼ liang)
Shi Gao 6 zhu (¼ liang)
Bai Zhu 6 zhu (¼ liang)
Gan Jiang 6 zhu (¼ liang)
Note: In one edition of Shang Han Lun, Wei Rui was replaced by Shi Chang Pu.

Ma Huang Tang
麻黄汤
Clause **35**, 36, 37, 46, 51, 52, 55, 232, 235
Ma Huang 3 liang
Gui Zhi 2 liang
Zhi Gan Cao 1 liang
Xing Ren 70 pieces

Ma Huang Xi Xin Fu Zi Tang
麻黄细辛附子汤
Clause **301**
Ma Huang 2 liang
Xi Xin 2 liang
Fu Zi 1 piece

Ma Huang Xing Ren Gan Cao Shi Gao Tang
麻黄杏仁甘草石膏汤
Clause **63,** 162
Ma Huang 4 liang
Xing Ren 50 pieces
Zhi Gan Cao 2 liang
Shi Gao ½ jin (8 liang)

Ma Zi Ren Wan
麻子仁丸
Clause **247**
Ma Zi Ren 2 sheng
Shao Yao ½ jin (8 liang)
Zhi Shi ½ jin (8 liang)
Da Huang 1 jin (16 liang)
Hou Po 1 chi (approx. 33 cm)
Xing Ren 1 sheng

Mu Li Ze Xie San
牡蛎泽泻散
Clause **395**
Equal parts of:
Mu Li (dry-fried)
Ze Xie
Shu Qi (washed in warm water to eliminate the fishy smell)
Ting Li Zi (dry-fried)
Shang Lu Gen (dry-fried)
Hai Zao (washed to eliminate the salt)
Gua Lou Gen (Tian Hua Fen)

Pig's Bile
猪胆汁
Clause **233**
Pig's bile
Vinegar

Qu Gui jia Bai Zhu Tang
去桂加白术汤
Clause 174
Fu Zi 3 pieces
Bai Zhu 4 liang
Sheng Jiang 3 liang
Zhi Gan Cao 2 liang
Da Zao 12 pieces

San Wu Bai San
三物白散
Clause **141B**
Jie Geng 3 fen (¾ liang)
Ba Dou 1 fen (¼ liang)
Bei Mu 3 fen (¾ liang)

Shao Kun San
烧裈散
Clause **392**
The crotch of a woman's pants scorched and charred.

Shao Yao Gan Cao Fu Zi Tang
芍药甘草附子汤
Clause **68**
Shao Yao 3 liang
Zhi Gan Cao 3 liang
Fu Zi 1 piece

Shao Yao Gan Cao Tang
芍药甘草汤
Clause 29, 30
Bai Shao 4 liang
Zhi Gan Cao 4 liang

Sheng Jiang Xie Xin Tang
生姜泻心汤
Clause **157**
Sheng Jiang 4 liang
Zhi Gan Cao 3 liang
Ren Shen 3 liang
Gan Jiang 1 liang
Huang Qin 3 liang
Ban Xia ½ jin (8 liang)
Huang Lian 1 liang
Da Zao 12 pieces

Shi Zao Tang
十枣汤
Clause **152**
Equal parts of:
Yuan Hua
Gan Sui
Da Ji
Da Zao (10 plump pieces)

Si Ni jia Ren Shen Tang
四逆加人参汤
Clause **385**
Zhi Gan Cao 2 liang
Fu Zi 1 piece
Gan Jiang 1½ liang
Ren Shen 1 liang

Si Ni San
四逆散
Clause **318**, 387, 388, 389
10 fen (2½ liang) each of:
Zhi Gan Cao
Zhi Shi
Chai Hu

Si Ni Tang
四逆汤
Clause 29, 91, 92, 277, **323**, 324, 353, 354, 372, 377, 389
Zhi Gan Cao 2 liang
Gan Jiang 1½ liang
Fu Zi 1 piece

Tao He Cheng Qi Tang
桃核承气
Clause **106**
Tao Ren 50 pieces
Da Huang 4 liang
Gui Zhi 2 liang
Zhi Gan Cao 2 liang
Mang Xiao 2 liang

Tao Hua Tang
桃花汤
Clause **306**, 307
Chi Shi Zhi 1 jin (8 liang): one-half used whole in the decoction and the other half crushed and sieved for use as a powder.
Gan Jiang 1 liang
Jing Mi 1 sheng

Tiao Wei Cheng Qi Tang
调胃承气汤
Clause 29, 70, 94, 123, **207**, 248, 249
Zhi Gan Cao 2 liang
Mang Xiao ½ jin (8 liang)
Da Huang 4 liang

Tong Mai Si Ni Tang
通脉四逆汤
Clause **317**, 370
Zhi Gan Cao 2 liang
Fu Zi 1 large piece
Gan Jiang 3 liang (for a person with a strong constitution, 4 liang can be given)

Tong Mai Si Ni jia Zhu Dan Zhi Tang
通脉四逆加猪胆汁汤
Clause **390**
Zhi Gan Cao 2 liang
Gan Jiang 3 liang (4 liang for a robust person)
Fu Zi 1 piece
Zhu Dan Zhi ½ ge (10mL)

Tu Gua Gen
土瓜根及猪胆汁
Clause **233**
Tu Gua Gen

Wu Ling San
五苓散
Clause **71**, 72, 74, 156, **386**
Zhu Ling 18 zhu (¾ liang)
Ze Xie 1 liang 6 zhu (1¼ liang)
Bai Zhu 18 zhu (¾ liang)
Fu Ling 18 zhu (¾ liang)
Gui Zhi ½ liang or 12 zhu

Wu Mei Wan
乌梅丸
Clause **338**
Wu Mei 300 pieces
Xi Xin 6 liang
Gan Jiang 10 liang
Huang Lian 16 liang
Dang Gui 4 liang
Fu Zi 6 liang
Shu Jiao 4 liang
Gui Zhi 6 liang
Ren Shen 6 liang
Huang Bai 6 liang

Wu Zhu Yu Tang
吴茱萸汤
Clause **243**, 309, 378
Wu Zhu Yu 1 sheng
Ren Shen 3 liang
Sheng Jiang 6 liang
Da Zao 12 pieces

Xiao Chai Hu Tang
小柴胡汤
Clause 37, **96**, 97, 98, 99, 100, 101, 103, 104, 144, 148, 149, 229, 230, 231, 266, 379, 394
Chai Hu ½ jin (8 liang)
Huang Qin 3 liang
Ren Shen 3 liang
Ban Xia ½ jin (8 liang)
Zhi Gan Cao 3 liang
Sheng Jiang 3 liang
Da Zao 12 pieces

Xiao Cheng Qi Tang
小承气汤
208, 209, **213**, 214, 250, 251, 374
Da Huang 4 liang
Hou Po 2 liang
Zhi Shi 3 large pieces

Xiao Jian Zhong Tang
小建中汤
Clause 100, **102**
Gui Zhi 3 liang
Zhi Gan Cao 2 liang
Da Zao 12 pieces
Shao Yao 6 liang
Sheng Jiang 3 liang
Yi Tang 1 sheng

Xiao Qing Long Tang
小青龙汤
Clause **40**, 213, 214, 250
Ma Huang 3 liang
Shao Yao 3 liang
Xi Xin 3 liang
Gan Jiang 3 liang
Zhi Gan Cao 3 liang
Wu Wei Zi ½ sheng
Ban Xia ½ sheng

Xiao Xian Xiong Tang
小陷胸汤
Clause **138**
Huang Lian 1 liang
Ban Xia ½ jin (8 liang)
Gua Lou Shi 1 large piece (approx. 30g)

Xuan Fu Dai Zhe Tang
旋复代赭汤
Clause **161**
Xuan Fu Hua 3 liang
Ren Shen 2 liang
Sheng Jiang 5 liang
Dai Zhe Shi 1 liang
Zhi Gan Cao 3 liang
Ban Xia ½ sheng
Da Zao 12 pieces

Yin Chen Hao Tang
茵陈蒿汤
Clause **236**, 260
Yin Chen Hao 6 liang
Zhi Zi 14 pieces
Da Huang 2 liang

Yu Yu Liang Wan
禹余粮丸
Clause 88
Unknown.

Zhen Wu Tang
真武汤
Clause **82**, **316**
Fu Ling 3 liang
Shao Yao 3 liang
Bai Zhu 2 liang
Sheng Jiang 3 liang
Fu Zi 1 piece

Zhi Gan Cao Tang
炙甘草汤
Clause **177**
Zhi Gan Cao 4 liang
Sheng Jiang 3 liang
Ren Shen 2 liang
Sheng Di Huang 1 jin (16 liang)
Gui Zhi 3 liang
E Jiao 2 liang
Mai Dong ½ jin (8 liang)
Ma Ren ½ jin (8 liang)
Da Zao 30 pieces

Zhi Shi Zhi Zi Chi Tang
枳实栀子豉汤
Clause **393**
Zhi Shi (mix-fried) 3 pieces
Zhi Zi (broken) 14 pieces
Xiang Chi 1 sheng

Zhi Zi Bai Pi Tang
栀子柏皮汤
Clause **261**
Zhi Zi 15 pieces
Zhi Gan Cao 1 liang
Huang Bai 2 liang

Zhi Zi Chi Tang
栀子豉汤
Clause **76**, 77, 78, 81, 221, 228, 375
Zhi Zi 14 pieces
Xiang Chi 4 ge

Zhi Zi Gan Cao Chi Tang
栀子甘草豉汤
Clause **76**
Zhi Zi 14 pieces
Zhi Gan Cao 2 liang
Xiang Chi 4 ge

Zhi Zi Gan Jiang Tang
栀子干姜汤
Clause **80**
Zhi Zi 14 pieces
Gan Jiang 2 liang

Zhi Zi Hou Po Tang
栀子厚朴汤
Clause **79**
Zhi Zi 14 pieces
Hou Po 4 liang
Zhi Shi 4 pieces

Zhi Zi Sheng Jiang Chi Tang
栀子生姜豉汤
Clause **76**
Zhi Zi 14 pieces
Sheng Jiang 5 liang
Xiang Chi 4 ge

Zhu Fu Tang
猪肤汤
Clause **310**
Zhu Fu (pig's skin) 1 jin (16 liang)

Zhu Ling Tang
猪苓汤
Clause **223**, 224, 319
1 liang each of:
Zhu Ling
Fu Ling
Ze Xie
E Jiao
Hua Shi

Zhu Ye Shi Gao Tang
竹叶石膏汤
Clause **397**
Zhu Ye 2 bundles
Shi Gao 1 sheng
Ban Xia ½ jin (8 liang)
Mai Dong 1 sheng
Ren Shen 2 liang
Zhi Gan Cao 2 liang
Jing Mi ½ jin (8 liang)

Appendix 6

Fu Zi Research

Concern about the use of Fu Zi *(aconiti radix lateralis)* is not entirely misplaced, but is nevertheless exaggerated. The ramifications for the Chinese medical profession are that it restricts or prohibits our use of a highly effective herb. This herb, when prescribed according to the principles of Chinese medicine, in regard to appropriate diagnosis, dosage, and proper preparation, has been used safely for centuries. Such extensive clinical observation should more than satisfy calls for evidence-based medicine, and yet it appears that the Western medical fraternity has been successful in lobbying for legislation preventing the use of this herb by the professional group which is most qualified to use it.

Traditionally, Fu Zi is prepared by cooking, usually with the addition of Gan Jiang, and Gan Cao, and it is also recommended to start with a small initial dose before gradually increasing to a dose of between 6 and 10 grams. Potential side effects are listed as numbness of the lips, or of the hands and feet, nausea, vomiting, diarrhoea, dizziness, and in extreme cases, palpitations, dyspnoea, tremor and hypotension. However, when prescribed according to the principles of differential diagnosis in an appropriate dose, and when prepared according to traditional methods, reports of side effects seem to be scarcer than reports of side effects for Gan Cao. Nevertheless, some outstanding trials have been conducted in China in recent years, showing that enormous doses can be taken by a healthy person, not exhibiting the pre-requisite cold signs, with no ill effect.

Pang Xin's Trial with Fu Zi in Large Doses

Dr Pang Xin is currently enrolled as a PhD student in the *Shang Han Lun* program at the Beijing University of Chinese Medicine. For five months, starting at the end of 2003, Pang Xin self-administered a formula containing an exceptionally large dose of Fu Zi. The base formula was: Fu Zi 30g, Gan Jiang 30g and Zhi Gan Cao 50g. In the first week, he had diarrhoea which stopped after one week. The second effect was a general sense of warmth and comfort in the area of Dan Tian, just below the umbilicus. Pang reported that when he meditated following the administration of the Fu Zi formula, there was a sense of freedom in the interior, as if all the network vessels were flowing freely. The third effect was a reduction in sensitivity to heat in the summer. He attributed this to the preservation of true yang. During the five-month trial, the dosage of Fu Zi was increased by 10g each week until a dosage of 500g was reached. Following that peak, the dosage was gradually reduced again to 30g.

It is important to note that the larger the dosage of Fu Zi, the longer the cooking time required. The cooking time in this trial ranged from 2 to 8 hours, and Fu Zi was decocted with Gan Jiang and Gan Cao. During the five-month trial, Pang sometimes alternated the base formula with Fu Zi Li Zhong Tang (Fu Zi 100g, Gan Jiang 200g, Bai Zhu 200g, Zhi Gan Cao 100g).

Pang Xin stated that his constitution was normal; there was no deficiency of kidney yang; and his appetite and sleep were also normal.

Important Considerations

1. The decoction time for Fu Zi has to be at least 2 hours. Research has shown that the cooking process eliminates the alkaloid contained in the Fu Zi which is believed responsible for negative side effects.

2. Prior to taking the formula, a drop should be taste-tested to ensure no numbness of the tongue occurs.
3. During the course of medication, the patient should refrain from sexual activity.
4. During the course of medication, any flu-like symptoms, such as body aches, stiffness, headache, aversion to cold and fever, or any worsening of an existing condition, are attributed to the source qi attacking the nidus of the disease, and are seen as the manifestation of the zheng qi prevailing over the pathogenic qi.

Using Fu Zi Li Zhong Tang, Dr Pang Xin has also successfully treated stubborn dermatological conditions in two patients, one with acne and one with urticaria.

Appendix 7

Index to Symptoms and Ailments

Appendix 8

Glossary

Translation of the terminology of Chinese medicine is fraught with problems and often, despite the best attempts, translated terms are less than satisfactory. It is the view of many (including the authors), providing there is no ambiguity, that the original terminology should be used as far as possible, in particular, for the most common terms. To that end, original Chinese terms have been used and supplemented by translations, rather than relying solely on translated terms. Nevertheless, where a translated term is useful and convenient, the authors have sought to find a term which reflects the sense of the Chinese as closely as possible in order to convey to the reader the flavour of the original text.

agitation 躁 *zao* Agitation is not the same as 'irritability' or 'annoyance'. In *Shang Han Lun* it refers to unconscious fidgeting associated with altered consciousness and is thus distinguished from vexation 心烦 *xin fan*, which refers to an emotional sensation, not an action.

ba gang bian zheng 八纲辩证 Eight principle pattern differentiation also known as the eight guiding principles of pattern differentiation.

bai yin 白饮 Literally: 'white fluid'. Rice water taken from the pot as the rice is cooking.

below the heart 心下*xin xia* This refers to the epigastric region.

ben tun 奔豚 An upsurge of qi from the lower jiao due to kidney cold with accumulated water qi. (See Clause 65: Discussion.)

bi syndrome *See* **bi zheng**

bi zheng 闭证 Bi pattern. Literally: 'obstruction pattern'. Often translated as 'painful obstruction syndrome'.

bian zheng 变证 Transmuted pattern. Literally: 'changed pattern'.

bian zheng 辩证 Pattern differentiation.

bian bing 辩病 Disease differentiation.

bing bing 并病 Lagover pattern. This term refers to the pathogen 'lagging over' in one channel whilst proceeding to the next.

bing yin bian zheng 病因辩证 Pattern differentiation according to the cause of illness.

blood amassment 蓄血 *xu xue* This refers to the accumulation of stagnant blood, usually in the lower abdomen.

bo qi zi 博棋子 *See* **qi zi**

bu geng yi 不更衣 No change of clothes. This refers to constipation. To change one's clothes is a euphemistic expression for going to the lavatory to pass a stool.

chen shi 辰时 This is the time according to the Han dynasty system of the twelve earthly branches, which covers the period from 7am to 9am. It represents the later part of the six-hour period when Shao Yang channel qi is at its peak.

chou shi 丑时 This is the time according to the Han dynasty system of the twelve earthly branches, which covers the period from 1am to 3am. It represents the middle part of the six-hour period when the Shao Yin channel qi is at its peak, and overlaps with the end of the Tai Yin peak period and the beginning of the Jue Yin peak period.

chu zhong 除中 Expiry of middle qi. This indicates a serious condition of depleted qi of the middle jiao. The text suggests it may be *xiao zhong,* which refers to *xiao ke,* meaning insatiable thirst and usually thought to parallel diabetes.

chuan bian Transmission and transmutation.

concurrent pattern 合病 *he bing* This term refers to the presence of disease in more than one channel.

cou li 腠理 The openings or interstices in the space running between the skin and muscles, which may include, but are not limited to, the pores of the skin. It is these interstices which provide a means for pathogens to pass into or out of the body. In modern terms it could be interpreted as the intercellular space.

defence 卫 *wei See* **defence yang**

defence yang 卫阳 *wei yang* This term refers to the yang qi which flows outside the blood vessels in the superficial layers of the body. Its functions include opening and closing the pores to regulate sweating, warming the skin and the exterior of the body, and defending it from exterior pathogens (cf *ying yin* or nutrient yin).

desertion 厥 *jue* The term desertion can refer to extreme devastation of a vital substance. However, when it is used as a translation of the term *jue*, it has two specific interpretations. The first meaning is sudden loss of consciousness. The second meaning, relevant in the reading of *Shang Han Lun,* is cold extremities due to the non-communication of yin and yang. The cause can be deficiency of yang, or obstruction due to heat, cold, worms, water or some other substance.

dou 斗 An ancient Han dynasty unit of capacity approximating 2L. It is not to be confused with the modern metric unit which equals 10L. *(For more detail refer to Appendix 9.)*

du mai 督脉 Governing vessel.

expiry of middle qi 除中 *chu zhong* This indicates a serious condition of depleted qi of the middle jiao. The text suggests it may be *xiao zhong,* which refers to *xiao ke,* meaning insatiable thirst and usually thought to parallel diabetes.

external bleeding 衄 *nǜ* This term does not refer to internal bleeding but to bleeding from external orifices and principally to bleeding from the nose.

fan 烦 *See* **xin fan**

fa re 发热 To have a fever. Literally: 'to emit heat'.

fang cun bi 方寸匕 A square-inch spoon with a capacity of about 5mL.

feather-warm fever 翕翕发热 *xi xi fa re* This refers to just a slight rise in temperature and is a feature of Tai Yang zhong feng.

fen 分 The ancient Han dynasty measure approximating 3.8g. It is not the same as the modern *fen* which equals 0.5g. *(For more detail refer to Appendix 9.)*

feng wen 风温 Wind warmth.

five heart heat 五心烦热 *wu xin fan re* This may be translated as vexation and heat in the five centres and refers to the sensation of heat in the soles of the feet, the palms of the hands and in the chest. It is a sign of heat due to yin deficiency.

fu yang mai 趺阳脉 Instep pulse. This refers to the pulse felt at the highest point of the instep coinciding with the acupuncture point Chong Yang (St 42).

gan lan shui 甘澜水 Literally: 'sweet rippled water'. This is water which has been 'worked' by pouring about 4L into a large pan and stirring continuously until thousands of water bubbles appear. Water is attributed with a salty flavour; the rationale of working the water is to render it sweet in order to benefit the spleen.

gan 感 Affect. In the context of *Shang Han Lun*, this refers to contraction of an illness.

gang jing 刚痉 Hard tetany. This refers to rigidity due to spasm and contraction of muscles or to convulsions, and is associated with an excess pattern, as opposed to soft or flaccid tetany which is characterised by spontaneous sweating and is associated with a deficiency pattern.

ge 合 An ancient Han dynasty unit of capacity. Dry measure equals a closed handful or fistful, and liquid measure is approximately 20mL. It is not to be confused with the modern metric unit which equals 100mL. *(For more detail refer to Appendix 9.)*

glomus 痞 *pi* Glomus is a sensation of fullness or blockage which can be soft, when it is a reflection of the knotting of qi, or hard, when there is a knotting of heat or qi with water, food stagnation or phlegm.

hai shi 亥时 This is the time according to the Han dynasty system of the twelve earthly branches, which covers the period from 9pm to 11pm and represents the earlier part of the six-hour period when Tai Yin channel qi is at its peak.

hard tetany 刚痉 *gang jing* This refers to rigidity due to spasm and contraction of muscles or to convulsions and is associated with an excess pattern, as opposed to soft tetany which is characterised by spontaneous sweating and is associated with a deficiency pattern.

he bing 合病 Concurrent pattern, where the disease is present in more than one channel.

hou zhong 后重 A heavy sensation in the rectum.

huo luan 霍乱 Sudden upheaval. Other translations include 'sudden rebellion' and 'sudden turmoil'. This disorder can refer to a range of acute stomach and intestinal disorders such as food poisoning or gastroenteritis. It must not be confused with the contemporary Chinese name for cholera.

huai bing 坏病 Transmuted pattern. Literally: 'deterioration of disease'.

huddled aversion to cold 啬啬恶寒 *se se wu han* This refers to the tendency of the person to huddle in order to keep warm and fend off the cold. It is one of the primary symptoms of Tai Yang zhong feng.

instep pulse 趺阳脉 *fu yang mai* This refers to the pulse felt at the highest point of the instep coinciding with the acupuncture point Chong Yang (St 42).

insubstantial vexation 虚烦 *xu fan* This is caused by a pathogen without substance such as heat which has not bound with a material substance and is deemed to be formless or intangible. It contrasts with vexation which arises from heat which is said to have formed because it has knotted with a substance such as phlegm, water, blood stasis, stagnant food, or bowel accumulation.

interstices 腠理 *cou li* This term refers to the openings or interstices in the layer running between the skin and muscle. These may include, but are not limited to, the pores of the skin. It is the interstices which provide a means for pathogens to pass into or out of the body. In modern terms *cou li* could be interpreted as the intercellular space.

jing luo 经络 Channels and network vessels, where the jing are the major channel pathways and the luo refer to the finer interconnecting branches.

jing mi 粳米 Sometimes mistakenly pronounced geng mi, is a variety of round grain non-glutinous rice.

jin 斤 The largest of the ancient Han dynasty units of weight approximating 250g. It is not the same as the modern *jin*, which equals 500g, and is also not to be confused with the term *gong jin* 公斤, which is the Chinese term for kilogram. *(For more detail refer to Appendix 9.)*

jiu ke bing 酒客病 Alcoholism.

jue 厥 The term *jue* as used in *Shang Han Lun* refers to cold extremities due to the non-communication of yin and yang. The cause can be deficiency of yang, or obstruction due to heat, cold, worms, water or some other substance. It can also refer to sudden loss of consciousness. It may be translated as 'final', 'ultimate', 'utmost', 'extreme', 'terminal' or 'desertion'.

jue ni 厥逆 This term refers to cold extremities due to deficient yang failing to flow to the extremities. This can be a result of the non-interaction of yin and yang or to obstruction to the flow of yang. *See also* **jue**

jue leng 厥冷 This term refers to cold extremities due to deficient yang failing to flow to the extremities. This can be a result of the non-interaction of yin and yang or to obstruction to the flow of yang. *See also* **jue**

Jue Yin 厥阴 This is the name of the sixth and final channel in the six channel system of *Shang Han Lun*. It incorporates the liver and pericardium channels and is sometimes translated as 'Terminal Yin' or 'Ultimate Yin'.

lagover pattern 并病 *bing bing* This term refers to the pathogen 'lagging over' in one channel whilst proceeding to the next.

lao fu 劳复 Taxation relapse. This is the term used in English to translate the Chinese word for over-exertion (*lao*) or exhaustion of energy by immoderate activity. This is relative to the individual. When recovering from illness, even those who are normally of robust constitution are at a low ebb, and are therefore prone to relapse (*fu*) of illness if a sensible aftercare regimen is not followed. Taxation relapse refers to relapse of illness in the recuperative period, when dietary and other protocols have not been complied with.

lesser abdomen 少腹 *shao fu* This term has two interpretations. The general definition is the lower abdomen. The more specific definition is the two sides of the lower abdomen relating to the foot Jue Yin liver channel. *See also* **small abdomen** 小腹 *xiao fu*

li ji hou zhong 里急后重 This is the term for tenesmus. *Li ji* refers to abdominal urgency and *hou zhong* refers to a heavy sensation in the rectum.

liang 两 An ancient Han dynasty unit of weight approximating 15.625g. The *liang* of *Shang Han*

Lun is not the same as the modern *liang*. For many centuries, a *liang* was equal to approximately 30g, with regional and periodic variations, and 16 *liang* equaled 1 *jin*. In the twentieth century, weights were decimalised: 1 *liang* was standardised to 50g and given the formal name of *shi liang* 市两 to differentiate it from the earlier measurement. The modern *liang* is $^1/_{10}$ of a modern *jin*, which is 500g. *(For more detail refer to Appendix 9.)*

lou han 漏汗 Leaking sweat. This describes a constant trickle of perspiration.

mao shi 卯时 This is the time according to the Han dynasty system of the twelve earthly branches, which covers the period from 5am to 7am. It represents the middle part of the six-hour period when Shao Yang channel qi is at its peak, and the later part of the peak period for Jue Yin.

muscle layer This is a common translation for the term *cou li* 腠理. It is sometimes also translated as 'skin pores' but more accurately refers to the layer running between the skin and the muscles, whose openings or interstices are generally accepted as including the pores of the skin, but not being limited to that concept. Some have proposed that it could refer to the interstitial spaces.

ni 逆 Reversal or reversed flow, found in such terms as *qi ni* 气逆 qi reversal; *shui ni* 水逆 reversed flow of water and sometimes translated as counterflow. It also has the sense of adverse or perverse in regard to treatment outcomes or unexpected symptoms.

no change of clothes 不更衣 *bu geng yi* This refers to constipation. To change one's clothes is a euphemistic expression for going to the lavatory to pass a stool.

noodles 索饼 *suo bing* This is an old word for noodles and literally means 'string pasta'. *Suo* means string, and *bing* refers to pastry made from flour. Today, *bing* most commonly refers to a pancake.

nǜ 衄 External bleeding. Refers to bleeding from an orifice, principally to bleeding from the nose.

nutrient 营 *See* **ying yin**

nutrient qi 营气 *See* **ying yin**

nutrient yin 营阴 *ying yin* This flows in the vessels with blood, nourishing blood and the interior (cf *wei yang* or defence yang).

pi 痞 This is translated as glomus and refers to a sensation of fullness or blockage which can be soft, when it is a reflection of the knotting of qi, or hard, when there is a knotting of heat or qi with water or phlegm.

pi yue 脾约 Spleen restraint. This refers to a pattern of spleen dysfunction causing constipation.

pi zheng 痞证 Glomus pattern.

pores *See* **interstices**

qi zi 棋子 These are the stones used in an ancient form of chess which enjoyed universal popularity in China. It was known as *wei qi* 围棋 or 'encircling chess' and was played on a board divided into 361 squares, using black and white stones as chessmen. The object was for one player to surround the opponent's stones with his and claim the squares thus occupied as his 'territory'. The stones measured about one inch in diameter. *Qian Jin Fang* records them as being the size of a 方寸匕 or 'square-inch spoon'. The *Shang Han Lun Da Ci Dian (The Complete Shang Han Lun Dictionary)* explains it is the equivalent of 10–12g in modern measurement. A reference to bigger stones used for chess pieces, known as *bo qi zi* (博棋子), as a form of measurement is found in Clause 393, where the footnote to Zhi Shi Zhi Zi Chi Tang reads: "If there is food stagnation, add Da Huang equalling the size of five or six bo qi zi, and recovery will follow after medication". *Qian Jin Fang* says: "The size of bo qi zi measure 2 inch by 1 inch square" (Clause 107).

qian 钱 A unit of measurement introduced in the Song dynasty, equaling $^1/_{10}$ of a *liang* or about 3 g. In the 20th century, it was standardised as 5g and given the formal appellation of *shi qian* 市钱, which might be translated as 'city qian' or 'metropolitan qian'. *(For more detail refer to Appendix 9.)*

qian bi 钱匕 A small teaspoon with a capacity of approximately 3mL.

re jie pang liu 热结旁流 This refers to constipation where the hard stool is accompanied by a foul watery discharge. A direct translation is 'knotting of heat with collateral flow'.

reversal cold *See* **jue, jue ni**

ri bu 日晡 Late afternoon. This is associated with *shen shi* or the period from 3pm to 5pm, and constitutes the early part of the period over which Yang Ming qi reaches its peak, which incorporates shen shi, you shi and xu shi, and lasts from 3pm to 9pm. During this time, the sun starts on its descending path, and its descent supports the descent of qi in the Yang Ming channel (Clauses 104, 212, 240).

rice water 白饮 *bai yin* This is the water taken from the pot as the rice is cooking.

rong qi 荣气 This is an alternative term for *ying qi* or nutrient qi.

running piglet *See* **ben tun**

san jiao 三焦 Triple burner. This concept incorporates the upper burner, the middle burner and the lower burner. The san jiao represents three segments of the body and is also a pathway for fire, qi and fluids.

san yin 三因 Three causes: the cause of season, the cause of region and the cause of the individual constitution (因时 *yin shi;* 因地 *yin di;* 因人 *yin ren*).

se se 啬啬 Huddled. *See* **se se wu han**

se se wu han 啬啬恶寒 Huddled aversion to cold. This refers to the tendency of the person to huddle in order to keep warm and fend off the cold, and is a feature of Tai Yang zhong feng.

separation of yin and yang 阴阳离决 This describes extreme instability of yin and yang leading to their separation, which means death.

sha zhen 砂疹 An externally contracted heat (febrile) disease pattern characterised by papules. *Sha* means sand and is descriptive of the distribution of papules in the skin.

shang 伤 Injury.

shang feng 伤风 Wind injury.

shang han 伤寒 Cold injury.

shao fu 少腹 This term has two interpretations. The general definition is the lower abdomen. The more specific definition is the two sides of the lower abdomen relating to the foot Jue Yin liver channel. *See also* **small abdomen** 小腹 *xiao fu*

Shao Yang 少阳 This is the name of the third of the yang channels in the six channel system of *Shang Han Lun*. It incorporates the gallbladder and san jiao channels and represents the connection between the exterior and interior. It can be translated as 'minor yang'.

Shao Yin 少阴 This is the name of the second of the yin channels in the six channel system of *Shang Han Lun*. It incorporates the kidney and heart channels and can be translated as 'minor yin'.

shen shi申时 This is the time according to the Han dynasty system of the twelve earthly branches, which covers the period from 3pm to 5pm. It represents the earlier part of the six-hour period when Yang Ming channel qi is at its peak.

sheng 升 An ancient Han dynasty unit of capacity equalling 200mL. It is not to be confused with the modern metric *sheng* which equals 1L. *(For more detail refer to Appendix 9.)*

shi 实 Fullness, excess. The opposite of deficiency.

shivering sweat 战汗 *zhan han* This describes aversion to cold accompanied by episodes of sweating, which is a manifestation of the zheng qi vying against the pathogen and indicates imminent recovery.

shui ni 水逆 Reversed flow of water.

si shi 巳时 This is the time according to the Han dynasty system of the twelve earthly branches, which covers the period from 9am to 11am. It represents the earlier part of the six-hour period when Tai Yang channel qi is at its peak.

si zhen 四诊 Four examinations.

small abdomen 小腹 *xiao fu* This refers to the centre of the lower abdomen between the umbilicus and the pubic bone. It relates to the foot Shao Yin kidney channel.

spleen restraint 脾约 *pi yue* This refers to a pattern of spleen dysfunction causing constipation.

spontaneous diarrhoea 自利 *zi li* This refers to diarrheoa not caused by purgation.

spontaneous sweating 自汗 *zi han* This refers to sweating which is not caused by diaphoretic therapy.

spontaneous urge to vomit 自欲呕 *zi yu tu* Urge to vomit not induced by emetics.

suo bing 索饼 An old term for noodles. This literally means 'string pasta'. *Suo* means string, and *bing* refers to pastry made from flour. Today, *bing* most commonly refers to a pancake.

suspended fluids 悬饮 *xuan yin* This refers to a pattern of accumulated phlegm fluids in the chest and hypochondrium.

Tai Yang 太阳 This is the name of the first of the yang channels in the six channel system of *Shang Han Lun* and as such is the most exterior. It incorporates the urinary bladder and small intestine channels and can be translated as 'great yang'.

Tai Yin 太阴 This is the name of the first of the yin channels in the six channel system of *Shang Han Lun*. It incorporates the spleen and lung channels and can be translated as 'great yin'.

tan shi 痰实 Phlegm excess.

tan yin 痰饮 Phlegm fluids.

taxation relapse 劳复 *lao fu* Taxation is the term used in English to translate the Chinese word for over-exertion (*lao*) or exhaustion of energy by immoderate activity. This is relative to the individual. When recovering from illness, even those who are normally of robust constitution are at a low ebb, and are therefore prone to relapse (*fu*) of illness if a sensible aftercare regimen is not followed. Taxation relapse refers to relapse of illness in the recuperative period, when dietary and other protocols have not been complied with.

three causes 三因 *san yin* The cause of season, the cause of region and the cause of the individual constitution (因时 *yin shi;* 因地 *yin di;* 因人 *yin ren*).

throbbing heart 心动悸 *xin dong ji* This is to be differentiated from palpitations 心悸 *xin ji* in that the throbbing is not subjective, as can be the case with palpitations, and furthermore, is not merely objectively palpable, but causes a visible movement of the chest.

transmuted pattern 坏病 *huai bing* This can be translated as 'deterioration of disease' and refers to the change of symptoms so the pattern is no longer characteristic of the channel. It is usually the result of incorrect treatment and is sometimes called *bian zheng* 变证 or 'changed pattern'.

vexation 心烦 *xin fan* This is not the same as 'irritability' or 'annoyance', as is the common modern translation, and it differs from *zao* 躁 'agitation' in that it refers to a sensation, not an action.

wei 卫 Defence. *See* **wei yang**

wei qi 卫气 Defence qi. *See* **wei yang**

wei shi 未时 This is the time according to the Han dynasty system of the twelve earthly branches, which covers the period from 1pm to 3pm. It represents the later part of the six-hour period when Tai Yang channel qi is at its peak.

wei yang 卫阳 Defence yang. This term refers to the yang qi which flows outside the blood vessels in the superficial layers of the body. Its functions include opening and closing the pores to regulate sweating, warming the skin and the exterior of the body, and defending it from exterior pathogens (cf *ying yin* or nutrient yin).

wei zheng 痿证 Wilting pattern characterised by weakness of the limbs.

wen bing 瘟病 Warm disease.

wen re 温热 Warm heat.

wetted aversion to wind 淅淅恶风 *xi xi wu feng* This refers to the increased susceptibility to wind when one is wet and is a feature of Tai Yang zhong feng.

wu shi 午时 This is the time according to the Han dynasty system, which covers the period from 11am to 1pm. It represents the middle part of the six-hour period when Tai Yang channel qi is at its peak.

xi xi 淅淅 Wetted. *See* **xi xi wu feng** *or* **wetted aversion to wind**

xi xi 翕翕 Feather-warm. *See* **xi xi fa re** *or* **feather-warm fever**

xi xi fa re 翕翕发热 Feather-warm fever. This refers to just a slight rise in temperature and is a feature of Tai Yang zhong feng.

xi xi wu feng 淅淅恶风 Wetted aversion to wind. This refers to the increased susceptibility to wind when one is wet and is a feature of Tai Yang zhong feng.

xian xiong 陷胸 Chest bind. Literally: 'stuffed chest'.

xiao fu 小腹 Small abdomen. This refers to the centre of the lower abdomen between the umbilicus and the pubic bone. It relates to the foot Shao Yin kidney channel.

xin dong ji 心动悸 This refers to a throbbing heart, which is to be differentiated from palpitations 心悸 *xin ji* in that the throbbing is not subjective, as can be the case with palpitations, and furthermore, is not merely objectively palpable, but causes a visible movement of the chest.

xin fan 心烦 vexation. This is not the same as 'irritability' or 'annoyance', as is the common modern translation, and it differs from *zao* 躁 'agitation' in that it refers to a sensation, not an action.

xin xia 心下 This is translated as below the heart and refers to the epigastric region.

xin xia pi 心下痞 Glomus below the heart. This refers to a sensation of fullness in the epigastric region.

xu fan 虚烦 Literally translated as ' deficiency vexation'. This term is sometimes misunderstood as meaning vexation due to deficiency. In fact, it refers to insubstantial vexation, which is the result of a pathogen without substance such as heat. It is deemed to be formless or intangible because it is not bound with a formed or tangible substance. This contrasts with vexation arising from heat which is said to have formed because it has knotted with a substance such as phlegm, water, blood stasis, stagnant food, or bowel accumulation.

xu 虚 Deficiency.

xu 蓄 Amassment.

xu shi 戌时 This is the time according to the Han dynasty system of the twelve earthly branches, which covers the period from 7pm to 9pm. It represents the later part of the six-hour period when Yang Ming channel qi is at its peak.

xu shui 蓄水 Water amassment.

xu xue 蓄血 Blood amassment.

xuan yin 悬饮 This is translated as suspended fluids and refers to a pattern of accumulated phlegm fluids in the chest and hypochondrium.

xun jing chuan 循经传 This describes pathogenic transmission according to the orthodox sequence of the six channels.

Yang Ming 阳明 This is the name of the second of the yang channels in the six channel system of *Shang Han Lun*. It incorporates the stomach and large intestine channels and could be translated as 'yang glory'.

yin shi 寅时 This is the time according to the Han dynasty system of the twelve earthly branches, which covers the period from 3am to 5am. It represents the middle part of the six-hour period when the Jue Yin channel qi is at its peak, overlapping with the end of the Shao Yin peak period and the beginning of the Shao Yang peak period.

ying 营 Nutrient. Sometimes also translated as 'nutritive'. *See* **ying yin**

ying qi 营气 Nutrient qi. Sometimes also translated as 'nutritive qi'. *See* **ying yin**

ying yin 营阴 Nutrient yin. It flows in the vessels with blood, nourishing blood and the interior (cf *wei yang* or defence yang).

you shi 时 This is the time according to the Han dynasty system of the twelve earthly branches, which covers the period from 5pm to 7pm. It represents the middle part of the six-hour period when Yang Ming channel qi is at its peak.

yu mao 郁冒 This refers to a foggy sensation in the head, dizziness and an oppressed sensation in the chest. It can precede blackout.

yue jing chuan 越经传 This describes pathogenic transmission which skips one or more channels.

za bing 杂病 Miscellaneous disease.

zang 脏、藏、臟 Zang or yin organ.

zang fu 臟腑、脏腑 Zang fu or organs (comprising both yin and yang organs).

zang zao 脏躁 Literally: 'organ agitation'. This refers to an ancient diagnosis comparable to 'hysteria'.

zao 躁 This refers to agitation which is not the same as 'irritability' or 'annoyance'. In *Shang Han Lun* it refers to unconscious fidgeting associated with altered consciousness and is thus distinguished from vexation 心烦 *xin fan,* which refers to an emotional sensation, not an action.

zhan han 战汗 Shivering sweat. This describes aversion to cold accompanied by episodes of sweating, which is a manifestation of the zheng qi vying against the pathogen and indicates imminent recovery.

zhen zang mai 真脏脉 True zang pulse.

zheng qi 正气 Antipathogenic qi. This refers to the aggregate of physiological qi which defends the body from pathogenic attack.

zheng 证 Pattern. This refers to a group of signs and symptoms which are the manifestation of a particular disease.

zheng 症 Disorder. This refers to a disease or syndrome.

zhi 制 Prepared or processed. This refers to any of several methods of herbal preparation.

zhi zhong 直中 Direct strike. This refers to the direct invasion of a pathogen into a channel other than Tai Yang.

zhong feng 中风 Wind strike. This refers to a pattern of exterior deficiency.

zhu 铢 The ancient Han dynasty measure approximating 0.651 grams. *(For more detail refer to Appendix 9.)*

zi han 自汗 Spontaneous sweating. This refers to sweating which is not the result of diaphoretic therapy.

zi li 自利 Spontaneous diarrhoea. This refers to diarrheoa not caused by purgation.

zi shi 子时 This is the time according to the Han dynasty system of the twelve earthly branches, which covers the period from 11pm to 1am. It represents the middle part of the period when Tai Yin channel qi is at its peak, and also the earlier part of the six-hour period when Shao Yin channel qi is at its peak.

zi yu tu 自欲呕 Spontaneous urge to vomit. An urge to vomit not induced by emetics.

zui shi 晬时 A period of twenty four hours.

Appendix 9

Weights and Measures

History of Weights and Measures used in China

Shang Han Lun was written in the Eastern Han period, approximately 200 AD. The system of weights and measures was similar to that of the Tang dynasty, and should not be confused with the measurement system introduced in the modern era. Both systems are compared in the tables below.

In early periods of Chinese history, the means of transport and communication between various regions was restricted. This resulted in considerable variation in the standard units of measurement, with records showing that the equivalent metric weight of a *jin* (斤) ranged from about 200 to 260g, with later eras designating 250g as a conversion for the purposes of expedience. In addition, there were two standard systems, a large measure known as *da cheng* (大称 also written 大秤) and a small measure known as *xiao cheng* (小称 also written 小秤), which was one-tenth the measure of *da cheng*. *Da cheng* was used for common goods, and *xiao cheng* was used specifically for measuring herbs (Tang Hui Yao唐会要). This is reminiscent of the many traditional systems of the West, amongst which there was the avoirdupois system for the measurement of common goods, the troy system for gold and silver, and the apothecaries' system for medicines.

The system of weights in use during the Eastern Han (东汉), which persisted through to the Later Jin (后晋) dynasty was as follows:

1 jin = 16 liang; 1 liang = 24 zhu or 4 fen;
1 fen = 6 zhu

The base unit of *da cheng* was *liang* (两), which is recorded variously as 13.92g and 15.625g. The smallest unit in common use was *zhu* (铢), which is recorded as being 0.65g. There were 24 *zhu* in a *liang* and 16 *liang* in a *jin*. Another measure in use was the *fen*, which was a measure of capacity, not of weight and was equal to 6 *zhu*. The apothecaries' measure, or *xiao cheng*, was $^1/_{10}$ that of the common measure or *da cheng*, where 1 *jin* was about 25g, and 1 *liang* is variously recorded as being equivalent to 13.92g and 15.625g. The capacity measure of 1 *fen* was similar to a small teaspoon.

This system was maintained over the next few hundred years, but was complicated by different systems being used in different kingdoms. The *liang* remained consistent in successive dynasties of some regions, but elsewhere tended to be much greater, with an equivalent weight of 20g in the Southern Qi (南齐), 27g in the Northern Qi (北齐), with both a smaller standard of 14 to 16g, and a second standard of 42g being used during the Sui dynasty (隋朝) of 581 to 618 AD. The standard measure for one *jin* varied from 250g to 600g and one *sheng* ranged from 200mL to 1L.

Further complications came as a result of taxation. Prior to and during the early part of the Tang dynasty, China's landlords levied land and grain tax on the peasants and, by reducing the base unit of weight, higher taxes could be exacted. Thus, *da cheng* (大称) came to be replaced for some time by *xiao cheng* (小称) in the measure of common goods for the purpose of exacting higher taxes.

Finally, in the Tang dynasty (唐朝) came a more unified system, where 1 *liang* was 37.3g. In the Song dynasty, the *qian* was introduced as a unit of measure which was $^1/_{10}$ of a *liang*, or 3.7g, and a new system was established which endured until the Chinese revolution in 1911. However, even in this relatively stable system, there is some conflict as to whether a *liang* was in fact 37.3g, as recorded in *The Concise Chinese Medical Dictionary* 简明中医辞典 (1979), or 31.25g, as recorded in many modern dictionaries. The Song dynasty system was recorded as follows:

1 jin = 16 liang; 1 liang = 10 qian; 1 qian = 10 fen; 1 fen = 10 li; 1 li = 10 hao

From the Song dynasty until the end of the Qing dynasty, there was no significant change in the system of weights and measures, thanks in part to improved transport and communications and also to the development of international commerce. After 1911, a modernised system was introduced, which was more easily converted into the metric system of the West. The standard unit was the *jin*, which was set at 500g, with the *liang* being 50g, a *qian* being 5g, and a *fen* being 0.5g Nevertheless, the Chinese medical community conserved the earlier standard.

Because of these many changes, there is much confusion about the equivalent gram dosage of the ancient dosages used by Zhang Zhong Jing. Confusion also arises because many of the formulas were intended to be used over a period of a few days, or discontinued once the desired effect was achieved. Additionally, today, a decoction is often administered in two larger, rather than three smaller doses, and there is also a variation in the decoction method, where the modern practice of re-decoction increases the extraction rate of essential components. Finally, in *Shang Han Lun*, the use of the unit 'fen' does not refer to a specific weight or measurement, but is used in the sense of the word 'part', as in 'one part powdered Gua Di and one part powdered Chi Xiao Dou'.

Eastern Han Da Cheng System Xiao Cheng measures are 1/10th of Da Cheng Gram equivalents are an approximation only					Modern System		
铢	1 zhu	0.651g			市分	1 fen	0.5g
分	1 fen	3.8g	= 6 zhu or 3.8mL		市钱	1 qian	5g
旧市两	1 old liang	15.625g	= 24 zhu or 4 fen		市两	1 liang	50g
市斤	1 jin	250g	= 16 old liang		市斤	1 jin	500g
(Ref: Ben Cao Jing Ji Zhu 本草经集注)							

Ancient Measures of Volume or Capacity Gram equivalents are an approximation only			Modern Equivalent
钱匕	1 qian bi or small teaspoon	3mL	
方寸匕	1 fang cun bi or square-inch spoon	5mL	
合	1 ge (dry measure)	1 fistful	
合	1 ge (liquid measure)	20mL	Modern ge = 100mL
升	1 old sheng	200mL	Modern sheng = 1L
斗	1 old dou	2L	Modern dou = 10L
(Ref: Han Shu: Lu Li Zhi 汉书律历志)			

The dosage of *Shang Han Lun* formulas may be adjusted according to individual circumstances. The factors affecting dosage are: (1) the patient's constitution; (2) the severity of the disease; and (3) the patient's response following administration.

1. *Patient's constitution.* An example is found in the dosage of Shi Zao Tang, which is 1 qian bi for a strong patient, and half a qian bi for a patient with a weak constitution. A second example is in the dose of Fu Zi in Si Ni Tang, where the recommended dose for a patient with a strong constitution, is a big piece, but otherwise a small piece should be used.
2. *Severity of the disease.* The dose is adjusted to be appropriate to the nature of the disease. In other words, where the condition is serious, the dose must be large enough to resolve the disease; if the condition is serious, too small a

dose will be ineffective. For example, Clause 29 advises that Tiao Wei Cheng Qi Tang should be taken a little at a time so as to harmonise the stomach qi; in contrast, Clauses 70, 212 and 250 advise that the decoction should be taken in one single dose, where a more potent draught is needed to address Yang Ming exuberant dryness heat bind.

3. *Patient's response to the initial dose.* Some formulas contain toxic herbs and the initial dose is small so as to assess the patient's tolerance; thereafter the size of the dose can be gradually increased.

Because of the complexity of the issue of weights and measures and the contentious nature of their conversion, this text does not venture to provide a simple and definitive equation. However, in modern China, the 'rule of thumb' conversion system for the calculation of doses in grams is: 1 old liang = 1 qian = 3.125g. Despite some uncertainty in the accuracy of conversion, it is generally the proportions which are most important, and the preservation of these proportions is demonstrated in the following comparison of the ancient and modern measures for Ma Huang Xing Ren Gan Cao Tang.

Ma Huang Xing Ren Gan Cao Tang

***Shang Han Lun* Dosage**		**Modern Dosage**	
Ma Huang	4 liang	Ma Huang	12g
Xing Ren	50 pieces	Xing Ren	9g
Zhi Gan Cao	2 liang	Zhi Gan Cao	6g
Shi Gao	½ jin (8 liang)	Shi Gao	24g

The information given in this section is not conclusive, but is proffered for the reader's consideration as we continue to seek an answer to the confusion surrounding the ancient measures.

Appendix 10

Han Dynasty Time: the Ebb and Flow of the Six Channels

Ebb and Flow of Qi in the Six Channels

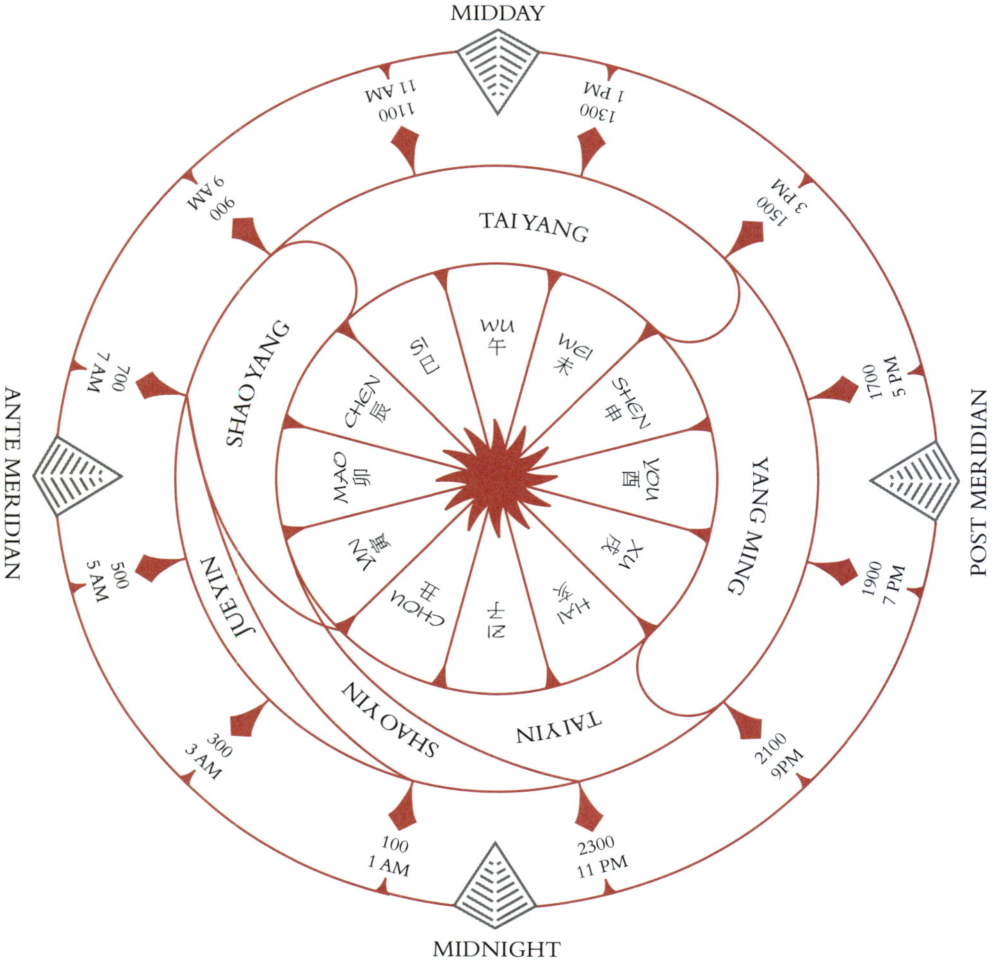

Overlapping of the six channels						
Zi 子 11pm–1am	Tai Yin	Shao Yin				
Chou 丑 1am–3am	Tai Yin	Shao Yin	Jue Yin			
Yin 寅 3am–5am		Shao Yin	Jue Yin	Shao Yang		
Mao 卯 5am–7am			Jue Yin	Shao Yang		
Chen 辰 7am–9am				Shao Yang		
Si 巳 9am–11am					Tai Yang	
Wu 午 11am–1pm					Tai Yang	
Wei 未 1pm–3pm					Tai Yang	
Shen 申 3pm–5pm						Yang Ming
You 酉 5pm–7pm						Yang Ming
Xu 戌 7pm–9pm						Yang Ming
Hai 亥 9pm–11pm	Tai Yin					

Peak periods of the six channels		
太阳 Tai Yang Channel	巳 午 未 Si Wu Wei	9am–3pm
阳明 Yang Ming Channel	申 酉 戌 Shen You Xu	3pm–9pm
少阳 Shao Yang Channel	寅 卯 辰 Yin Mao Chen	3am–9am
太阴 Tai Yin Channel	亥 子 丑 Hai Zi Chou	9pm–3am
少阴 Shao Yin Channel	子 丑 寅 Zi Chou Yin	11pm–5am
厥阴 Jue Yin Channel	丑 寅 卯 Chou Yin Mao	1am–7am

Relationship between the Twelve Earthly Branches and the Six Channels

子 zi	丑 chou	寅 yin	卯 mao
11pm–1am Tai Yin Shao Yin	1am–3am Tai Yin Shao Yin Jue Yin	3am–5am Shao Yin Jue Yin Shao Yang	5am–7am Jue Yin Shao Yang

辰 chen	巳 si	午 wu	未 wei
7am–9am Shao Yang	9am–11am Tai Yang	11am–1pm Tai Yang	1pm–3pm Tai Yang

申 shen	酉 you	戌 xu	亥 hai
3pm–5pm Yang Ming	5pm–7pm Yang Ming	7pm–9pm Yang Ming	9pm–11pm Tai Yin

Appendix 11

Heavenly Stems and Earthly Branches

The Heavenly Stems can be used for a series like 'a', 'b', 'c' and are combined with the Earthly Branches to denote years, months, days and hours. The Earthly Branches were used in the Han Dynasty to mark two-hour periods in a 24-hour system of measuring time, and appear in *Shang Han Lun* to refer to the period of time in which the qi each of the six channels comes to its peak. They are also found in the system of *zǐ wǔ liú zhù* 子午流注 or Midnight to Midday Flow and Fill, famously used in the Ming dynasty to explain and understand the flow of qi and xue in the channels at particular times.

HEAVENLY STEMS 天干 tiān gān			EARTHLY BRANCHES 地支 dì zhī		
甲	jiǎ	1st heavenly stem	子	zǐ	1st earthly branch
乙	yǐ	2nd heavenly stem	丑	chǒu	2nd earthly branch
丙	bǐng	3rd heavenly stem	寅	yín	3rd earthly branch
丁	dīng	4th heavenly stem	卯	mǎo	4th earthly branch
戊	wù	5th heavenly stem	辰	chén	5th earthly branch
己	jǐ	6th heavenly stem	巳	sì	6th earthly branch
庚	gēng	7th heavenly stem	午	wǔ	7th earthly branch
辛	xīn	8th heavenly stem	未	wèi	8th earthly branch
壬	rèn	9th heavenly stem	申	shēn	9th earthly branch
癸	guǐ	10th heavenly stem	酉	yóu	10th earthly branch
			戌	xū	11th earthly branch
			亥	hài	12th earthly branch

Appendix 12

Chinese Dynasties and Historical Periods

夏	**XIA DYNASTY**			2100 – 1600 BC
商	**DYNASTY**			1600 – 1100 BC
周	**ZHOU DYNASTY**	西周	WESTERN ZHOU	1100 – 771 BC
		东周	EASTERN ZHOU	770 – 256 BC
		春秋	SPRING & AUTUMN	770 – 476 BC
		战国	WARRING STATES	475 – 221 BC
秦	**QIN DYNASTY**			221 – 206 BC
汉	**HAN DYNASTY**	西汉	WESTERN HAN	206 BC – 24 AD
		东汉	EASTERN HAN	25 – 220 AD
三国	**THREE KINGDOMS**	魏	WEI	220 – 265 AD
		蜀汉	SHU HAN	221 – 263 AD
		吴	WU	222 – 280 AD
西晋	**WESTERN JIN DYNASTY**			265 – 316 AD
东晋	**EASTERN JIN DYNASTY**			317 – 420 AD
南北朝	**SOUTHERN & NORTHERN DYNASTIES:**			
南朝	SOUTHERN DYNASTIES			
		宋	SONG	420 – 479 AD
		齐	QI	479 – 502 AD
		梁	LIANG	502 – 557 AD
		陈	CHEN	557 – 589 AD
北朝	NORTHERN DYNASTIES			
		北魏	NORTHERN WEI	386 – 534 AD
		东魏	EASTERN WEI	534 – 550 AD
		北齐	NORTHERN QI	550 – 577 AD
		西魏	WESTERN WEI	535 – 556 AD
		北周	NORTHERN ZHOU	557 – 581 AD
隋	**SUI DYNASTY**			581 – 618 AD
唐	**TANG DYNASTY**			618 – 907 AD

五代	**FIVE DYNASTIES**			
		后梁	LATER LIANG	907 – 923 AD
		后唐	LATER TANG	923 – 936 AD
		后晋	LATER JIN	936 – 946 AD
		后汉	LATER HAN	947 – 950 AD
		后周	LATER ZHOU	951 – 960 AD
宋	**SONG DYNASTY**			
		北宋	NORTHERN SONG	960 – 1127
		南宋	SOUTHERN SONG	1127 – 1279
辽	**LIAO DYNASTY**			916 – 1125
金	**JIN DYNASTY**			1115 – 1234
元	**YUAN DYNASTY**			1271 – 1368
明	**MING DYNASTY**			1368 – 1644
清	**QING DYNASTY**			1644 – 1911
中华民国	**REPUBLIC OF CHINA**			1912 – 1949
中华人民共和	**PEOPLE'S REPUBLIC OF CHINA**			1949 – present day

Appendix 13

Notable Figures in Chinese Medicine

For clarification and for the reader's interest, we have provided an alphabetical list of the authors named in this book in pinyin accompanied by the Chinese characters of the names. Where a name adopted by an author later in life is relatively well known, it appears in brackets following the birth name.

Bian Que 扁鹊 (Qin Yue Ren 秦越人) 407–310 BC
Cao Ying Fu 曹颖甫 1866–1938
Chao Yuan Fang 巢元方 581–618
Chen Ping Bo 陈平伯 1809–?
Chen Rui Chun 陈瑞春 1936–
Chen Shen Wu 陈慎吾 1897–1972
Chen Xiu Yuan陈修圆 1766–1833
Chen Yan 陈言 12th century
Chen Yi 臣亿 Unknown
Chen Zhi 陈治 Qing dynasty
Chen Zi Ming 陈自明 1190–1270
Cheng Dan An 承淡安1899–1957
Cheng Ying Mao 程应旄 (Cheng Jiao Qian) Qing dynasty
Cheng Wu Ji 成无己 1066–1156?
Dai Yuan Li 戴原礼 1324–1405
Du Ben 杜本 1271–1368
Fang You Zhi方有执 1523–?
Fu Qing Zhu 傅青主 1607–1684
Gao Wu 高武 (Gao Mei Gu) 16th century
Ge Hong 葛洪 (Ge Zhi Chuan 葛稚川) 261–341 AD
Guo Zi Guang 郭子光1932–
He Lian Chen 何廉臣 1860–1929
Hu Xi Shu 胡希恕 1899–1984
Hua Tuo 华佗 ?–208 AD
Huang Fu Mi 皇甫谧 214–282 AD
Huang Yuan Yu 黄元御 (Huang Kun Zai) Qing dynasty
Ke Yun Bo 柯韵伯 1662–1735
Li Gao 李杲 (Li Dong Yuan, Li Ming Zhi) 1180–1251
Li Shi Zhen 李时珍 (Li Dong Bi, Li Bin Hu) 1518–1593
Li Zhong Zi 李中梓 1588–1655
Lin Yi 林亿 1057–?
Liu Du Zhou刘渡舟 1917–2001
Liu He Jian刘河间 1120–1200
Liu Zheng Cai 刘正才 Unknown
Lu Jiu Zhi 陆九芝 1815–1887
Luo Tian Yi 罗天益 1200–1290
Pang An Shi 庞安时 1042–1099
Qian Huang 钱潢 (Tian Lai) Qing dynasty
Qian Yi 钱亿 1035–1117
Qin Yue Ren 秦越人 407–310 BC
Shen Ming Zong 沈明宗 Qing dynasty
Shen Jin Ao 沈金鳌 (Qian Lu) 1717–1776
Song Yun Gong 宋云公 Jin-Yuan period
Sun Si Miao 孙思邈 590–682 AD
Tang Rong Chuan 唐容川 1862–1918
Tao Hong Jing 陶弘景 (Tao Tong Ming 陶通明) 456–536 AD
Wang Hu 汪琥 (Ling You) circa 1680
Wang Jin Zhi 王进之 (Wang Hao Gu王好古) Yuan dynasty
Wang Ken Tang 王肯堂 Ming dynasty
Wang Qing Ren 王清任 (Wang Xun Chen 王勋臣) 1768–1831
Wang Ri Xiu 王日休 Ming dynasty

Wang Shu He 王叔和 (Wang Xi 王熙) 210–285 AD
Wang Wei Yi 王惟一 (Wang Wei De 王惟德) 987–1067 AD
Wei Li Tong 魏荔彤 Qing dynasty
Wu Kun An 吴坤安 Qing dynasty
Wu Tang 吴瑭 (Wu Ju Tong 吴鞠通) 1758–1836
Wu You Ke 吴又可 (Wu You Xing 吴有性) Ming dynasty
Xu Chun Fu 徐春甫 16th century
Xu Hong 许宏 1341–?
Xu Ling Tai 徐灵胎 1693–1771
Xu Shu Wei 许叔微 1080–1154
Xue Sheng Bai 薛生白 1681–1770
Yang Ji Zhou 杨继洲 1522–1621
Yang Jie 杨介 11th century
Ye Gui 叶桂 (Ye Tian Shi 叶天士) 1667–1746
Ye Ju Quan 叶橘泉 1896–1989
Ye Tang Bo 叶堂伯 13th century
You Zai Jing 尤在泾 ?–1749
Yu Gen Chu 俞根初 1734–1799
Yu Jia Yan 俞嘉言山 1585–1664
Yue Mei Zhong 岳美中 1900–1982
Zhao Kai Mei 赵开美 1563–1624
Zhang Bo Zu 张伯祖East Han; Zhang Zhong Jing's teacher
Zhang Jie Bin 张介宾 (Zhang Jing Yue 张景岳) 1563–1640
Zhang Lu Yu 张路玉 1617–1699
Zhang Zhi Cong 张志聪 1644–1722
Zhang Xi Chun张锡纯 1860–1933
Zhang Xu Gu 章虚谷 1825
Zhang Yin An 张隐庵 Qing dynasty
Zhang Zhong Jing 张仲景 (Zhang Ji 张机) 142–220 AD
Zhu Gong 朱肱 12th Northern Song dynasty
Zhu Zhen Heng 朱震亨 (Zhu Dan Xi 朱丹溪) 1281–1358

Appendix 14

References

Ba Shi Yi Nan 八十一难 *(Eighty-One Difficult Issues)*. Attributed to Qin Yue Ren 秦越人 also known as Bian Que 扁鹊. Eastern Han dynasty. People's Medical Publishing House, Beijing 2002.

Ben Cao Gang Mu 本草纲目 *(Compendium of Materia Medica)*. Li Shi Zhen 李时珍. First published 1596.

Ben Cao Jing Ji Zhu 本草经集注 *(Collection of Commentaries on the Classic of the Material Medica.)* Tao Hong Jing 陶弘景. Qi dynasty 494 AD.

Ben Cao Zheng Yi 本草正义 *(Rectification of the Meaning of the Materia Medica)*. Zhang Shan Lei 1914.

Bian Mai Fa Extracted from *Shang Han Lun*. Zhang Zhong Jing. First published 300 AD. People's Medical Publishing House, Beijing 2005.

Chen Rui Chun Lun Shang Han 陈瑞春论伤寒 (*Chen Rui Chun's Cold Injury)*. Hunan Ke Xue Ji Shu Chu Ban She湖南科学技术出版社 (Hunan Science & Technology Publishing House), Hunan 2002.

Chong Ding Tong Su Shang Han Lun 重订通俗伤寒论 *(Revised Popular Guide to the Treatise of Cold Damage Diseases)*. Yu Gen Chu 俞根初 (1734–1799). The original manuscript was never published. In 1934, the book was edited by Cao Bing Zhang and published by Shanghai Liu Ye Tang Shu Ju. Later, in 1956, it was compiled and edited by Xu Rong Zai and published by Shanghai Medical Press, Shanghai 1956.

Fu Jian Zhong Yi Yao 福建中医药 (Fujian Journal of Traditional Chinese Medicine) 1961; (433) 3:1.

Fu Jian Zhong Yi Yao 福建中医药 (Fujian Journal of Traditional Chinese Medicine) 1964;Vol 5.

Fu Ren Liang Fang Da Quan 妇人良方大全 *(Compendium of Effective Prescriptions for Women)*. Chen Zi Ming 陈自明. First published 1237.

Gu Ben Shang Han Za Bing Lun 古本伤寒杂病论 *(Ancient Edition of the Discourses on Cold Damage and Miscellaneous Diseases)*. Ed Liu Zhong Mai 刘仲迈 1932. This text is also known as *Chang Sha Gu Ben* 长沙古本 (*The Ancient Text from Changsha)*.

Gu Jin Yi An An 古今医案 *(Ancient and Modern Medical Cases)*. Yu Zhen Zuan 海科技出版社. Shanghai Science and Technology Press, Shanghai 1959.

Gu Jin Yi Tong Da Quan 古今医统大全 *(Compendium of Ancient and Modern Medical Systems)*. Xu Chun Fu 徐春甫. First published 1566.

Guang Dong Yi Xue 广东医学 (Guangdong Medical Journal) 1982; 9:26.

Guang Dong Zhong Yi 广东中医 (Guangdong Journal of Traditional Chinese Medicine) 1959; 4:163.

Guang Dong Zhong Yi 广东中医 (Guangdong Journal of Traditional Chinese Medicine) 1960; 6:305.

Guang Dong Zhong Yi 广东中医 (Guangdong Journal of Traditional Chinese Medicine) 1963; 2:38.

Guang Dong Zhong Yi 广东中医 (Guangdong Journal of Traditional Chinese Medicine) 1963; 3:39.

Guang Ming Zhong Yi 光明中医 (Guang Ming

Journal of Traditional Chinese Medicine) 1988; 3:17.
Gui Yang Zhong Yi Xue Bao 贵阳中医学报 (Journal of Guiyang College of Traditional Chinese Medicine 1991; (1).
Han Shu: Lu Li Zhi 汉书律历志 *(Book of Han: Gazette of Standard Measurements)*. Ban Gu (班固). Collection of Ancient Chinese Measurements. Compiled by Wang Pu Zhuan. Song dynasty.
Han Yao Shen Xiao Fang 汉药神效方 *(Miraculous Han Herbal Formulas)*. Qin dynasty (author unknown).
Harbin Zhong Yi 哈尔滨中医 (Harbin Journal of Traditional Chinese Medicine) 1960; 2:2.
Hebei Xin Yi Yao 河北新医药 (Hebei New Herbal Medicine) 1973; 3.
He Tu Luo Shu 河图洛书 *(River Charts and the Book of Luo)*. Early Qin dynasty.
Henan Zhong Yi 河南中医 (Henan Journal of Traditional Chinese Medicine) 1978; (4):1
Henan Zhong Yi 河南中医 (Henan Journal of Traditional Chinese Medicine) 1983; (3):33.
Henan Zhong Yi 河南中医 (Henan Journal of Traditional Chinese Medicine) 1986; (3):18.
Henan Zhong Yi 河南中医 (Henan Journal of Traditional Chinese Medicine) 1986; (5):8–10.
Hu Bei Zhong Yi Za Zhi 湖北中医杂志 (Hubei Journal of Traditional Chinese Medicine) 1981; 6:30.
Hu Bei Zhong Yi Za Zhi 湖北中医杂志 (Hubei Journal of Traditional Chinese Medicine) 1986; 3:36.
Hu Bei Zhong Yi Za Zhi 湖北中医杂志 (Hubei Journal of Traditional Chinese Medicine) 1983; 4:31.
Hu Nan Yi Yao Wei Sheng Ke Ji 湖南医药卫生科技 (Hunan Medical Technology) 1971; 11.
Hu Nan Yi Xue Za Zhi 湖南医学杂志 (Hunan Medical Magazine) 1977; June issue.
Huang Di Nei Jing 黄帝内经 *(The Yellow Emperor's Internal Classic)*. Anonymous. 400–200 BC.
Huang Han Yi Xue: Tang Ben Qiu Zhen 皇汉医学: 汤本求真. *(Chinese Medicine Series: Seeking the Truth of the Basis of Decoction)*. Originally published 1927. Shanghai Zhong Yi Xue Yuan Chu Ban She上海中医学院出版社(Shanghai College of Traditional Chinese Medicine Publishing House), Shanghai 1993.
Huang Han Yi Xue: Yan Ke Jin Nang 皇汉医学: 眼科锦囊. *(Chinese Medicine Series: Brocade Purse of Ophthalmology)*. Compiled by Chen Cun Ren in 1936, Shanghai Zhong Yi Xue Yuan Chu Ban She 上海中医学院出版社 (Shanghai College of Traditional Chinese Medicine Publishing House), Shanghai 1993.
Huang Wen Dong Yi An 黄文东医案 *(Huang Wen Dong Medical Cases)*. 上海科技出版社 Shanghai Science and Technology Press, Shanghai 1977.
Huo Ren Shi Zheng Fang Hou Ji: Qian Jin Bao Yao 活人事证方后集: 千金宝要 *(Patterns and Formulas to Safeguard Life: Essential Thousand Ducat Treasure)*. Compiled by Guo Si郭思 and Liu Xin Fu 刘信甫 Song dynasty. 上海科学技术出版社 Shanghai Science and Technology Press, Shanghai 2003.
Ji Sheng Fang 济生方 *(Formulas to Aid the Living)*. Yan Yong He (嚴用和). First published 1253.
Ji Yang Gang Mu 济阳纲目 *(Guide to Saving Yang)*. Wu Zhi Wang 武之望. First published 1626.
Jiang Su Zhong Yi 江苏中医 (Jiang Su Journal of Traditional Chinese Medicine) 1990; 10:29.
Jiang Su Zhong Yi 江苏中医 (Jiang Su Journal of Traditional Chinese Medicine) 1996; 7: 33.
Jiang Xi Zhong Yi Yao 江西中医药 (Jiangxi Journal of Traditional Chinese Medicine) 1990; 3:25.
Jiang Xi Zhong Yi Yao 江西中医药 (Jiangxi Journal of Traditional Chinese Medicine) 1980; 4:29.
Jiang Xi Zhong Yi Yao 江西中医药 (Jiangxi Journal of Traditional Chinese Medicine) 1990; 3:25 (580).
Jiang Xi Yi Yao 江西医药 (Jiangxi Medical Journal) 1983; 3:67.
Jiang Su Zhong Yi 江苏中医 (Jiang Su Journal of Traditional Chinese Medicine) 1997; 3:18.
Jiang Su Zhong Yi 江苏中医 (Jiang Su Journal of Traditional Chinese Medicine) 1963; 6:15.
Jilin Zhong Yi Yao 吉林中医药 (Jilin Journal of Traditional Chinese Medicine) 1997; (2):20.
Jin Gui Yao Lue 金匮要略 *(Essentials of the Golden Chamber)*. Zhang Zhong Jing张仲景. First published circa 210 AD.
Jin Gui Yao Lue Qian Zhu Bu Zheng 金匮要略浅注补正 *(Supplementary Overview to Essentials of the Golden Chamber)*. Tang Rong Chuan 唐容川. First published 1894.
Jin Gui Yu Han Jing 金匮玉函经 *(Classic of the Golden Chamber and Jade Sheath)*. Zhang Zhong Jing 张仲景. First published circa 210 AD.
Jin Jing Nei Tai Fang Yi 金镜内台方义 *(Golden Mirror of the Imperial Pharmacy)*. Xu Hong 许宏. 1422.
Jing Fang Shi Yan Lu 经方实验录 *(A Record of Tried and True Classic Formulas)*. Cao Ying Fu 曹颖甫. First published 1937. Shanghai Science and Technology Press, Shanghai 1979.

Jing Yue Quan Shu 岳全书 (Complete Works of Jing Yue). Zhang Jing Yue 张景岳. 1640.

Jiu Juan 九卷 *(The Nine Fascicles)*. Anonymous. (Alternative title for *Ling Shu* or *Miraculous Pivot.)* Circa 200 BC.

Lan Shi Mi Cang 兰室秘藏 *(Secret Records of the Orchid Chamber)*. Li Gao. First published 1276.

Lei Ju Fang Guang Yi 类聚方广义 *(Overview of Formulas according to Category)*. Wei Tai Rong Tang 尾台 榕堂 Zhu Shi Hui She Da An Press 株式会社大安, Tokyo 1962.

Lei Zheng Huo Ren Shu 类证活人书 *(Book to Safeguard Life)*. Zhu Gong 朱肱. First published 1108. Tian Jin Ke Xue Ji Shu Chu Ban She 天津科学技术出版社 (Tianjin Science & Technology Press), Tianjin 2003. Later renamed *Nan Yang Huo Ren Shu* 南阳活人书 *Nan Yang Book to Safeguard Life*. Zhu Gong 朱. First published 1118.

Liao Ning Zhong Yi Za Zhi 辽宁中医杂志 (Liaoning Journal of Traditional Chinese Medicine) 1980; (5):35

Liao Ning Zhong Yi Za Zhi 辽宁中医 (Liaoning Journal of Traditional Chinese Medicine) Feb 2003; Vol 30: No 2.

Liao Ning Zhong Yi Za Zhi 辽宁中医杂志 (Liaoning Journal of Traditional Chinese Medicine) 1980; (3):22.

Lin Zheng Zhi Nan Yi An 临证指南医案 *(Guide to Clinical Cases)*. Ye Tian Shi 叶天士. First published 1746.

Ling Shu 灵枢 *(Miraculous Pivot)*. Second volume of *Huang Di Nei Jing*. Anonymous. Circa 200 BC.

Liu Du Zhou Yi Xue Quan Ji 刘渡舟医学全集 *(Complete Works of Liu Du Zhou)*. Qi Ye Shu Ju 启业书局 Enterprise Books, Taiwan 1998.

Liu Jing Bian Zheng Shi Yong Jie 六经辨证实用解 *(Practical Explanation of Six Channel Pattern Differentiation)*. Compiled by Jia Xiu Lin 贾秀林 and Jia Fang 贾芳. Ren Min Wei Sheng Chu Ban She 人民卫生出版社 People's Medical Publishing House. Beijing 2002.

Ming Yi Jing Yan Lu 名医经验录 *(Record of Medical Experience)*. Compiled by Jing Lu Xian 景录先. Zhong Guo Yi Yao Ke Ji Chu Ban She中国医药科技出版社 China Medical-Pharmaceutical Science and Technology Press, Beijing 1996.

Nan Jing 难经 *(Classic of Difficult Issues)*. Attributed to Qin Yue Ren 秦越人 also known as Bian Que 扁鹊. Eastern Han. People's Medical Publishing House, Beijing 2002.

Nan Yang Huo Ren Shu 南阳活人书 *(Nan Yang Book to Safeguard Life)*. Zhu Gong 朱. First published 1118.

Pu Ji Ben Shi Fang 普济本事方 *(Formulas of Universal Benefit)*. Xu Shu Wei 1132.

Qian Jin Fang 千金方 *(Thousand Ducat Formulas)*. (Includes *Qian Jin Yao Fang* 千金要方 and *Qian Jin Yi Fang* 千金翼方). Sun Si Miao 孙思邈. Tang dynasty, 7th century.

Ri Yong Ben Cao 日用本草 *(Household Materia Medica)*. Wu Rui (吴瑞). Circa 1350.

San Ding Tong Su Shang Han Lun 三丁通俗伤寒论 *(Revised Popular Guide to the Treatise of Cold Damage Diseases)*. Yu Gen Chu 俞根初. Edited by Lian Jian Wei. 中医古籍出版社Chinese Medicine Ancient Book Publications, Beijing 2002.

San Yin Fang 三因方 *(Formulas for the Three Causes)*. Chen Yan 陈言, 1174.

Shaanxi Zhong Yi 陕西中医 (Shaanxi Journal of Traditional Chinese Medicine)1976; Vol 2:22.

Shanghai Zhong Yi Yao Za Zhi 上海中医药杂志 (Shanghai Journal of Traditional Chinese Medicine) 1955; 11:1.

Shanghai Zhong Yi Za Zhi 上海中医药杂志 (Shanghai Journal Of Traditional Chinese Medicine) 1979; 6:37.

Shanghai Zhong Yi Yao Za Zhi 上海中医药杂志 (Shanghai Journal Of Traditional Chinese Medicine) 1965; 8:19.

Shang Han Bai Wen 伤寒百问 *(One Hundred Questions on Shang Han)*. Zhu Gong朱肱. 1108 AD.

Shang Han Bao Ming Ji 伤寒保命集 *(Preserving Life from Cold Damage Collection)*. Zhang Bi 张璧. Yuan dynasty.

Shang Han Bu Wang Lun 伤寒补亡论 *(Discourse on Supplementing Desertion in Cold Damage)*. Guo Yong 郭雍. 1181 AD.

Shang Han Da Bai 伤寒大白 *(Clarification of Shang Han Lun)*. Qin Zhi Zhen 秦之桢. 1714.

Shang Han Fa Wei Lun 伤寒发微论 *(Elaboration on Cold Damage)*. Xu Shu Wei 许叔微. Song dynasty, 12th century.

Shang Han Fu Yi 伤寒附翼 *(Supplement to Shang Han)*. Ke Yun Bo 柯韵伯. Qing dynasty. (Part of *Collected Writings on Renewal of the Discussion of Cold Damage.)*

Shang Han Guan Zhu Ji 伤寒贯珠集 *(Collected Pearls on Cold Damage)*. You Zai Jing 尤在泾. 1729.

Shang Han Jiu Shi Lun 伤寒九十论 *(Nineteen Discourses on Cold Injury)*. Xu Shu Wei 许叔微. 1132.

Shang Han Lai Su Ji 伤寒来苏集 *(Shang Han Revival Compendium)*. Ke Yun Bo 柯韵伯. Qing dynasty.

Shang Han Lei Fang 伤寒类方 *(Categorised Formulas in Cold Damage)*. Xu Ling Tai 徐灵胎. 1759.

Shang Han Lei Zheng 傷寒类証 *(Categorised Patterns of Shang Han)*. Song Yun Gong 宋云公. Jin-Yuan period.

Shang Han Li Xin Zhu 伤寒例新注 *(New Illustrated Edition of Shang Han)*. Lu Jiu Zhi 陆九芝 (1815-1887).

Shang Han Liu Shu 伤寒六书 *(Six Texts on Cold Damage)*. Tao Hua 陶华. 1445 AD.

Shang Han Lun Fang Yun Yong Fa 伤寒方运用法 *(Application of Shang Han Lun Formulas)*. Zhejiang Ke Ji Chu Ban She浙江科技出版社 (Zhejiang Science & Technology Publishing House), Zhejiang 1985.

Shang Han Lun 伤寒论 *(Treatise on Cold Damage Disease)*. Zhang Zhong Jing 张仲景. Circa 200 AD.

Shang Han Lun Ben Zhi 伤寒论本旨 *(The Basic Meaning of Shang Han Lun)*. Zhang Xu Gu 章虚谷. 1835.

Shang Han Lun Bian Zheng Guang Zhu 伤寒论辩证广注 *(Overview of the Differential Diagnosis of Shang Han Lun)*. Wang Hu 汪琥. First published Qing dynasty. Shanghai Ke Ji Chu Ban She上海科技出版社 (Shanghai Science & Technology Publishing House), Shanghai 1959.

Shang Han Lun Chan Shi 伤寒论阐释. *(Shang Han Lun Explained)*. Cheng You Ren. Shaanxi Science and Technology Press, Shaanxi 1983.

Shang Han Lun Fang Yi An Xuan Bian 伤寒论方医案选编 *(Selected Medical Cases Using Shang Han Formulas)*. Gao De (Ed.) 高德编. Hunan Ke Ji Chu Ban She 湖南科技出版社 (Hunan Science & Technology Publishing House), Hunan 1981.

Shang Han Lun Gang Mu 伤寒论纲目 *(Guide to Shang Han Lun)*. Shen Jin Ao 沈金鳌. First published 1773.

Shang Han Lun Jiang Yi 伤寒论讲义 *(Discussion of Shang Han Lun)*. Compiled by Nie Hui Min 聂惠民. Xue Yuan Chu Ban She学苑出版社 (Academy Press), Beijing 1995.

Shang Han Lun Hui Yao Fen Xi 伤寒论汇要分析 *(Collection of Important Analyses of Shang Han Lun)*. Yu Chang Rong 俞长荣. Fujian Ren Min Chu Ban She 福建人民出版社 (Fujian People's Publishing House), Fujian 1964.

Shang Han Lun Lin Chuang Shi Yan Lu 伤寒论临床实验录 *(A Record of Shang Han Lun Clinically Tried and True Formulas)*. Compiled by Xing Xibo 邢锡波. Tianjin Ke Ji Chu Ban She天津科技出版社 (Tianjin Science & Technology Publishing House), Tianjin 1984.

Shang Han Lun Lin Chuang Ying Yong Wu Shi Lun 伤寒论临床应用五十论 *(Fifty Clinical Applications of Shang Han Lun)*. Pei Yong Qing 裴永清. Xue Yuan Chu Ban She学苑出版社 (Academy Press), Beijing 1995.

Shang Han Lun Tang Zheng Lun Zhi 伤寒论汤证论治 *(Patterns, Theory and Treatment Using Shang Han Lun Decoctions)*. Edited by Li Wen Rui 李文瑞 and Li Qiu Gui 李秋贵. Zhong Guo Ke Xue Ji Shu Chu Ban She 中国科学技术出版社 (China Science and Technology Press), Beijing 2000.

Shang Han Lun Tang Zheng Xin Pian 伤寒论汤证新篇 *(New Edition of Shang Han Lun Decoction Patterns)*. Guo Zi Gang et al. Shanghai Science and Technology Press, Shanghai 1983.

Shang Han Lun Tiao Bian 伤寒论条辩 *(Systematic Differentiation in Shang Han Lun)*. Fang You Zhi 方有执. Ren Min Wei Sheng Chu Ban She 人民卫生出版社 (People's Medical Publishing House), Beijing 1957.

Shang Han Lun Xin Zhu 伤寒论新注 *(New Annotations on Shang Han Lun)*. Cheng Dan An (承淡安). 20th century.

Shang Han Lun Yan Jiu Da Ci Dian 伤寒论研究大辞典 *(Large Shang Han Lun Research Dictionary)*. Fu Yan Ling et al (Ed.). Shandong Ke Xue Ji Shu Chu Ban She山东科学技术出版社 (Shandong Science & Technology Publishing House), Shandong 1994.

Shang Han Lun Yi An Xuan Ping 伤寒论医案选評 *(Evaluation of Selected Cases from Shang Han Lun)* 伤寒论医案选评 : *Guangdong Zhong Yi* 广东中医 (Guangdong Journal of Traditional Chinese Medicine) 1963; 3:39.

Shang Han Lun Yi Shi 伤寒论译释 *(Interpretation of Shang Han Lun)*. 南京中医学院 Nanjing University of Chinese Medicine, Shanghai Ke Ji Chu Ban She 上海科技出版社 (Shanghai Science & Technology Publishing House), Shanghai 1992.

Shang Han Lun Yu Lin Chuang 伤寒论与临床 *(Clinical Application of Shang Han Lun)*. Nie Hui Min 聂惠民 Guang Dong Ke Ji Chu Ban She 广东科技出版社 (Guangdong Science & Technology Publishing House), Guangdong 1993.

Shang Han Qie Yao 伤寒挈要 *(Essentials of Shang Han)* by Liu Duzhou 刘渡舟. Ren Min Wei Sheng Chu Ban She 人民卫生出版社 (People's Medical Publishing House), Beijing 1983.

Shang Han Shi Jian Lun 伤寒实践论 *(Discourse on Practical Experience with Shang Han)*. Chen

Rui Chun 陈瑞春. Ren Min Wei Sheng Chu Ban She 人民卫生出版社(People's Medical Publishing House), Beijing 2003.

Shang Han Shi Si Jiang 伤寒十四讲 *(Fourteen Lectures on Shang Han)*. Liu Du Zhou刘渡舟. Tianjin Ke Xue Ji Shu Chu Ban She天津科学技术出版社 (Tianjin Science & Technology Publishing House), Tianjin 1982.

Shang Han Shuo Yuan Ji 伤寒溯源集 *(Tracing Shang Han to its Source)*. Qian Tian Lai钱天来 (Qian Huang 钱璜). Shanghai Ke Ji Chu Ban She 上海科技出版社 (Shanghai Science & Technology Publishing House), Shanghai 1959.

Shang Han Xu Lun 伤寒绪论 *(Introduction to Shang Han)*. Zhang Lu Yu 张路玉. First published 1699. 1899 edition stored in the library of Shandong University of Traditional Chinese Medicine.

Shang Han Yi Fang Ji Zhu 伤寒医方集注 *(Collection of Shang Han Medical Formulas)*. Chen Xiu Yuan 陈修园. First published Qing dynasty.

Shang Han Za Bing Lun 伤寒杂病论 *(Treatise on Cold Damage and Miscellaneous Diseases)*. Zhang Zhong Jing 張仲景. 210 AD.

Shang Han Zheng Zhi Zhun Sheng 伤寒证治准绳 *(Shang Han Standards of Pattern Identification and Treatment)*. Wang Ken Tang 王肯堂. 1602.

Shang Han Zhi Ge 伤寒直格 *(The Proper Standards of Shang Han)*. Liu Wan Su 刘完素. Ren Min Wei Sheng Chu Ban She 人民卫生出版社 (People's Medical Publishing House), Beijing 1982.

Shang Han Zong Bing Lun 伤寒总病论 庞安时 *(Complete Discourse on Shang Han Disease)*. Pang An Shi 庞安时. First published 1098. Ren Ming Wei Sheng Chu Ban She 人民卫生出版社 (People's Medical Publishing House), Beijing 2007.

Shang Lun Pian 尚论篇 *(Dissertation on the Esteemed Discourse)*. Yu Jia Yan 喻嘉. First published 1763. Zhong Guo Zhong Yi Yao Chu Ban She 中国中医药出版社 (China Press of Traditional Chinese Medicine), Beijing 2003.

Shen Nong Ben Cao Jing 神农本草经 *(Shen Nong's Materia Medica Classic)*. Anonymous. Han dynasty, circa 220 AD.

Sheng Ji Zong Lu 圣济总录 *(Complete Record of Sacred Benevolence)*. First published 1117. Compiled by Zhao Ji 赵佶 et al. Ren Min Wei Sheng Chu Ban She 人民卫生出版社 (People's Medical Publishing House), Beijing 1998.

Shi Bian Liang Fang 十便良方 *(Ten Convenient Fine Formulas)*. Guo Tan 郭坦. 1195.

Shi Re Bing Pian 湿热病篇 *(Writings on Damp Heat Disease)*. Xue Sheng Bai 薛生白. 18th century.

Shi Yong Zhong Xi Yi Jie He Za Zhi 实用中西医结合杂志 (The Journal of the Application of Integrated Chinese and Western Medicine) 1991; (4):280-281.

Shou Shi Bao Yuan 寿世保元 *(Preservation of Life and Longevity)*. Gong Ting Xian 龔廷賢. First published 1615. Shanxi Science & Technology Publishing House, Shanxi 2006.

Si Chuan Zhong Yi 四川中医 (Journal of Si Chuan Traditional Chinese Medicine) 1987; 1:18.

Si Chuan Zhong Yi 四川中医 (Journal of Si Chuan Traditional Chinese Medicine) 1993; 12:45.

Si Chuan Zhong Yi 四川中医 (Journal of Si Chuan Traditional Chinese Medicine) 1994; 10:52.

Su Wen 素问 *(Plain Questions)*. First volume of *Huang Di Ne Jing*. Anonymous. Circa 200 BC.

Su Wen: Bing Ji Qi Yi Bao Ming Ji (416) 素问病机气宜保命集 *(Plain Questions: Mechanism of Disease and Qi for the Preservation of Life Collection)*. Liu Wan Su 刘完素. 1186. 中国中医药出版社 (China Press of Traditional Chinese Medicine), Beijing, 2007.

Tai Ping Sheng Hui Fang 太平圣惠方 *(Tai Ping Blessed Formulas)*. First published 992. Ren Min Wei Sheng Chu Ban She 人民卫生出版社 (People's Medical Publishing House), Beijing 1980.

Tai Ping Hui Ming He Ji Ju Fang 太平惠民和剂局方 *(Prescriptions from the Tai Ping Imperial Grace Pharmacy)*. Revised by Chen Shi Wen 陈诗文. First published 1107.

Tang Hui Yao 唐会要.Wang Pu Zhuan 王浦撰. Song dynasty.

Tianjin Yi Yao 天津医药 (Tianjin Medical Journal) 1973; 1:10.

Tong Su Shang Han Lun 通俗伤寒论 *(Revised Popular Guide to the Treatise of Cold Damage Diseases)*. Yu Gen Chu 俞根初. The original by Yu Gen Chu was written in the 18th century and re-published in the *Shao Xing Chinese Medical Monthly* journal around 1929. The revised edition known as *Zhong Ding Tong Su Shang Han Lun* was compiled and edited by Xu Rong Zai in 1956 and published by Shanghai Technology Press. The *San Ding Tong Su Shang Han Lun* was edited by Lian Jian Wei and published by Zhong Yi Gu Ji Chu Ban She 中医古籍出版社 (Chinese Medicine Ancient Book Publications), Beijing 2002.

Wang Shi Jian Yi Fang 王氏简易方 *(Master Wang's Simple Formulas)*. 王清任. Late 18th–early 19th century.

Wai Gan Wen Bing Pian 外感温病篇 *(Dissertation on Externally Contracted Warm Disease)*. Chen Bo Ping 陈平伯. From Wen Re Jing Wei 温热经纬 *(The Warp and Weft of Warm Heat Disease)*. Compiled by Wang Meng Ying 1852. 人民卫生出版社 (People's Medical Publishing House), Beijing 2005.

Wai Gan Wen Re Bing Pian 外感温热病篇 *(Dissertation on Externally Contracted Febrile Disease)*. Ye Tian Shi 叶天士. From 温热经纬 *(The Weft and Woof of Warm Diseases)*. Compiled by Wang Meng Ying 1852. 人民卫生出版社 (People's Medical Publishing House), Beijing 2005.

Wai Tai Mi Yao 外台秘要 *(Essential Secrets from the Imperial Library)*. Wang Tao 王焘. 752 AD. Ren Min Wei Sheng Chu Ban She 人民卫生出版社 (People's Medical Publishing House), Beijing 1982.

Wan Bing Hui Chun 万病回春 *(Myriad Diseases and the Return of Spring)*. Gong Ting Xian 龚廷贤. 1587. 人民卫生出版社 (People's Medical Publishing House), Beijing, 2007.

Wei Sheng Bao Jian Bu Yi 卫生宝鉴补遗 *(Supplement to the Mirror of Medical Treasures)*. Luo Tian Yi罗天益. Originally published Yuan dynasty. Zhong Guo Zhong Yi Yao Chu Ban She 中国中医药出版社 (China Press of Traditional Chinese Medicine), Beijing 2007.

Wei Sheng Bao Jian Shi Yi 卫生宝鉴拾遗 *(The MissingSection of the Mirror of Medical Treasures)*. Luo Tian Yi 罗天益. Originally published Yuan dynasty. Zhong Guo Zhong Yi Yao Chu Ban She 中国中医药出版社 (China Press of Traditional Chinese Medicine), Beijing 2007.

Wen Bing Tiao Bian 温病条辨 *(Systematic Differentiation of Warm Diseases)*. Wu Tang 吴塘. First published 1798. 人民卫生出版社 (People's Medical Publishing House), Beijing 1972.

Wen Re Jing Wei 温热经纬 *(The Warp and Weft of Warm Heat Diseases)*. Compiled by Wang Meng Ying. 1852. 人民卫生出版社 (People's Medical Publishing House), Beijing 2005.

Wen Yi Lun 温疫论 *(Discourse on Febrile Epidemic Disease)*. Wu You Ke. Ming dynasty.

Wu Pei Heng Yi An 吴佩衡医案 *(Wu Pei Heng's Medical Cases)*. Yun Nan Ren Min Chu Ban She 云南人民出版社 (Yunnan People's Publishing House), Yunnan 1979.

Xiao Er *Yao Zheng Zhi Jue* 小儿药证直诀 *(Key to Childhood Medicinal Patterns)*. Qian Yi 钱乙. 1119. 人民卫生出版社 (People's Medical Publishing House) Beijing, 2006.

Xin Bian Shang Han Lun Lei Fang 新编伤寒论类方 *(New Edition of Categorised Shang Han Lun Formulas)*. Liu Du Zhou 刘渡舟. 山西人民出版社 (Shanxi People's Publishing House), Taiwan 1984.

Xin Zhong Yi 新中医 (New Journal of Traditional Chinese Medicine) 1981; 1:49.

Xin Zhong Yi 新中医 (New Journal of Traditional Chinese Medicine) 1983; (4).

Xin Zhong Yi 新中医 (New Journal of Traditional Chinese Medicine) 1995; 2:14.

Xin Zhong Yi 新中医 (New Journal of Traditional Chinese Medicine) 1975; 3:24.

Xin Yi Yao Xue Za Zhi 新医药学杂志 (New Journal of Herbal Medicine) 1977; 7:30.

Xu Shu Wei Shang Han Lun Zhu San Zhong 许叔微伤寒论著三种 *(Xu Shu Wei's Three Works on Shang Han Lun)*. Xu Shu Wei 许叔微. Song dynasty.

Xue Zheng Lun 血证论 *(Treatise on Blood Patterns)*. Tang Rong Chuan 唐容川. 1884. Zhong Guo Zhong Yi Yao Chu Ban She中国中医药出版社 (China Press of Traditional Chinese Medicine), Beijing 1996.

Yi Fang Ji Jie 医方集解 *(Collected Explanations of Medical Formulas)*. Wang Ang 汪昂. First published 1682. Ren Min Wei Sheng Chu Ban She 人民卫生出版社 (People's Medical Publishing House), Beijing 2006.

Yi Fang Xin Xian 医方新鲜 *(Medical Formulas Renewed)*. Ma You Du 马有度. Shanghai Ke Ji Chu Ban She上海科技出版社 (Shanghai Science & Technology Publishing House), Shanghai 1996.

Yi Guan 医贯 *(Thorough Knowledge of Medicine)*. Zhao Xian Ke 赵献可. 1687. 学苑出版社 (Academy Press), Beijing 2005.

Yi Jing Hui Yuan 医经会元 *(Medical Classic of a First-class Scholar)*. Wu Jia Yan 吴嘉言. Yuan Hu Zhong Yi College: Shang Han Lun Supplement: 80.

Yi Men Bang He 医门棒喝 *(Medical Warnings)*. Zhang Xu Gu 章虚谷. Zhong Yi Gu Ji Chu Ban She 中医古籍出版社 (Ancient Chinese Medical Texts Publishing House), Beijing 1999.

Yi Xue Gang Mu 医学纲目 *(Compendium of Medicine)*. Lou Ying 楼英. Ming dynasty, between 1332 and 1400. Zhong Guo Zhong Yi Yao Chu Ban She 中国中医药出版社 (China Press of Traditional Chinese Medicine), Beijing 1996.

Yi Xue Ru Men 医学入门 *(Introduction to Medicine)*. Li Chan 李梴. First published 1575. Ren Min Wei Sheng Chu Ban She 人民卫生出版社

(People's Medical Publishing House), Beijing 2006.

Yi Xue Ru Men Liang Fang 医学入门良方 *(Introduction to Fine Formulas in Medicine).* Edited by Wan Biao 万表. 中国古籍出版社 (China Ancient Text Publishing House), Beijing 2000.

Yi Xue Xin Wu 医学心悟 *(Medical Insights.)* Cheng Guo Pang 程国彭. First published 1732. Ren Min Wei Sheng Chu Ban She 人民卫生出版社 (People's Medical Publishing House), Beijing 2006.

Yi Xue Zhong Zhong Can Xi Lu 医学衷中参西录 *(Genuine Medical Records with Reference to the West).* Zhang Xi Chun 张锡纯. Between 1918 and 1934. Hebei Ke Xue Ji Shu Chu Ban She 河北科学技术出版社 (Hebei Science & Technology Publishing House), Hebei 2002.

Yi Zong Bi Du 医宗必读 *(Required Readings from Medical Ancestors).* Li Zhong Zi 李中梓. First published 1637. Ren Min Wei Sheng Chu Ban She (People's Medical Publishing House), Beijing 2006.

Yi Zong Jin Jian 医宗金鉴 *(Golden Mirror of Medical Tradition).* Wu Qian 吴谦. First published 1742. Ren Min Wei Sheng Chu Ban She 人民卫生出版社 (People's Medical Publishing House), Beijing 2005.

Yin Yang Da Lun 阴阳大论 *(The Great Treatise on Yin and Yang).* Pre-Han dynasty.

Yin Zheng Lue Li 阴证略例 *(An Outline of Yin Patterns).* Wang Hao Gu 王进之. First published Yuan dynasty. Shang Wu Yin Shu Guan 商务印书馆 (The Commercial Press), Shanghai 1956.

You Ke Fa Hui 幼科发挥 *(Giving Rein to the Study of the Young).* Wan Quan 万全. First published Ming dynasty. Zhong Guo Zhong Yi Yao Chu Ban She 中国中医药出版社 (China Press of Traditional Chinese Medicine), Beijing 2006.

Yue Mei Zhong Yi An 岳美中医案 *(Yue Mei Zhong's Chinese Medical Cases).* Compiled by Chinese Academy of Traditional Chinese Medicine. Ren Min Wei Sheng Chu Ban She 人民卫生出版社 (People's Medical Publishing House), Beijing 1978.

Zhang Shi Yi Tong 张氏医通 *(Master Zhang's Medical Expertise).* Zhang Lu Yu 张璐玉. 1695. Ren Min Wei Sheng Chu Ban She 人民卫生出版社 (People's Medical Publishing House), Beijing 2006.

Zhang Zhong Jing Yao Fa Yan Jiu 张仲景药法研究 *(Zhang Zhong Jing's Medicinal Investigations).* Compiled by Wang Zhan Xi 王占玺 et al. Ke Xue Ji Shu Wen Xian Chu Ban She 北京：科学技术文献出版社 (Science and Technology Literature Publishing House), Beijing 1984, p 656.

Zhejiang Zhong Yi Za Zhi 浙江中医杂志 (Zhejiang Journal of Traditional Chinese Medicine) 1957; 6:242.

Zhejiang Zhong Yi Za Zhi 浙江中医杂志 (Zhejiang Journal of Traditional Chinese Medicine) 1960; 6:269.

Zhejiang Zhong Yi Za Zhi 浙江中医杂志 (Zhejiang Journal of Traditional Chinese Medicine) 1964; 8:14.

Zhejiang Zhong Yi Za Zhi 浙江中医杂志 (Zhejiang Journal of Traditional Chinese Medicine) 1965; 8:7.

Zhejiang Zhong Yi Za Zhi 浙江中医杂志 (Zhejiang Journal of Traditional Chinese Medicine) 1979; 5:12.

Zheng Zhi Yao Jue 证治要诀 *(Essential Verses in Patterns of Treatment).* Dai Yuan Li 戴原礼. Yuan dynasty. Ren Min Wei Sheng Chu Ban She 人民卫生出版社 (People's Medical Publishing House). Beijing 2006.

Zheng Zhi Da Huan 证治大还 *(Great Reward of Patterns and Treatment).* Chen Zhi 陈治. Late 17th century.

Zheng Zhi Zhun Sheng 证治准绳 *(Standards of Patterns and Treatment).* Wang Ken Tang 王肯堂. First published 1602. Ren Min Wei Sheng Chu Ban She 人民卫生出版社 (People's Medical Publishing House), Beijing 2001.

Zhi Zhi Fang 直指方 *(Indicated Formulas).* Yang Shi Yin 杨士瀛. Fujian Ke Xue Ji Shu Chu Ban She 福建科学技术出版社 (Fujian Science & Technology Publishing House), Fujian 1989.

Zhong Guo Gu Dai Du Liang Heng Tu Ji 中国古代度量衡图集 *Illustrated Collection of Ancient Measurements in China.* 国家计量总局主编. Compiled by the National Bureau of Weights and Measures. 文物出版社 Cultural Relics Press, Beijing 1984.

Zhong Hua Yi Xue Za Zhi 中华医学杂志 (Chinese Medical Journal) 1980; 1:57.

Zhong Xi Yi Jie He Za Zhi 中西医结合杂志 (Chinese Journal of Integrated Chinese and Western Medicine) 1982; 2:90.

Zhong Yi Nian Jian 中医年鉴 *(Year Book of Traditional Chinese Medicine)* Ren Min Wei Sheng Chu Ban She 人民卫生出版社 (People's Medical Publishing House), Beijing 1983.

Zhong Yi Yan Jiu 中医研究 (Chinese Medicine Research) 1995; 1:23.

Zhong Yi Yan Jiu Tong Xin 中医研究通信 (Chinese Medicine Research Newsletter) 1962; 3:42.
Zhong Yi Yao Za Zhi 中医药杂志 (Journal of Chinese Herbal Medicine) 1982; 6:33.
Zhong Yi Za Zhi 中医杂志 (Journal of Traditional Chinese Medicine) 1955; 4:25.
Zhong Yi Za Zhi 中医杂志 (Journal of Traditional Chinese Medicine) 1962; 2:14.
Zhong Yi Za Zhi 中医杂志 (Journal of Traditional Chinese Medicine) 1966; 3:23.
Zhong Yi Zha Zhi 中医杂志 (Journal of Traditional Chinese Medicine) 1980; 1:23.
Zhong Yi Za Zhi 中医杂志 (Journal of Traditional Chinese Medicine) 1983; 4:31.
Zhong Yi Za Zhi 中医杂志 (Journal of Traditional Chinese Medicine) 1985; 4:44.
Zhong Yi Za Zhi 中医杂志 (Journal of Traditional Chinese Medicine) 1986; 4:283.
Zhong Yi Za Zhi 中医杂志 (Journal of Traditional Chinese Medicine) 1986; 5:347.
Zhong Yi Za Zhi 中医杂志 (Journal of Traditional Chinese Medicine) 1990; 3:21.
Zhong Yi Za Zhi 中医杂志 (Journal of Traditional Chinese Medicine) 1993; 3:145.
Zhou Hou Bei Ji Fang 肘后备急方 *(Emergency Formulas to Keep up One's Sleeve)*. Ge Hong 葛洪. First published 341 AD. Anhui Ke Xue Ji Shu Chu Ban She 安徽科学技术出版社 (Anhui Science & Technology Publishing House), 1996.
Zhu Bing Yuan Hou Lun 诸病源候论 *(Treatise on the Pathogenesis and Manifestations of All Diseases).* Chao Yuan Fang 巢元方. First published 610 AD. 人民军医出版社 (People's Military Medical Press), Beijing 2006.
Zhu Jie Shang Han Lun 注解伤寒论 *(Annotations to Shang Han Lun)* by Cheng Wu Ji成无己. First published 12th–13th century. Ren Min Wei Sheng Chu Ban She 人民卫生出版社 (People's Medical Publishing House), Beijing1963.
Zhu Shi Ji Yan Fang 朱氏集验方 *(Master Zhu's Collected Empirical Formulas).* Zhu Jun Fu 朱君辅. Ren Min Wei Sheng Chu Ban She 人民卫生出版社 (People's Medical Publishing House), Beijing 1983.

Appendix 15

Herb Names: Cross-reference of Chinese and Pharmaceutical Names

Ai Ye	艾叶	Artemisiae Argyi Folium
Ba Dou	巴豆	Crotonis Semen
Ba Ji Tian	巴戟天	Morindae Officinalis Radix
Bai Bu	百部	Stemonae Radix
Bai Dou Kou	白豆蔻	Amomi Fructus Rotundus
Bai Fu Zi	白附子	Typhonii Rhizoma Preparatum
Bai Guo	白果	Ginkgo Semen
Bai He	百合	Lilii Bulbus
Bai Hua She She Cao	白花蛇舌草	Hedyotis Diffusae Herba
Bai Ji	白芨	Bletillae Rhizoma
Bai Ji Li	白蒺藜	Tribuli Fructus
Bai Jiang Can	白僵蚕	Bombyx Batryticatus
Bai Jiang Cao	败酱草	Patriniae Herba
Bai Jie Zi	白芥子	Sinapis Semen
Bai Mao Gen	白茅根	Imperatae Rhizoma
Bai Qian	白前	Cynanchi Stauntonii Rhizoma
Bai Shao	白芍	Paeoniae Radix Alba
Bai Tou Weng	白头翁	Pulsatillae Radix
Bai Wei	白薇	Cynanchi Atrati Radix
Bai Xian Pi	白鲜皮	Dictamni Cortex
Bai Zhi	白芷	Angelicae Dahuricae Radix
Bai Zhu	白术	Atractylodis Macrocephalae Rhizoma
Bai Zi Ren	柏子仁	Platycladi Semen
Ban Lan Gen	板蓝根	Isatidis/Baphicacanthis Radix
Ban Xia	半夏	Pinellia Rhizoma
Ban Zhi Lian	半支莲	Scutellariae Barbatae Herba
Bei Mu	贝母	Fritillariae Bulbus
Bei Sha Shen	北沙参	Glehniae Radix
Bi Ba	荜茇	Piperis Longi Fructus
Bi Cheng Qie	荜澄茄	Litseae Fructus
Bi Xie	萆薢	Dioscoreae Hypoglaucae Rhizoma

Bian Xu	萹蓄	Polygoni Avicularis Herba
Bie Jia	鳖甲	Trionycis Carapax
Bing Lang	槟榔	Arecae Semen
Bing Pian	冰片	Borneolum
Bo He	薄荷	Menthae Haplocalycis Herba
Bu Gu Zhi	补骨脂	Psoraleae Fructus
Can Sha	蚕沙	Bombycis Faeces
Cang Er Zi	苍耳子	Xanthii Fructus
Cang Zhu	苍术	Atractylodis Rhizoma
Ce Bai Ye	侧柏叶	Platycladi Cacumen
Chai Hu	柴胡	Bupleuri Radix
Chan Tui	蝉蜕	Cicadae Periostracum
Che Qian Zi	车前子	Plantaginis Semen
Chen Pi	陈皮	Citri Reticulatae Pericarpium
Chen Xiang	沉香	Aquilariae Lignum Resinatum
Chi Fu Ling	赤茯苓	Poria Rubra
Chi Shao	赤芍	Paeoniae Radix Rubra
Chi Shi Zhi	赤石脂	Halloysitum Rubrum
Chi Xiao Dou	赤小豆	Phaseoli Semen
Chong Wei Zi	茺蔚子	Leonuri Fructus
Chuan Bei Mu	川贝母	Fritillariae Cirrhosae Bulbus
Chuan Lian Zi	川楝子	Toosendan Fructus
Chuan Niu Xi	川牛膝	Cyathulae Radix
Chuan Shan Jia	穿山甲	Manitis Squama
Chuan Xin Lian	穿心莲	Andrographitis Herba
Chuan Xiong	川芎	Chuanxiong Rhizoma
Chui Pen Cao	垂盆草	Sedi Herba
Chun Pi	椿皮	Ailanthi Cortex
Ci Shi	磁石	Magnetitum
Ci Wu Jia	刺五加	Acanthopanacis Senticosi Radix Et Caulis
Cong Bai	葱白	Allii Fistulosi Bulbus
Da Dou Juan	大豆卷	Sojae Semen Germinatum
Da Fu Pi	大腹皮	Arecae Pericarpium
Da Huang	大黄	Rhei Radix Et Rhizoma
Da Ji	大蓟	Cirsii Japonici Herba Sive Radix
Da Ji	大戟	Knoxiae/Euphorbiae Radix
Da Qing Ye	大青叶	Isatidis Folium
Da Suan	大蒜	Allii Sativi Bulbus
Da Zao	大枣	Jujubae Fructus
Dai ZheShi	代赭石	Haematitum
Dan Dou Chi	淡豆豉	Sojae Semen Preparatum
Dan Nan Xing	胆南星	Arisaema Cum Bile
Da Shen	丹参	Salviae Miltiorrhizae Radix
Dan Zhu Ye	淡竹叶	Lophateri Herba
Dang Gui	当归	Angelicae Sinensis Radix
Dang Shen	党参	Codonopsis Radix
Deng Xin Cao	灯心草	Junci Medulla
Di Fu Zi	地肤子	Kochiae Fructus
Di Gu Pi	地骨皮	Lycii Cortex
Di Long	地龙	Pheretima
Di Yu	地榆	Sanguisorbae Radix
Ding Xiang	丁香	Caryophylli Flos
Dong Chong Xia Cao	冬虫夏草	Cordyceps
Dong Gua Pi	冬瓜皮	Benincasae Exocarpium
Dong Gua Ren	冬瓜仁	Benincasae Semen
Du Huo	独活	Angelicae Pubescentis Radix
Du Zhong	杜仲	Eucommiae Cortex
E Bu Shi Cao	鹅不食草	Centipedae Herba
E Jiao	阿胶	Asini Corii Colla

E Zhu	莪术	Curcumae Rhizoma
Fan Xie Ye	番泻叶	Sennae Folium
Fang Feng	防风	Saposhnikoviae Radix
Fo Shou	佛手	Citri Sarcodactylis Fructus
Fu Ling Pi	茯苓皮	Poriae Cutis
Fu Ling	茯苓	Poria
Fu Pen Zi	覆盆子	Rubi Fructus
Fu Ping	浮萍	Spirodelae Herba
Fu Shen	茯神	Poriae Sclerotium Pararadicis
Fu Xiao Mai	浮小麦	Tritici Fructus Levis
Fu Zi	附子	Aconiti Radix Lateralis
Gan Cao	甘草	Glycyrrhizae Radix
Gan Jiang	干姜	Zingiberis Rhizoma
Gan Song	甘松	Nardostachydis Radix Seu Rhizoma
Gao Ben	藁本	Ligustici Rhizoma
Gao Liang Jiang	高良姜	Alpiniae Officinarum Rhizoma
Ge Gen	葛根	Puerariae Radix
Ge Jie	蛤蚧	Gecko
Gou Ji	狗脊	Cibotii Rhizoma
Gou Qi Zi	枸杞子	Lycii Fructus
Gou Teng	钩藤	Uncariae Ramulus Cum Uncis
Gu Sui Bu	骨碎补	Drynariae Rhizoma
Gu Ya	谷芽	Oryzae Fructus Germinatus
Gua Di	瓜蒂	Melo Pedicellus
Gua Lou Pi	瓜蒌皮	Trichosanthis Pericarpium
Gua Lou Ren	瓜蒌仁	Trichosanthis Semen
Gua Lou	瓜蒌	Trichosanthis Fructus
Guan Zhong	贯众	Cyrtomii Rhizoma
Guang Fang Ji	广防己	Aristolochiae Fangchi Radix
Gui Ban	龟板	Testudinis Plastrum
Gui Zhi	桂枝	Cinnamomi Ramulus
Hai Dai	海带	Laminariae Thallus
Hai Feng Teng	海风藤	Piperis Kadsurae Caulis
Hai Fu Shi	海浮石	Pumex
Hai Jin Sha	海金沙	Lygodii Spora
Hai Piao Xiao	海螵蛸	Sepiae Endoconcha
Hai Tong Pi	海桐皮	Erythrinae Cortex
Hai Zao	海藻	Sargassum
Han Fang Ji	汉防己	Stephaniae Tetrandrae Radix
Han Shui Shi	寒水石	Glauberitum
He Huan Pi	合欢皮	Albiziae Cortex
Han Lian Cao	旱莲草	Ecliptae Herba
He Shou Wu	何首乌	Polygoni Multiflori Radix
He Tao Ren	核桃仁	Juglandis Semen
He ye	荷叶	Nelumbinis Folium
He Zi (Ke Zi)	诃子	Chebulae Fructus
Hei Zhi Ma	黑芝麻	Sesami Semen Nigrum
Hong Hua	红花	Carthami Flos
Hou Po	厚朴	Magnoliae Officinalis Cortex
Hu Huang Lian	胡黄连	Picrorhizae Rhizoma
Hu Ji Sheng	槲寄生	Visci Herba
Hu Jiao	胡椒	Piperis Fructus
Hu Po	琥珀	Succinum
Hu Zhang	虎杖	Polygoni Cuspidati Rhizoma
Hua Jiao	花椒	Zanthoxyli Pericarpium
Hua Rui Shi	花蕊石	Ophicalcitum
Hua Shi	滑石	Talcum
Huang Bai	黄柏	Phellodendri Cortex
Huang Jing	黄精	Polygonati Rhizoma

Huang Lian	黄连	Coptidis Rhizoma
Huang Qi	黄芪	Astragali Radix
Huang Qin	黄芩	Scutellariae Radix
Huang Yao Zi	黄药子	Dioscoreae Bulbiferae Rhizoma
Huo Ma Ren	火麻仁	Cannabis Semen
Huo Xiang	藿香	Pogostemonis/ Agastaches Herba
Ji Nei Jin	鸡内金	Gigeriae Galli Endothelium Corneum
Ji Xue Teng	鸡血藤	Spatholobi Caulis
Jiang Huang	姜黄	Curcumae Longae Rhizoma
Jiang Xiang	降香	Dalbergiae Odoriferae Lignum
Jie Geng	桔梗	Platycodi Radix
Jin Qian Cao	金钱草	Lysimachiae Herba
Jin Yin Hua	金银花	Lonicerae Flos
Jin Ying Zi	金樱子	Rosae Laevigatae Fructus
Jing Jie	荆芥	Schizonepetae Herba
Jing Jie Sui	荆芥穗	Schizonepetae Spica
Jiu Cai Zi	韭菜子	Allii Tuberosi Semen
Ju He	橘核	Citri Reticulatae Semen
Ju Hong	橘红	Citri Reticulatae Exocarpium Rubrum
Ju Hua	菊花	Chrysanthemi Flos
Jue Ming Zi	决明子	Cassiae Semen
Ku Lian Pi	苦楝皮	Meliae Cortex
Ku Shen	苦参	Sophorae Flavescentis Radix
Kuan Dong Hua	款冬花	Farfarae Flos
Kuan Jin Teng	宽筋藤	Tinosporae Sinensis Caulis
Kun Bu	昆布	Eckloniae Thallus
Lai Fu Zi	莱菔子	Raphani Semen
Li Zhi He	荔枝核	Litchi Semen
Lian Qiao	连翘	Forsythiae Fructus
Lian Xu	莲须	Nelumbinis Stamen
Lian Zi	莲子	Nelumbinis Semen
Lian Zi Xin	莲子心	Nelumbinis Plumula
Ling Yang Jiao	羚羊角	Saigae Tataricae Cornu
Ling Zhi	灵芝	Ganoderma
Liu Huang	硫黄	Sulfur
Liu Ji Nu	刘寄奴	Artemisiae Anomalae Herba
Long Dan Cao	龙胆草	Gentianae Radix
Long Gu	龙骨	Fossilia Ossis Mastodi
Long Yan Rou	龙眼肉	Longan Arillus
Lu Gan Shi	炉甘石	Calamina
Lu Gen	芦根	Phragmitis Rhizoma
Lu Jiao	鹿角	Cervi Cornu
Lu Jiao Jiao	鹿角胶	Cervi Cornus Colla
Lu Jiao Shuang	鹿角霜	Cervi Cornu Degelatinatum
Lu Lu Tong	路路通	Liquidambaris Fructus
Lu Rong	鹿茸	Cervi Cornu Pantotrichum
Luo Shi Teng	络石藤	Trachelospermi Caulis
Ma Bian Cao	马鞭草	Verbenae Herba
Ma Chi Xian	马齿苋	Portulacae Herba
Ma Dou Ling	马兜铃	Aristolochiae Fructus
Ma Huang	麻黄	Ephedrae Herba
Ma Huang Gen	麻黄根	Ephedrae Radix
Mai Men Dong	麦门冬	Ophiopogonis Radix
Mai Ya	麦芽	Hordei Fructus Germinatus
Man Jing Zi	蔓荆子	Viticis Fructus
Mang Xiao	硭硝	Natrii Sulfas
Meng Chong	虻虫	Tabanus
Méng Shí	礞石	Chloriti Lapis
Mi Meng Hua	蜜蒙花	Buddlejae Flos

Mo Han Lian	墨旱莲	Ecliptae Herba
Mo Yao	没药	Myrrha
Mu Dan Pi	牡丹皮	Moutan Cortex
Mu Gua	木瓜	Chaenomelis Fructus
Mu Hu Die	木蝴蝶	Oroxyli Semen
Mu Li	牡蛎	Ostreae Concha
Mu Tong	木通	Akebiae Caulis
Mu Xiang	木香	Aucklandiae Radix
Mu Zei	木贼	Equiseti Hiemalis Herba
Nan Gua Zi	南瓜子	Cucurbitae Moschatae Semen
Niu Bang Zi	牛蒡子	Arctii Fructus
Niu Huang	牛黄	Bovis Calculus
Niu Xi	牛膝	Achyranthis Bidentatae Radix
Nu Zhen Zi	女贞子	Ligustri Lucidi Fructus
Nuo Dao Gen	糯稻根	Oryzae Glutinosae Radix
Ou Jie	藕节	Nelumbinis Nodus Rhizomatis
Pang Da Hai	胖大海	Sterculiae Lychnophorae Semen
Pao Jiang	炮姜	Zingiberis Rhizoma Preparatum
Pei Lan	佩兰	Eupatorii Herba
Pi Pa Ye	枇杷叶	Eriobotryae Folium
Pu Gong Ying	蒲公英	Taraxaci Herba
Pu Huang	蒲黄	Typhae Pollen
Qian Cao	茜草	Rubiae Radix
Qian Hu	前胡	Peucedani Radix
Qian Niu Zi	牵牛子	Pharbitidis Semen
Qian Shi	芡实	Euryales Semen
Qiang Huo	羌活	Notopterygii Rhizoma Seu Radix
Qin Jiao	秦艽	Gentianae Macrophyllae Radix
Qin Pi	秦皮	Fraxini Cortex
Qing Dai	清黛	Indigo Naturalis
Qing Hao	青蒿	Artemisiae Annuae Herba
Qing Pi	青皮	Citri Reticulatae Viride Pericarpium
Qu Mai	瞿麦	Dianthi Herba
Quan Gua Lou	全瓜蒌	Trichosanthis Fructus
Quan Xie	全蝎	Scorpio
Ren Dong Teng	忍冬藤	Lonicerae Caulis
Ren Shen	人参	Ginseng Radix
Rou Cong Rong	肉苁蓉	Cistanches Herba
Rou Dou Kou	肉豆蔻	Myristicae Semen
Rou Gui	肉桂	Cinnamomi Cortex
Ru Xiang	乳香	Olibanum
San Leng	三棱	Sparganii Rhizoma
San Qi	三七	Notoginseng Radix
Sang Bai Pi	桑白皮	Mori Cortex
Sang Ji Sheng	桑寄生	Taxilli Herba
Sang Piao Xiao	桑螵蛸	Mantidis Oötheca
Sang Shen	桑椹	Mori Fructus
Sang Ye	桑叶	Mori Folium
Sang Zhi	桑枝	Mori Ramulus
Sha Ren	砂仁	Amomi Fructus
Sha Shen	沙参	Glehniae/Adenophorae Radix
Sha Yuan Zi	沙苑子	Astragali Complanati Semen
Shan Ci Gu	山慈姑	Cremastrae/Pleiones Pseudobulbus
Shan Dou Gen	山豆根	Sophorae Tonkinensis Radix
Shan Yao	山药	Dioscoreae Rhizoma
Shan Zha	山楂	Crataegi Fructus
Shan Zhu Yu	山茱萸	Corni Fructus
She Chuang Zi	蛇床子	Cnidii Fructus
She Gan	射干	Belamcandae Rhizoma

She Xiang	麝香	Moschus
Shen Qu	神曲	Massa Medicata Fermentata
Sheng Di Huang	生地黄	Rehmanniae Radix
Sheng Jiang	生姜	Zingiberis Rhizoma Recens
Sheng Ma	升麻	Cimicifugae Rhizoma
Shi Chang Pu	石菖蒲	Acori Tatarinowii Rhizoma
Shi Gao	石膏	Gypsum Fibrosum
Shi Hu	石斛	Dendrobii Herba
Shi Jue Ming	石决明	Haliotidis Concha
Shi Liu Pi	石榴皮	Granati Pericarpium
Shu Di Huang	熟地黄	Rehmanniae Radix Preparata
Shui Niu Jiao	水牛角	Bubali Cornu
Shui Zhi	水蛭	Hirudo
Si Gua Luo	丝瓜络	Luffae Fructus Retinervus
Su Geng	苏更	Perillae Caulis
Su Zi	苏子	Perillae Fructus
Suan Zao Rn	酸枣仁	Ziziphi Spinosae Semen
Suo Yang	锁阳	Cynomorii Herba
Tai Zi Shen	太子参	Pseudostellariae Radix
Tao Ren	桃仁	Persicae Semen
Tian Hua Fen	天花粉	Trichosanthis Radix
Tian Ma	天麻	Gastrodiae Rhizoma
Tian Men Dong	天门冬	Asparagi Radix
Tian Nan Xing	天南星	Arisaematis Rhizoma Preparatum
Ting Li Zi	葶苈子	Lepidii/Descurainiae Semen
Tu Bie Chong	土鳖虫	Eupolyphaga/Steleophaga
Tu Fu Ling	土茯苓	Smilacis Glabrae Rhizoma
Tu Si Zi	菟丝子	Cuscutae Semen
Wa Leng Zi	瓦楞子	Arcae Concha
Wang Bu Liu Xing	王不留行	Vaccariae Semen
Wei Ling Xian	威灵仙	Clematidis Radix
Wu Bei Zi	五倍子	Galla Chinensis
Wu Gong	蜈蚣	Scolopendra
Wu Jia Pi	五加皮	Acanthopanacis Cortex
Wu Ling Zhi	五灵脂	Trogopterori Faeces
Wu Mei	乌梅	Mume Fructus
Wu Wei Zi	五味子	Schisandrae Fructus
Wu Yao	乌药	Linderae Radix
Wu Zhu Yu	吴茱萸	Evodiae Fructus
Xi Jiao	犀角	Rhinocerotis Cornu
Xi Xian Cao	豨莶草	Siegesbeckiae Herba
Xi Xin	细辛	Asari Herba
Xi Yang Shen	西洋参	Panacis Quinquefolii Radix
Xia Ku Cao	夏枯草	Prunellae Spica
Xian He Cao	仙鹤草	Agrimoniae Herba
Xian Mao	仙茅	Curculiginis Rhizoma
Xiang Fu	香附	Cyperi Rhizoma
Xiao Hui Xiang	小茴香	Foeniculi Fructus
Xiao Ji	小蓟	Cirsii Herba
Xie Bai	薤白	Allii Macrostemi Bulbus
Xin Yi Hua	辛荑花	Magnoliae Flos
Xing Ren	杏仁	Armeniacae Semen Amarum
Xiong Huang	雄黄	Realgar
Xu Chang Qing	徐长卿	Cynanchi Paniculati Radix
Xu Duan	续断	Dipsaci Radix
Xuan Fu Hua	旋复花	Inulae Flos
Xuan Shen	玄参	Scrophulariae Radix
Xue Yu Tan	血余炭	Crinis Carbonisatus
Yan Hu Suo	延胡索	Corydalis Rhizoma

Ye Jiao Teng	夜交藤	Polygoni Multiflori Caulis
Ye Ju Hua	野菊花	Chrysanthemi Indici Flos
Ye Ming Sha	夜明沙	Vespertilionis Faeces
Yi Mu Cao	益母草	Leonuri Herba
Yi Tang	饴糖	Maltosum
Yi Yi Ren	薏苡仁	Coicis Semen
Yi Zhi Ren	益智仁	Alpiniae Oxyphyllae Fructus
Yin Chai Hu	银柴胡	Stellariae Radix
Yin Chen	茵陈	Artemisiae Scopariae Herba
Yin Yang Huo	淫羊藿	Epimedii Herba
Yu Jin	郁金	Curcumae Radix
Yu Li Ren	郁李仁	Pruni Semen
Yu Xing Cao	鱼腥草	Houttuyniae Herba
Yu Yu Liang	禹余粮	Limonitum
Yu Zhu	玉竹	Polygonati Odorati Rhizoma
Yuan Hua	芫花	Genkwa Flos
Yuan Zhi	远志	Polygalae Radix
Zao Jia	皂甲	Gleditsiae Fructus
Zao Jiao Ci	皂角刺	Gleditsiae Spina
Zao Xin Tu	灶心土	Terra Flava Usta
Ze Lan	泽兰	Lycopi Herba
Ze Xie	泽泻	Alismatis Rhizoma
Zhe Bei Mu	浙贝母	Fritillariae Thunbergii Bulbus
Zhe Chong	蛰虫	Eupolyphaga/Steleophaga
Zhen Zhu Mu	珍珠母	Margaritiferae Concha Usta
Zhen Zhu	珍珠	Margarita
Zhi Gan Cao	炙甘草	Glycyrrhizae Radix Preparata
Zhi Mu	知母	Anemarrhenae Rhizoma
Zhi Qiao (Zhi Ke)	枳壳	Aurantii Fructus
Zhi Shi	枳实	Aurantii Fructus Immaturus
Zhi Zi	栀子	Gardeniae Fructus
Zhu Li	竹沥	Bambusae Succus
Zhu Ling	猪苓	Polyporus
Zhu Ru	竹茹	Bambusae Caulis In Taeniam
Zhu Sha	朱砂	Cinnabaris
Zi Cao	紫草	Arnebiae/Lithospermi Radix
Zi He Che	紫河车	Hominis Placenta
Zi Hua Di Ding	紫花地丁	Violae Herba
Zi Ran Tong	自然铜	Pyritum
Zi Shi Ying	紫石英	Fluoritum
Zi Su Ye	紫苏叶	Perillae Folium
Zi Wan	紫菀	Asteris Radix

Appendix 16

Bibliography

Beijing Chinese Medicine College. *Nei Jing Shi Yi* 内经释义. Shanghai People's Publishing House, 1972.

Bensky D, Clavey S et al. *Chinese Herbal Medicine Materia Medica*. 3rd Edition. Eastland Press, 2004.

Cai Xin Pei. *Shao Pai Shang Han Xue Shuo Yan Jiu* 绍派伤寒学说研究. www.ssreader.com

Ceng Xian Ling (Editor). *Pocket English-Chinese Medical Dictionary*. Shanghai Science & Technology Press, 1993.

Chen Wei Yi (Editor). *Ying Han Yi Xue Ci Dian* 英汉医学辞典. Shanghai Science & Technology Press, 1996.

Chen Rui Chun. *Shang Han Shi Jian Lun* 伤寒实践论. People's Medical Publishing House, 2003.

Chen Yi Ren, *Shang Han Lun Qiu Shi* 伤寒论求是. People's Medical Publishing House, 1987.

Cheng Wu Ji, *Shang Han Ming Li Lun* 伤寒明理论. Yue Lu Book Publications, 1990.

Cheng Wu Ji (Annotations). *Zhu Jie Shang Han Lun* 注解伤寒论. People's Medical Publishing House, 1963.

Cheng Jiao Qian, *Shang Han Hou Tiao Bian* 伤寒后条辩. China's Ancient Texts Publishing Press, 1990.

Cheng Zhong Ling, *Yi Xue Xin Wu* 医学心悟. www.ssreader.com.

Collier J et al. *Oxford Handbook of Clinical Specialties*. Oxford University Press, 1998.

Dorland I & Newman W. *Dorland's Illustrated Medical Dictionary*. WB Saunders Company, 1994.

Editorial Board. *Jian Ming Zhong Yi Ci Dian* 简明中医辞典. People's Medical Publishing House, 1979.

Edwards C et al. *Davidson's Principles and Practice of Medicine*. Seventeenth Edition. Churchill Livingstone, 1995.

Ellis A et al. *Fundamentals of Chinese Acupuncture*. Paradigm Publications, 1995.

Fang You Zhi. *Shang Han Lun Tiao Bian* 伤寒论条辩. People's Medical Publishing House, 1957.

Fu Yan Ling et al (Editors). *Shang Han Lun Yan Jiu Da Ci Dian* 伤寒论研究大词典. Shandong Science & Technology Press, 1994.

Guo Ai Chun et al (Editors). *Huang Di Nei Jing Ci Dian* 黄帝内经词典. Tianjin Science & Technology Press, 1991.

He Lian Chen. *Chong Ding Guang Wen Re Lun* 重订广温热论. People's Medical Publishing House, 1960.

He Lian Chen. *Chong Yin Quan Guo Ming Yi Yan An Lei Bian* 重印全国名医验案类编. Shanghai Science & Technology Press, 1959.

Hubei Chinese Medicine College. *Shang Han Lun Selected Readings* 伤寒论选读. Shanghai Science & Technology Press, 1979.

Jiang Ren An (Editor). *Xu Ling Tai Yi Shu Quan Ji* 徐灵胎医书全集. Wu Zhou Chu Ban She, 1969.

Ke Qin. *Shang Han Lai Su Ji* 伤寒来苏集. Yue Lu Book Publications, 1990.

Li Ren Qian et al (Editors). *Zhong Yi Zhen Duan Zhi Liao Xue* 中医诊断治疗学. Guangdong Science & Technology Press, 1996.

Li Wen Rui et al (Editors). *Shang Han Lun Tang Zheng Lun Zhi* 伤寒论汤证论治. Zhong Guo Ke Xue Ji Shu Chu Ban She, 2000.

Lian Jian Wei (Editor). *San Ding Tong Su Shang Han Lun* 三订通俗伤寒论. Chinese Ancient Texts Publishing Press, 2002.

Lin Hui Guang (Editor). *Chen Xiu Yuan Yi Xue Quan Shu* 陈修园医学全书. China's Chinese Medicine Publishing Press, 1999.

Liu De Lai (Chief Editor). *Nei Jing Shi Yi* 黄帝内经. The Times Literature and Art Press: Beijing, 2001.

Liu Du Zhou. *Liu Du Zhou Yi Xue Quan Ji* 刘渡舟医学全集. Qi Ye Publishing Press, 1998.

Liu Zhu Yi et al (Editors). *Zhong Guo Li Dai Ming Yi Ming Shu* 中国历代名医名术. Chinese Ancient Texts Publishing Press, 1999.

Mang Shu Jiang (Editor). *Wen Bing Xue* 温病学. Shanghai Science & Technology Press, 1985.

Mitchell C et al. *Shang Han Lun: On Cold Damage*. Paradigm Publications, 1999.

Nie Hui Ming. *Shang Han Lun Yu Lin Chuang* 伤寒论与临床. Guangdong Science & Technology Press, 1993.

Pan Hua Xin. *Ye Tian Shi Yi An Da Quan* 叶天士医案大全. Shanghai Chinese Medicine University Press, 1994.

Pang An Shi. *Shang Han Zong Bing Lun* 伤寒总病论. People's Medical Publishing House, 1989.

Pei Yong Qing. *Shang Han Lun Lin Chuang Ying Yong Wu Shi Lun* 伤寒论临床应用五十论. Xue Yuan Publishing Press, 1995.

Tortora G, Derrickson B. *Principles of Anatomy and Physiology*. 11th Edition. Wiley, 2006.

Wang Hong Tu et al (Editors). *Huang Di Nei Jing Yan Jiu Da Cheng* 黄帝内经研究大成. Beijing Publishing Press, 2000.

Wang Hong Tu. *Huang Di Yi Shu Lin Zheng Qie Yao* 黄帝内经临证切要. Hua Xia Publishing Press, 1993.

Wang Mang Ying, *Hui Chun Lu Xin Quan* 回春录新诠. Hunan Science & Technology Press, 1982.

Wu Ju Tong. *Wen Bin Tiao Bian* 温病条辩. People's Medical Publishing House, 1963.

Wu Kun An. *Shang Han Zhi Zhang* 伤寒指掌. Shanghai Science & Technology Press, 1985.

Wu Qian et al (Editors). *Yi Zhong Jin Jian* 医宗金鉴. People's Medical Publishing House, 2005.

Wu Qian et al (Editors). *Yi Zong Jin Jian* 医宗金鉴. People's Medical Publishing House, 1979.

You Yi. *Shang Han Guan Zhu Ji* 伤寒贯珠集. Yue Lu Book Publications, 1990.

Yu Gen Chu, edited by He Lian Chen. *Chong Ding Tong Su Shang Han Lun* 重订通俗伤寒论. Shang Hai Liu Ye Tang Pharmaceutical Texts Press, 1932.

Zeng Xian Ling (Editor). *Ying Han Yi Xue Xiao Ci Dian* 英汉医学小词典. Shanghai Science & Technology Press, 1993.

Zhang Yan Mo et al (Editors). *Han Ying Shuang Jie Zhong Yi Xiao Ci Dian* 汉英双解中医小辞典. People's Medical Publishing House, 2003.

Zhao Xiao Qing (Editor). *Jiang Xue Yuan Gu Fang Xuan Zhu* 绛雪园古方选注. China's Chinese Medicine Publishing Press, 1993.

Zhu Gong. *Lei Zheng Huo Ren Shu* 类证活人书. People's Medical Publishing House, 1993.

Websites

http://www.plantnames.org/calp747.html

http://www.plantnames.unimelb.edu.au